# THORACIC SURGICAL TECHNIQUES

To our surgical trainees past, present and future who are, or one day will be, our colleagues.

# THORACIC SURGICAL TECHNIQUES

F. C. Wells MS, FRCS
*Consultant Cardiothoracic Surgeon*
*Papworth Hospital*
*Papworth Everard*
*Cambridgeshire, UK*

B. B. Milstein MA, FRCS
*Formerly Consultant Cardiothoracic Surgeon*
*Papworth Hospital*
*Papworth Everard*
*Cambridgeshire, UK*

*Illustrated by*
Gillian Lee and Kevin Marks

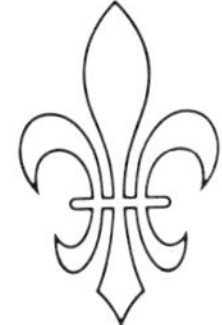

Baillière Tindall Limited
London Philadelphia Toronto Sydney Tokyo

This book is printed on acid free paper. ♾

*Bailliere Tindall* 24–28 Oval Road
W. B. Saunders London NW1 7DX

The Curtis Center
Independence Square West
Philadelphia, PA 19106-3399

55 Horner Avenue
Toronto, Ontario M8Z 4X6, Canada

Harcourt Brace Jovanovich (Australia) Pty Ltd,
30–52 Smidmore St
Marrickville, NSW 2204, Australia

Harcourt Brace Jovanovich Japan Inc.
Ichibancho Central Building, 22–1 Ichibancho
Chiyoda-ku, Tokyo 102, Japan



First published 1990

**British Library Cataloguing in Publication Data**
Wells, F. C.
Thoracic surgical techniques.
1. Chest. Surgery
I. Title II. Milstein, B. B.
617'.54059

ISBN 0–7020–1239–4



Typeset by Photo·graphics Ltd.,
and printed in Great Britain by Thomson Litho Ltd, East Kilbride, Scotland.

# Contents

# Preface

Over the last twenty years the rapid expansion in cardiac surgery has led to something of an eclipse of the status of non-cardiac thoracic surgery, particularly its teaching. In many ways good thoracic surgical technique is more difficult to learn than cardiac surgery, most of which is limited in range. These observations led us to produce a book of thoracic surgical techniques which unashamedly emphasizes the practical steps in the more frequently performed procedures, and some less common operations which trainees may never see, yet may need to have recourse to in their subsequent careers.

In some cases we have given alternatives, but in the main have chosen techniques that we have found reliable. We appreciate, however, that established thoracic surgeons may prefer other techniques. In particular there will be considerable variation in suture techniques. The materials that are available are continuously changing, allowing greater variety in technique. The introduction of stapling devices has had a profound effect on the practice of some surgeons. Although we have included description of the use of staples we have concentrated on conventional suture techniques. We believe that a good grounding in these methods is essential for all trainee thoracic surgeons before they move on to the use of the staple gun in its various forms.

We have deliberately omitted sections on thoracic trauma and on paediatrics for fear that the size of the book would become excessive. We hope that this book may be of value to the apprentice thoracic surgeon, to the established consultant who is faced with an unfamiliar operation and to the general surgeon who finds the occasional need to stray into the thorax in the absence of experienced help.

F. C. WELLS
B. B. MILSTEIN

# SECTION 1

# INVESTIGATIVE AND MINOR THORACIC SURGICAL PROCEDURES

# 1 Bronchoscopy

Bronchoscopy, in combination with a plain chest radiograph, is fundamental to the management of patients with disease involving the lung and major airways. Two basic instruments are available: the fibre-optic bronchoscope and the rigid bronchoscope. Each has its own merits and indications.

The rigid instrument is more suitable for the removal of foreign bodies and the aspiration of secretions. It allows safer biopsy of vascular tumours because it is easier to control bleeding. This is accomplished by direct application of a 1:10 000 adrenaline solution to the bleeding area with a cotton wool bud. The rigid nature of the instrument allows the endoscopist an assessment of the fixity of a tumour by proprioception. The extent of vision is shown in **Fig. 1.1.**

The flexible endoscope can penetrate much further into the bronchial tree, and allows brushings and biopsies of very peripheral lesions. It has a wider angle of vision, particularly in the upper lobes. It is the instrument of choice for patients with cervical spine problems or with a fixed small bite, because of its flexibility. In addition it can be passed easily through an endobronchial or tracheostomy tube. The extent of vision by flexible bronchoscopy is shown in **Fig. 1.2**.

**Figure 1.2**

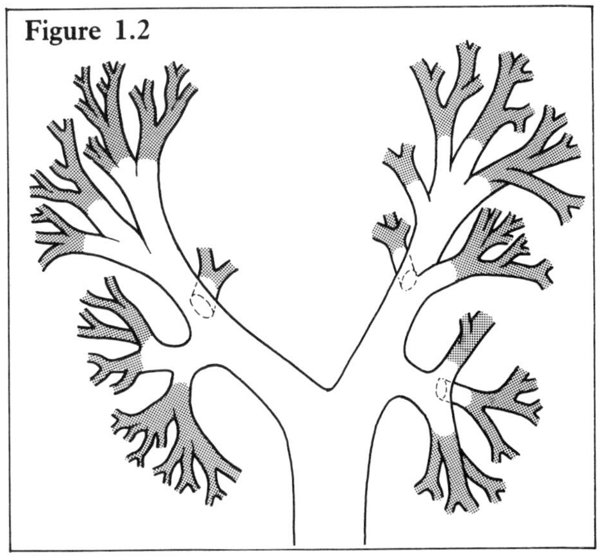

**Figure 1.1**

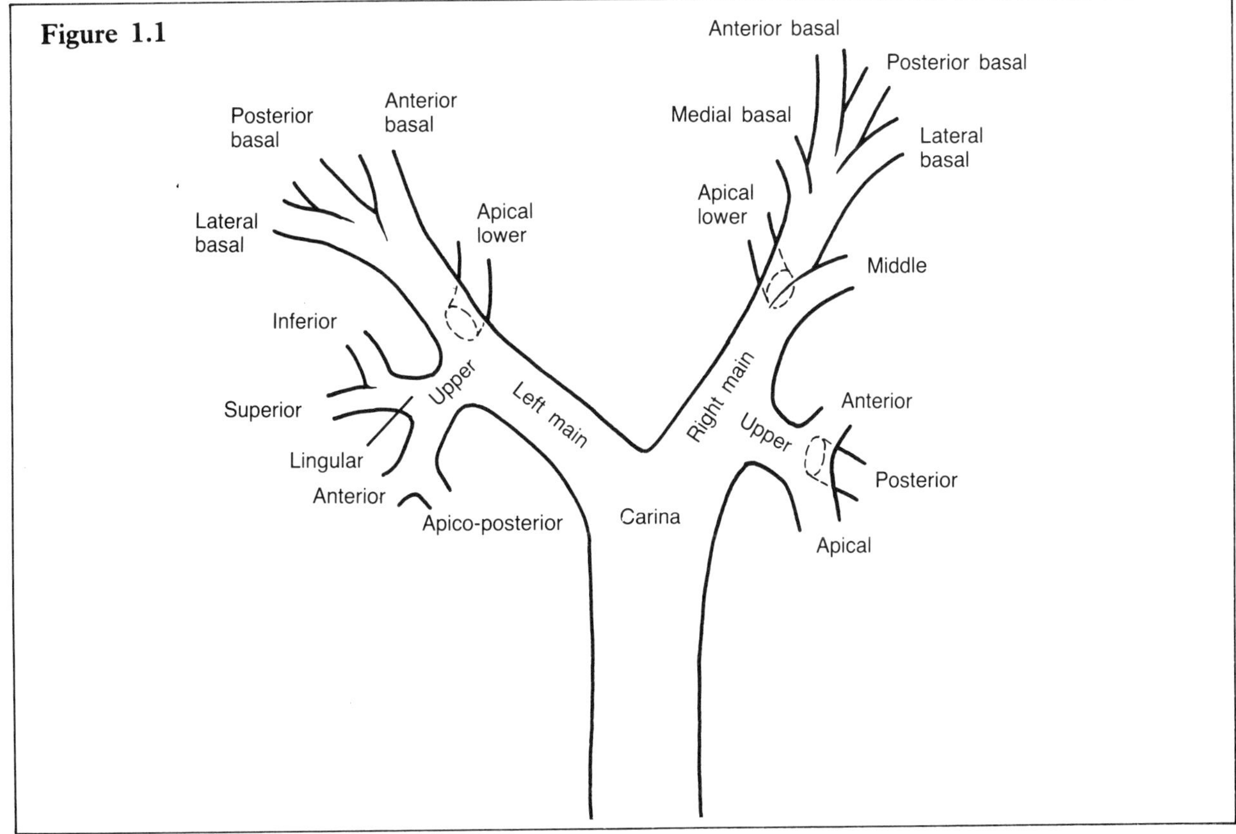

The techniques involved in the use of each instrument are quite different. The thoracic surgeon in training should endeavour to become expert in the handling of both of them.

## The instruments

### Rigid bronchoscope

The Negus bronchoscope is most frequently used in clinical practice, a variety of sizes being available for various age groups. Fibre-optic light cables are the best source of illumination, and an attachment for both the bronchoscope and a range of telescopes should be available. Three principal telescopes are used: direct vision, 90-degree angled and 60-degree angled. The combined use of these allows inspection of all lobar bronchi and their segmental divisions. Additional necessary instruments include straight and angled Brock's biopsy forceps, Chevalier-Jackson forceps for foreign bodies, and a straight metal sucker. Some form of bronchial blocker is necessary in case of bleeding that cannot be easily controlled. Specifically designed bronchus blockers are available, but a suitably sized Fogarty catheter is an acceptable alternative.

To ventilate the patient the inspired gas is administered by a Venturi system. Oxygen is injected under pressure through a nozzle in the side of the bronchoscope. Air is entrained through the open proximal end of the bronchoscope, creating an oxygen-air mixture.

### Fibre-optic bronchoscope

Several models are now available. All are delicate and expensive instruments, and careful handling by trained staff is essential. The operating head of the endoscope has an adjustable eyepiece and a finger-and-thumb control lever or knob to direct the distal end of the instrument. A channel for the introduction of biopsy forceps, brush or Dormier basket is present on most current models. There is a further port for suction to one side.

For optimal performance careful cleaning at the conclusion of an investigation is essential.

**Figure 1.3**

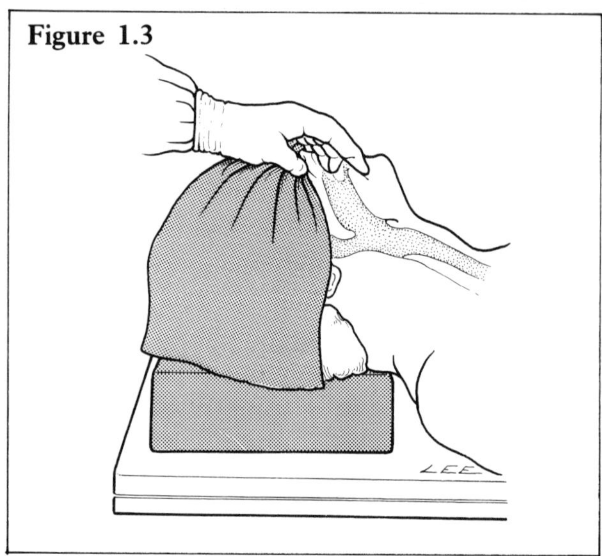


**Figure 1.4**

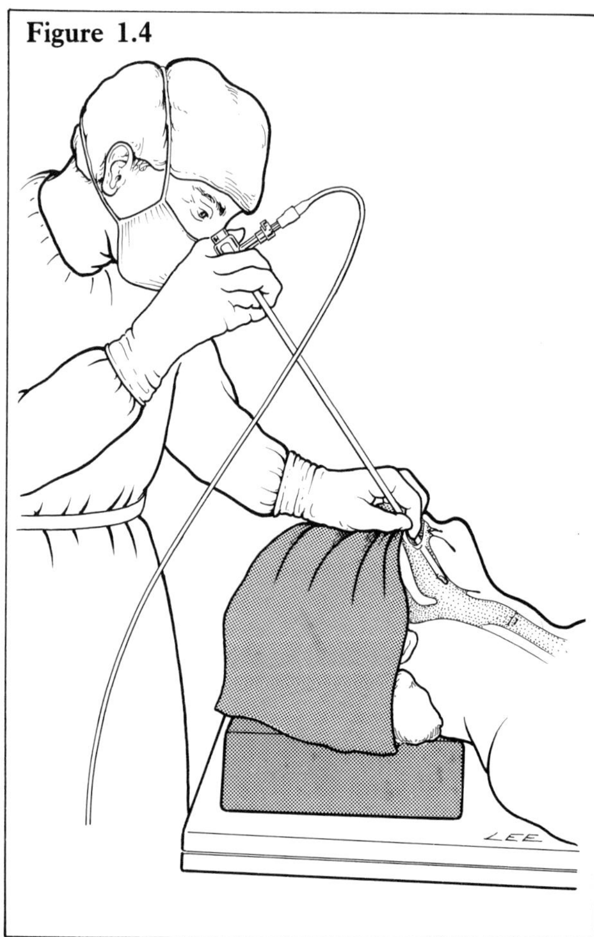


## Rigid bronchoscopy

The patient's head is rested on a foam pillow and wrapped in a clean towel to protect the eyes and face (**Fig. 1.3**). The surgeon's left hand retracts the patient's upper lip and grasps the maxilla with the middle and ring fingers, leaving the index finger and thumb free to control the endoscope.

The bronchoscope is then inserted through the right side of the mouth, resting against the palmar surface of the thumb, not against the upper lip or teeth of the patient. The bronchoscope at this point is vertical. The tongue is then pushed forwards and the bronchoscope advanced until the posterior wall of the oropharynx is reached. At this point the bronchoscope is angled backwards until the epiglottis comes into view (**Fig. 1.4**). Keeping the bronchoscope in the midline, the epiglottis is elevated and the bronchoscope advanced until the vocal cords and corniculate tubercles come into view (**Fig. 1.5**). A note is made of the anatomical

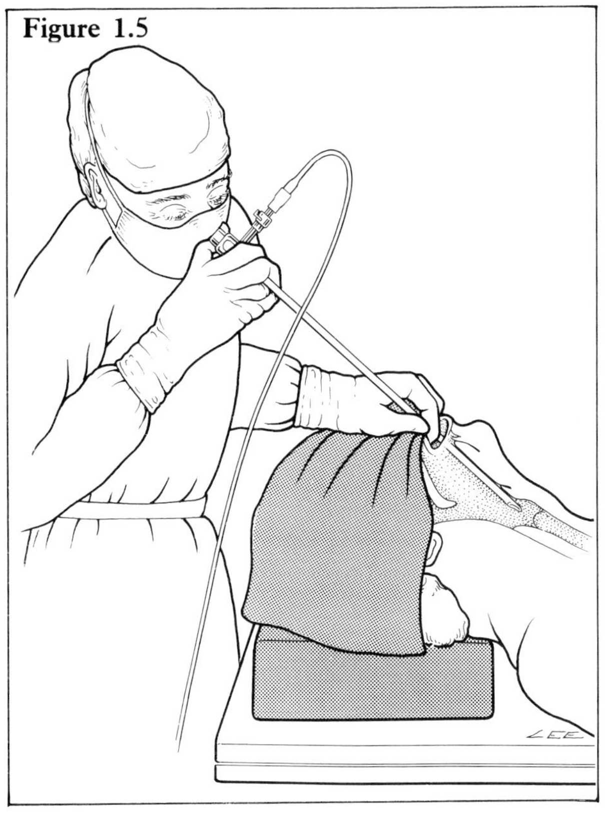
Figure 1.5

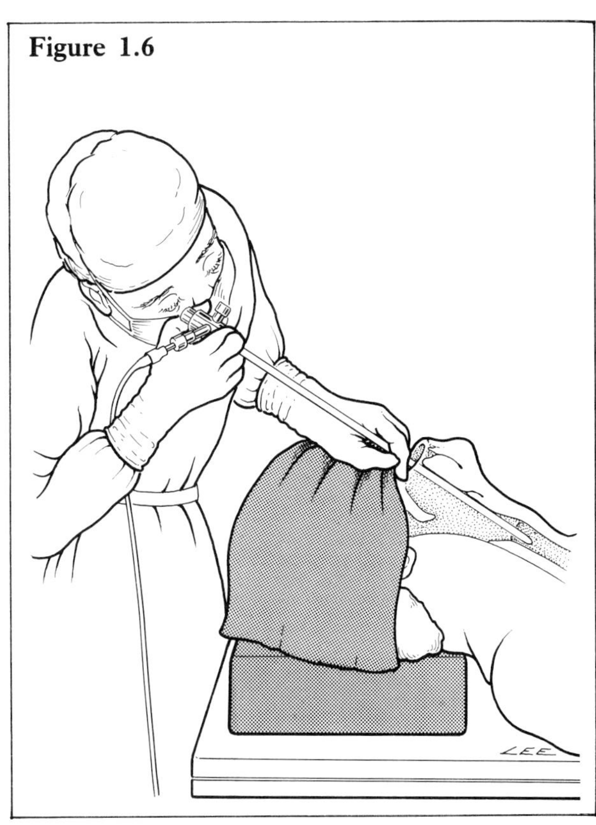
Figure 1.6

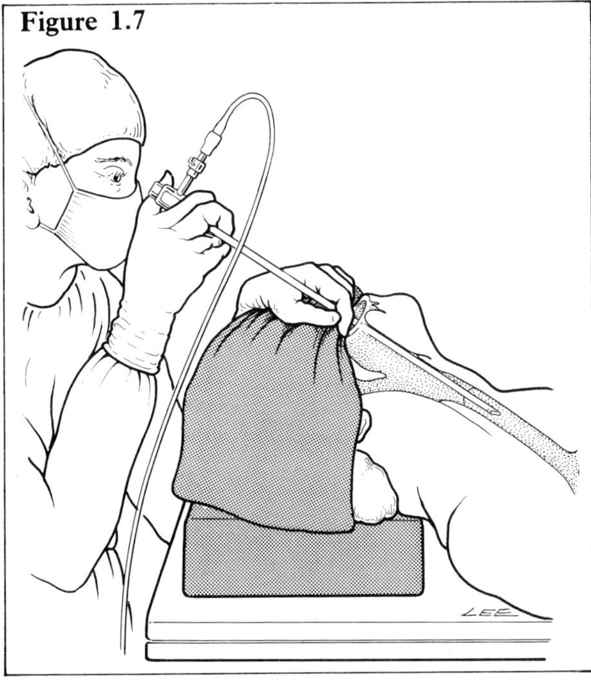
Figure 1.7

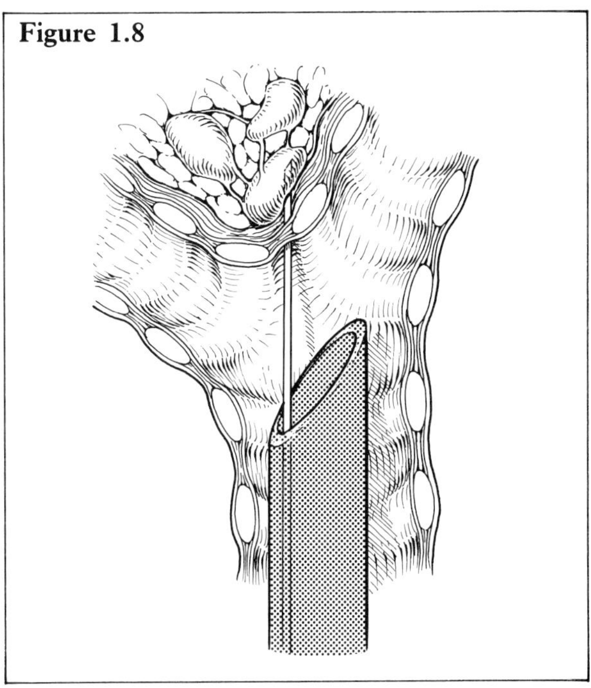
Figure 1.8

position of the cords. The bronchoscope is then turned through 90 degrees so that its beak is parallel with the opening between the vocal cords. It is then slid through the cords into the upper trachea (**Fig. 1.6**). The instrument is then rotated back through 90 degrees to its original position and the inspection of the major airways may begin (**Fig. 1.7**).

Any compression or deviation of the trachea is noted as well as any mucosal abnormality. The bronchoscope is passed further into the trachea until the carina can be clearly seen. Significant enlargement of the subcarinal lymph nodes will result in splaying of the carina. Specimens of these nodes may be obtained for cytological examination by transcarinal needle biopsy (**Fig. 1.8**).

For meaningful interpretation of the remainder of the examination, a sound knowledge of the anatomy of the bronchopulmonary segments is essential (**Figs. 1.9, 1.10**).

**Figure 1.9a**

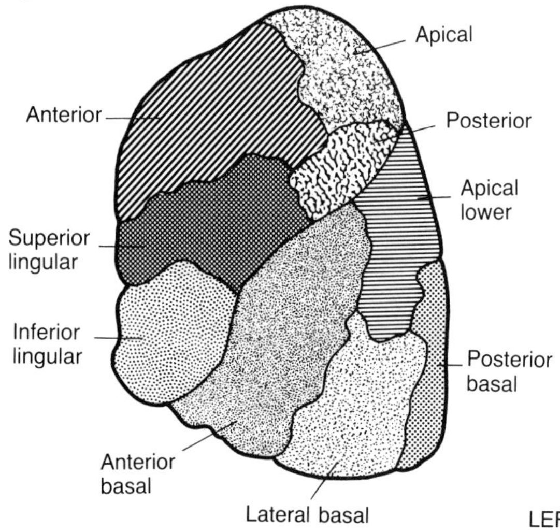

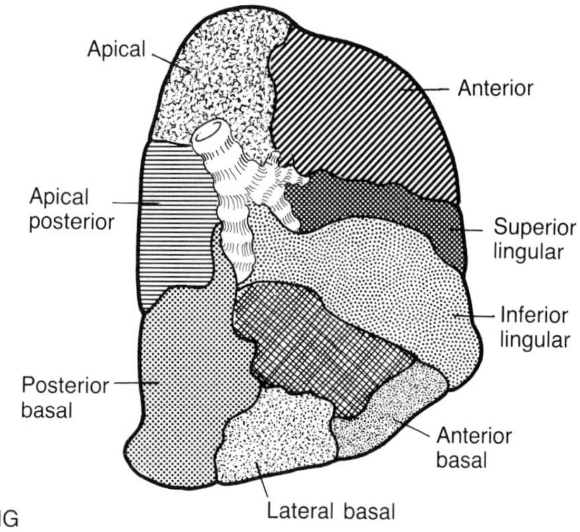

Apical
Anterior
Posterior
Apical lower
Superior lingular
Inferior lingular
Posterior basal
Anterior basal
Lateral basal

**Figure 1.9b**

Apical
Anterior
Apical posterior
Superior lingular
Inferior lingular
Posterior basal
Anterior basal
Lateral basal

LEFT LUNG

**Figure 1.10a**

Apical
Posterior
Anterior
Apical lower
Medial
Middle lobe
Posterior basal
Lateral
Lateral basal
Anterior basal

**Figure 1.10b**

Apical
Posterior
Anterior
Apical lower
Medial
Posterior basal
Medial basal
Anterior basal

RIGHT LUNG

**Figure 1.11a**

**Figure 1.11b**

Basal orifices
Lingular branch
Upper division orifice
Apical lower orifice

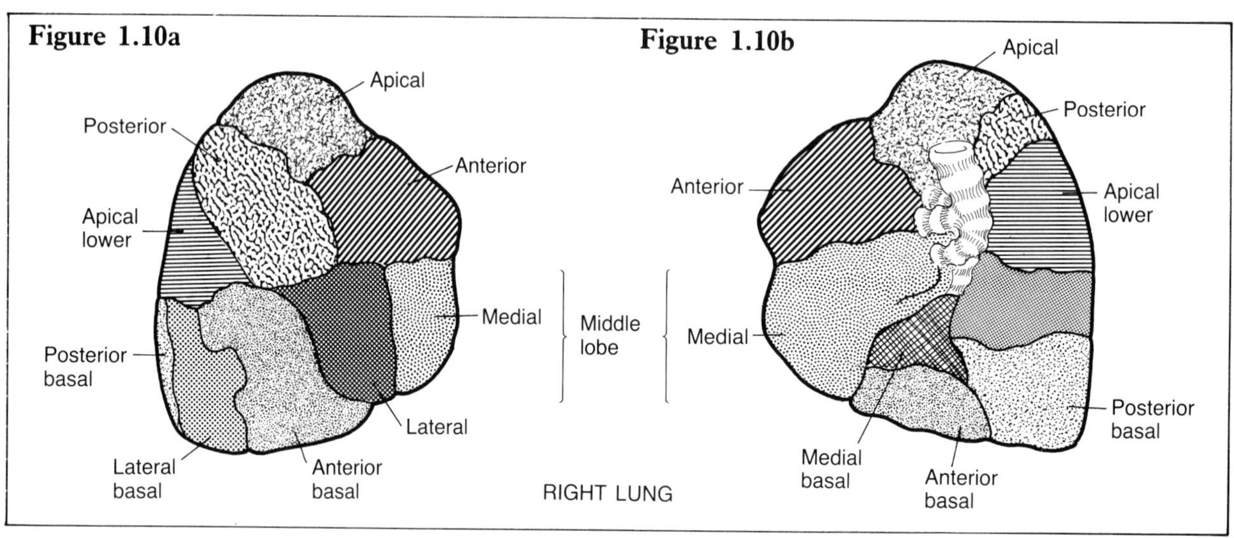

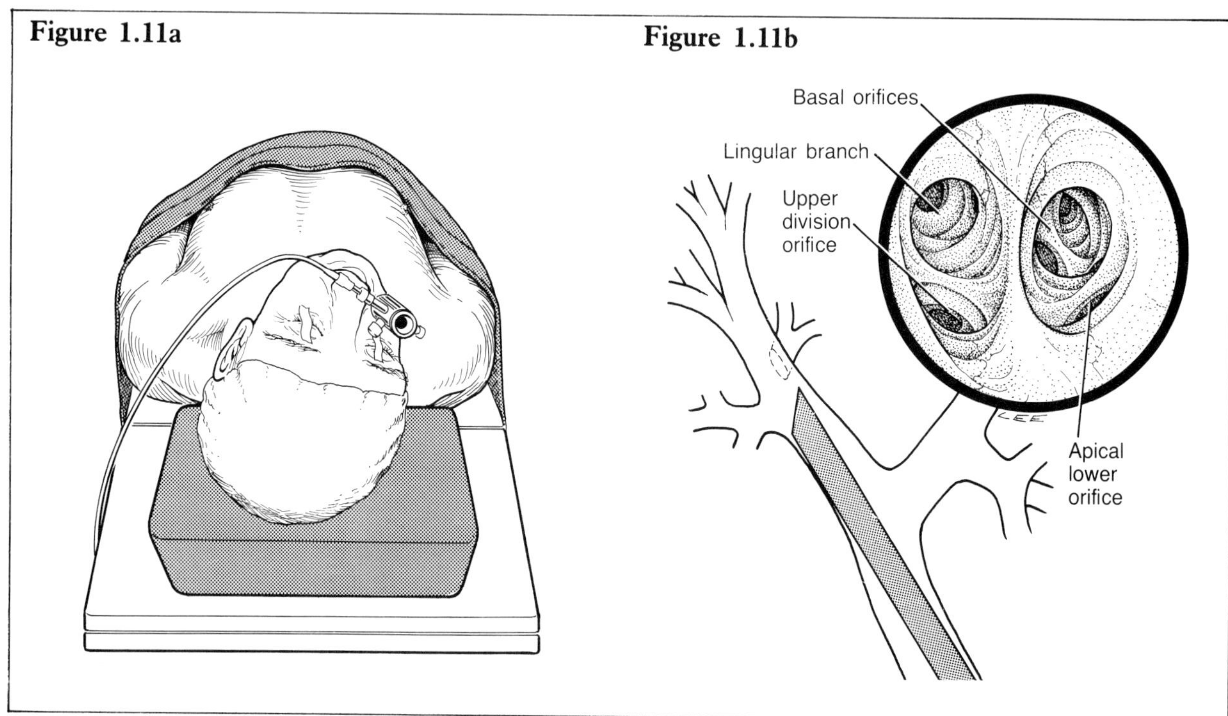

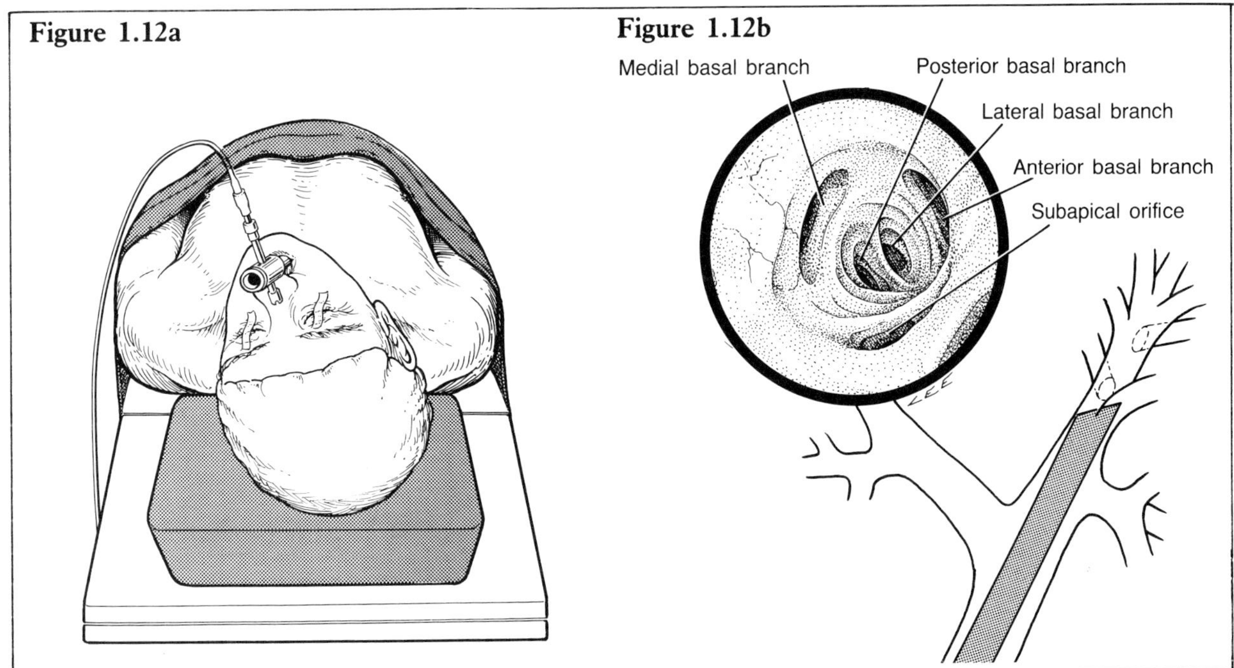


Figure 1.12a

Figure 1.12b

If the pathology for which bronchoscopy is being carried out is unilateral, then we advise that the detailed examination of the airways should begin on the contralateral side. This will ensure that a complete examination is accomplished, and that any blood or cellular debris will not be carried over to the normal side in error.

To introduce the bronchoscope into either of the main bronchi, the head must be turned to the opposite side, bringing the long axes of the instrument and bronchus into line (**Figs. 1.11, 1.12**). Each of the lobar and segmental bronchi is then carefully examined.

## Collection of specimens and biopsies

All aspirated material is collected in a sputum trap and sent for culture and cytology. It is essential to separate specimens from the right and left bronchial trees. If secretions are scant, lavage with 50 ml normal saline which is then aspirated will often yield sufficient cells to allow a diagnosis to be made.

Biopsies are best taken with the integral biopsy forceps and telescope (**Fig. 1.13**). Any resulting bleeding may be controlled by applying a 1:10 000 adrenaline solution on a cottonwool bud held with the long biopsy forceps. If bleeding is uncontrolled, then occlusion of the lobar or segmental bronchus with a bronchial blocker may be all that is possible prior to immediate thoracotomy.

## Removal of foreign bodies

Two principal groups of foreign bodies are encountered. The first is irritant vegetable matter such as a peanut. This causes rapid swelling of the mucosa which may envelop the peanut, making removal very difficult. After a comparatively short time the peanut may denature to the extent that it will break up on even the gentlest contact. Both of these reasons are sufficient to encourage endoscopic examination of the patient at even the slightest suspicion of inhalation of this type of object.

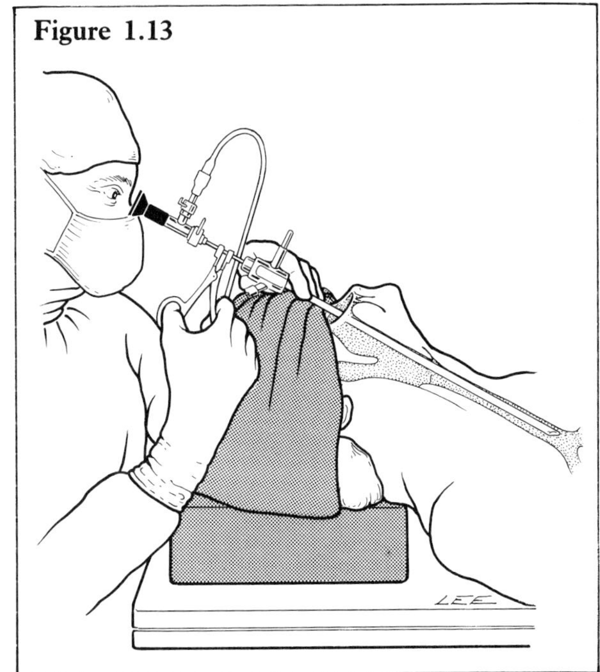

Figure 1.13

The second group of foreign bodies comprises inert objects such as pieces of plastic from toys, small ballbearings, etc. Each object can represent its own small challenge to the endoscopist for removal. The choice of instrument to remove the offending object will depend upon its site, size and

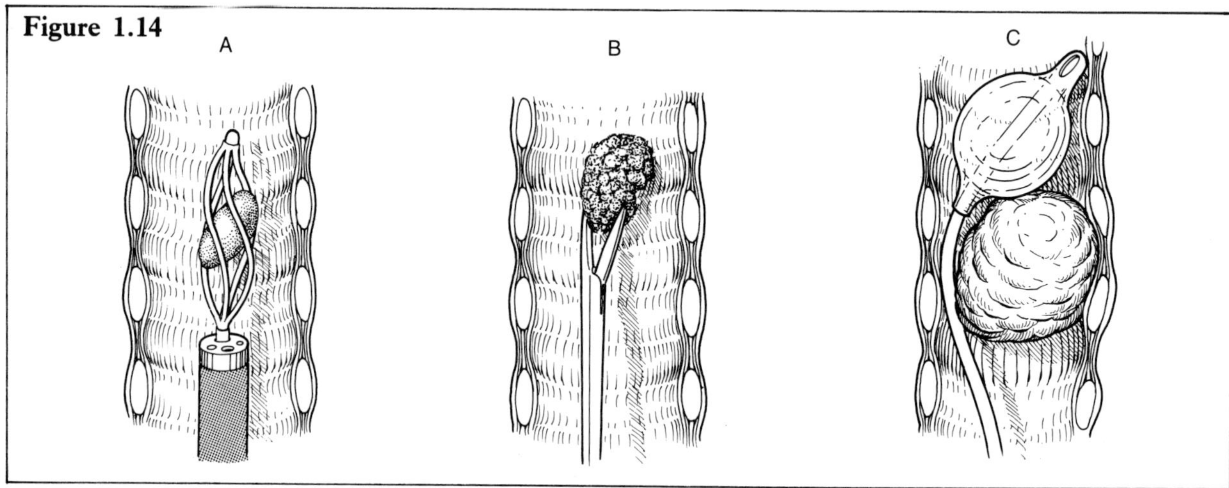


**Figure 1.14**

consistency. Generally speaking, the first attempt to grasp the object is the easiest, as repeated manipulation will cause the surrounding mucosa to swell. Three different methods are demonstrated in **Fig. 1.14**.

Often the diameter of the foreign body is greater than that of the bronchoscope. To allow removal of the object under these circumstances, the bronchoscope must be removed at the same time as the foreign body. Following removal, the bronchoscope should be reintroduced to check for further debris and allow careful endobronchial toilet. During removal, there is a danger of the foreign body becoming impacted between the vocal cords. For this reason a laryngoscope and laryngeal forceps must be to hand, and if the object cannot be speedily grasped and removed, it must be pushed downwards into the trachea to avoid the patient becoming asphyxiated.

## Fibre-optic bronchoscopy

The patient should be given 0.6 mg of atropine as a premedication to reduce oropharyngeal secretions. An intravenous sedative such as diazepam may be used if the patient is very anxious. The judicious use of local anaesthetic spray and cream on the external nares, the pharynx and vocal cords is essential.

The patient should be seated at 45 degrees, facing the operator, or lie in a supine position. The operator's right hand controls the operating head of the bronchoscope, holding the tip of the instrument in the neutral position. The tip is then passed into the more widely patent side of the nose and guided with the utmost care into the nasopharynx (**Fig. 1.15**). From here, further progress is facilitated by forward angulation of the tip. The epiglottis is identified.

The next part of the procedure is the most delicate: 2 ml of 4% lignocaine is injected into the

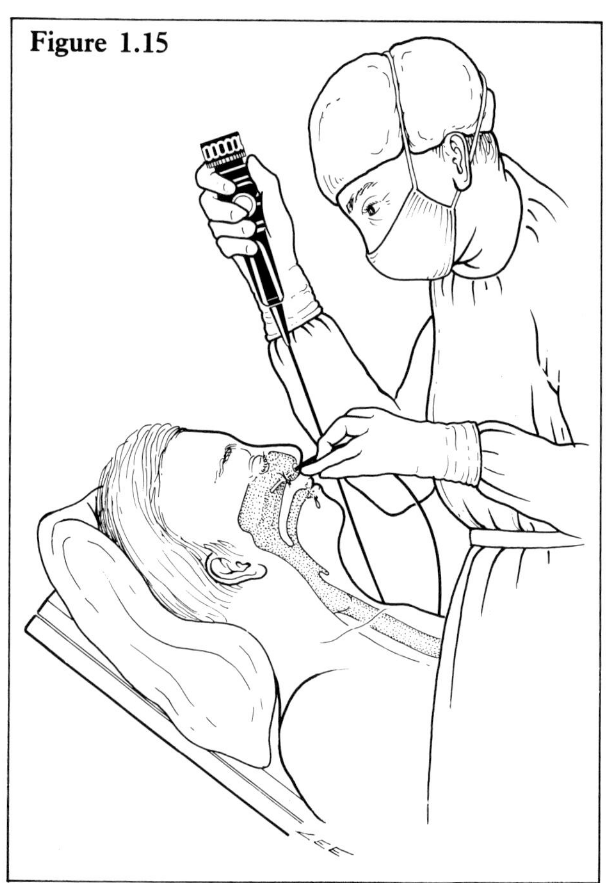

**Figure 1.15**

epiglottis and the entrance to the larynx while the patient takes a deep breath. This will cause the patient to cough, but rapid anaesthesia of the larynx is achieved. The operator should now wait for two or three minutes while the local anaesthetic takes effect. The tip of the bronchoscope is then very cautiously passed between the vocal cords and into the upper trachea (**Fig. 1.16**). Patients vary in their needs for further local anaesthetic from this point, but some is likely to be needed at regular intervals.

Following careful examination of the lobar and segmental airways, biopsy under direct vision may be undertaken (**Fig. 1.17**).

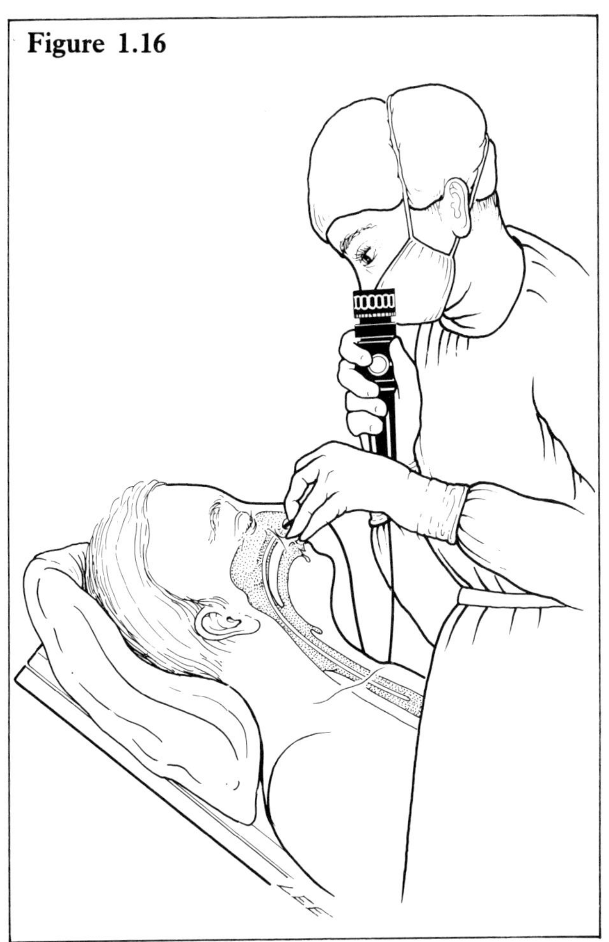


Figure 1.16

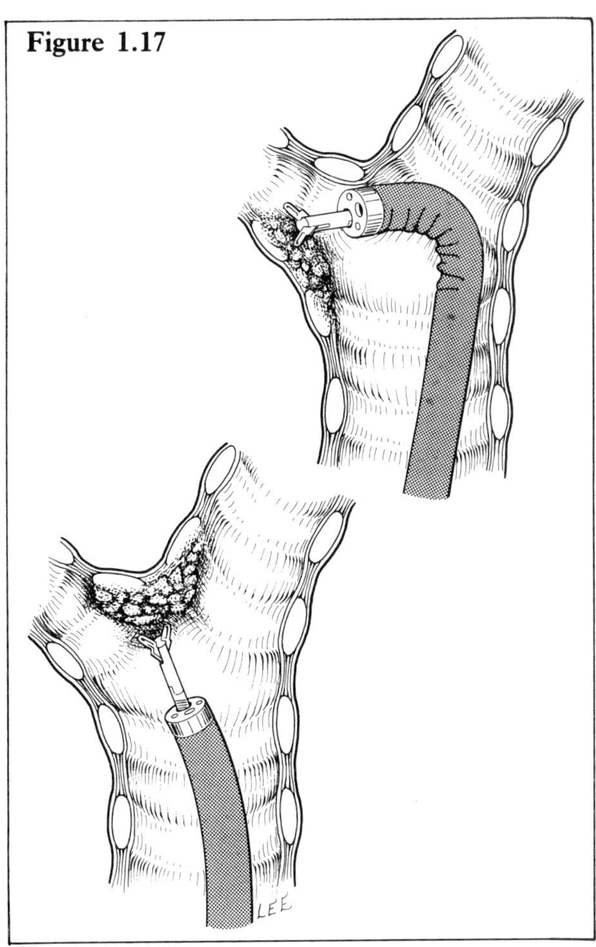


Figure 1.17

# 2 Thoracoscopy

## Indications

1. The evaluation of a pleural effusion, to establish or exclude a malignant cause.
2. Evaluation and management of empyema cavities.
3. Assessment of mediastinal tumours.
4. Assessment of chest wall tumours.

## Contraindications

1. Coagulopathies.
2. Recent myocardial infarction (within six weeks).
3. Severe impairment of pulmonary function (although this is not an absolute contraindication, great care must be taken).
4. Absence of a pleural space.

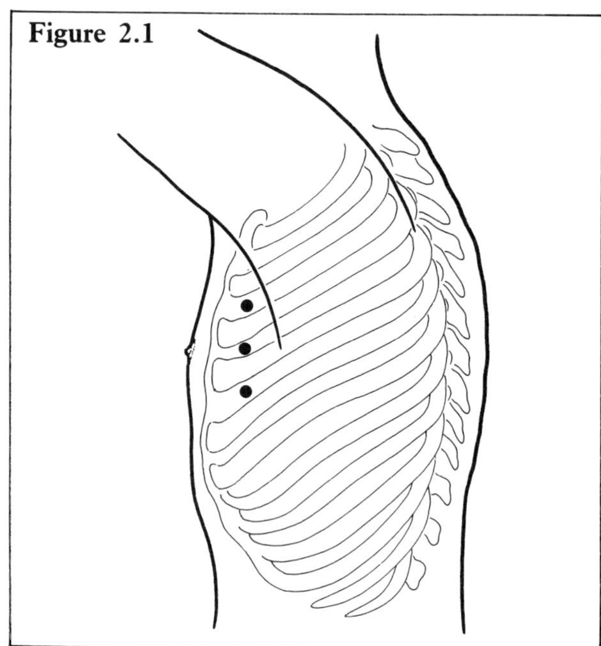
Figure 2.1

## Procedure

After premedication, the patient is anaesthetized and positioned on the appropriate side. First a pneumothorax is induced. Apparatus is available to control the rate and degree of pneumothorax that is to be created.

The induction and monitoring of the pneumothorax varies a little according to the intrathoracic conditions (pleural effusion, previous pneumothorax, etc.). Ultrasound is invaluable to localize the site of fluid collections. In the presence of an effusion a wide-bore needle is introduced and the pleural fluid will usually pour out spontaneously until atmospheric pressure is reached. Conversely, if the intrapleural pressure is negative, air will be heard to rush into the chest, and if there is a pneumothorax under tension air will rush out. If air does not enter the chest, it can be introduced using the pneumothorax device referred to above. The typical sites for inducing a pneumothorax are the same as for the thoracoscopy (**Fig. 2.1**).

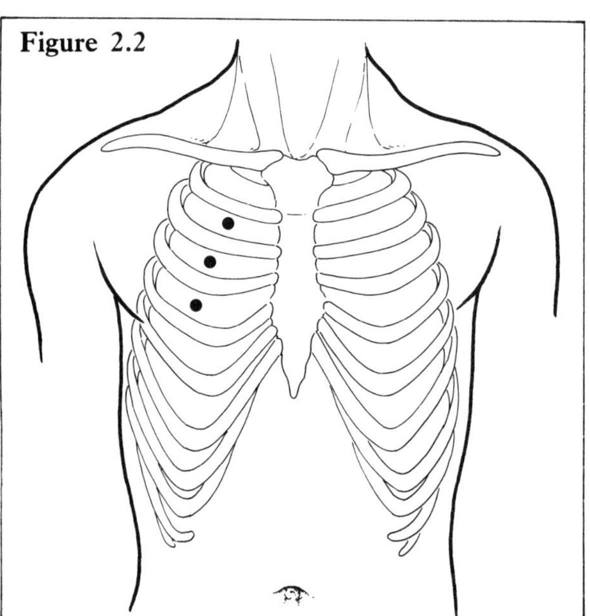
Figure 2.2

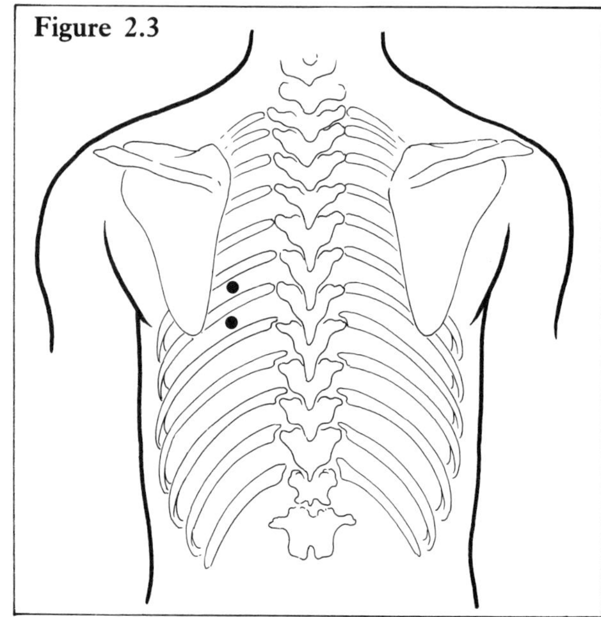
Figure 2.3

Once the pneumothorax has been induced the thoracoscope can be introduced. Typical safe areas are illustrated in **Figs. 2.2** and **2.3**. The actual site chosen will be predetermined by the site and extent of the pathology.

The patient should be positioned to allow the best visualization of the area under suspicion. The prone position is best for examining the posterior mediastinum, the vertebral column, and lung and chest wall lesions that lie in the posterior paravertebral region. The lateral position provides the best approach for pleural effusions and parenchymal lung disease. A good site for ease of insertion is the auscultatory triangle, where there is often no muscle between the skin and chest wall. The dorsal position is best for anteriorly placed lesions.

To introduce the trocar, the sheath of which will allow passage of the thoracoscope, an incision approximately 15–20 mm long is made through the skin. The trocar is slid into the pleural cavity. The trocar sheath is valved so that when the trocar is removed the pneumothorax previously created is maintained.

The thoracoscope is then introduced. Pleural effusions can then be completely drained, biopsies taken and a thorough inspection made. A sucker with a diathermy tip should be available to stem any minor haemorrhage that might ensue.

## Drainage

On completion of the procedure a pleural drain should be inserted. This may be through the examination site, or lower if, for example, the former would be uncomfortable. The drain should be maintained on suction at 75–90 mmHg (10–12 kPa) attached to an underwater seal. Further management of the drain is described on p. 17.

# 3 Mini-tracheostomy

Sputum retention in the early postoperative period may be life-threatening. Repeated bronchoscopy culminating in intubation and ventilation was the former management of this problem.

Recently, suction through a cricothyroidostomy tube (a mini-tracheostomy) has been shown to be very effective for aspirating sputum and obviating the need for intubation and ventilation. The complications following the insertion of such a tube are very few as long as it is inserted carefully and accurately. There are now commercially available kits with full insertion details accompanying them.

Early intervention while the patient still has adequate spontaneous ventilation will usually result in rapid improvement in the patient's condition and obviate the need for bronchoscopy or ventilation. Therefore insertion at the earliest sign of sputum retention, or pre-emptively in the operating theatre in a patient at high risk, is desirable.

## Procedure

The patient is positioned supine, with the head fully extended and a sandbag placed under the shoulders (**Fig. 3.1**). It is possible to carry out the procedure with the patient sitting at 45 degrees with the head extended over a pillow. To prevent undue reflex movement of the larynx during the procedure an assistant holds the chin firmly. The skin is cleansed and the site of the cricothyroid membrane identified (**Fig. 3.1**).

The skin and tissues over this area are infiltrated with 1% local anaesthetic. The infiltration should extend through the cricothyroid membrane and a small amount of anaesthetic should be dribbled into the trachea. This will cause the patient to cough, which will diffuse the anaesthetic agent over the local tracheal epithelium and render it anaesthetized.

**Figure 3.1**

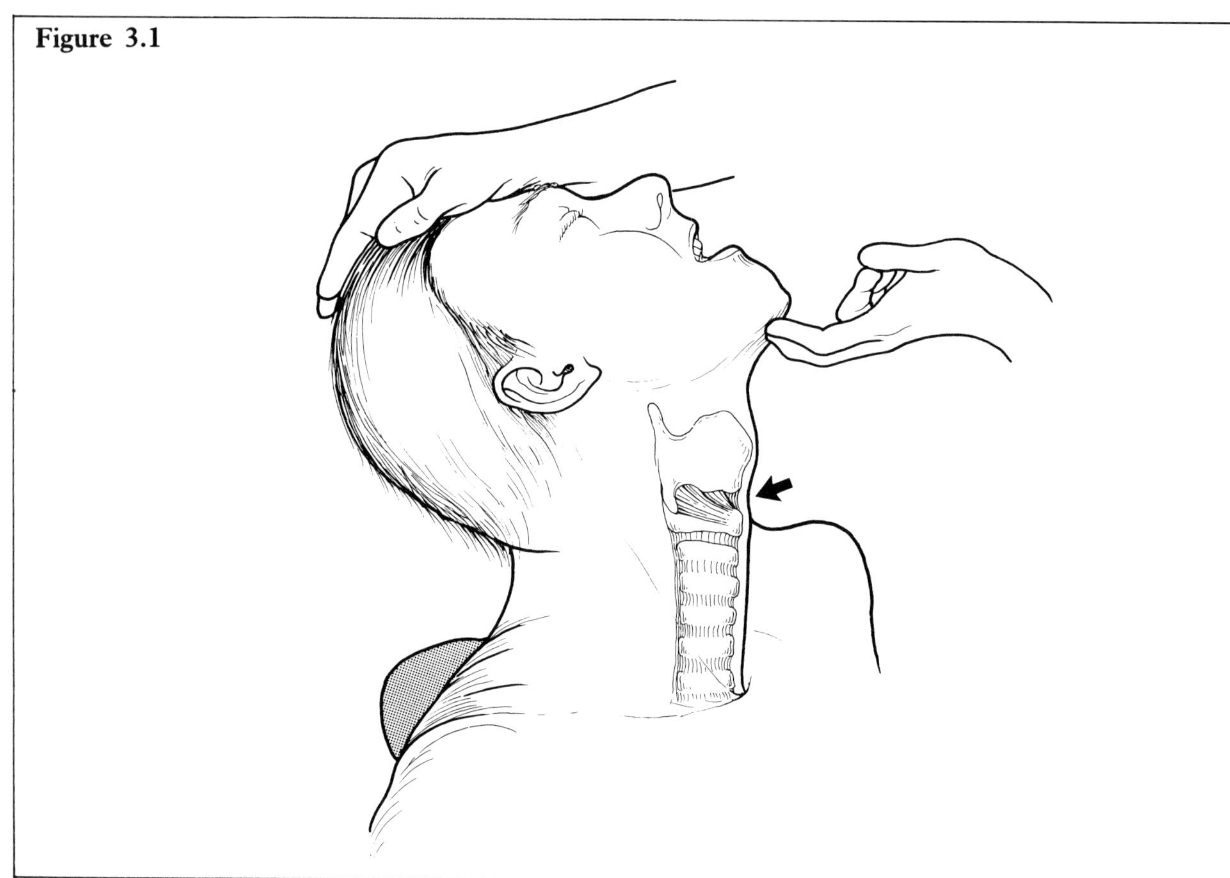

Figure 3.2

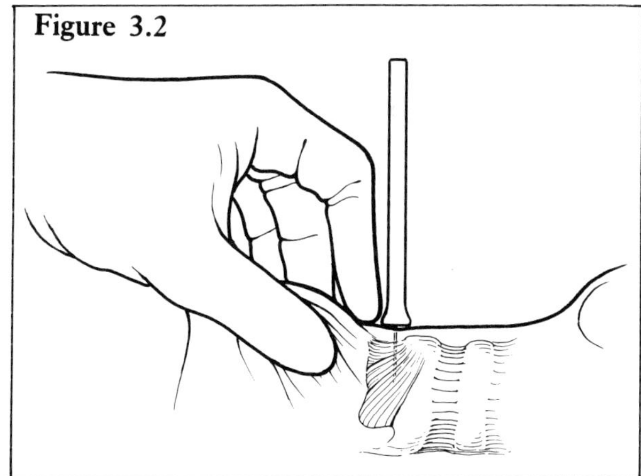

Figure 3.3

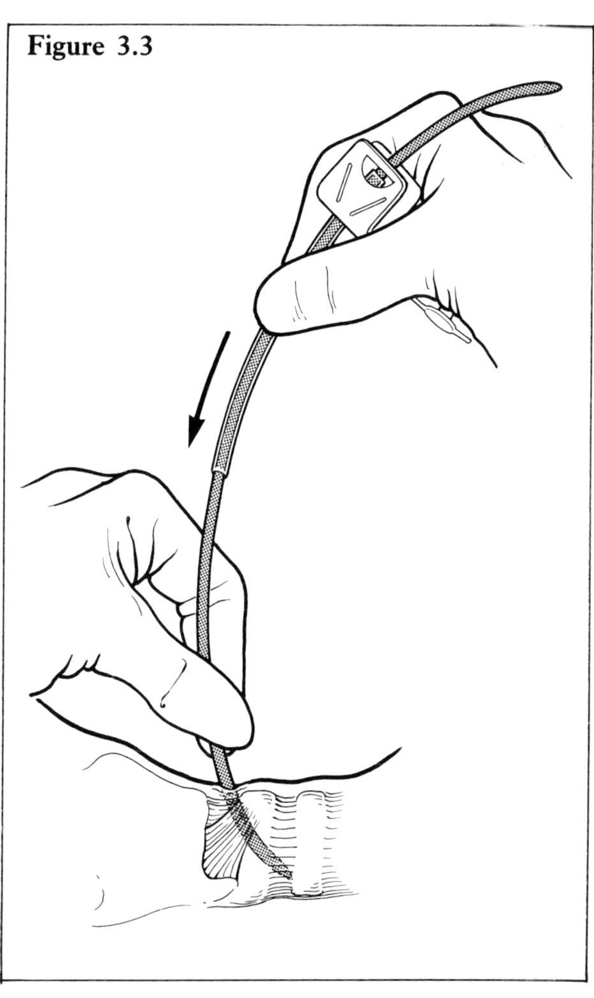

A transverse stab incision is made through the skin and underlying structures until the cricothyroid membrane has been punctured (**Fig. 3.2**). A scalpel with a guarded blade is useful for this part of the procedure, and is supplied with the commercially available kit.

An introducer is then passed through the wound and into the trachea. The cannula (which has an internal diameter of 4.0 mm) is passed over the introducer and into the trachea (**Fig. 3.3**); the introducer is withdrawn. There is a flange attached to the edge of the cannula which allows its secure attachment to the surrounding skin with sutures (**Fig. 3.4**). Suction is performed with a 10 Fr suction cannula (**Fig. 3.5**).

Figure 3.4

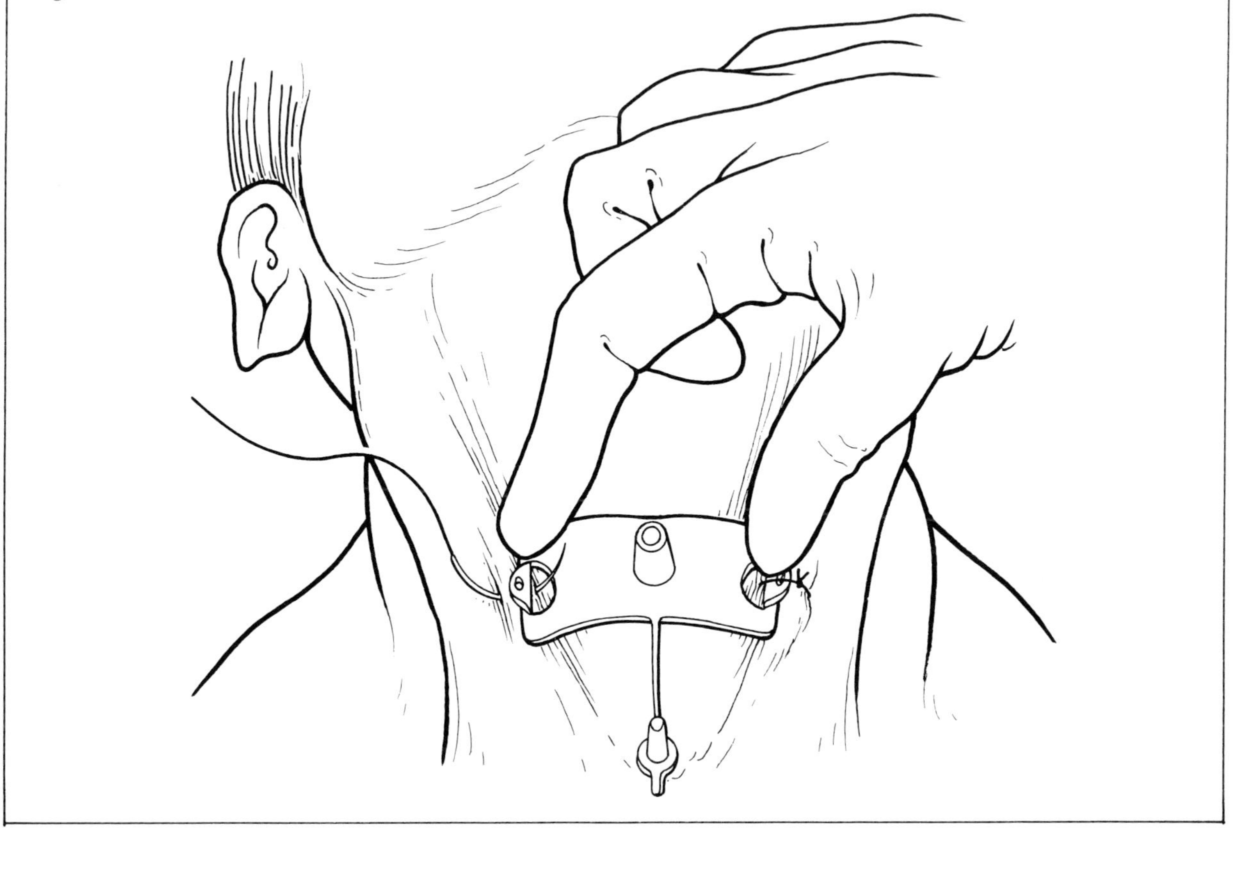

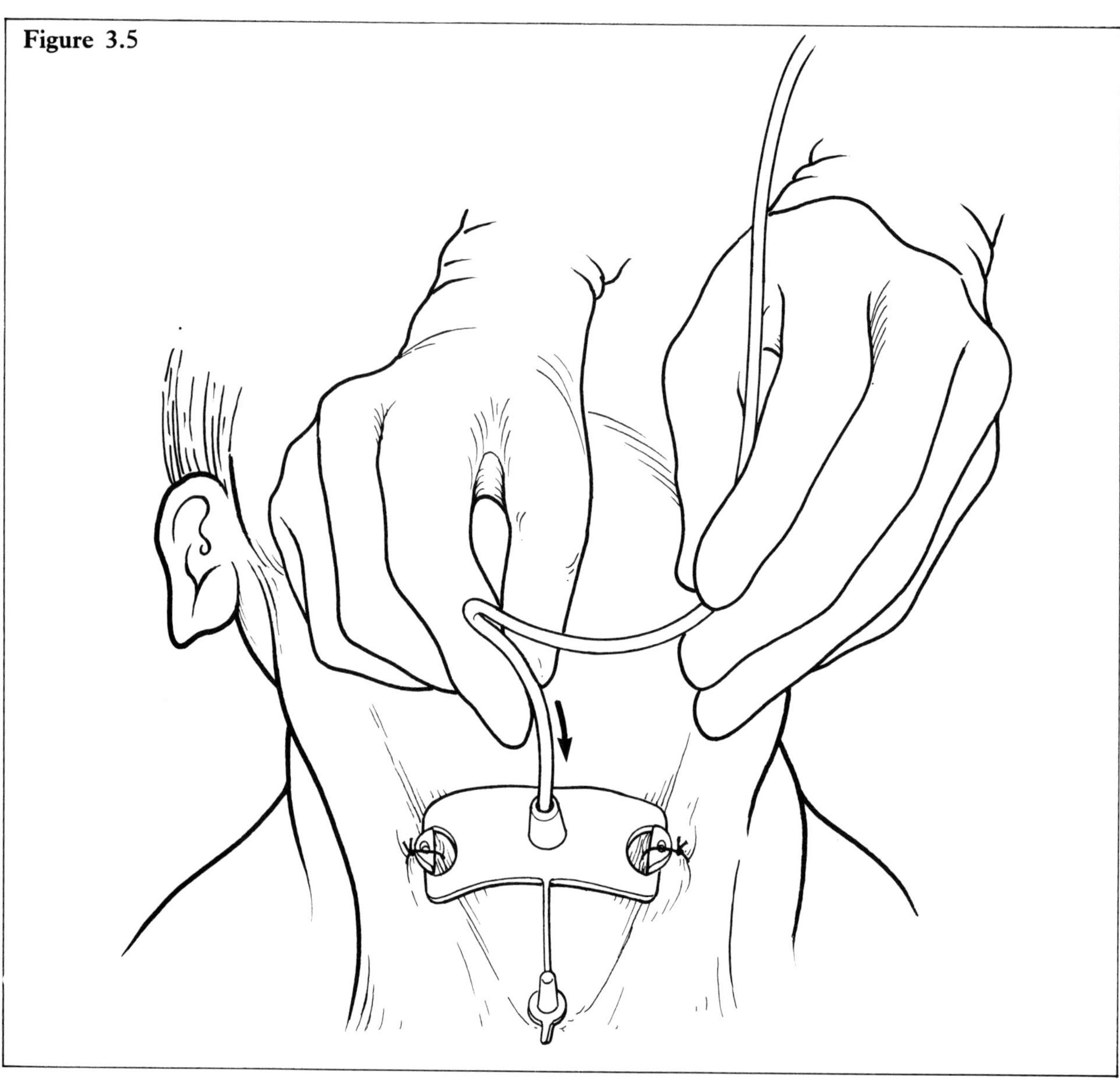
**Figure 3.5**

### Removal

To remove the mini-tracheostomy tube, simply pull it out and place a light dressing over the wound. It will close securely in two to three days. No sutures are required.

# 4 Insertion of a chest drain

The teaching of this common minor surgical procedure would appear to be confused and inadequate, judging by the frequency of subsequent complications that require the attention of a thoracic specialist unit. A simple and safe method is described here.

## Indications

1. Spontaneous pneumothorax. Although small pneumothoraces may be allowed to resolve without intervention, or by simple aspiration, those that are greater than 10% of the volume of the hemithorax ought to be treated by the insertion of a chest drain.
2. Tension pneumothorax (an absolute indication).
3. The presence of a significant pleural effusion, or empyema (see Chapter 16). Many specialists would now choose to drain such fluid collections initially by the insertion of a small-bore catheter introduced under ultrasonic or fluoroscopic control in the department of radiology. The argument persists, however, between some surgeons as to the relative merits of a fine-bore versus a large-bore tube for fluid collections within the thorax.
4. Post-traumatic haemothorax. In this situation a large-bore tube is to be preferred because of the likelihood of a blood clot obstructing a small catheter.

In each of these situations the attending physician should have a safe and practised method for the insertion of a chest drain. If the doctor who is to insert the drain lacks experience, it is imperative that he or she is supervised, as this procedure badly performed is very dangerous.

## Procedure

First, the site for insertion of the drain should be chosen. Usually the best site is through the fourth or fifth intercostal space in the mid-axillary line. The axilla is bounded anteriorly by the pectoralis major muscle, and posteriorly by the latissimus dorsi muscle. Between these two the only structures overlying the chest wall are skin and fat, and the uppermost part of the serratus anterior muscle (see p. 38). For the drainage of specific air or fluid collections, the appropriate site on the chest wall should be chosen.

If the patient is in a comfortable and relaxed position the procedure will be more easily accomplished. For most situations the patient may be allowed to sit on the edge of the bed with the bedside table in front and elevated to its maximum height. Place a pillow on top such that the patient may relax with arms crossed on the pillow and head resting on the arms. This will maintain the arms abducted from the chest wall to 90 degrees.

Adequate analgesia is essential. If the patient is extremely anxious an oral dose of benzodiazepine may be given 20 minutes before the procedure; if the situation is more pressing then a small intravenous dose is preferable. After preparing the skin with an antiseptic (chlorhexidine is to be preferred), 0.5% plain bupivacaine or lignocaine is infiltrated into the skin, muscles and finally (and very importantly) the pleura, at the chosen site. There is no need to use a stronger solution of local anaesthetic as it is no more effective and indeed reduces the volume that can be administered. Wait for 5 to 10 minutes for the anaesthetic effect to be achieved. During this time the equipment to be used should be checked and all the connections for the tubing and bottles inspected to ensure that they are of appropriate size and that they will fit together. This is the responsibility of the doctor carrying out the procedure, and the nurse who is helping should not be blamed if the equipment is faulty or inappropriate.

Next, an incision is made in the skin overlying the centre of the chosen intercostal space. This should be long enough to accept comfortably the diameter of the selected drain. The incision is deepened to the fat layer; any troublesome bleeding encountered should be dealt with at this stage. A pair of sharp, pointed scissors or short artery clips should then be used with a spreading action to develop a hole through the intercostal muscles down to the pleural layer (**Fig. 4.1**). The pleura is opened in a similar fashion. Final dissection into the pleural space is made with a finger (**Fig. 4.2**). If this procedure is uncomfortable for the patient, more local anaesthetic is inserted. Open the

Figure 4.1

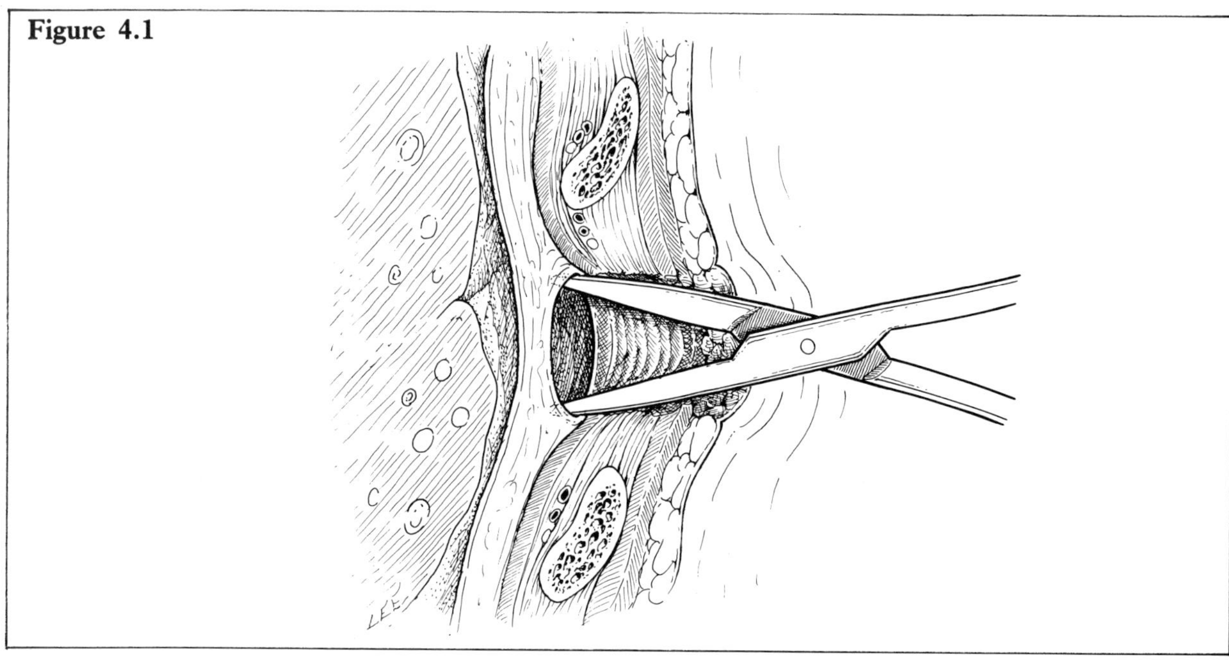

Figure 4.2

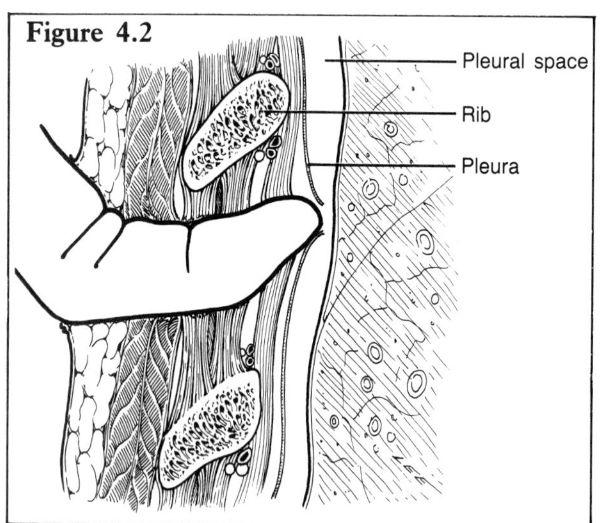


instrument widely in two directions at 90 degrees to each other. If there is a tension pneumothorax this action will be met with a rush of air and instant relief for the patient. If the underlying lung is collapsed no harm can be done. If the lung is only partially collapsed, the fact that it may collapse further is irrelevant because the drain will be introduced and connected to the underwater seal allowing complete re-expansion.

Next, sutures are inserted to hold the drain in place and to secure the hole when the drain is removed in due course. These should be strong, non-absorbable sutures—preferably not silk, which can be very irritant to the skin, and may weaken with time if the drain has to be in place for long. The suture to hold the drain in place is sited to one side of the incision, and the one for future closure of the incision should be a vertical or horizontal mattress suture in the centre of the wound. A purse-string suture is counterproductive, as it will tend to convert the longitudinal incision into a circle when it is pulled up and hence may hold the incision open.

The chest drain is then inserted through the chest wall. If the dissection has been adequate, little or no force will be required to enter the pleural space, hence removing the risk of damaging any of the underlying vital structures. The sharply pointed metal trocar within the tube may be withdrawn so that it does not protrude from the end but merely acts as a stent over which the drain may be advanced (**Fig. 4.3**). This allows the catheter to be placed in the appropriate position (**Fig. 4.4**).

The drain should be positioned so that the tip is 20–30 mm from the apex of the pleural space. It is secured in place with the stitch which has already been sited as described above. Heavy strapping should be avoided as it will tend to kink the drain and prevents ready inspection. The connections of the drainage tube to the underwater seal bottle should not be taped; a properly fitting connector is all that is necessary. In our opinion, in almost all situations the drain should be connected to suction. Wall suction of high flow and low pressure is optimal. The pressure that we usually advocate is 100 mmHg (13 kPa).

## Removal of a chest drain

A chest drain should be removed when all air and fluid leak has ceased. The lung should be fully expanded and there should not be a large ‘swing’ in the fluid level in the drainage tube. This acts as a water manometer and reflects the changes in the intrapleural pressure on breathing. A large excursion in the fluid level reflects significant

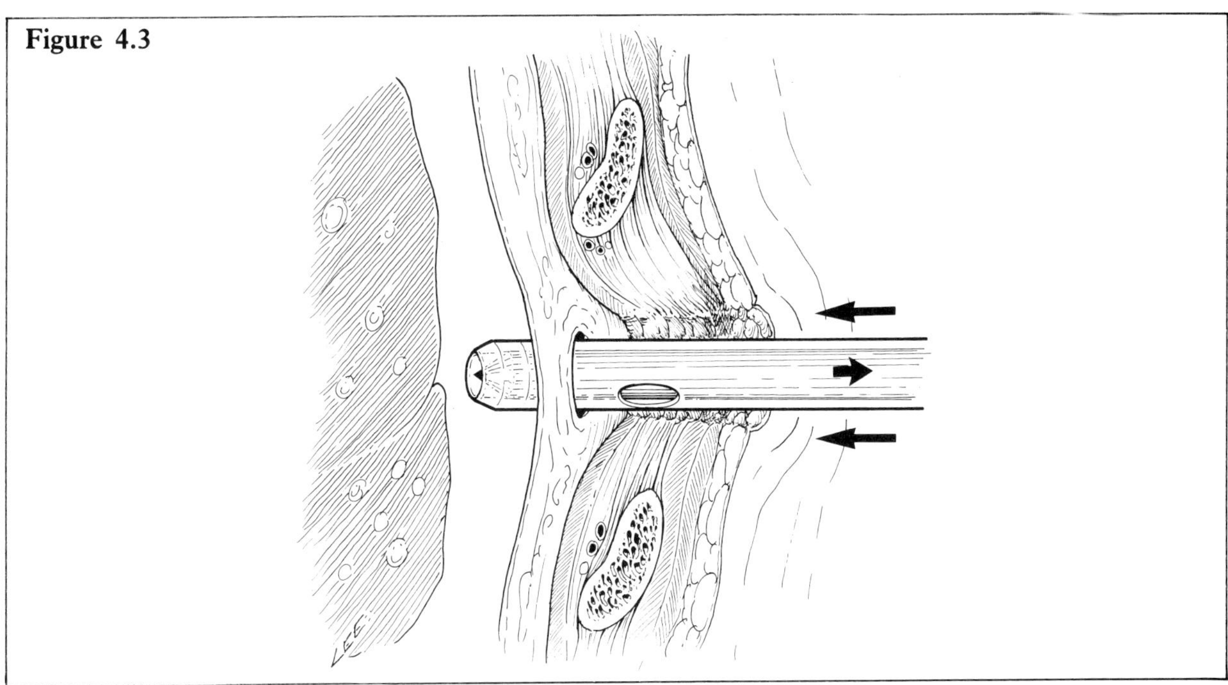


Figure 4.3

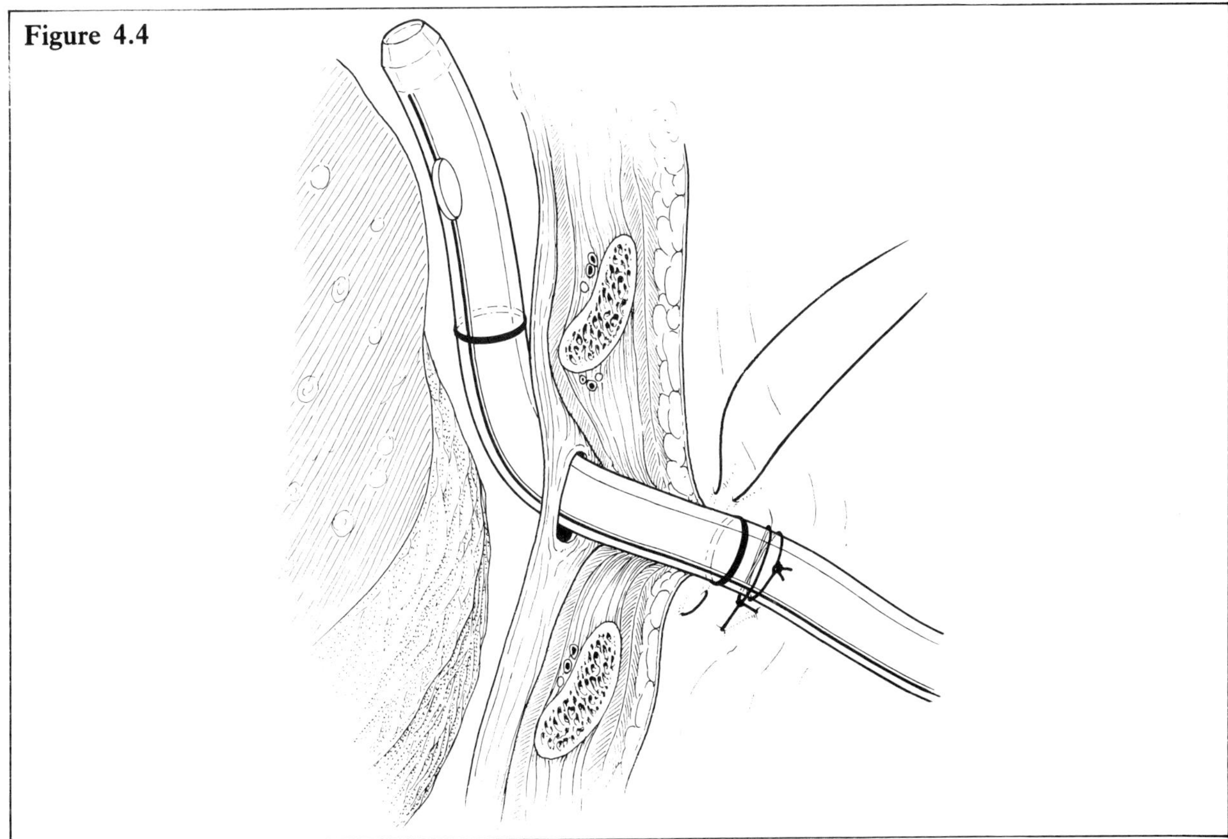

Figure 4.4

pressure changes in the pleural space with the movements of breathing. This occurs as a result of decreased compliance in the underlying lung. As complete re-aeration of the lung occurs, its compliance will return to normal and the swing in the fluid level will reduce. If the tube is removed too early while the lung is still very stiff there will be a tendency for it to collapse away from the chest wall, and any visceral pleural defect may reopen and a further pneumothorax occur.

Removal of the chest drain is best effected by asking the patient to breathe out maximally, while the drain is briskly withdrawn, and the previously sited suture tied.

SECTION 2

# ANATOMY OF THE CHEST WALL AND THORACIC INCISIONS

# 5 Surgical anatomy of the chest wall

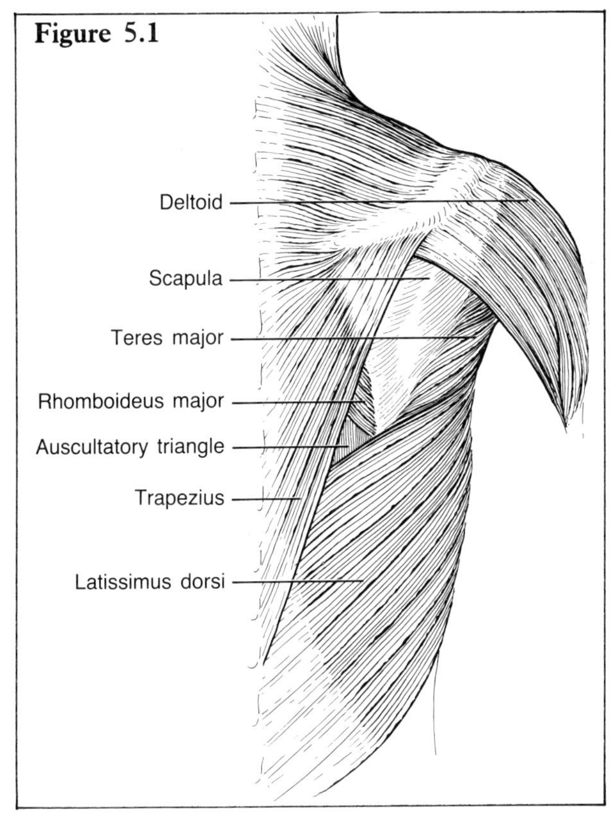


**Figure** 5.1

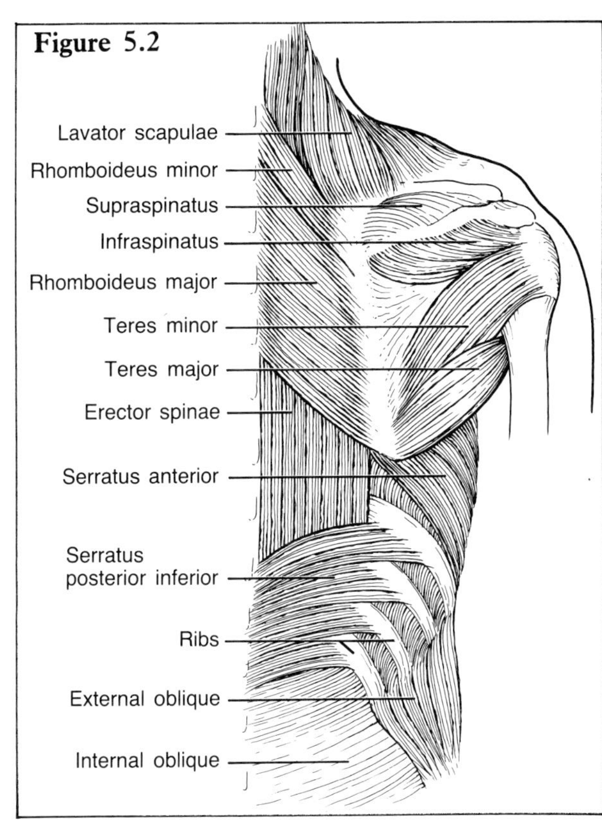


**Figure** 5.2

A clear understanding of the anatomy of the chest wall is essential to enable the surgeon to enter the thorax safely and in such a way that when the incision is closed it leaves an ultimately comfortable and cosmetically acceptable scar for the patient.

There are two layers of muscles overlying the chest wall. These are responsible for the control of movement of the arm and the shoulder. The largest muscles in the outer layer are the trapezius and latissimus dorsi muscles (**Fig. 5.1**). In lateral and posterolateral thoracotomy incisions the lower part of the trapezius and the whole of the latissimus dorsi muscles are transected. The nerve supply of the latissimus dorsi is via the long thoracic nerve which enters the muscle from in front and above. The lower the transection of this muscle, therefore, the less that will be denervated. The pectoralis major muscle lies in the same plane anteriorly and an anterior thoracotomy incision will pass through it.

Beneath this layer are the muscles that control the movements of the scapula (**Fig. 5.2**). These muscles can usually be preserved at thoracotomy. In operations such as thoracoplasty, however, the rhomboid muscles are divided (see p. 58).

## Intercostal spaces

There are three layers of muscle between the ribs. These are the external, internal and innermost intercostal muscles. The intercostal neurovascular bundle and its collateral branches are found between the inner and innermost layers (**Figs. 5.3, 5.4**).

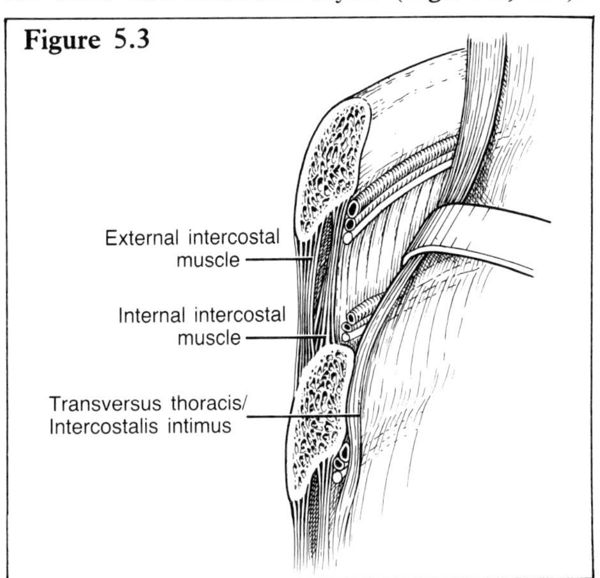


**Figure** 5.3

**Figure 5.4**

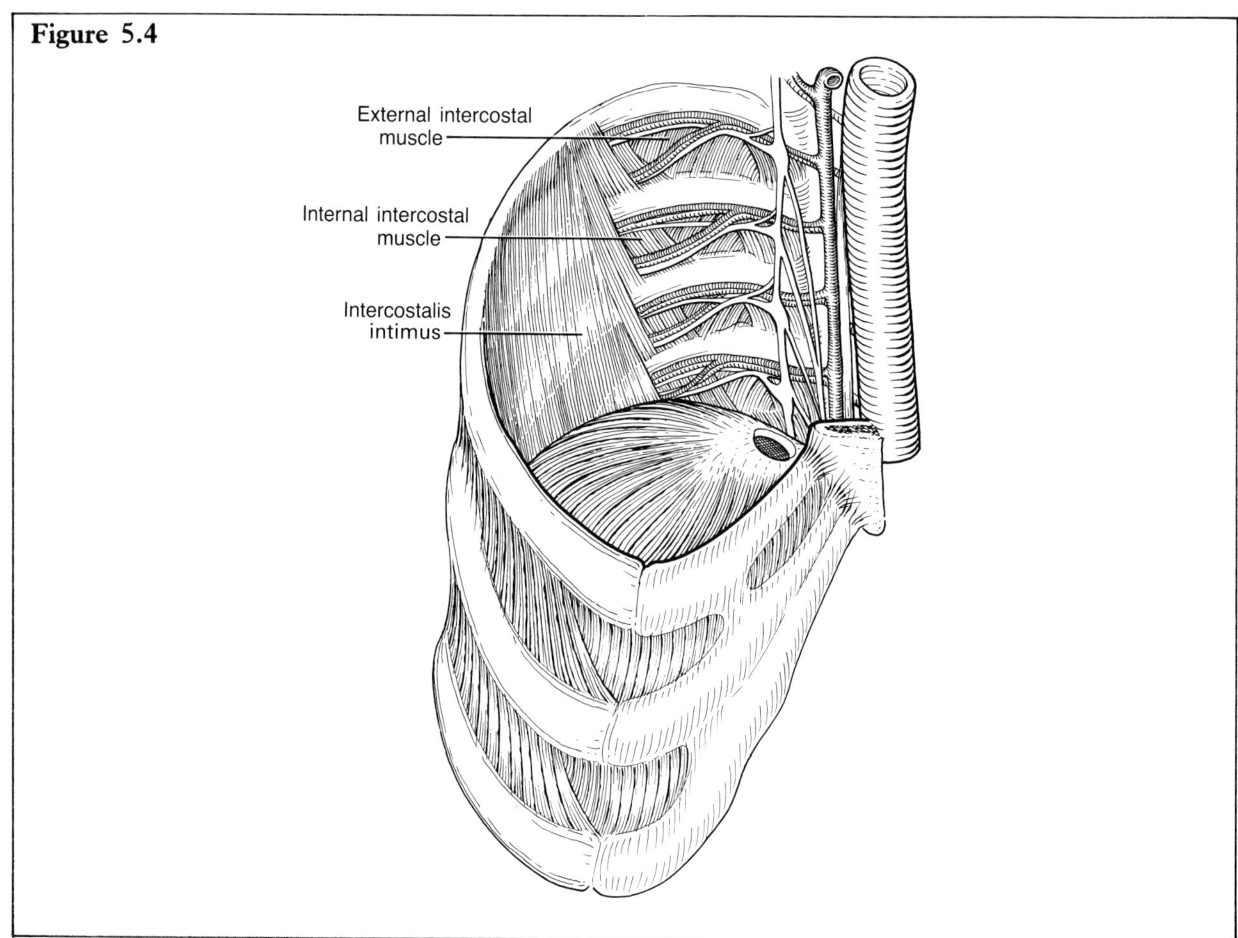


The innermost layer is made up of three elements. The transversus thoracis muscle anteriorly is in continuity with the innermost intercostal muscle laterally via a fascial membrane. Posteriorly are the slips of the subcostalis muscle. These arise from the inner surface of one rib near its angle, and are inserted into the inner surface of the second or third rib below. They are well developed only in the lower part of the thorax.

## Diaphragm

This large muscle separates the two great body cavities, the thorax and abdomen. It is an important muscle of respiration, innervated bilaterally by the phrenic nerves. These nerves radiate into the muscle from their point of departure from the pericardium. If the diaphragm is to be opened it should be cut radially between the nerves, or circumferentially approximately 25 mm from the costal attachment, to allow resuture at the end of the procedure. This will prevent paralysis due to complete denervation.

The diaphragm is a dome-shaped muscle with the concavity forming the roof of the abdomen. The posterior portion is almost vertical, forming a deep costophrenic recess. The muscle fibres insert into the central tendon through which the inferior vena cava passes at the level of the tenth thoracic vertebra. The attachment of the inferior vena cava at this point means that when the diaphragm contracts in inspiration the vessel is held open, aiding venous return.

The oesophagus traverses the diaphragm at the level of the tenth thoracic vertebra and is slung between two condensations of muscle, the right and left crura (**Fig. 5.5**). Although the aorta passes through the diaphragm at the level of the twelfth thoracic vertebra, because the diaphragm is so vertical at this point it is only a few centimetres behind and below the oesophagus.

## Thoracic outlet

The thoracic outlet is an important junctional area. It is bounded anteriorly by the manubrium and anterolaterally by the first ribs. Posteriorly the first thoracic vertebra and the posterior angles of the first ribs bound the space (**Fig. 5.6**).

Through this space the great vessels of the head, neck and arm pass to their destinations. They have a complex relationship with the scalene muscles and the first rib and clavicles. Compression of these structures gives rise to an important group of problems collectively referred to as the thoracic outlet syndrome (see p. 54).

**Figure 5.5**

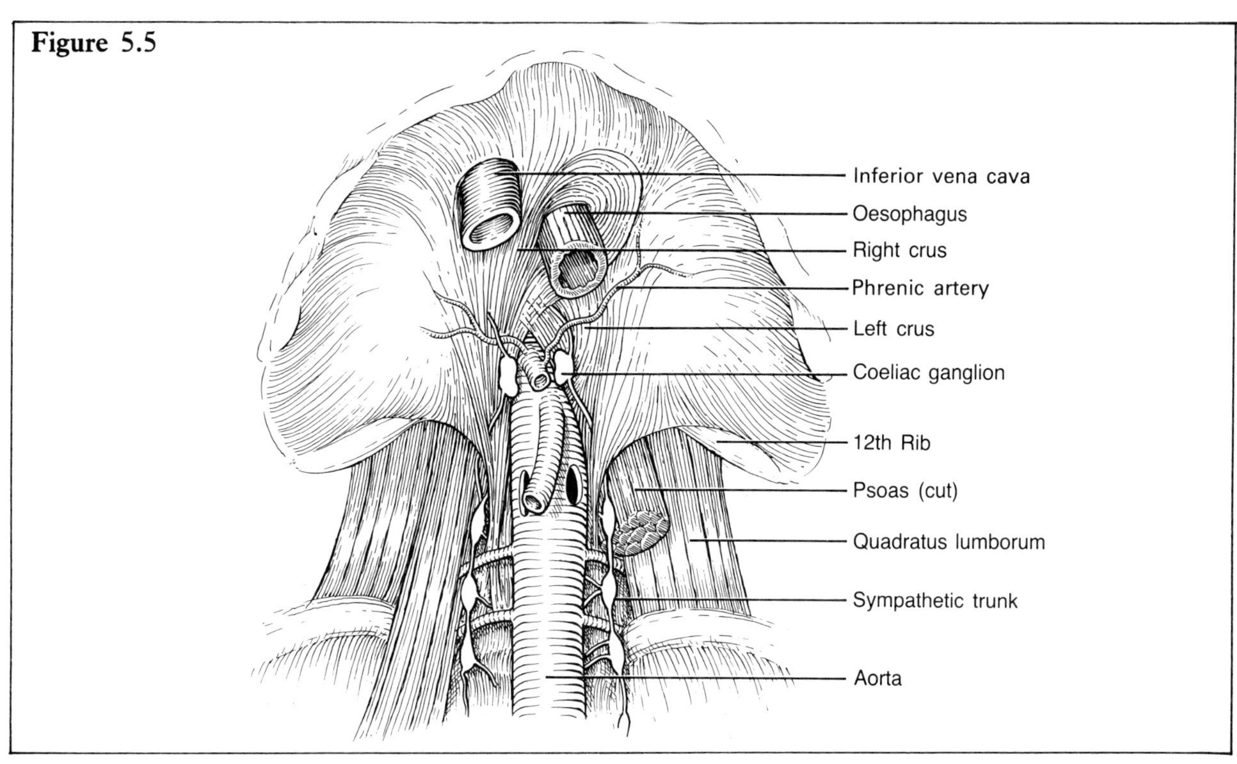


**Figure 5.6**

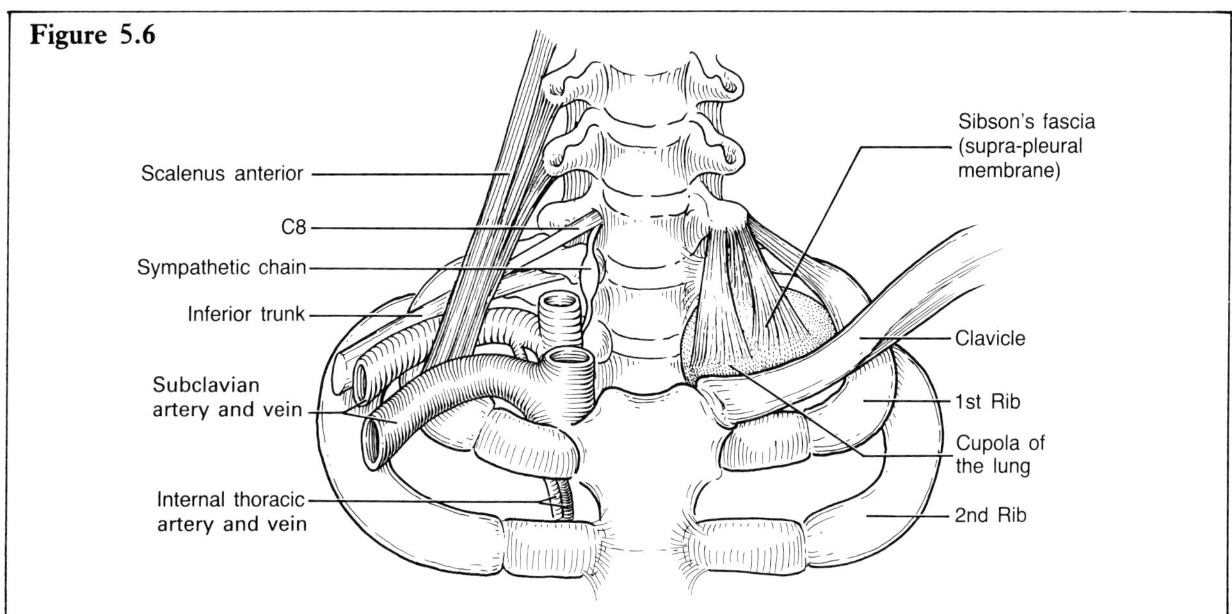

# 6 Posterolateral thoracotomy

The patient should be positioned on the contralateral side with the thoracic spinous processes vertically above the edge of the operating table so that the patient's back is vertical. The lower leg is flexed at both hip and knee and the upper leg is kept straight. The knees are separated by a pillow. A strap, carefully padded where it passes over the lateral aspect of the hip and buttocks, holds the lower half of the body in position (**Fig. 6.1**). A more rigid fixation is obtained if this strap passes over a pelvic support which is fixed anterior to the pubis. An anterior chest support is unnecessary, but additional fixation of the upper half of the body can be obtained by attaching the outer aspect of the upper arm and forearm to the operating table with adhesive plaster. The upper arm is flexed to a right angle at the elbow and shoulder to rotate the scapula forward away from the midline.

The incision starts at the midpoint between the thoracic spinous processes and the medial border of the scapula (**Fig. 6.2**, right inset). The upper limit of the incision depends on the particular intercostal space which is to be approached. For the common approach to the fifth rib, a point halfway between the spine of the scapula and its

**Figure 6.1**

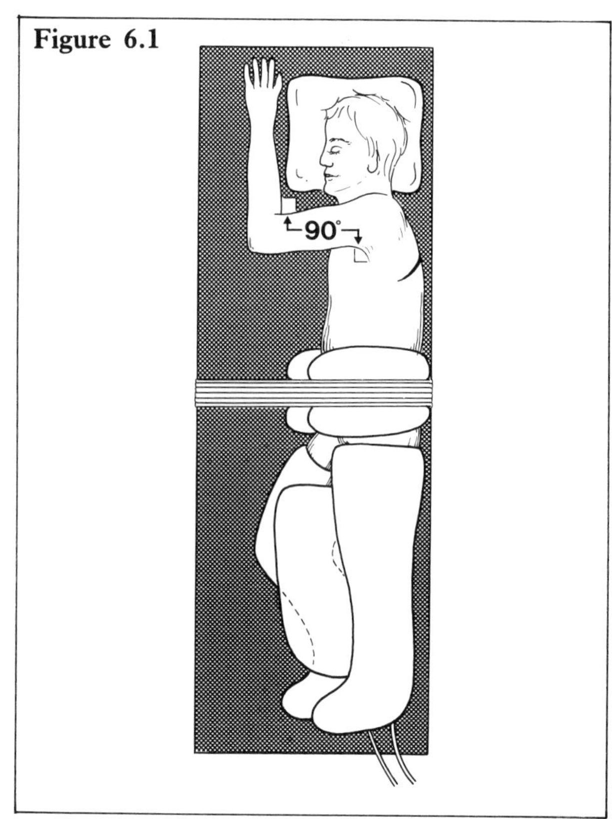


**Figure 6.2**

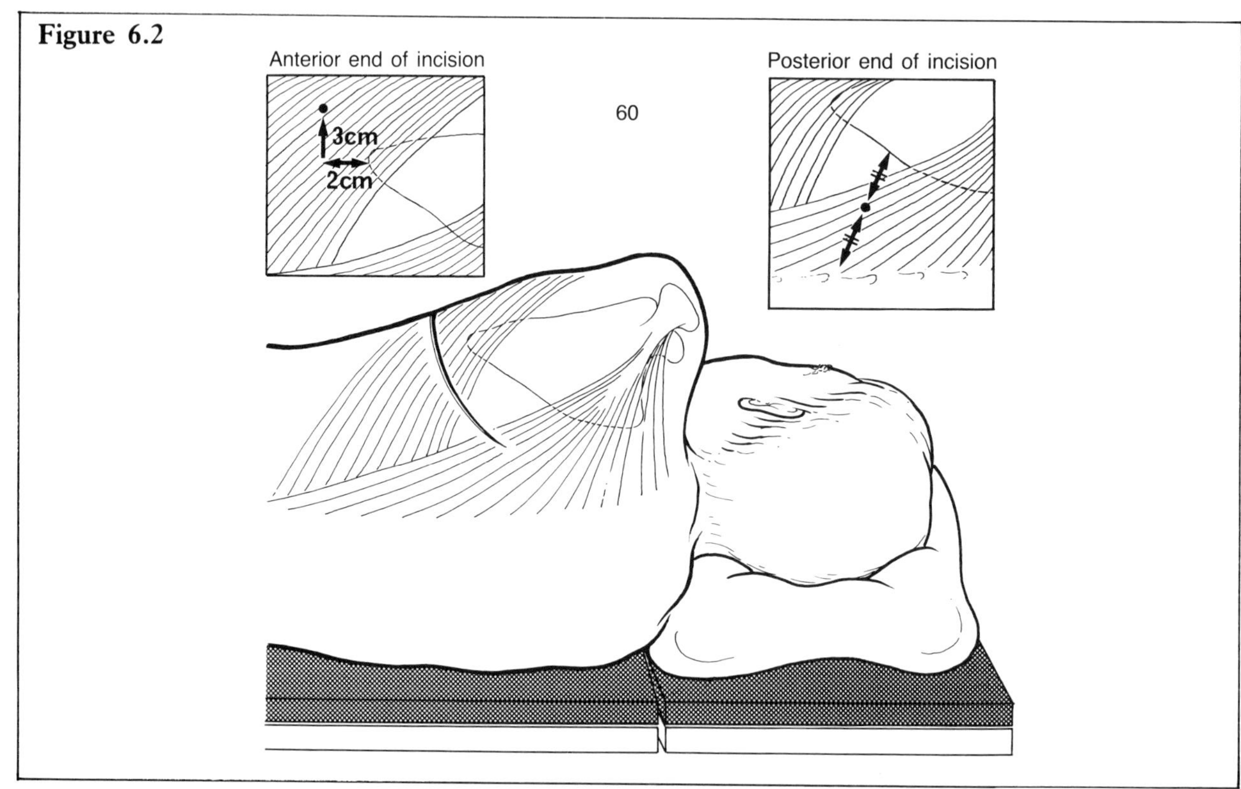

**Figure 6.3**

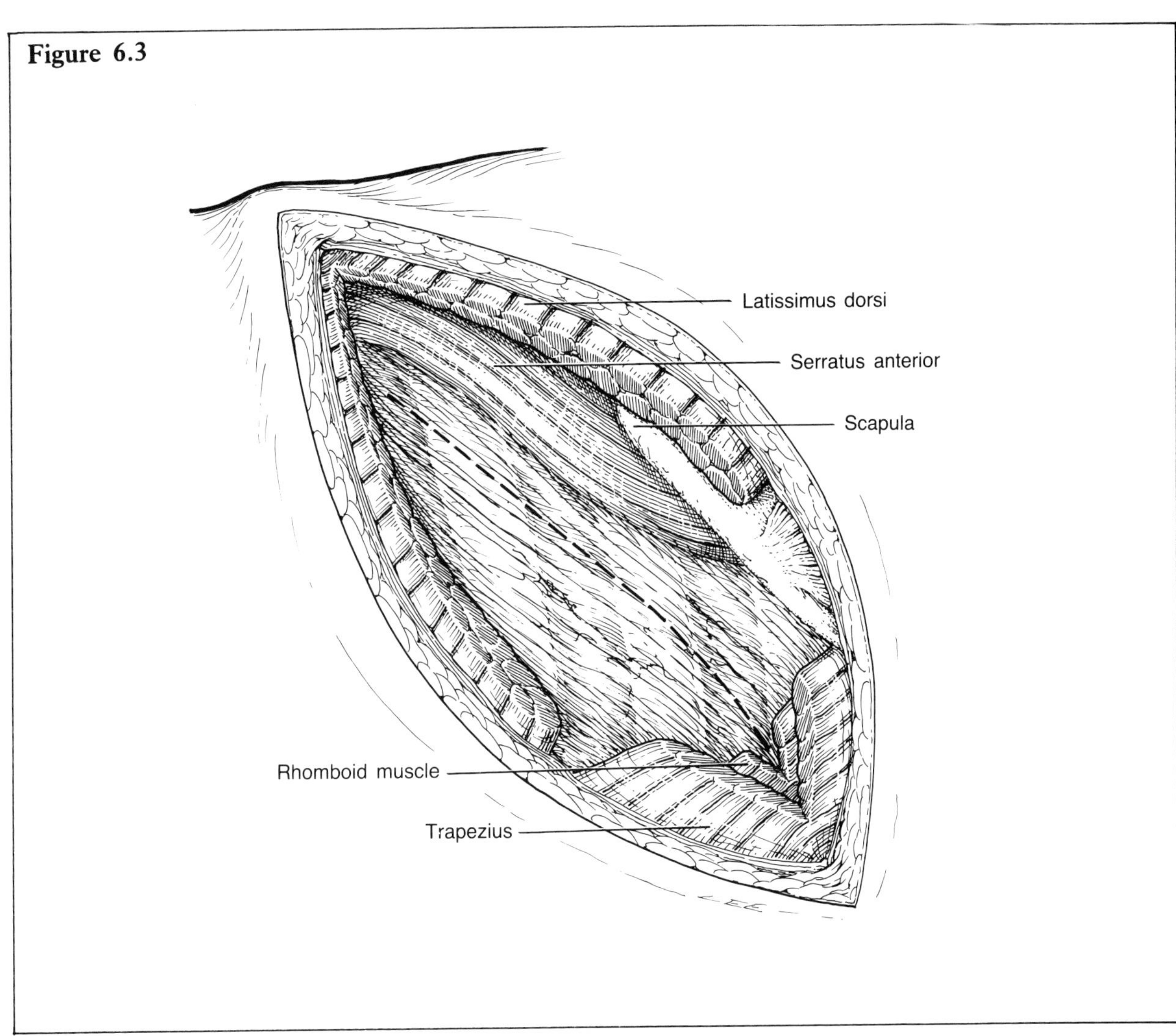


inferior angle is chosen. The anterior end of the incision is extended to 2 cm below and 3 cm in front of the inferior angle of the scapula (**Fig. 6.2**, left inset). The skin incision is made with a knife and all further cutting is done with diathermy.

In the posterior part of the incision a small part of the trapezius muscle is divided and at the centre and anterior end the whole of the latissimus dorsi muscle is divided (**Fig. 6.3**). Between these two muscles is a layer of fascia which unites them. This is incised down to the periosteum and the ribs. The rhomboid muscle and an extensive sheet of fibrofatty tissue anterior to it are divided as far forward as the serratus anterior muscle. The incision is extended along the posterior margin of the serratus anterior (**Fig. 6.3**). If extensive exposure is required, the serratus anterior is divided or detached from the ribs. Haemostasis is secured using diathermy.

By elevating the posteroinferior free margin of the serratus anterior muscle with a pair of strong toothed forceps, the fascia between it and the chest wall is stretched making it easier to incise with diathermy. The plane of the ribs and intercostal muscles is then reached. Working in this plane makes for a more haemostatic wound.

A scapula retractor is used to retract the scapula away from the chest wall. The ribs are counted by passing the hand, palm downwards, beneath and behind the scapula in the paravertebral region. In this way it is possible to identify the first rib and to count downwards. The second rib has attached to it a large digitation of the serratus anterior muscle, and the outer margin of the first rib can just be felt with the tips of the fingers above and behind this. The lowest digitation of the serratus posterior superior muscle commonly arises from the fifth rib, but occasionally from the fourth or sixth, so that it is not as good a means of identifying an individual rib (**Fig. 6.4**).

The pleural cavity is entered through the periosteal bed of a rib. It is hardly ever necessary to resect the rib. Resection is usually reserved for decortication of the lung and for dealing with very large tumours.

The periosteum is incised along the upper or lower margin of the selected rib (**Fig. 6.5**) from the sacrospinalis muscle behind, to the level of

**Figure 6.4**

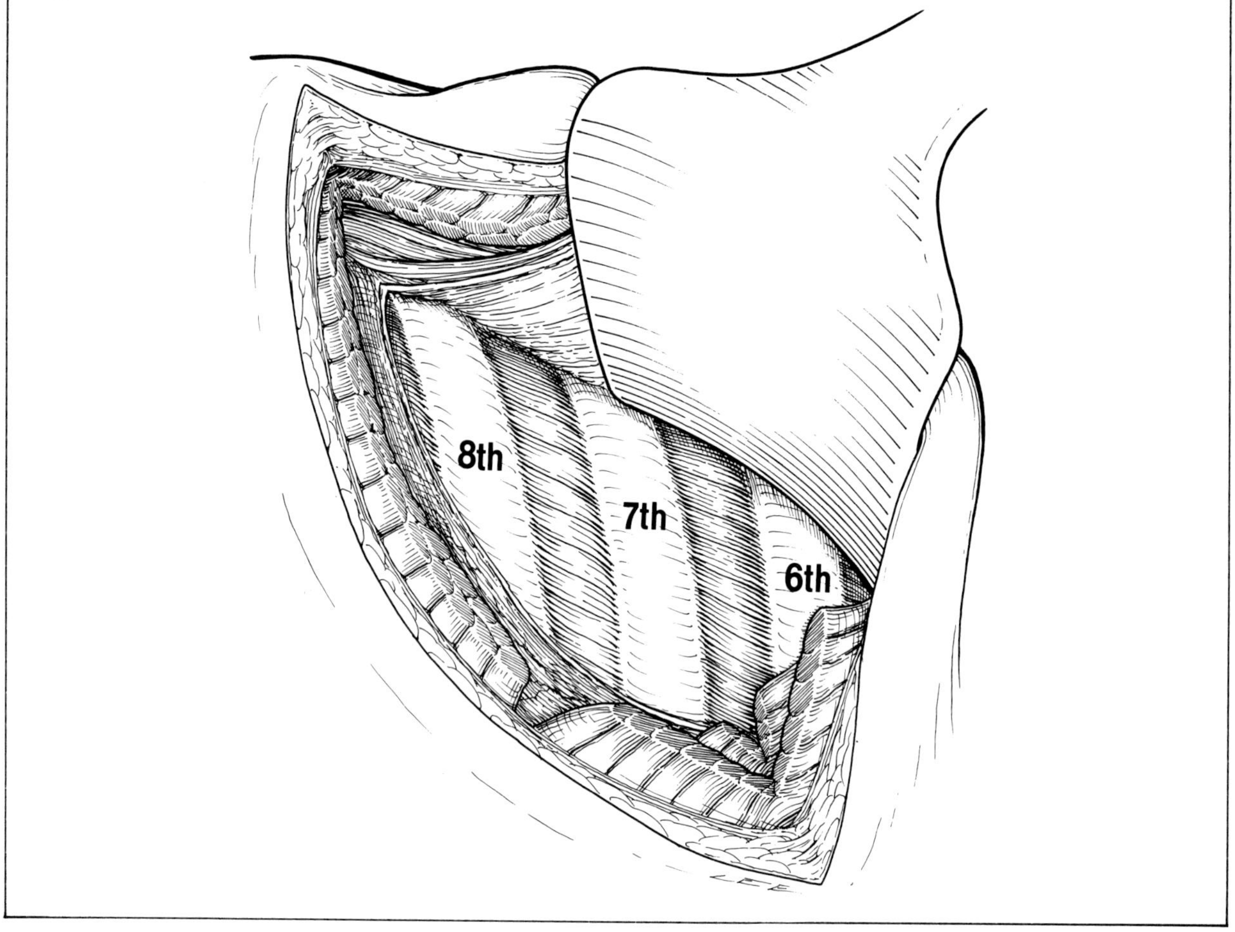

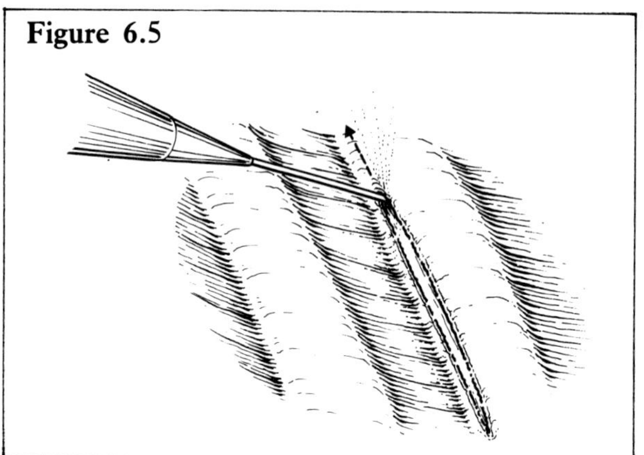

**Figure 6.5**

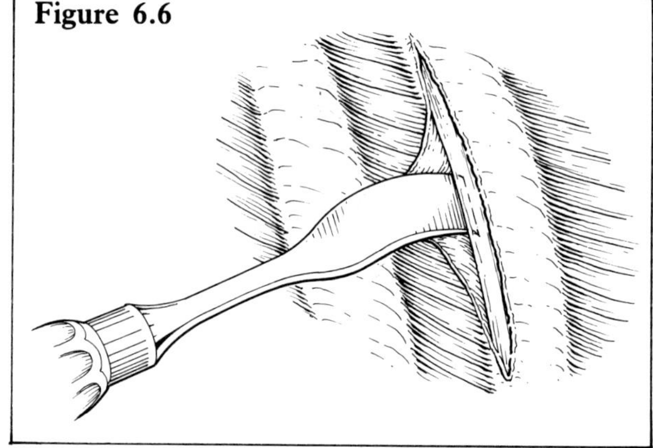

**Figure 6.6**

the anterior axillary line. Posteriorly it aids closure if the incision is carried for a distance of about 3 cm behind the sacrospinalis muscle. A curved raspatory is then used to free the periosteum from the outer surface of the rib, and then completely from its deep surface (**Fig. 6.6**). For a clean detachment of the periosteum the raspatory should be directed from behind forward along the lower margin of the rib (**Fig. 6.7**). The costotransverse ligament between the rib and transverse process may now be divided with the Semb chisel (**Fig. 6.8**). The ligament is reached by advancing the chisel medially along the outer and

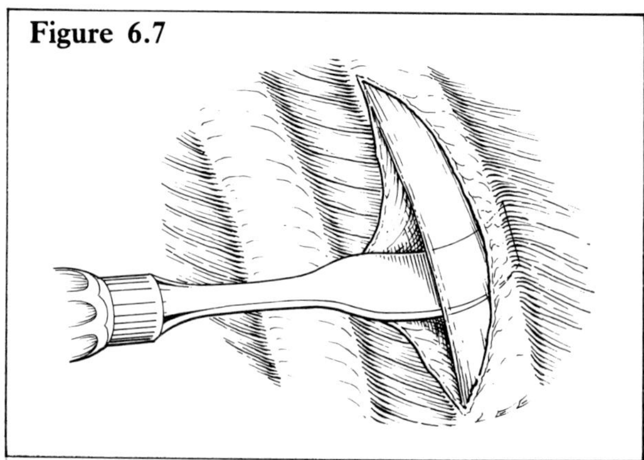

**Figure 6.7**

**Figure 6.8**

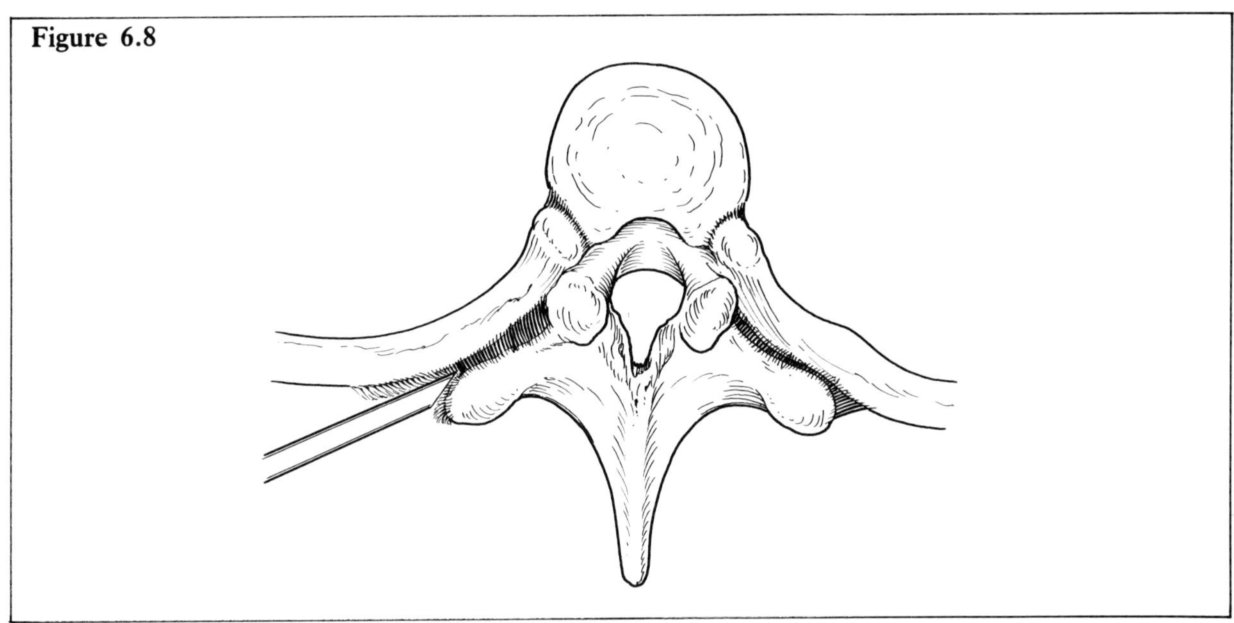

**Figure 6.9**

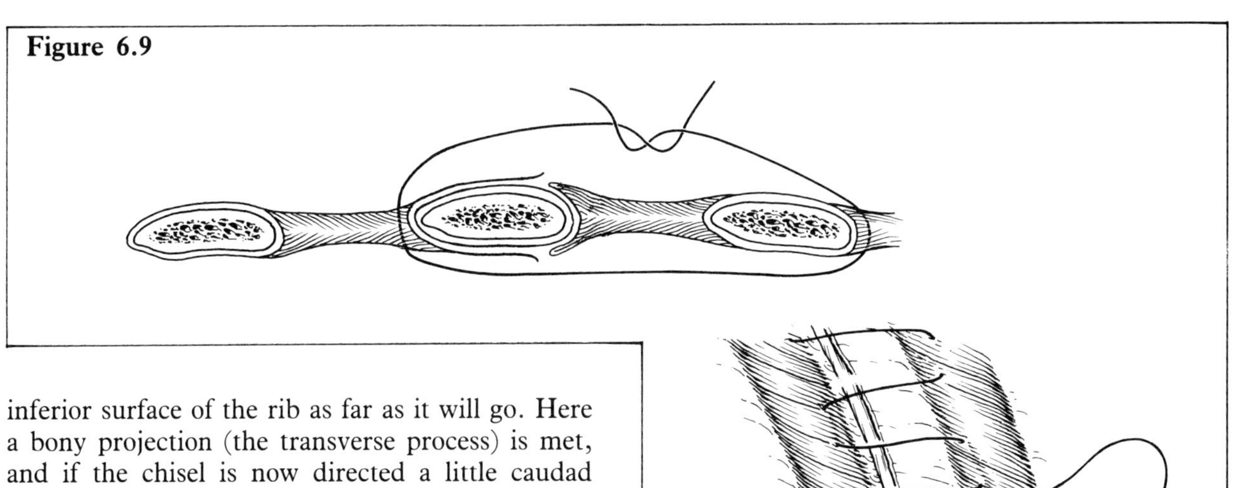

inferior surface of the rib as far as it will go. Here a bony projection (the transverse process) is met, and if the chisel is now directed a little caudad and gently rotated about its long axis with the application of pressure the ligament will be heard to disrupt. The manoeuvre can be made easier by introducing a rib spreader and opening it a little so that the ligament is under tension when it is cut. Alternatively a 1-cm length of rib may be removed posteriorly beneath the erector spinae muscle. This obviates the need to disrupt the costotransverse ligament and in our opinion leads to less late postoperative pain. It also removes the small but ever-present risk of damage to the spinal cord by diathermy to retracted bleeding vessels near the spinal foramina.

The pleural cavity is entered by incising with a knife the periosteum and pleura separated from the deep surface of the rib. The lung will then fall away from the parietal pleura, which can be incised throughout the length of the incision with diathermy or scissors without risk of damage.

Great care should be taken not to over-distract the ribs when the retractor is inserted, as this is another contributory factor to postoperative neuralgia.

Closure of the intercostal incision is achieved with a continuous suture of no. 1 nylon. The ribs on either side of the incision may be approximated with a rib approximator, although this is rarely necessary. The suture may be a continuous over-and-over stitch which passes over the rib above the incision and through the intercostal muscle below it (**Fig. 6.9a**), or a continuous, horizontal mattress suture traversing the intercostal muscles above and below the incision (**Fig. 6.9b**). The intercostal suture is started anteriorly as less tension is needed to approximate the ribs due to the lever effect. The partly mobilized sacrospinalis muscle can be used to complete the closure of the pleural space posteriorly. Alternatively six strong, interrupted pericostal sutures may be used to approximate the ribs.

Continuous nylon sutures are used to approximate the two muscle layers—the first layer comprising the rhomboideus major, the fascia and the serratus anterior, and the second, the trapezius and latissimus dorsi. Absorbable sutures are used for the subcutaneous tissue and also as a subcuticular suture to approximate the skin.

If there is a high risk of wound infection, interrupted monofilament inert sutures such as nylon or polypropylene are recommended to close the skin.

## Postoperative pleural drainage

The pleural space should be drained after any thoracotomy to prevent the development of a tension pneumothorax and to allow immediate detection of intrapleural haemorrhage. However, many thoracic surgeons do not insert a drain into the pleural space after pneumonectomy and rely on needle aspiration of the pleural cavity when necessary to adjust the intrapleural pressure and volume. In our opinion this adds a small, unnecessary risk to the operation.

A single tube suffices after pneumonectomy, most operations on the mediastinum, closed heart operations and lung biopsies.

Two tubes should be inserted after any major lung resection other than a pneumonectomy. This is to ensure early and complete expansion of the remaining lung to obliterate the pleural space as rapidly as possible. Multiple drains will ensure that air can continue to drain from the pleural cavity even if one tube becomes obstructed, and also allow for strategic placement. One tube may be placed at the apex and the other at the base of the thorax. Two tubes are recommended after oesophageal resections.

After partial lung resection it is advisable that the tubes should be located anteriorly and posteriorly to ensure drainage of all areas of the pleural cavity. The posterior drain will usually remain in position by virtue of the progressive expansion of the remaining lung. However, the anterior tube is liable to become displaced, and it is best to attach it by a single absorbable stitch to the posterior surface of the second or third intercostal muscle.

In cases where a large amount of oozing may be expected in the postoperative period (for example after decortication of the lung and drainage of an empyema), three drains are advisable.

### Insertion of drainage tubes

Drainage tubes are inserted into the pleural cavity below the line of the incision. Above the incision the scapula interferes with placement. After the rib spreader has been removed the pleural aspects of the two ends of the incision are inspected to ensure there is no bleeding after the release of tension on the wound edges. The latissimus dorsi muscle in the lower half of the wound is then pulled up to its anatomical position with the aid of two tissue forceps to overcome its retraction; 15-mm skin incisions are then made in the appropriate intercostal space. This is determined with one hand palpating the rib spaces from within (**Fig. 6.10**). The most dependent spaces are chosen. Two skin sutures are inserted at the site of each incision: one to the side of the incision which is to be used to secure the tube, and a second across the middle of the incision which will be used to close the incision when the drainage tube is removed.

A long, curved forceps is passed into the pleural cavity via the incision until the tip shows in the wound (**Fig. 6.11**). A 15-mm rubber or plastic tube is then grasped with the forceps and drawn outwards through the chest wall. Drains should run from base to apex and should have several side holes. Each drain will then remove both air and fluid.

Before the chest is closed the tubes are connected to underwater seal bottles.

After pneumonectomy the drain is clamped and released for one minute every hour. In this way some fluid is retained in the pleural cavity. Suction is never applied to the tube draining a pneumonectomy space since it would result in extreme mediastinal displacement. The tube is removed the morning after operation once a chest radiograph has shown that the mediastinum is central.

In all other cases suction of 50–100 mmHg (7–13 kPa)—100 mmHg being our preference for almost all cases—is applied to the exit tube of the underwater seal. The tubes remain *in situ* until drainage and any air leak have ceased completely.

The tubes are removed when there is no movement of the fluid level in the underwater end of the tubing, indicating that the tube is blocked, or minimal movement of the fluid level with respiration is observed, indicating a return towards normal compliance of the remaining lung, and a chest radiograph shows that the lung is fully expanded.

If the drain is clearly blocked but there is a persistent air space or fluid collection, a new drain should be inserted at the appropriate site. This can most accurately be accomplished with radiological screening and ultrasound guidance. For patient comfort a fine-bore pig-tail catheter may be used.

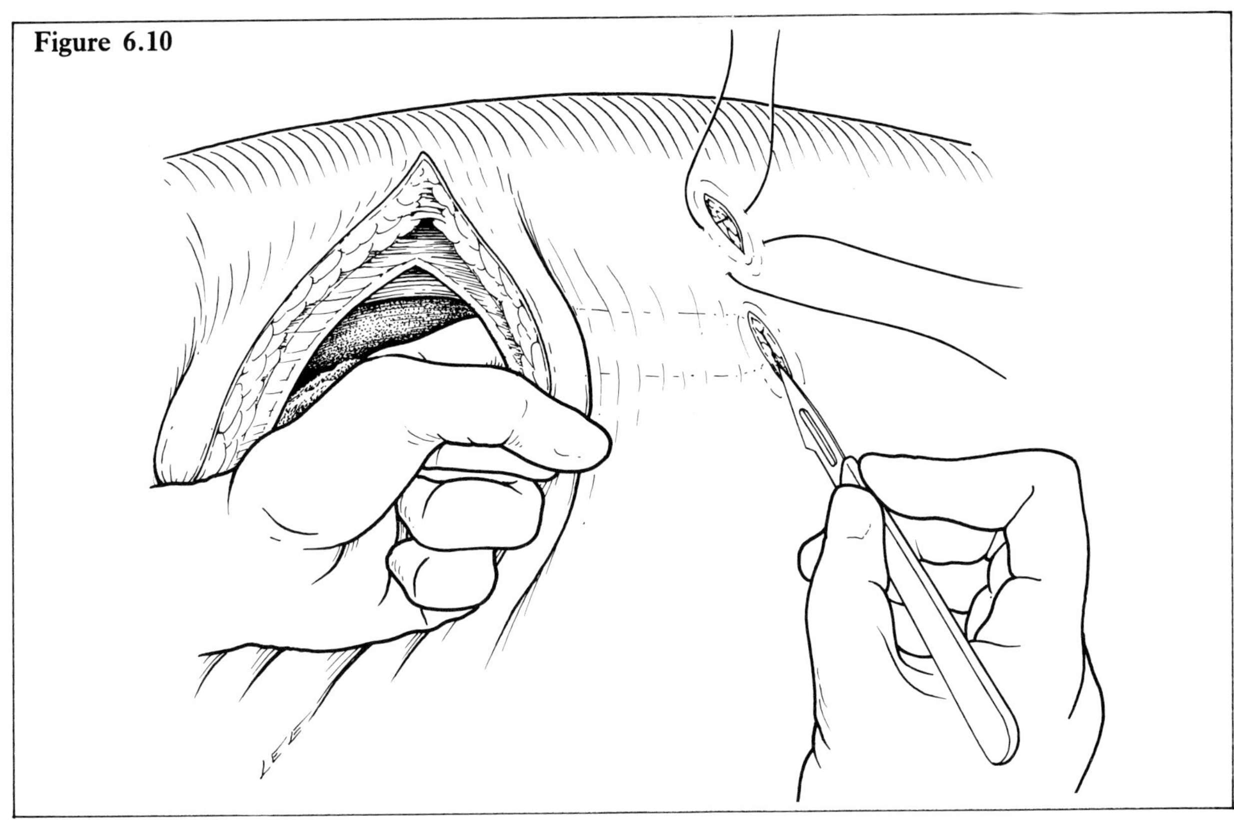

Figure 6.10

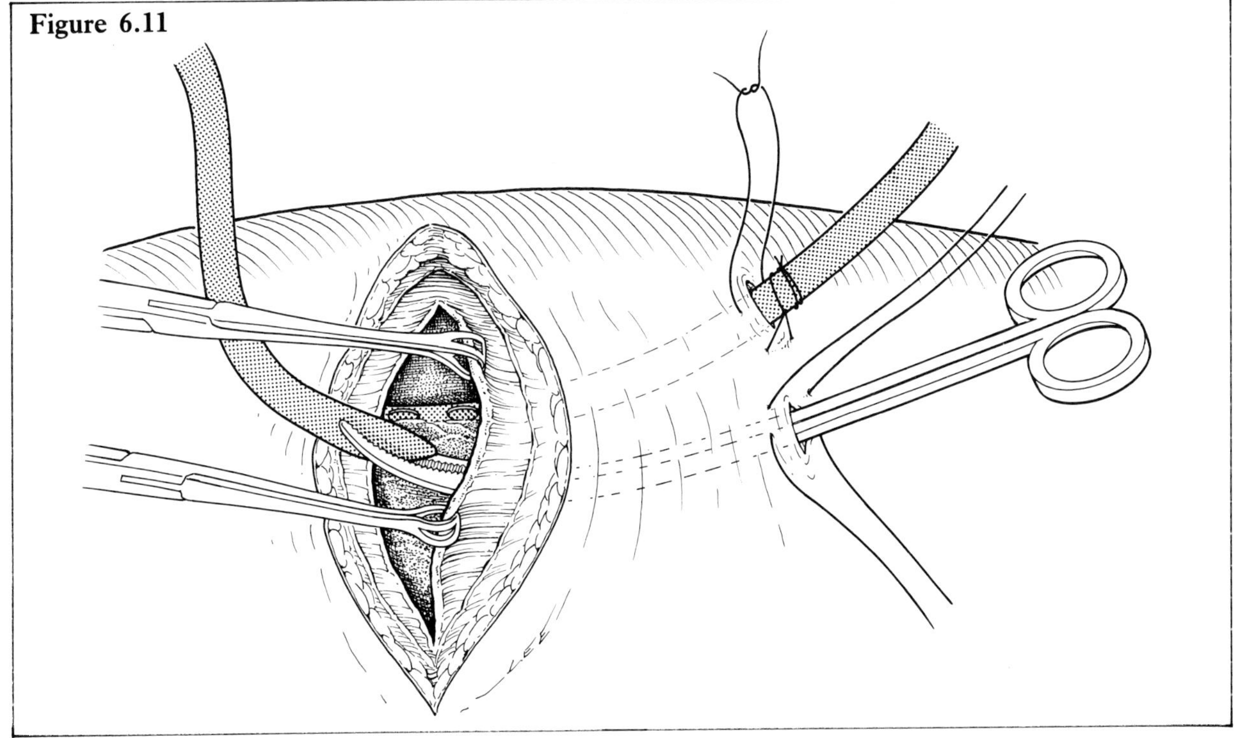

Figure 6.11

# 7 Anterolateral thoracotomy

## Indications

The following are some of the more common indications for this incision:

1. Closed mitral valvotomy.
2. Some operations in the anterior mediastinum, e.g. for bronchogenic cyst.
3. Simple operations on the anterior half of the upper or middle lobe or lingula.

## Procedure

The patient is placed supine on the operating table with the side to be operated upon tilted 30 degrees from the table (**Fig. 7.1**). The shoulder and elbow are flexed at right angles and the forearm is attached to the anaesthetic screen, protected by a foam pad. The pelvis is fixed in the position of 30-degree rotation with a strap (**Fig. 7.2**).

The incision extends from the midline in a slight curve just below the breast along the line of the anterior end of the fifth rib. It then continues as a straight line to a point 25 mm below and behind the inferior angle of the scapula (**Fig. 7.2**). The incision is deepened to expose the fascia over the pectoralis major and external oblique muscles anteriorly, and the latissimus dorsi muscle behind. The latissimus dorsi muscle is divided completely

**Figure 7.1**

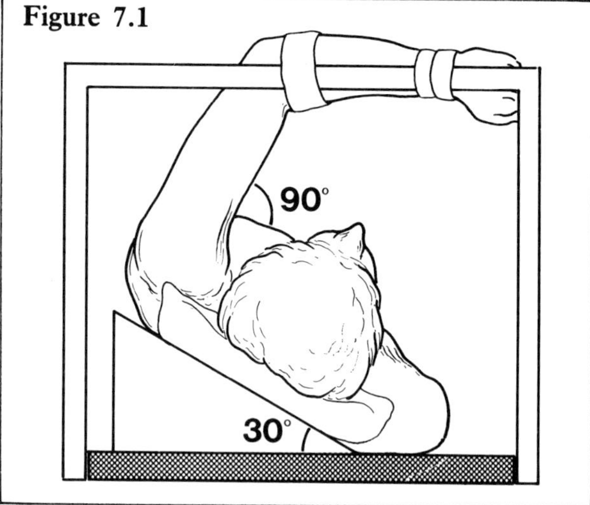


**Figure 7.2**

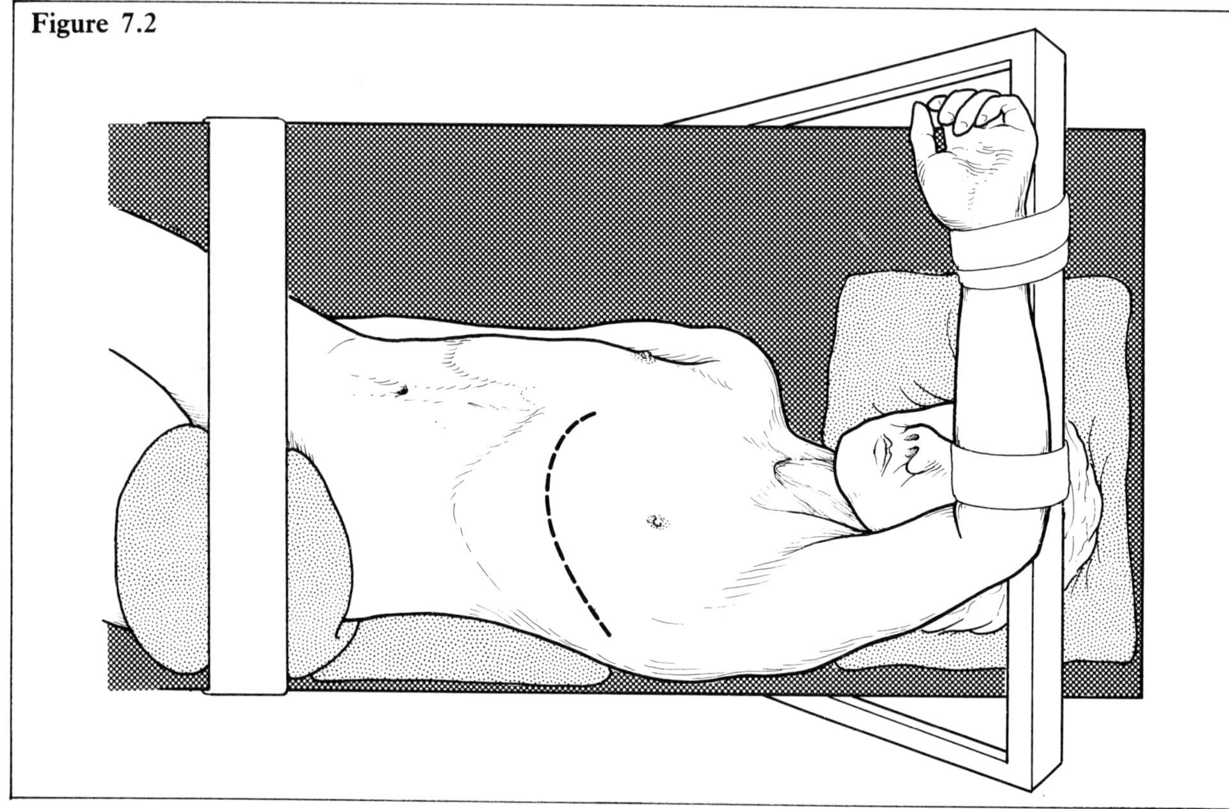

**Figure 7.3**

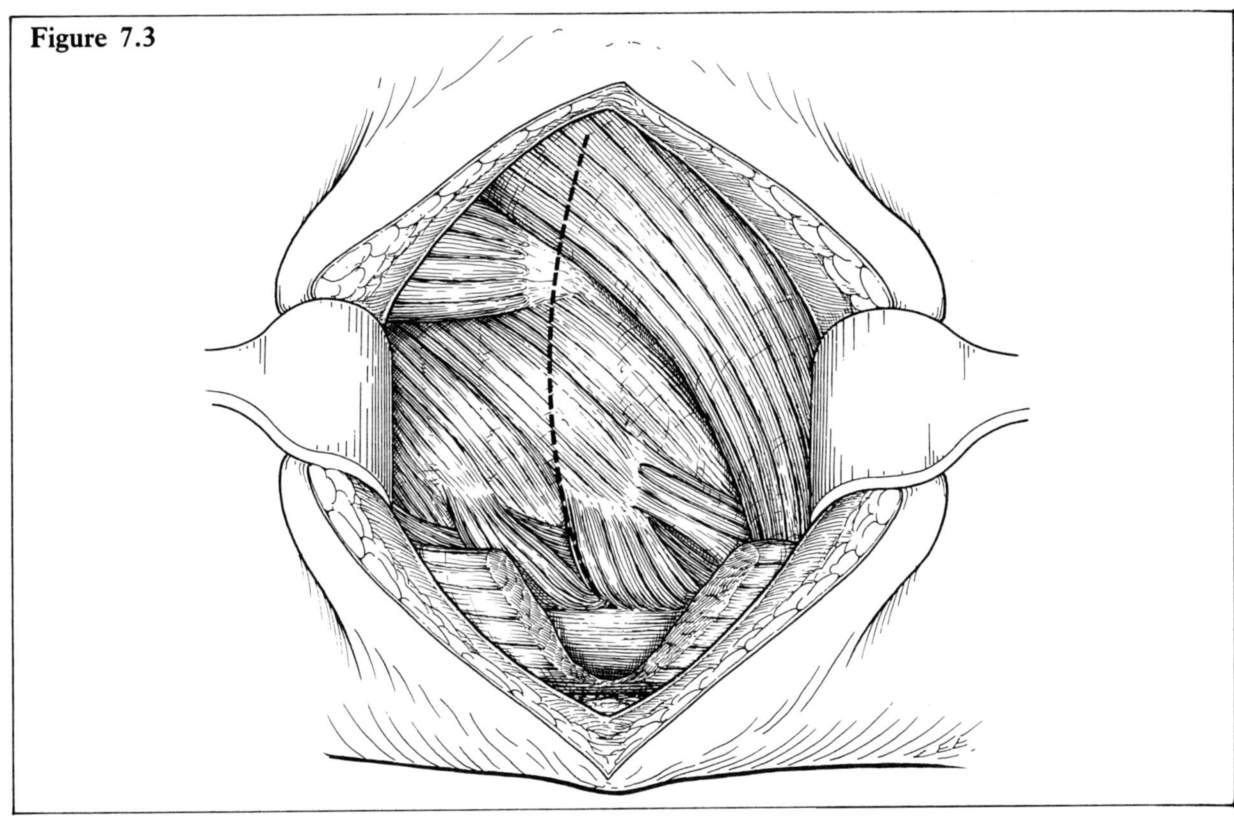

in the line of the incision to expose the free posteroinferior margin of the serratus muscle (**Fig. 7.3**).

The fascia extending backwards from the free margin of the serratus anterior is incised to expose the underlying rib. The line of this incision is made parallel to the free posterior margin of the serratus anterior muscle. The muscle is then lifted by retraction at the free posterior border. The digitations of the serratus anterior muscle are then revealed and divided along a line running upwards and forwards towards the midline, thus

**Figure 7.4**

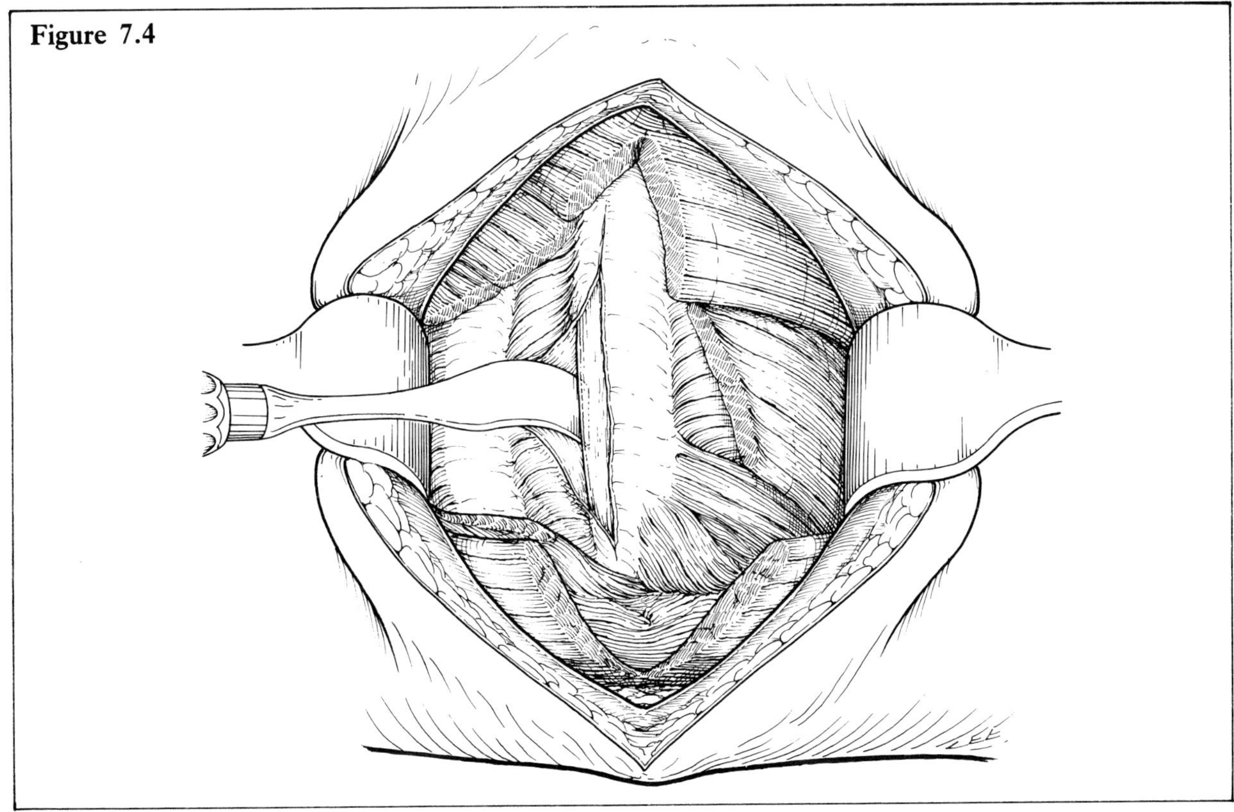

detaching the body of the muscle from the portion of the serratus muscle attached to the sixth, seventh and eighth ribs. The incision continues upwards to the fifth rib. This rib must be identified accurately by counting from above. An extra safeguard in identification is a very prominent vein lying on the rib beneath the serratus anterior digitations.

From this point the incision in the muscle continues up to the midline along the lower border of the anterior part of the fifth rib and costal cartilage through the pectoralis major muscle.

The periosteum is now stripped from the lower border of the fifth rib (**Fig. 7.4**). The periosteal elevator is then turned and introduced beneath the rib so that the concavity of the instrument lies against the underside. The notched Semb stripper is used for the posterior half.

It is not uncommon for the fifth and sixth costal cartilages to be fused together over a short distance at their front ends, in which case separation may be effected by freeing the perichondrium from the fifth costal cartilage both medial and lateral to the fused area. The periosteal stripper will usually find a line of cleavage in the area of fusion.

The deep surface of the periosteum and the pleura are incised and this incision is extended backwards as far as the angle of the rib and forwards to the midline.

A rib spreader is inserted at the junction of the anterior third and posterior two-thirds of the incision. As the space is widened the internal mammary artery and vein will be seen in the anterior end of the incision close to the surface (**Fig. 7.5**). These vessels are likely to be torn as the spreading progresses and they should therefore be secured at this stage. Simple ligatures are not adequate as it is difficult to obtain a sufficient distance between them. A suture ligature should therefore be put around the vessels and adjacent intercostal muscle above and below the incision. These ligatures should be at least 1 cm apart; it will then be safe to cut between them.

A single drain is adequate if the operation has been a mediastinal procedure or a closed mitral valvotomy. Two drains are advisable if a procedure has been carried out on the lung. See p. 28 for drainage procedure.

Closure is performed in three layers, using continuous nylon. The first layer approximates the anterior two-thirds of the rib to the intercostal muscle below it (**Fig. 7.6**). The second repairs the incision in the lumbar fascia running downwards and forwards in the posterior part of the incision, then the serratus anterior running upwards and forwards in the middle third, and finally the incision in the pectoralis major in the anterior third. The third layer is a repair of the latissimus dorsi muscle (**Fig. 7.7**). The subcutaneous layer and skin are closed as described on p. 28.

**Figure 7.5**

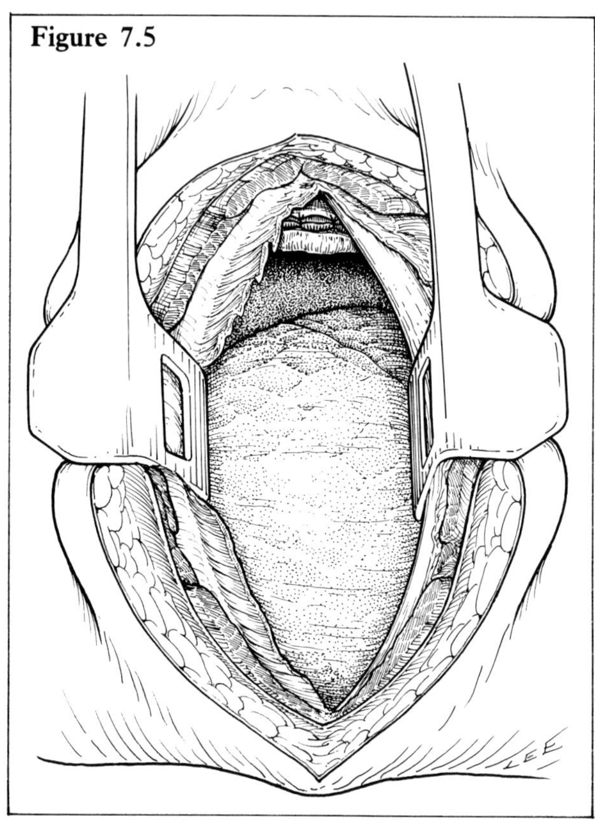

**Figure 7.6**

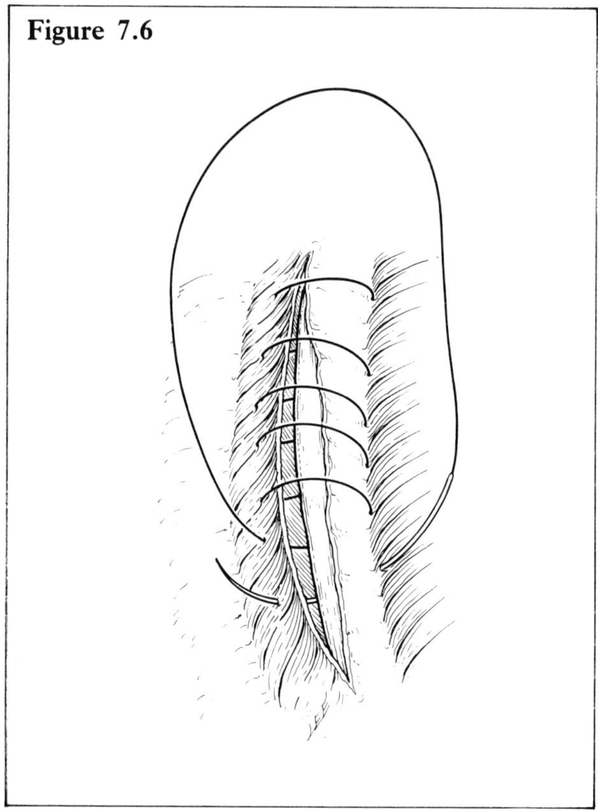

**Figure 7.7**

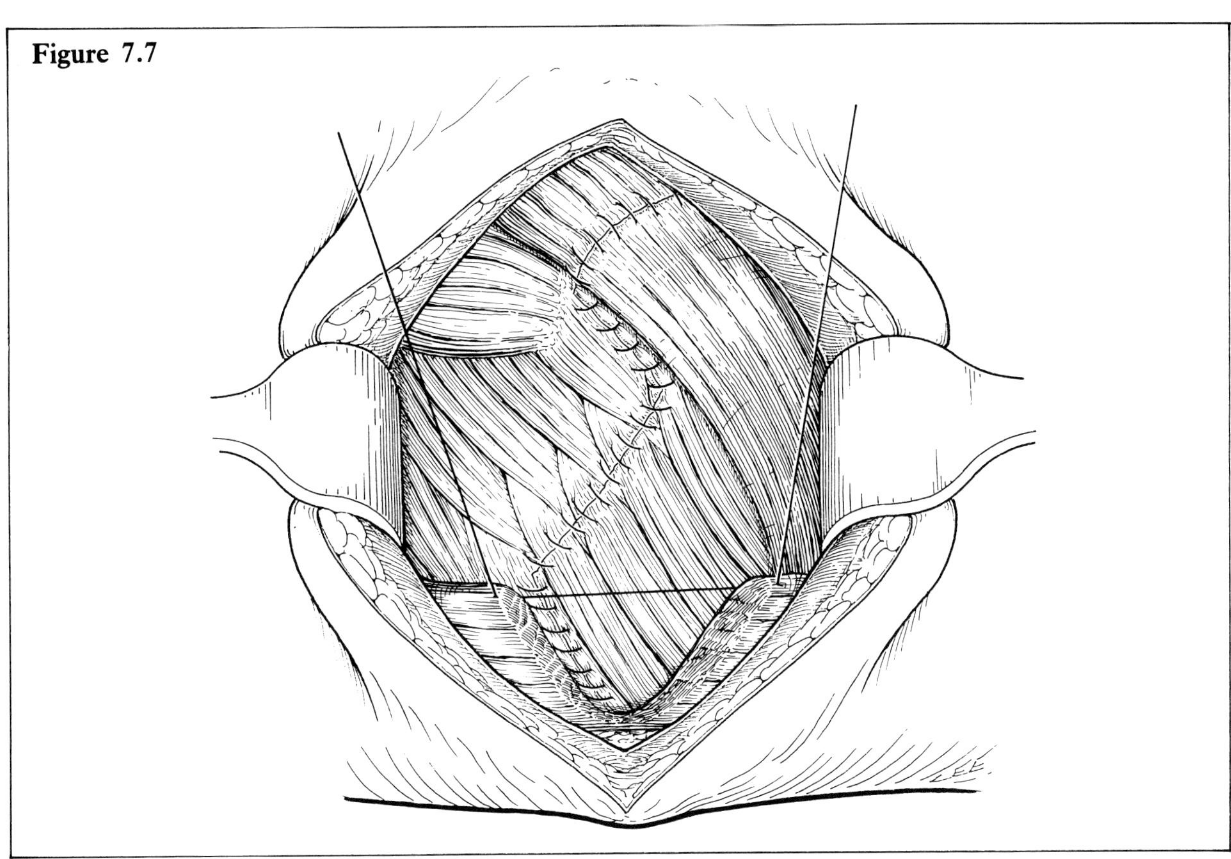

# 8 Anterior thoracotomy

Anterior thoracotomy gives limited but satisfactory access to the anterior mediastinum and pericardium. The patient is placed supine and the ipsilateral arm is flexed at the shoulder and elbow and fixed to the anaesthetist's screen. The forearm should be well padded where secured. A curved inframammary incision is made in the submammary skin crease, starting close to the midline and extending to the mid-axilla (**Fig. 8.1**). By counting from the manubriosternal junction, the third, fourth or fifth rib can be identified (**Fig. 8.2**). The incision is deepened through the pectoralis major muscle down to the periosteum of the rib. The flap of skin and pectoralis major muscle is then drawn upwards (**Fig. 8.3**). Continuation of the periosteal incision backwards results in a partial division of the pectoralis minor muscle and separation of the fibres of the serratus anterior in the direction of its digitations. The periosteum is stripped from the lower border of the selected rib (**Fig. 8.3**). The separation is continued backwards

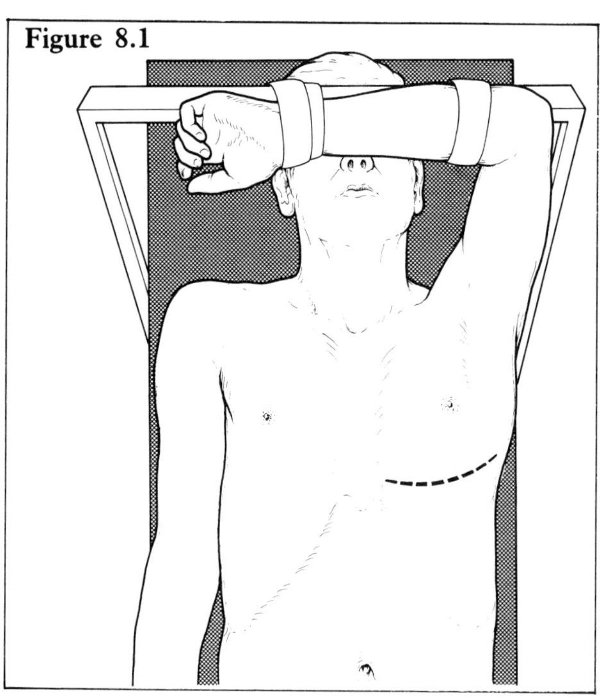

**Figure 8.1**

**Figure 8.2**

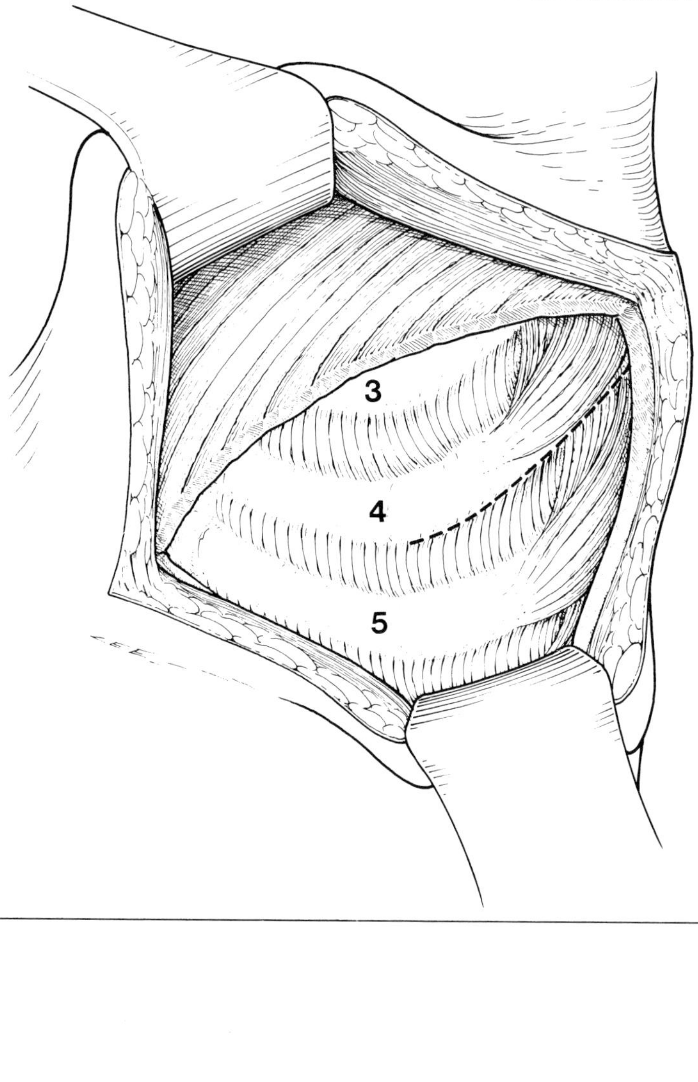

**Figure 8.3**

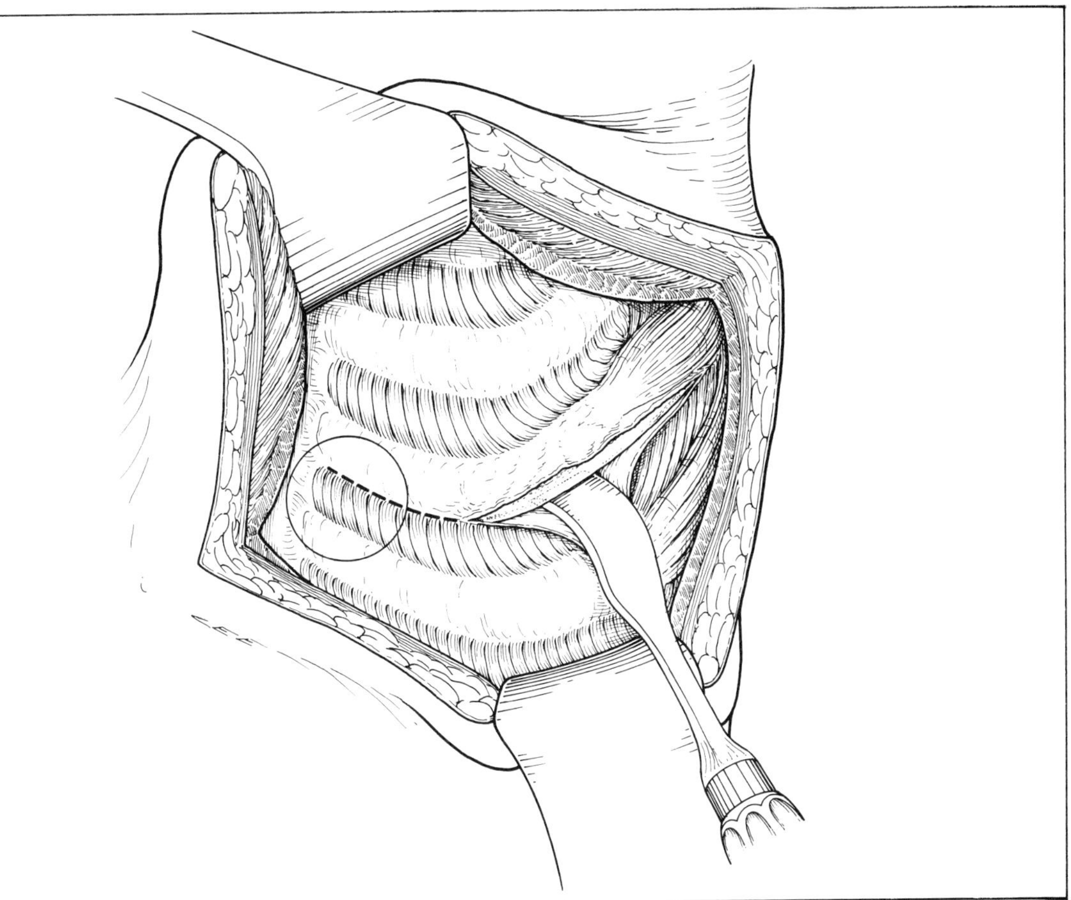

from within the pleural cavity at least as far as the posterior axillary line. The pleura is incised and a rib spreader inserted.

As the incision is opened the chondrosternal junction may dislocate, and the internal mammary vessels may be torn. It is advisable therefore to underrun these vessels with a stitch above and below the intercostal space (**Fig. 8.4**).

Satisfactory closure is obtained by a continuous suture, inserted loosely, passing around the costal cartilage and rib above and the intercostal muscle below. Once completed the suture will tighten without tearing when pulled. Closure of the incision may be difficult if the periosteum has been stripped from the upper margin of the rib. A second nylon suture approximates the muscle layer, and two layers of absorbable sutures are used for the subcutaneous fat and skin.

The pleural space should be drained as described on p. 28.

**Figure 8.4**

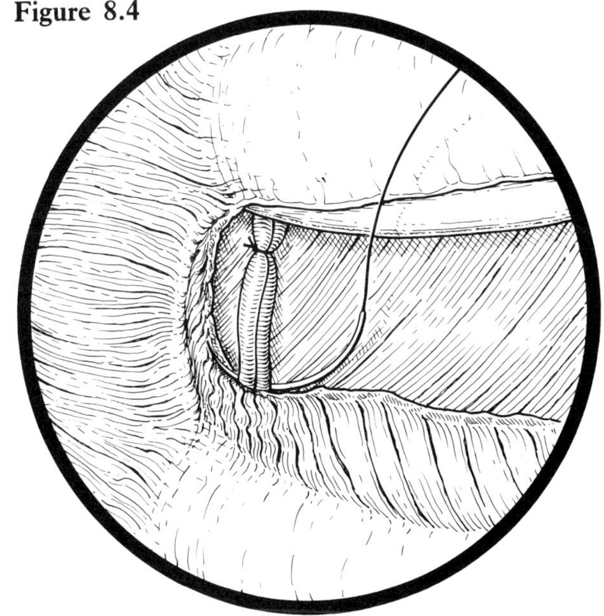

# 9 Median sternotomy

Median sternotomy is currently most frequently used for operations on the heart and mediastinum. It may be used when access to both lungs is necessary at the same operation. Practically all lung resections are possible through the midline, but lower lobectomy, especially on the left side, is difficult.

## Procedure

The patient is positioned supine on the operating table. The arms are placed by the patient's side and the bony prominences protected with foam sheets. In some institutions the anaesthetists prefer to have one or both arms abducted from the trunk to 90 degrees for access to venous and arterial lines. If this position is adopted extreme caution must be exercised to prevent over-abduction, and injury to the shoulder joint or over-stretching the nerves that supply the arm.

The incision is made from just below the suprasternal notch to 2 cm below the xiphisternum (**Fig. 9.1**). The skin is incised with a knife and the subcutaneous fat with diathermy. The incision is carried down between the interdigitations of the pectoralis major muscles and periosteum to the outer table of the sternum (**Fig. 9.2**). The periosteum may bleed profusely, and care should be taken over haemostasis. The subxiphisternal space is opened by incising the linea alba. The xiphisternum may be divided longitudinally with a knife or with a saw. The suprasternal space is developed with a finger and the interclavicular ligament divided with diathermy.

A compressed air-driven saw is then used to divide the sternum in the midline (**Fig. 9.3**). If such a saw is not available then a Gigli saw or a Lebsche knife may be used instead. Bleeding from the marrow cavity of the sternum is controlled with bonewax, and further haemostasis of the periosteum of both tables of the sternum obtained with diathermy.

The edges of the sternum may be protected with large packs or wound towels. The sternal edges are then distracted with a Finochietto retractor. Over-distraction should be avoided to prevent traction injury to the lower cords of the brachial plexus and damage to the first rib.

**Figure 9.1**

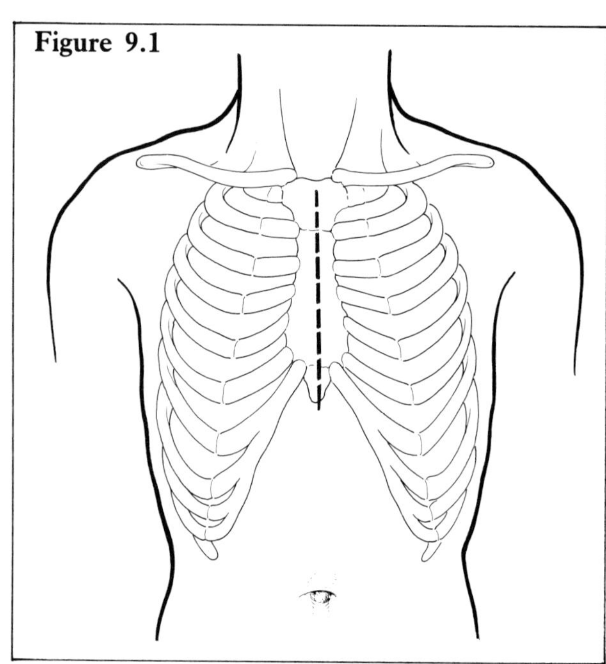

**Figure 9.2**

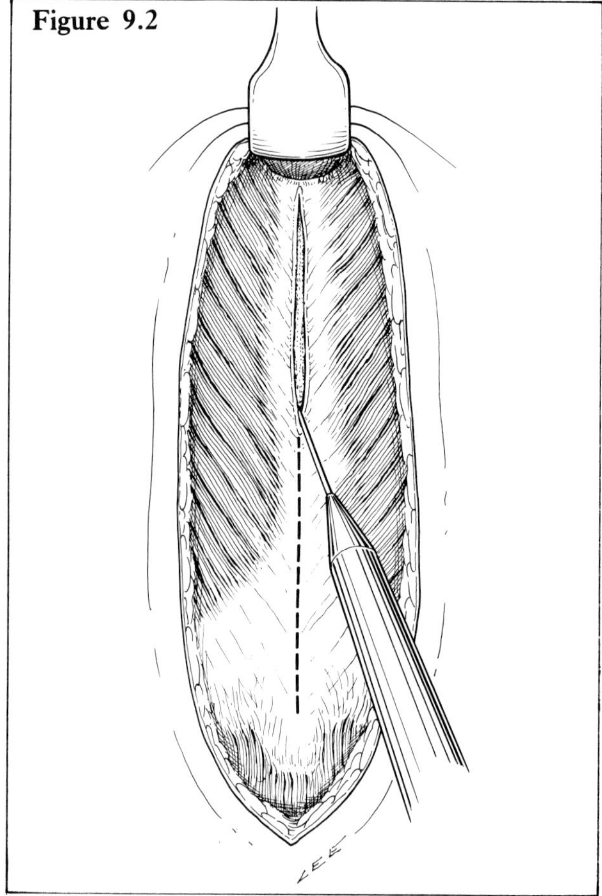

Figure 9.3

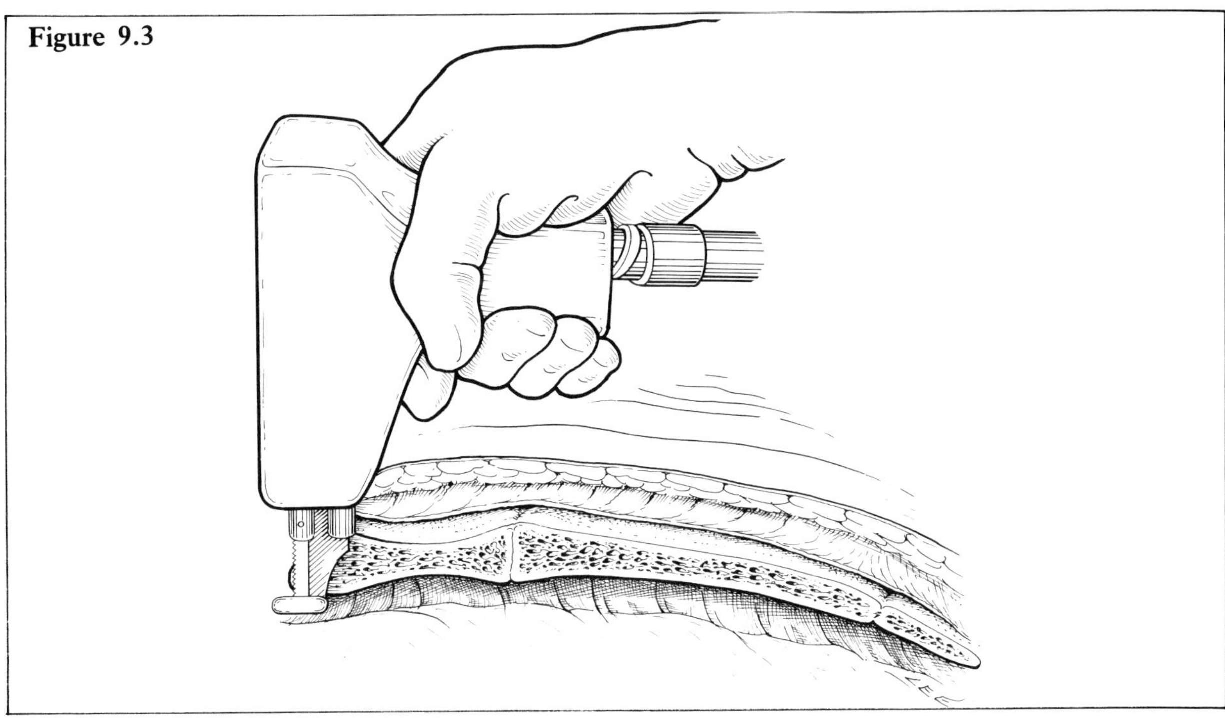

Figure 9.4

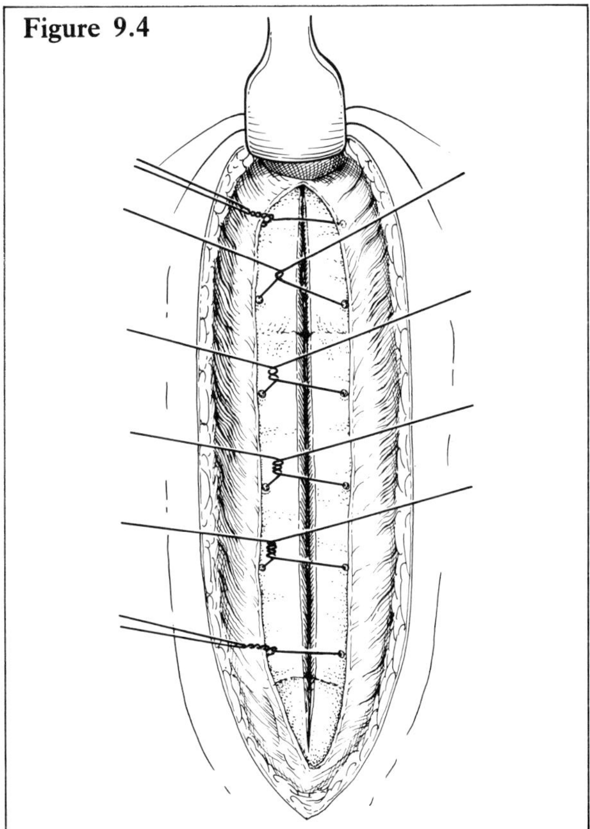

## Closure

When the procedure has been completed the sternum is reapproximated with six stainless steel wires passed through each edge of the sternum. The deep surface of the sternum must be inspected for bleeding at the sites of the penetration of the wires. This can be controlled by diathermy or mattress sutures. The wires are twisted together with some force to hold the edges firmly together (**Fig. 9.4**). As with all fractures, healing of the bone is more satisfactory and discomfort is less if there is a degree of compression. The rectus sheaths, the periosteum and the pectoralis muscles superficially are closed with a continuous 3/0 nylon suture. The fat and skin may be closed with absorbable sutures.

Drainage tubes should be placed as dictated by the procedure that has been carried out. If one or other of the pleural spaces has been opened, it should be drained. The drains may be brought out through the most dependent intercostal space. If the operation has been on the heart or the pericardium, it will be necessary to place one or two drains in the pericardial sac to prevent the development of postoperative cardiac tamponade. The drains are brought through the skin on either side of the lowest point of the incision. All the drainage tubes should be connected to one single underwater seal bottle.

# 10 Axillary thoracotomy

Axillary thoracotomy may be used for the following procedures:

1. Upper thoracic sympathectomy.
2. Monaldi–McArthur drainage procedure for an emphysematous bulla.
3. Apical pleurectomy.

## Procedure

With the patient in the lateral position, an incision is made with a knife in the lowest axillary skin crease (**Fig. 10.1**). The incision is deepened through the fat using diathermy until the chest wall is reached. With this approach the incision enters the axillary space between the pectoralis and latissimus dorsi muscles, there being no need to cut either.

The chest is entered through the third intercostal space. The periosteum over the third rib is incised with diathermy and the intercostal muscle stripped from the rib with a rugine (**Fig. 10.2**). The underlying periosteum and pleura are incised with a knife. The incision is carried as far forwards as is necessary to obtain satisfactory exposure. Usually a smaller rib spreader than a Finochietto is required.

**Figure 10.1**

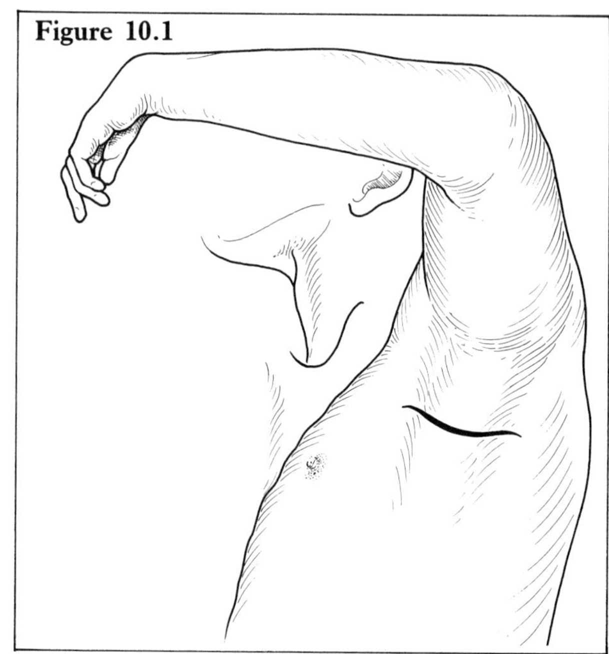

The wound is closed with a nylon stitch for the intercostal muscle layer, and absorbable sutures for the fat layer and the skin.

The pleural space should be drained as described on p. 28.

**Figure 10.2**

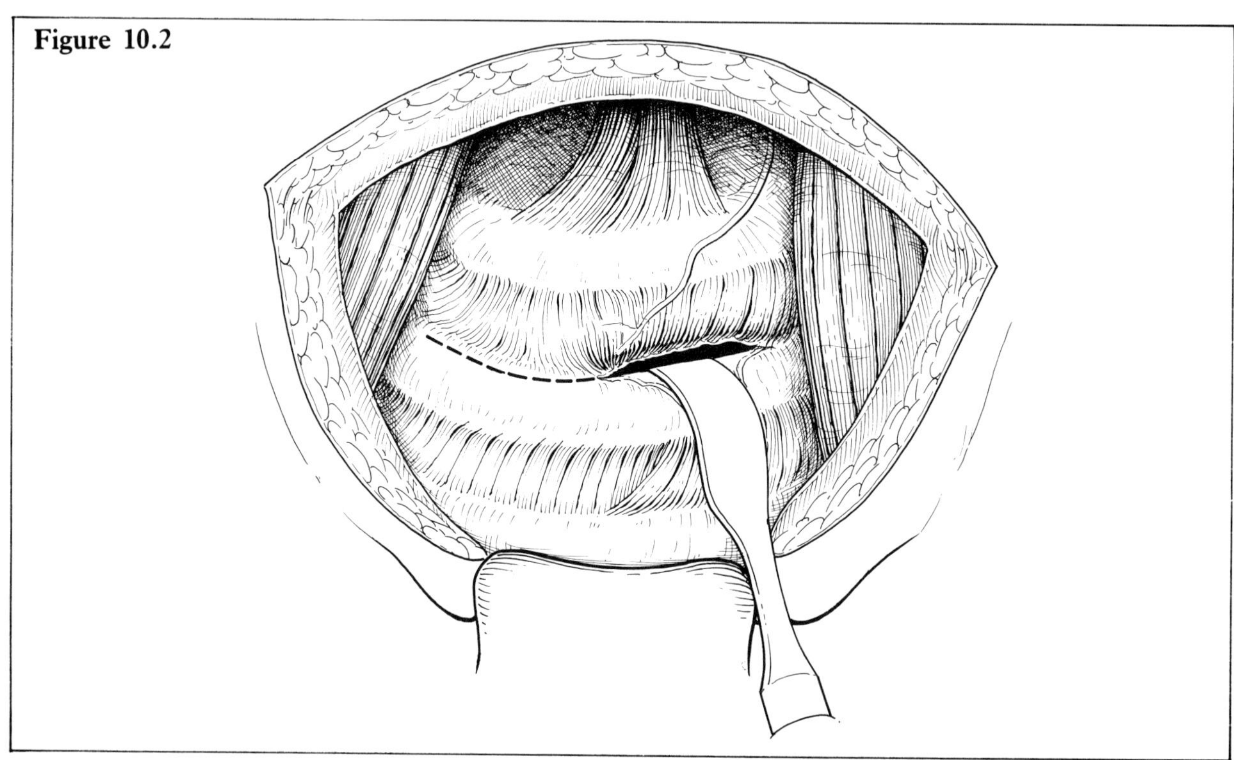

SECTION 3

# CHEST WALL PROCEDURES

# 11 Pectus excavatum

The deep depression at the lower half of the sternum for which patients seek treatment is usually associated with kyphosis (**Figs. 11.1, 11.2**). Although impaired cardiorespiratory function has been demonstrated in a few cases, in the majority surgical treatment is entirely cosmetic. The fact that the operation will remove one blemish at the expense of another (the scar) must be made clear to the patient and the parent. The operation may be required in infancy but is more commonly performed at the age of 10 or 11 years when children are embarrassed at having to undress in front of their peers, or a few years later when they come into close contact with members of the opposite sex.

Many different techniques have been used for the treatment of this condition but in recent years it has become obvious that without rigid fixation, what appears initially to be an excellent cosmetic result may ultimately be disappointing because of progressive retraction of the sternum. Long-term rigid fixation is therefore desirable, and can be achieved with a metal bar placed behind the sternum resting on the anterior end of the ribs.

## Procedure

The patient lies supine. A vertical midline incision is made from the level of the manubrium to a point just below the xiphisternum (**Fig. 11.1**). A flap of skin and pectoral muscle is then raised on either side by detaching the origins of the pectoral muscles from the sternum and costal cartilages. The flaps are progressively elevated with retractors until normal rib is encountered beyond the deformed costal cartilages. The origins of the rectus abdominis muscles are dissected off the lower end of the

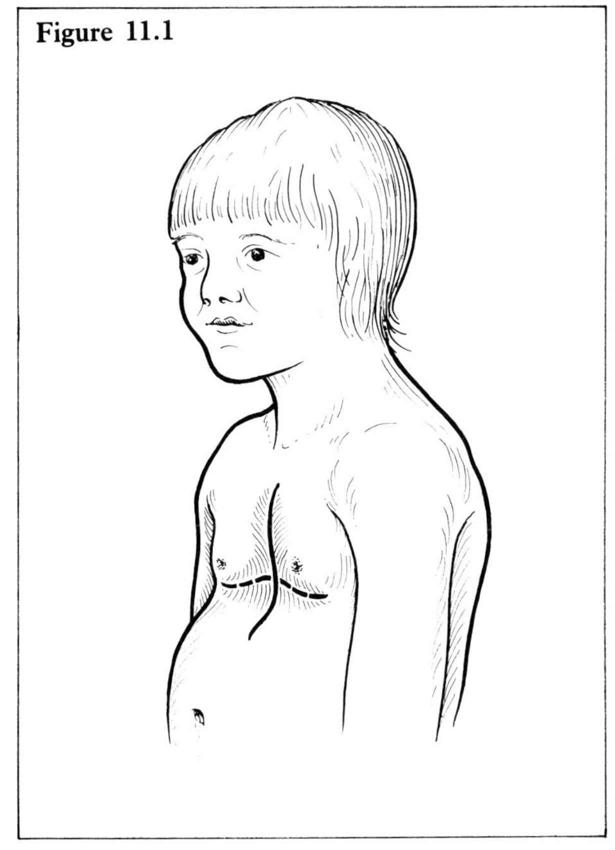

**Figure 11.1**

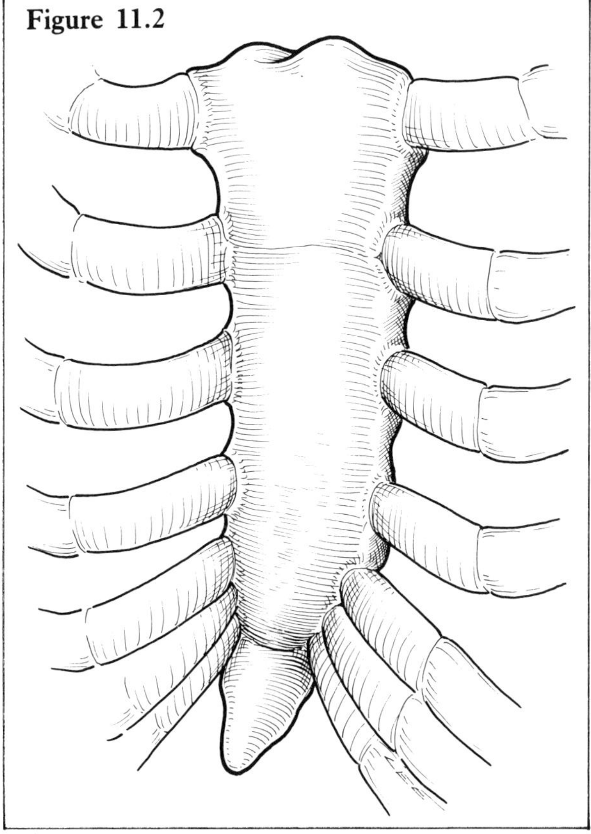

**Figure 11.2**

sternum and costal margins (**Fig. 11.3**) and retracted downwards (**Fig. 11.4**).

Alternatively, a bilateral submammary incision arching upwards over the lower sternum (**Fig. 11.1**) certainly gives a better cosmetic result, but necessitates dissecting the skin flaps off the muscle. The upper part of the distal skin flap then has an uncertain blood supply which may lead to necrosis and an unpleasant keloid scar across the midline, and we do not recommend this approach.

The deformed costal cartilages are now removed completely, preserving the perichondrium. A longitudinal incision is made with the diathermy point along the length of the perichondrium of each cartilage, and a second incision is made at right angles to each end of the longitudinal incision (**Fig. 11.5**). The perichondrium is then carefully stripped off both upper and lower borders with a periosteal elevator. The stripping is readily achieved in younger patients, but in older patients the perichondrium may be firmly adherent and painstaking efforts are required.

**Figure 11.3**

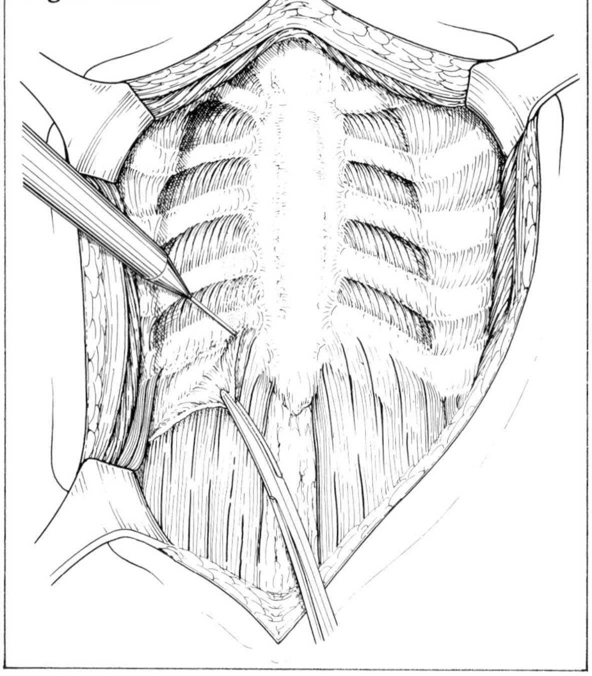

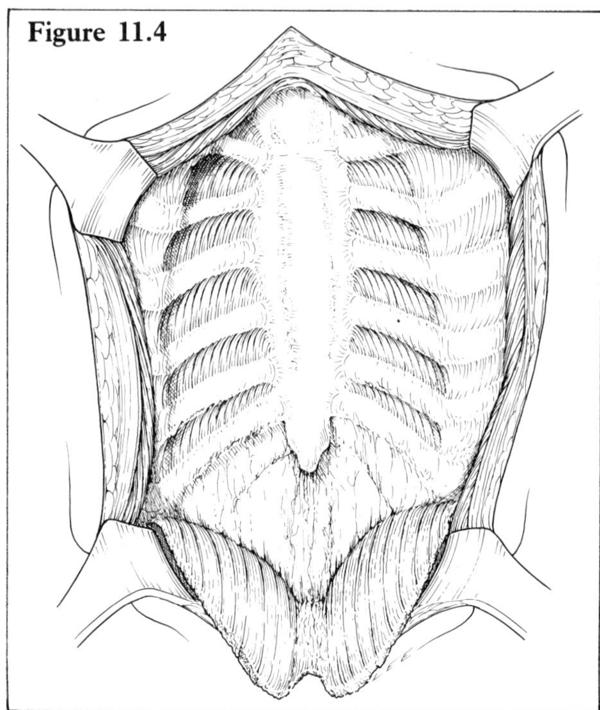

**Figure 11.4**

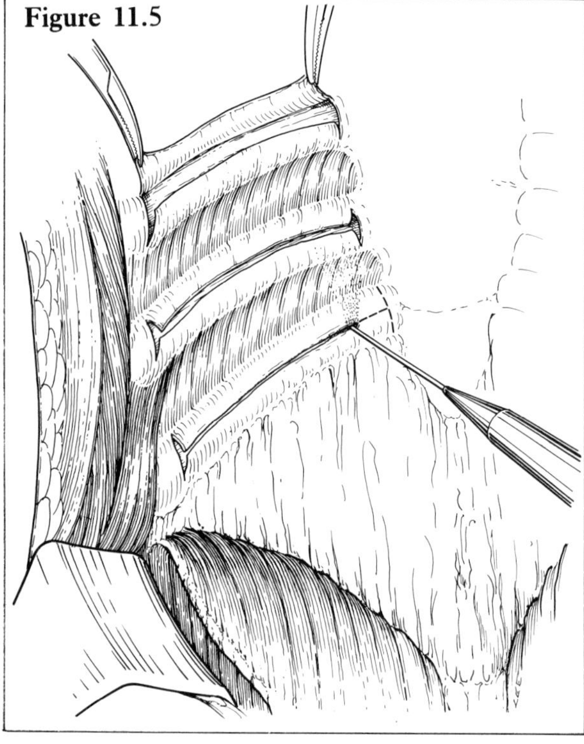

**Figure 11.5**

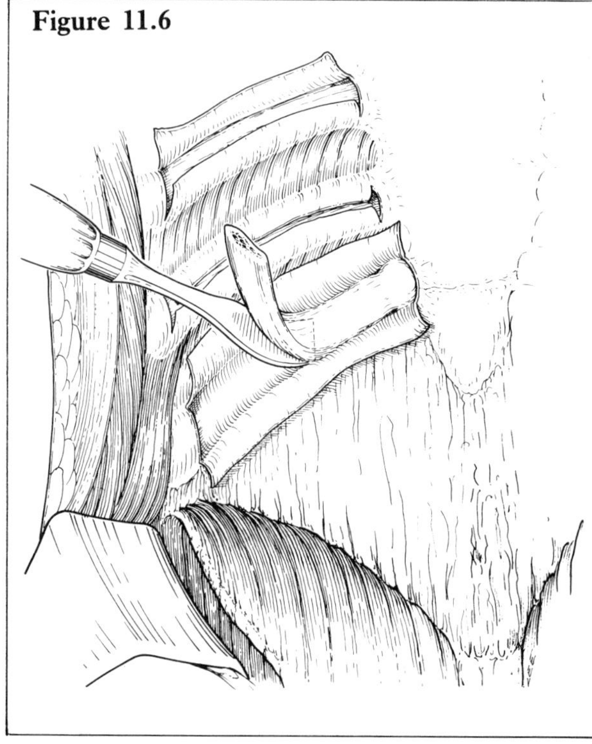

**Figure 11.6**

Figure 11.7

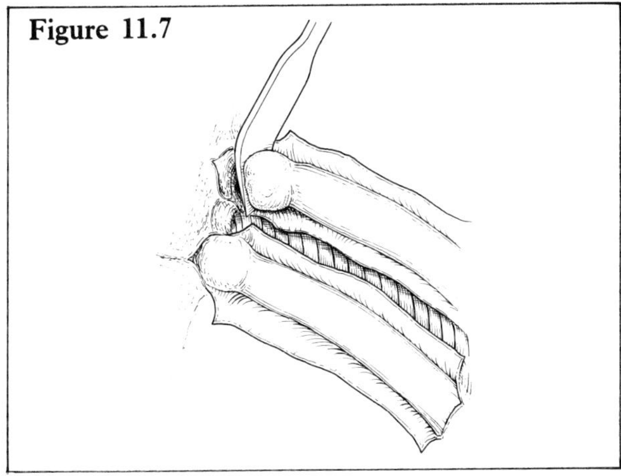

Figure 11.8

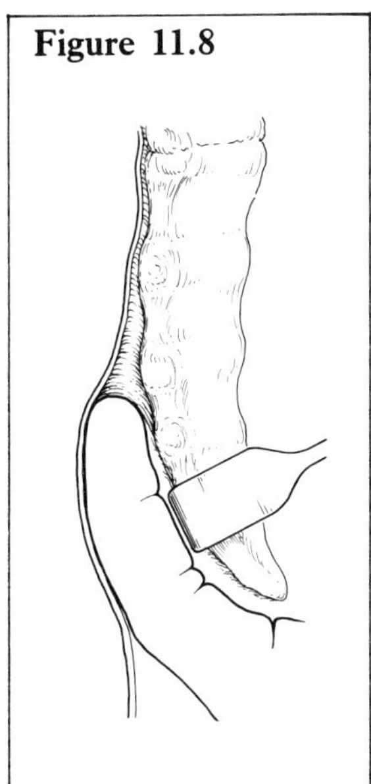

Figure 11.9

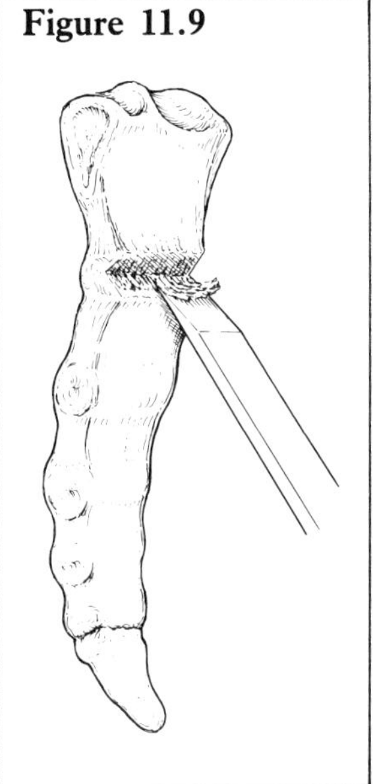

Figure 11.10

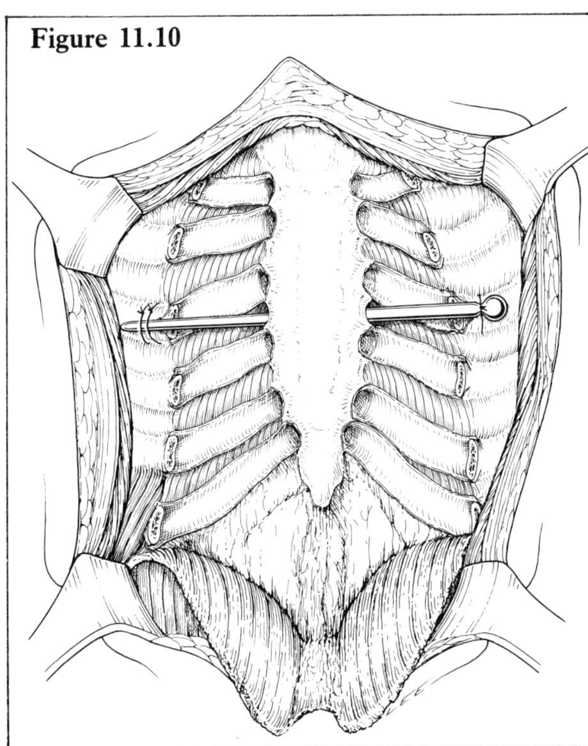

When the perichondrium has been freed from the outer surface of the cartilage the dissection is continued round the upper and lower margins until a curved periosteal elevator can be passed beneath the cartilage. The cartilage is then divided at its junction with the rib and elevated (**Fig. 11.6**). It is important to separate the costal cartilage from the sternum cleanly through the joint (**Fig. 11.7**). This sternal end of the cartilage has a smooth convex articular surface.

All cartilages attached to the sternum, excluding the first and second, must be removed, leaving the sternum free of cartilaginous attachments.

### Elevation of the sternum

The lower end of the sternum is elevated with a retractor and its deep surface cleared from the mediastinal structures and pleura by blunt dissection with the finger (**Fig. 11.8**). As each portion is freed, the corresponding perichondrial and intercostal attachments are divided at each side close to the sternum in order to avoid the internal mammary vessels.

### Sternal osteotomy

A transverse osteotomy is now made through the anterior cortex of the sternum at the point where in its descent it begins to angulate backwards. The osteotomy should take the form of a V-shaped gutter (**Fig. 11.9**). It should then be possible to elevate the sternum into a grossly over-corrected position. If this cannot be achieved it may be necessary to divide one more cartilage close to the sternum at the upper end. It is unnecessary to place sutures at the site of osteotomy to maintain the corrected position, since this is achieved by the metal fixation.

### Insertion of Abrams' bar

An Abrams' bar of suitable length is placed behind the sternum at about the level of the anterior end of the fourth rib. It should rest comfortably on the ribs and project a short distance laterally so that the blunt end will be just palpable when the skin has been closed (**Fig. 11.10**). The pointed end is fixed by two nylon sutures passing round the bar and the adjacent rib. The rounded end is fixed by a similar suture passing around the rib seated in the groove provided on the bar.

### Closure

A vacuum drain is passed into the anterior mediastinal space beneath the xiphisternum and brought out to one side of the lower end of the incision (**Fig. 11.11**). The rectus muscles are then carefully sutured back to the perichondrium and to the lower end of the sternum. It may be necessary to drill holes through the lower end of

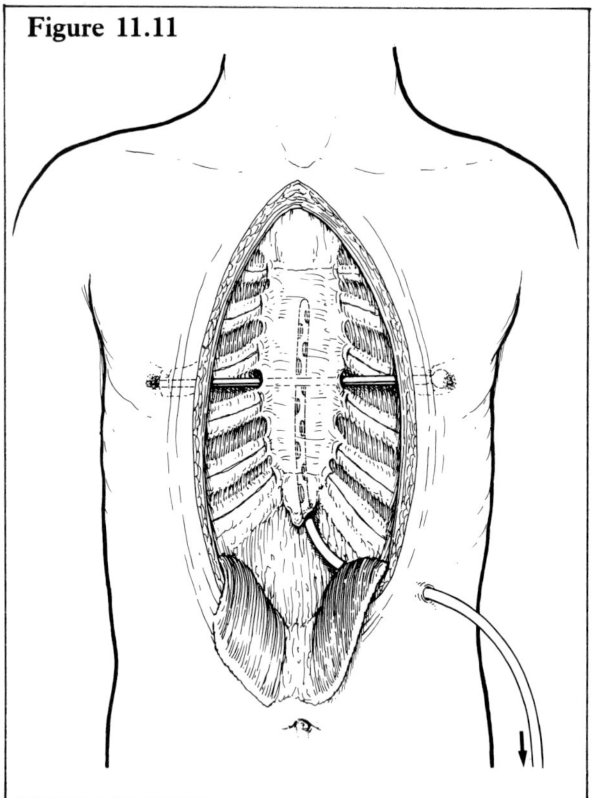
Figure 11.11

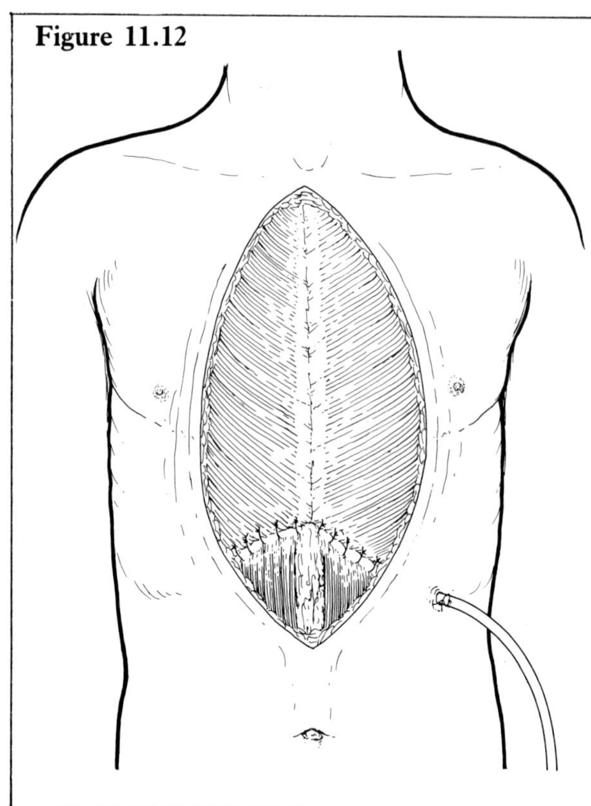
Figure 11.12

the sternum for the passage of sutures in order to achieve this. The pectoral muscles are sutured together in the midline and to the periosteum of the sternum to avoid leaving a dead space (**Fig. 11.12**).

Because of the risk of infection and subsequent sinus formation it is advisable to use a long-lasting absorbable suture. A subcuticular suture gives a good cosmetic result (**Fig. 11.13**).

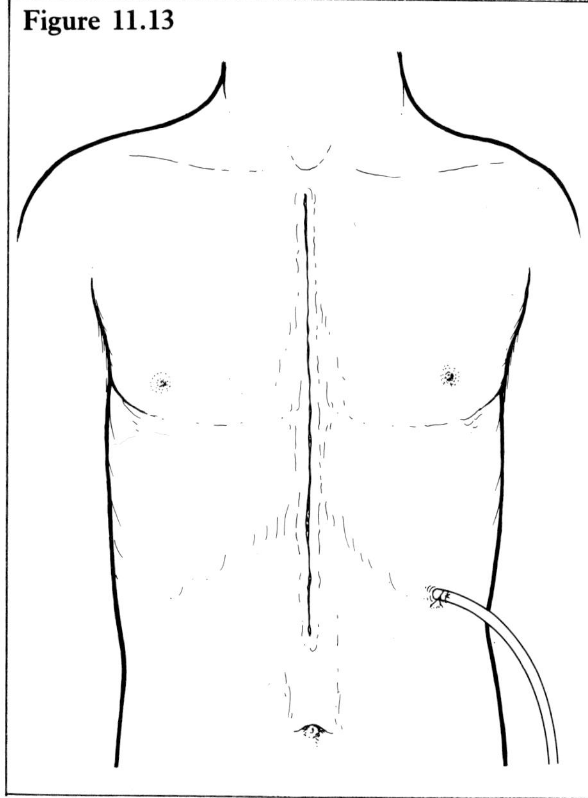
Figure 11.13

## Postoperative management

Good control of pain is the mainstay of postoperative management. Relatively pain-free patients will be able to clear their secretions and mobilize freely, and should be encouraged to get out of bed during the first postoperative day. The drains are removed when there is no further collection. The patient can leave hospital when freely mobile and comfortable. No restrictions are placed on subsequent activities. The Abrams' bar, which should be left in place for at least six months and preferably a year, is removed under local anaesthesia via a small incision (1 cm) in the skin, overlying the end that is more easily palpable.

# 12 Pectus carinatum

Pectus carinatum is a more complex condition than pectus excavatum, and is frequently asymmetrical. There are many varieties, the main ones being:

1. A transverse ridge at the level of the manubrium involving a forward projection of the sternum and costal cartilages at this level (**Fig. 12.1**).

**Figure 12.1**

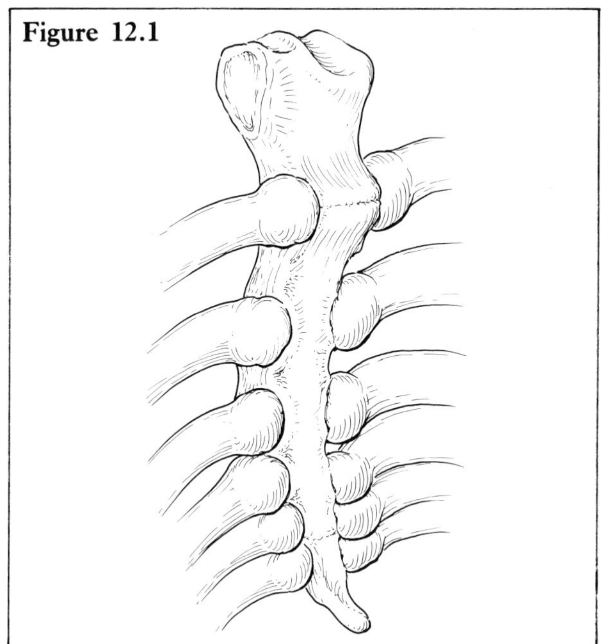

**Figure 12.2**

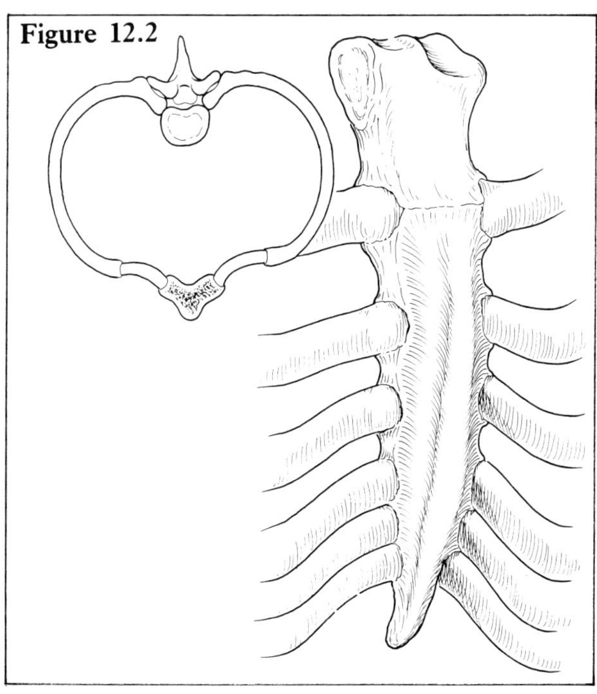

2. A vertical ridge affecting the lower half of the sternum (**Fig. 12.2**).
3. Retraction of the anterior thirds of the lower ribs which occurs in most cases (**Fig. 12.3**).
4. In asymmetrical cases there is usually a scoliosis, and the transverse section of one half of the hemithorax is much smaller than the other.
5. Rotation of the sternum of 45 degrees or more about its vertical axis (**Fig. 12.4**).
6. A deep depression affecting the second and third costal cartilages on one side may also occur in asymmetrical cases.

The anatomical variants imply that the operation must be tailored to suit the individual deformity.

**Figure 12.3**

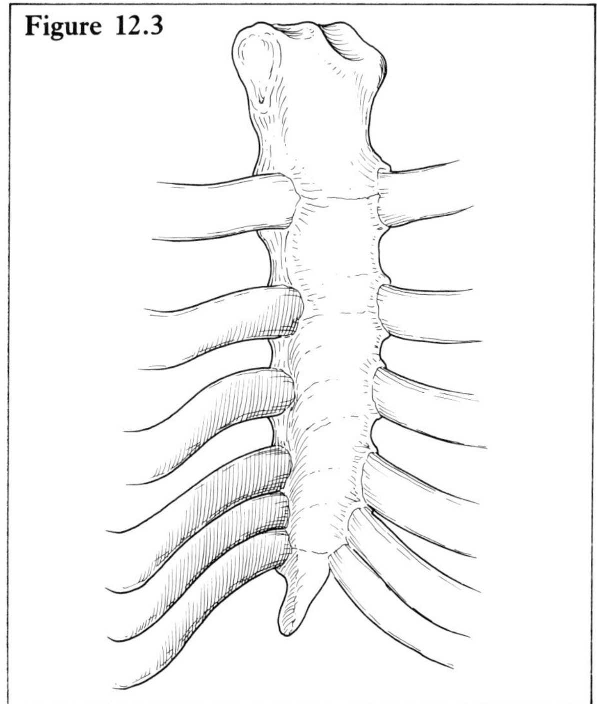

**Figure 12.4**

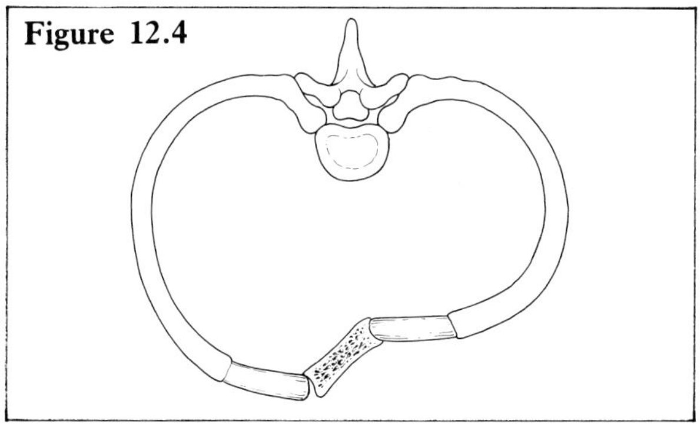

## Procedure

For the reasons described on p. 42 we prefer a midline incision from 5 cm below the suprasternal notch to just below the xiphisternum. This incision must be strictly in the midline and should not follow the line of the deformed sternum. In more severe cases a longer incision may be necessary. The pectoral and rectus muscles are dissected off the sternum and the deformed costal cartilages. If there is recession of the anterior ends of the lower ribs, the mobilization beneath the muscles should extend sufficiently far out to expose it.

### Removal of chondrosternal projection

In the simpler deformity, removal of the sternal prominence with an osteotome and shaving the projecting costal cartilages with a knife may give an acceptable result (**Fig. 12.5**).

### Dissection of costal cartilages

In more severe cases all the deformed costal cartilages should be resected as described on p. 42. The deformity usually extends as far as the corresponding rib, which is the lateral limit of the resection.

### Correction of sternal deformities

If the sternum is rotated more than 30 degrees about its vertical axis, its position is corrected by a transverse osteotomy at the level of the highest resected costal cartilage. A rugine is passed behind the sternum at this level, keeping close to the bone and emerging at its opposite edge. With this instrument protecting the underlying structures, the sternum is divided transversely with an osteotome and rotated into a slightly over-corrected position (**Fig. 12.6**). Two drill holes are then made with an awl about 1 cm from each side of the cut margin. The two halves of the sternum are then united with nylon sutures passed through the drill holes (**Fig. 12.7**). Tying the sutures will maintain the sternum in the corrected position.

As a result of this correction the perichondrium

**Figure 12.5**

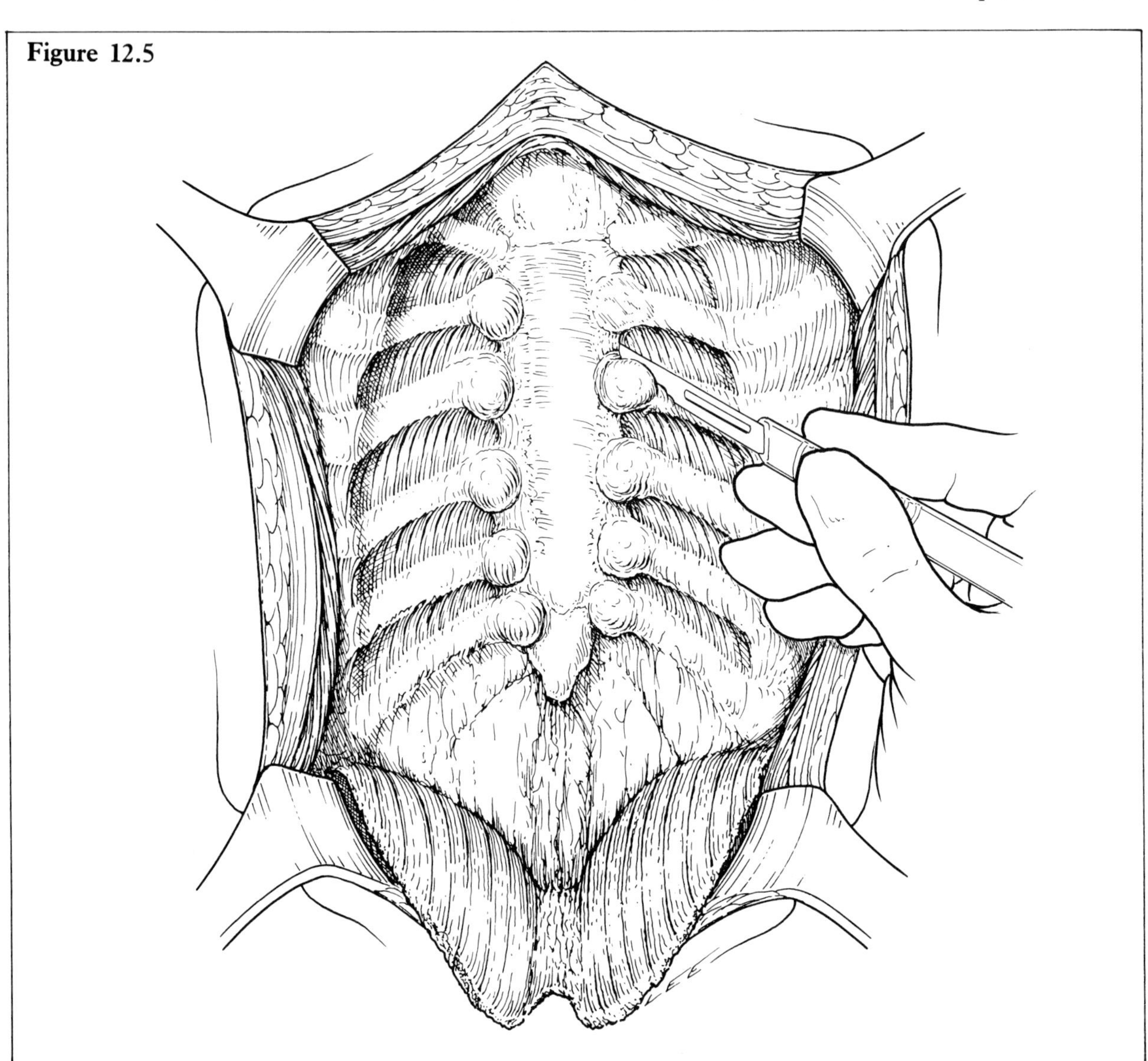

**Figure 12.6**

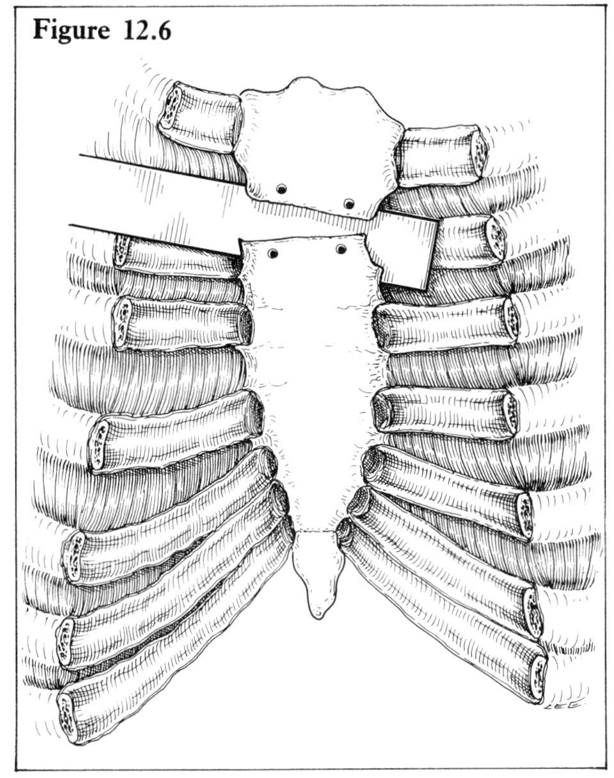

**Figure 12.7**

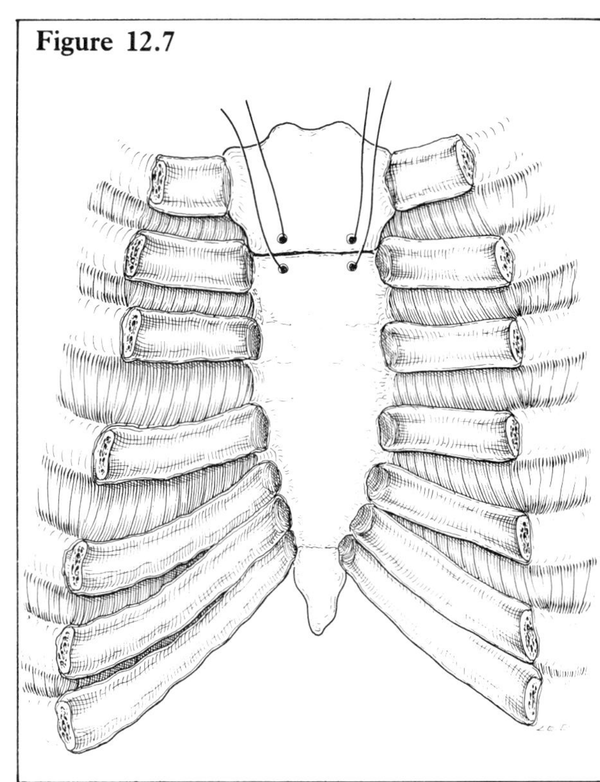

on one or both sides of the sternum will be quite lax where the cartilages were removed. A series of imbricating sutures are therefore placed so as to render the strips of perichondrium taut (**Fig. 12.8**).

### Correction of rib deformity

If the indrawing of the lower end of the anterior ribs persists, the cosmetic result can be greatly improved by elevating them. This is done by passing a series of heavy sutures round the anterior ends of the lower ribs and again round the first or second rib above this level and tying them tightly. Three or four such sutures may be inserted on each side and the improvement in the cosmetic appearance can be observed as the sutures are tied (**Fig. 12.9**).

### Closure

Haemostasis is secured and the whole area sprayed with antibiotic powder. A vacuum drain is left beneath the muscles and brought out to one side of the lower end of the wound. The rectus muscles are carefully reattached to the sternum, perichondrium and pectoral muscles. The pectoral muscles are sutured together in the midline and to the periosteum of the sternum. The skin incision is closed in two layers, the superficial layer with a subcuticular absorbable stitch.

## Postoperative management

Postoperative management is similar to that for pectus excavatum (p. 44).

**Figure 12.8**

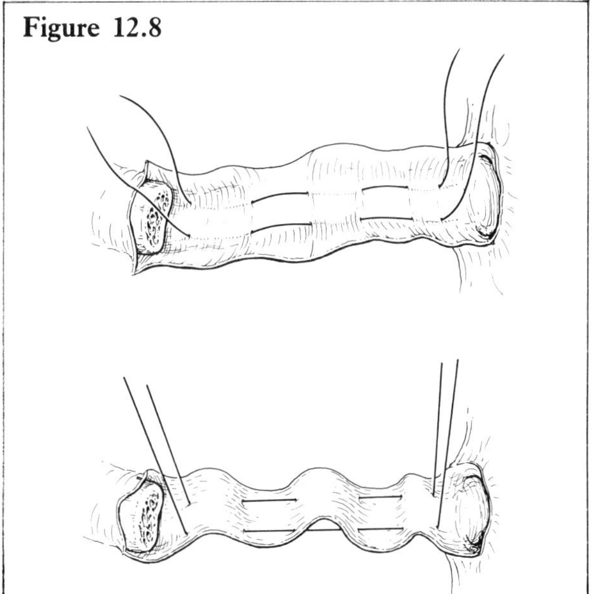

**Figure 12.9**

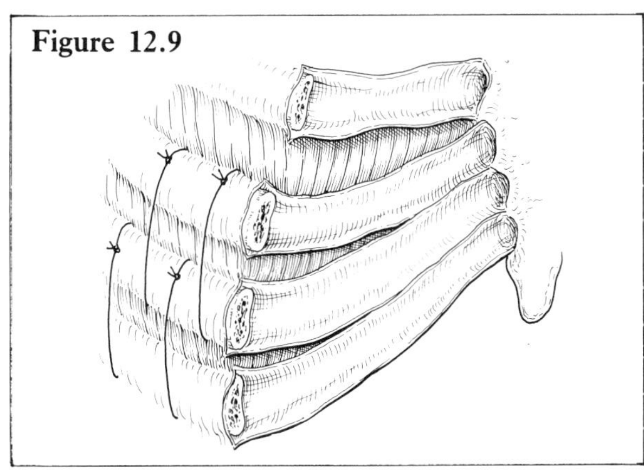

# 13 Resection of chest wall tumours and methods of reconstruction

The majority of primary tumours arising in the chest wall are malignant. Therefore, in the absence of metastases, radical local resection may be indicated.

Some tumours, however, respond well to contemporary chemotherapeutic regimens. For this reason histological diagnosis is important, but this is often extremely difficult. Frozen sections should therefore never be used. A formal open biopsy is essential and paraffin section technique is the only one acceptable.

The shape and amount of chest wall that is to be removed is dictated by the size, position and extent of the tumour. The resection determines the method of reconstruction that will be necessary. As a general principle at least one normal rib with its accompanying intercostal muscles above and below the tumour should be removed (**Fig. 13.1**). If the tumour is infiltrating the underlying pleura, lung or pericardium, this tissue should be resected *en bloc*. Similarly, if the overlying skin is involved it must be removed with a wide margin.

**Figure 13.1**

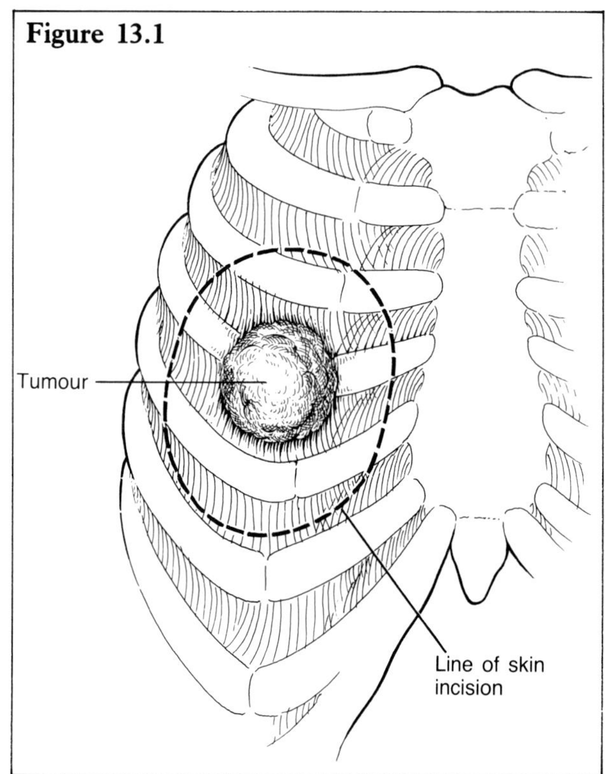


## Resection of tumours that do not infiltrate the overlying skin

A standard thoracic incision centred over the tumour should be used (**Fig. 13.2**). The plane between the subcutaneous tissues and chest wall muscles is then developed to reveal the extent of the tumour. Occasionally there may be no palpable tumour on the surface, all the tumour being on the inside of the chest wall. If this is the case the radiological appearances are used to plan the point of entry into the thorax. If the overlying muscles are freely mobile over the tumour, they may be dissected and divided in the classical way. For example, if the tumour is on the lateral chest wall, dissection may proceed as for a standard lateral thoracotomy (**Fig. 13.3**)—see p. 24.

The intercostal muscles are next separated from the upper border of the first uninvolved rib above the tumour (**Fig. 13.4**). This rib is then divided anteriorly and posteriorly giving a wide clearance from the edge of the tumour (**Fig. 13.5**). Next, the

**Figure 13.2**

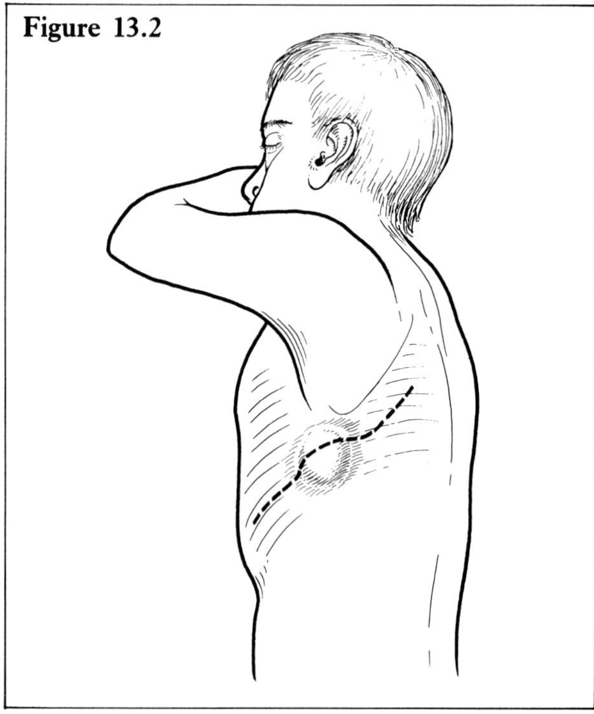

Figure 13.3

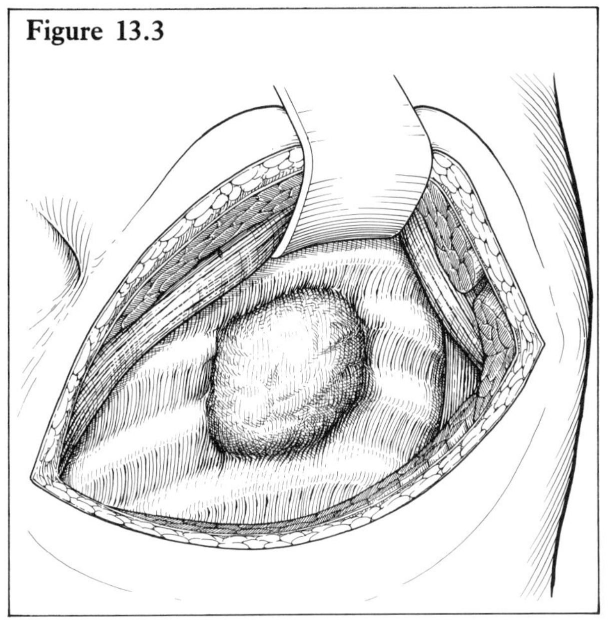

Figure 13.4

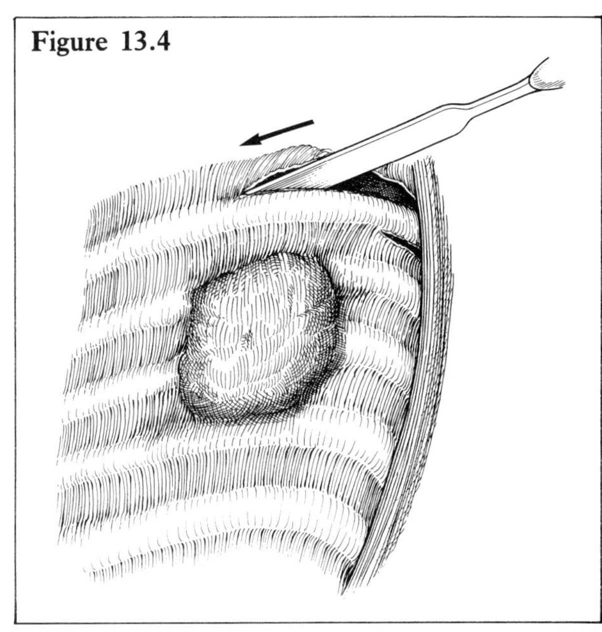

Figure 13.5

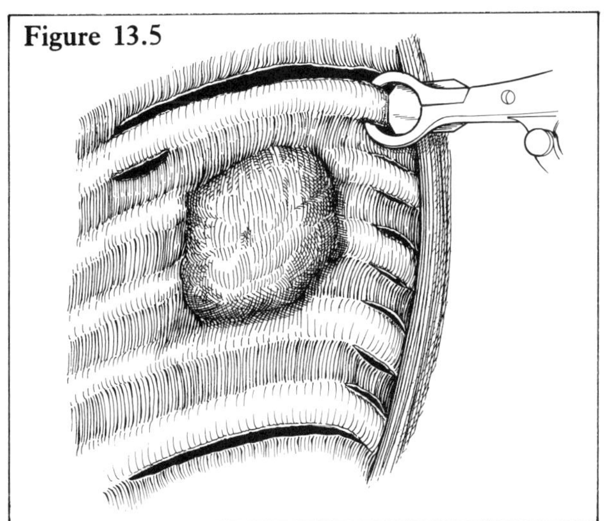

Figure 13.6

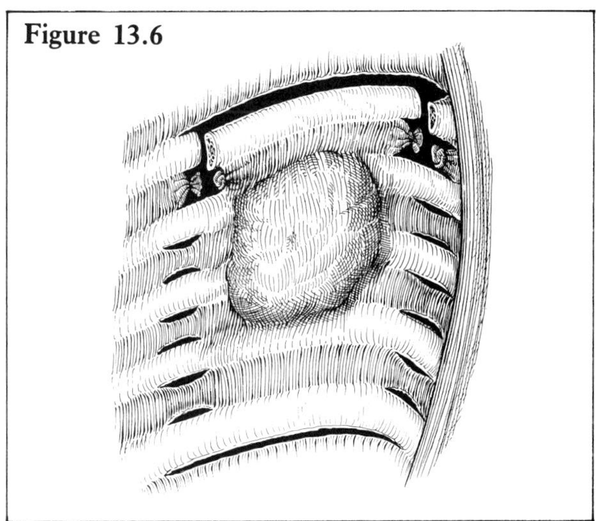

Figure 13.7

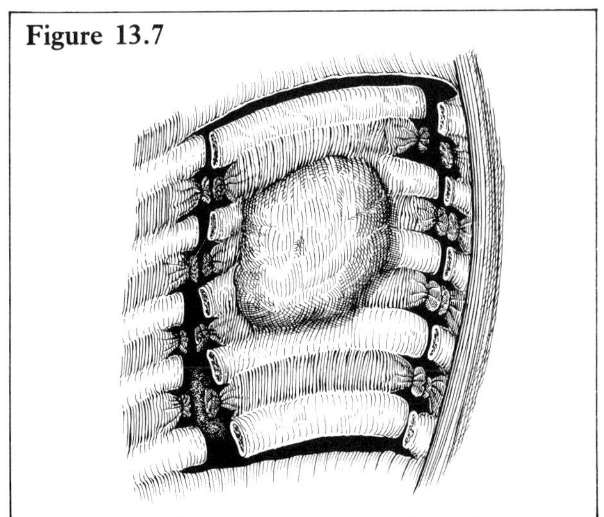

Figure 13.8

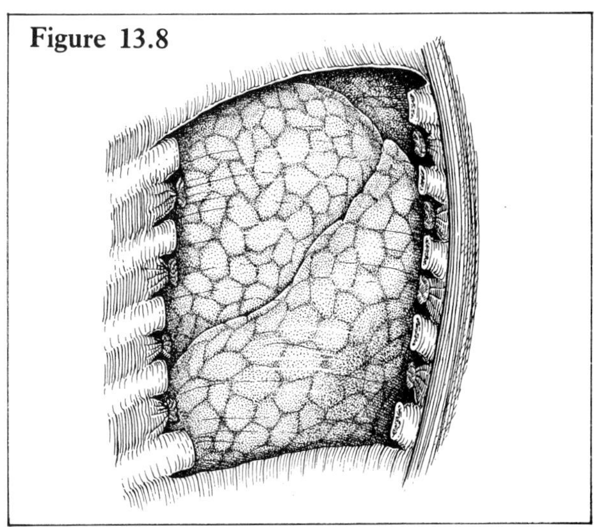

intercostal muscle bundle beneath it is divided between clamps and tied (**Fig. 13.6**). The next rib down (the first one to be involved with the tumour) is divided in a similar fashion, using the rib shears.

This process is repeated until the section of chest wall from which the tumour has arisen is completely free, with a wide margin of normal structures (**Figs. 13.7, 13.8**).

## Reconstruction of the chest wall

If the area of chest wall that has been resected lies beneath the scapula or at the apex of the thorax it is not necessary to fill the defect. The layers of chest wall muscles are simply closed over it. A single intrathoracic drain is maintained on suction at 100 mmHg (13 kPa). The defect will neither be apparent, nor of any potential risk to the patient.

### Repair with prosthetic material

If the resultant defect is in the lateral or anterior chest wall and extends over more than one rib space, then it should be repaired. Marlex (a strong nylon mesh) is the most commonly used material. Other materials are available, such as extra-thickness Goretex (expanded PTFE). The patch material is cut to the appropriate shape and size. If Marlex is to be used we suggest that the edge of the patch is folded over to give extra strength for the sutures. These folds can be tacked in position before sewing the patch to the chest wall (**Fig. 13.9**). The patch must be sewn in under tension (**Fig. 13.10**) to provide the support that is necessary for a good result.

If the defect is larger than two rib spaces, or is on the anterior chest, it should be reinforced. This can be done by making a 'sandwich' of methyl methacrylate bone cement between two layers of Marlex sheets. The Marlex patches are cut to the appropriate shape with an extra margin of 25 mm all around, on both sheets (**Fig. 13.11**). The bone cement is mixed to a thick paste and spread on the first Marlex patch, on which an outline of the defect has been marked. The second piece of Marlex is then placed over the cement and pressed firmly on to it (**Fig. 13.12**). The whole patch can then be moulded into the shape of the chest wall,

**Figure 13.9**

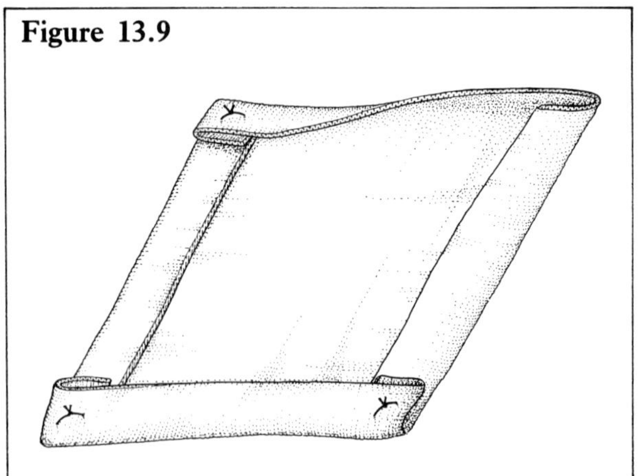

**Figure 13.11**

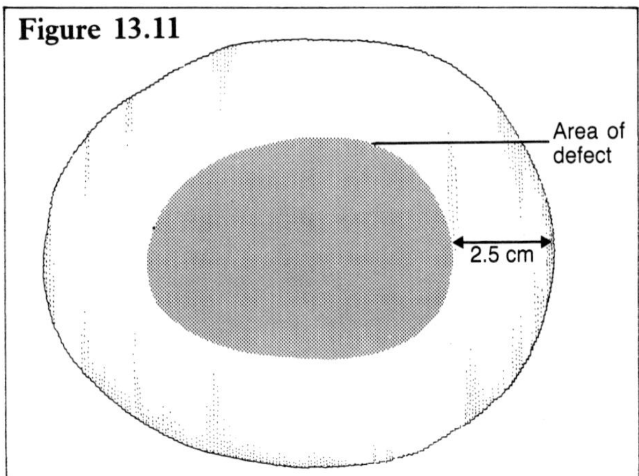


**Figure 13.10**

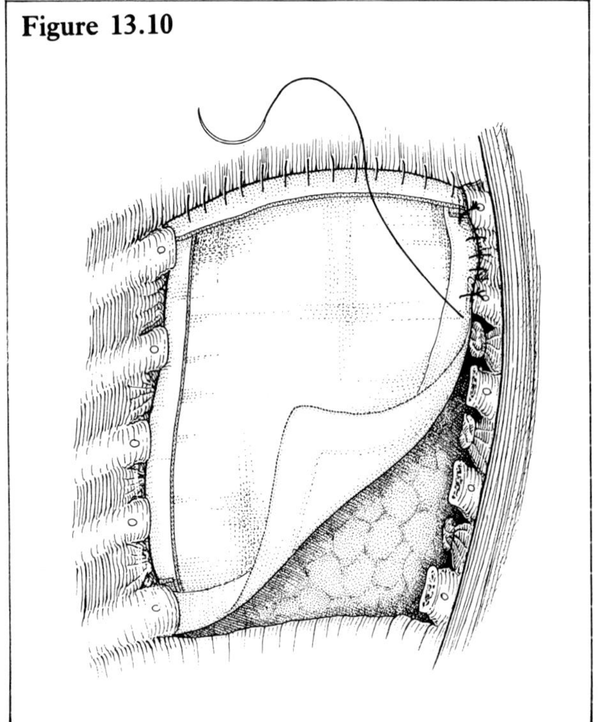

**Figure 13.12**

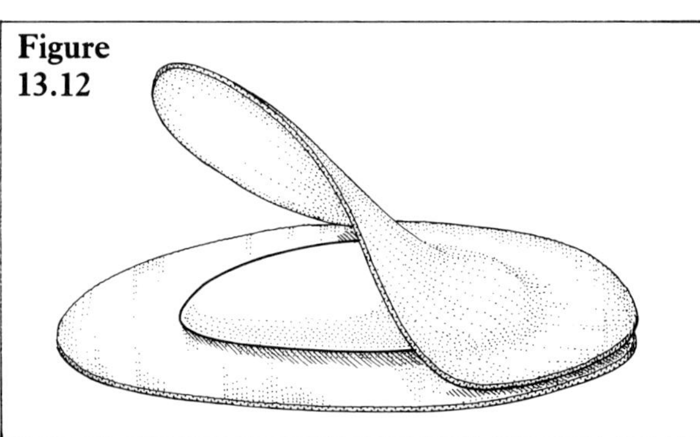

**Figure 13.13**

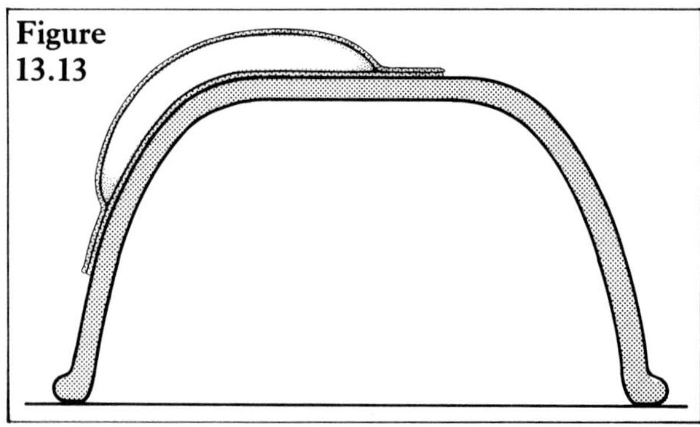

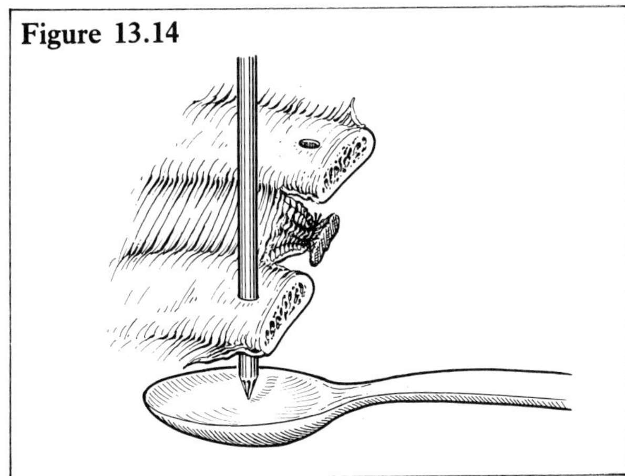
Figure 13.14

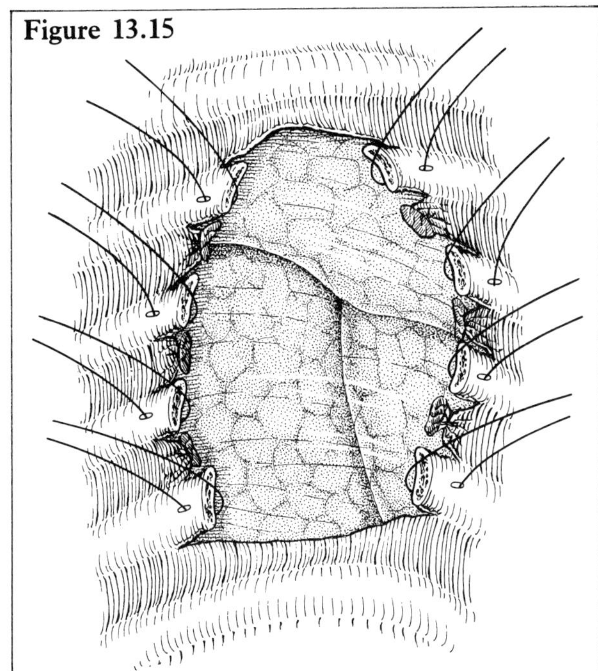
Figure 13.15

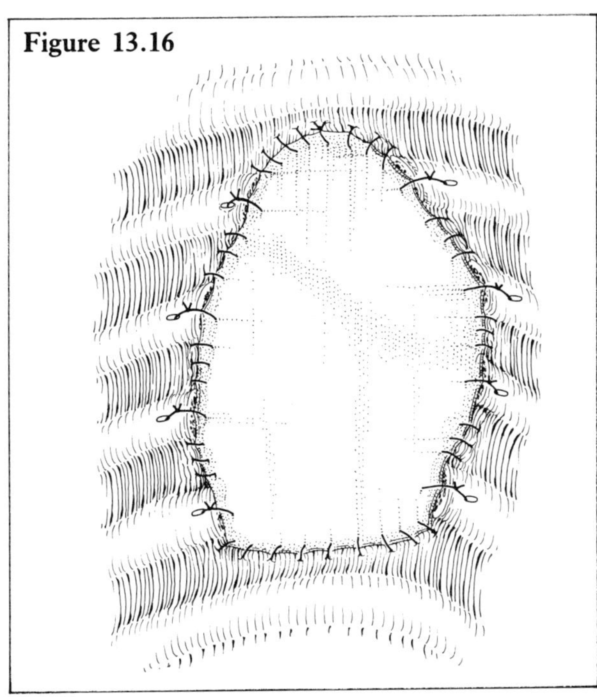
Figure 13.16

either on the back of the surgeon's hand or over the outside of a metal basin (**Fig. 13.13**).

Holes are drilled through the rib ends using an awl. A metal spoon may be used to protect the underlying structures (**Fig. 13.14**). Interrupted, heavy gauge non-absorbable sutures with needles at both ends are then placed through these holes (**Fig. 13.15**). The Marlex–methyl methacrylate patch can then be sewn into place using the free edge of Marlex. The patch should be sewn in as tightly as possible (**Fig. 13.16**).

If a myocutaneous flap is to be placed over the patch, it is helpful to suture the patch in such a way that it lies either within or below the defect. This will create a hollow for the subcutaneous fat of the flap to lie in and hence reduce tension on the surrounding skin edge sutures.

## Sternal resections

If the tumour has arisen within the sternum, the principles are the same. A wide local excision is carried out, dividing the ribs on either side sufficiently far away to give a good clearance (25–30 mm). The sternum is transected with a reciprocating saw and the underlying anterior mediastinal structures are separated using diathermy (**Figs. 13.17, 13.18**). If a myocutaneous

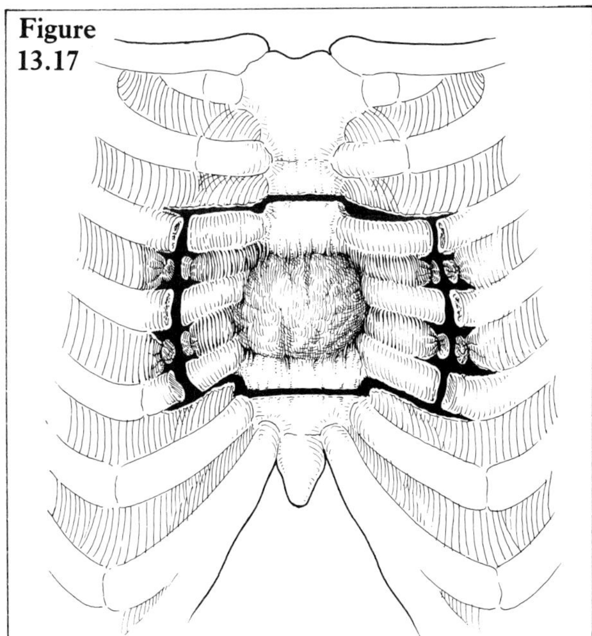
Figure 13.17

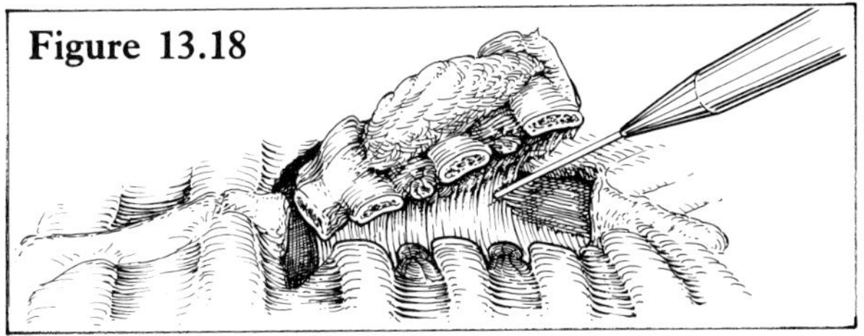
Figure 13.18

pedicled flap is necessary to close the defect, it is helpful to retain the internal mammary arteries if possible as this will allow the use of the rectus abdominis muscle flap.

## Resection of tumours that have invaded the overlying integuments

These procedures require a multidisciplinary approach, and are best performed in conjunction with a plastic surgeon. The same principles apply, except that in addition it will be necessary to circumscribe the lesion with the skin incision, leaving a clear margin of 25–50 mm (**Fig. 13.19**). The width of this margin will depend upon the type of tumour. For uncomplicated tumours such as a basal cell carcinoma a smaller margin is sufficient.

If the skin overlying the lesion is ulcerated, it is prudent to suture an antiseptic-soaked swab over it to reduce contamination of the wound (**Fig. 13.20**).

**Figure 13.19**

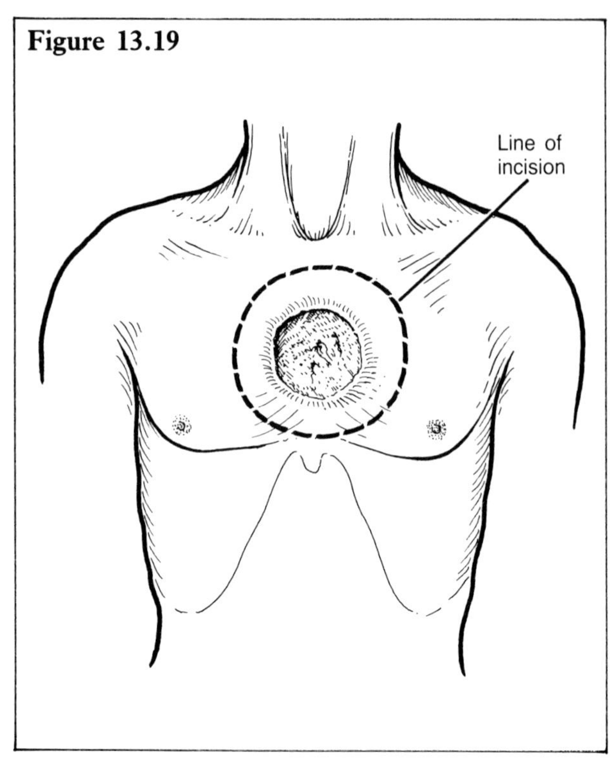


**Figure 13.20**

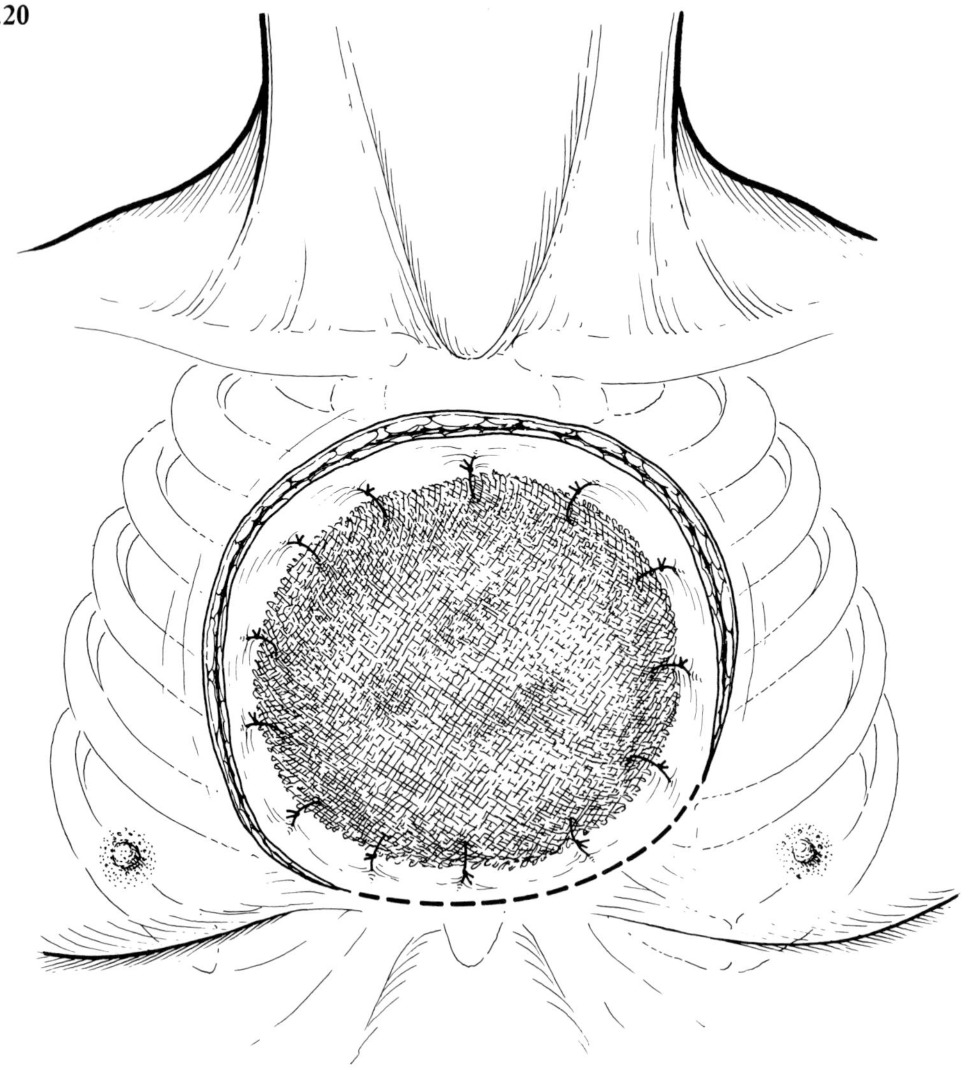

The incision is continued vertically downwards through the muscle layer until the chest wall is reached. The chest wall resection then follows the principles already described.

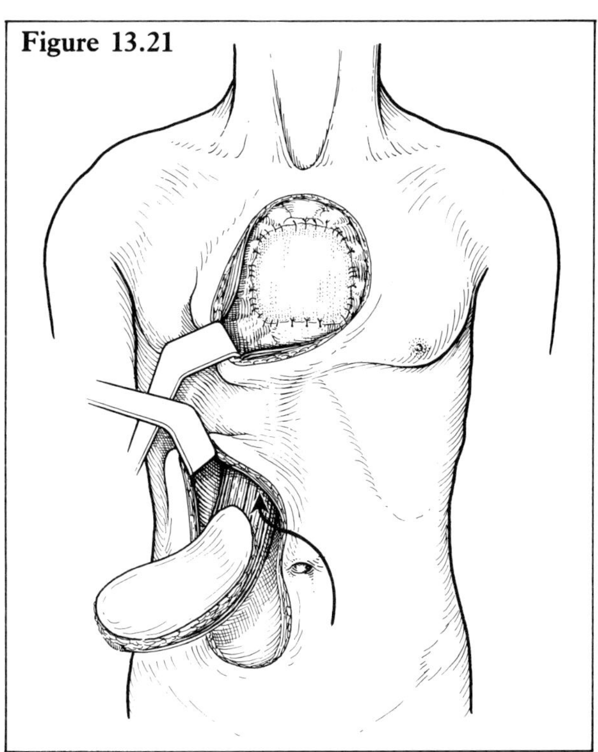

**Figure 13.21**

## Reconstruction of the chest wall

The large, full-thickness chest wall defect that results from this resection requires a more complex repair. First the chest wall defect is closed as described above, using a Marlex–methyl methacrylate sandwich. The myocutaneous defect usually cannot be closed directly, and therefore a vascularized myocutaneous flap is needed. The services of a plastic surgeon are invaluable here, as sometimes the more common rectus abdominis or latissimus dorsi flaps are not viable due to interference with their blood supply during resection of the tumour.

A complete review of the possible types of myocutaneous flaps is beyond the scope of this book. However, one type—the rectus abdominis flap—is illustrated (**Figs. 13.21–23**).

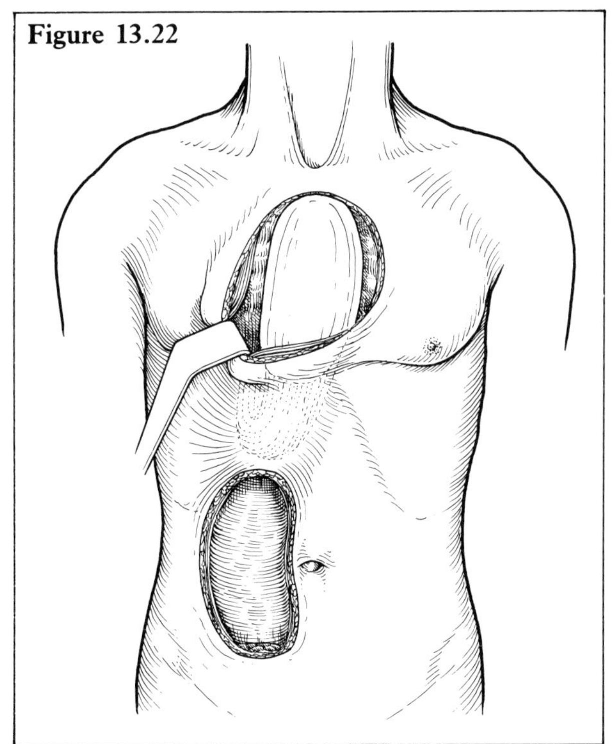

**Figure 13.22**

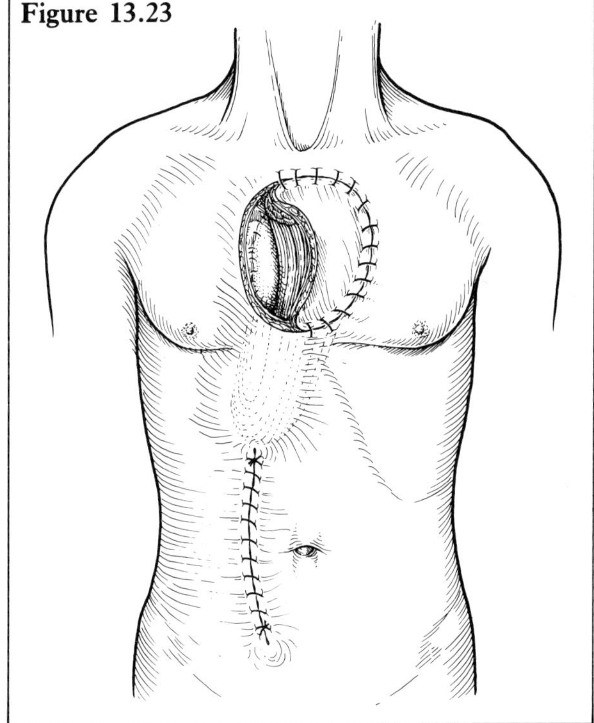

**Figure 13.23**

# 14 Excision of first rib

Neurovascular compression at the thoracic outlet may give rise to one of the thoracic outlet compression syndromes. It is generally accepted that all these compression syndromes have one common problem: compression of the nervous or vascular structures, or both, in the gap between the first rib and the clavicle. It seems probable that evolutionary progress to an erect posture has advanced more quickly than the adaptation by the thoracic outlet to accommodate the resultant change in position of the shoulder girdle.

## Anatomy

The thoracic outlet contains the subclavian artery, subclavian vein and brachial plexus (**Fig. 14.1**). There is sufficient space around these structures to allow full movement of the arm without compression.

### Variants

Various skeletal abnormalities may lead to compression of the contents of the thoracic outlet. These are:

1. Cervical rib (**Fig. 14.2**).
2. Elongated transverse process from C7 vertebra.
3. Fibrous band from C7 transverse process to the first rib (**Fig. 14.2**).
4. Excrescences and anomalies of the first rib.
5. Developmental abnormalities of the clavicle may reduce the costoclavicular space (**Fig. 14.3**).
6. Compression by the scalene muscles (**Fig. 14.4**).

Removal of the first rib decompresses the floor of the osseous 'scissors' of rib and clavicle and perforce ensures detachment of the scalene muscles and fibrous bands, thus relieving any compression that they may have caused.

**Figure 14.1**

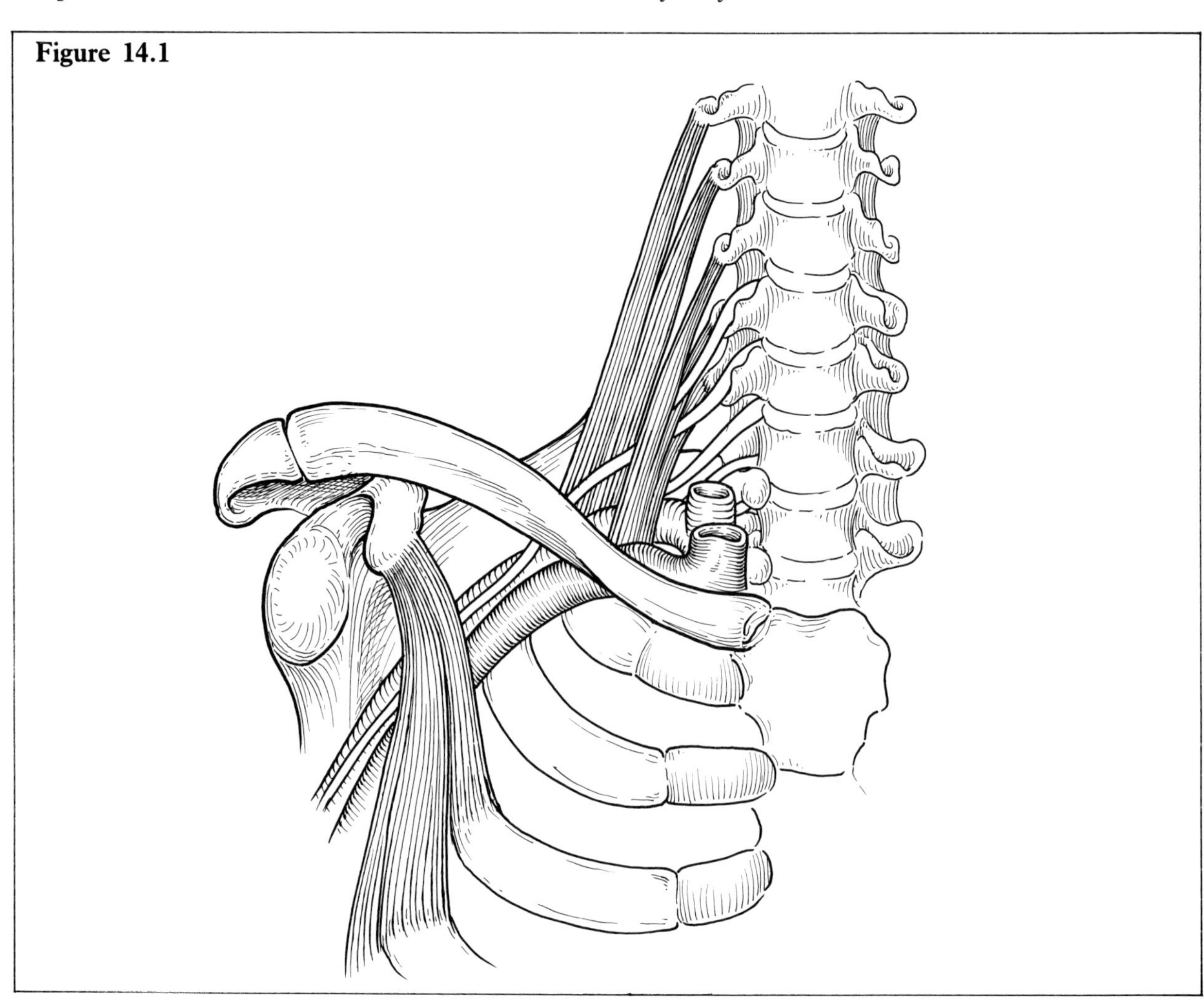

**Figure 14.2**

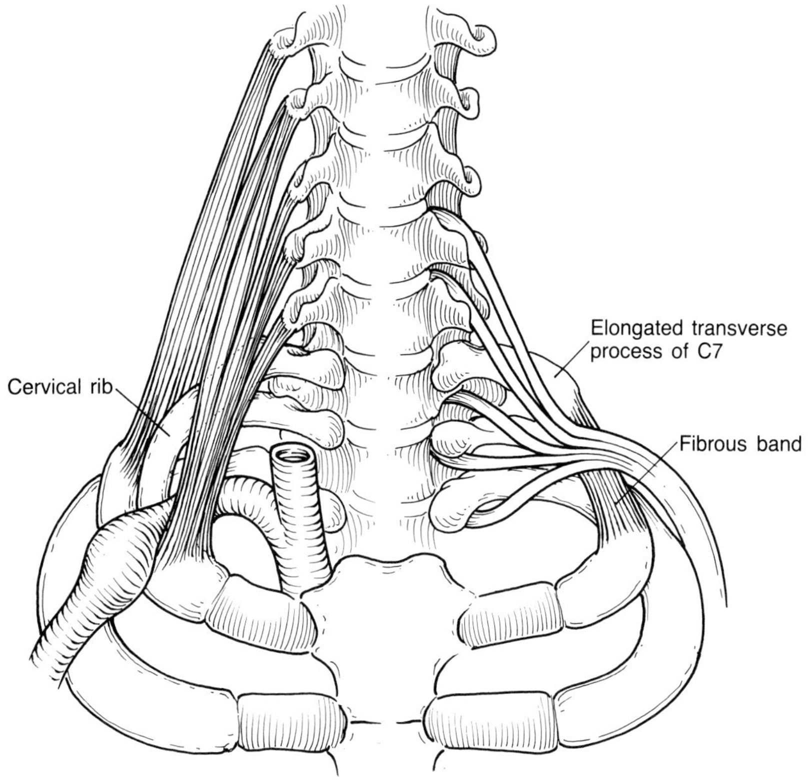

**Figure 14.3**

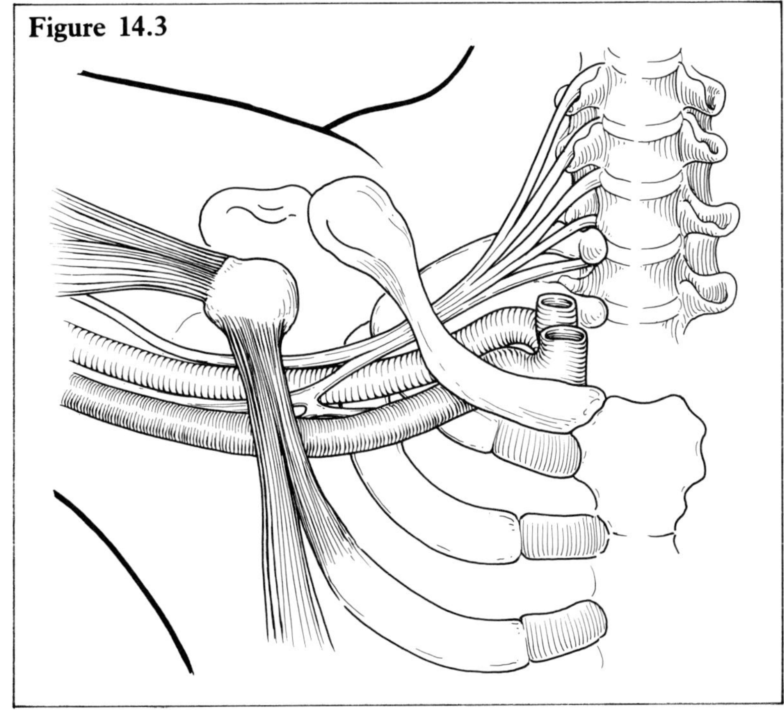

**Figure 14.4**

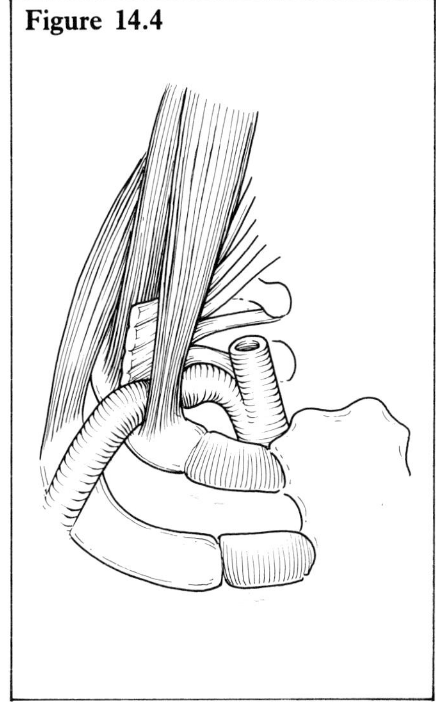

## Transaxillary approach

Several approaches have been used, but only the transaxillary approach developed by Roos is described here as we believe it to be the most satisfactory. The advantages of this method are:

1. It is easier.
2. It provides clear exposure of the first rib, major vessels and nerves.
3. Blood loss is minimal.
4. No muscles are cut other than those attached to the first rib.
5. The scar is cosmetic and hidden.

Figure 14.5

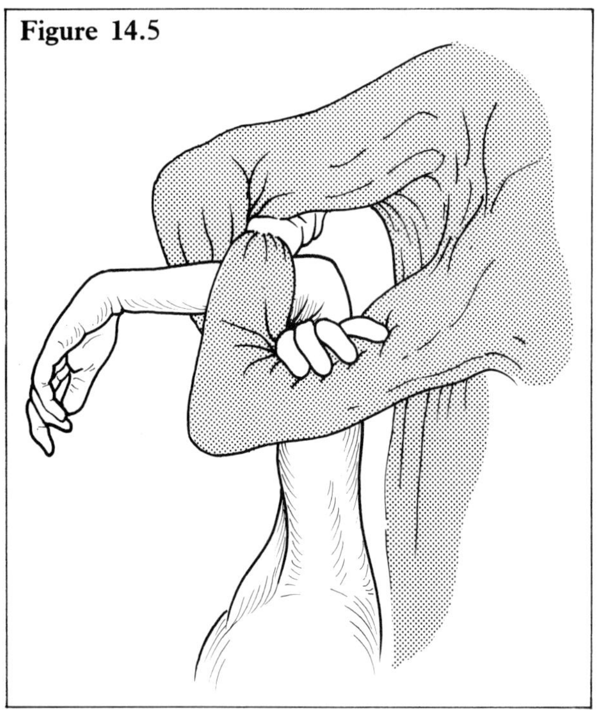

Figure 14.6

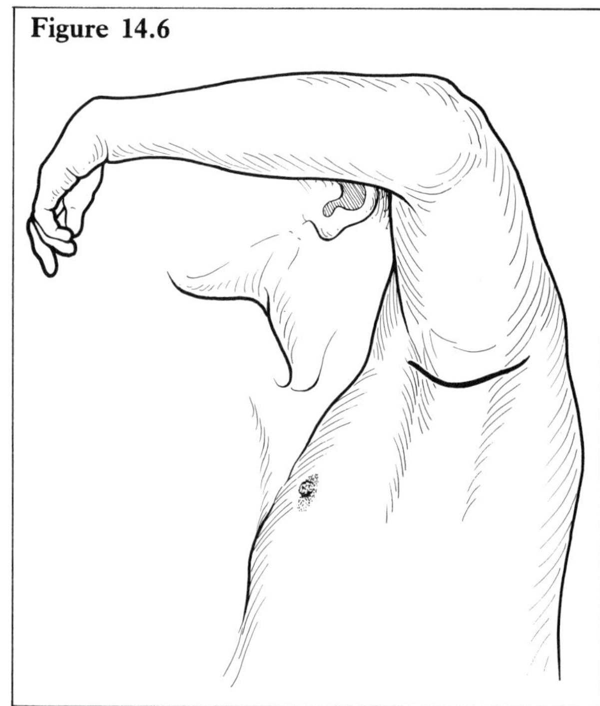

## Procedure

The patient is placed in the lateral position, and the arm is raised at 90 degrees to the body and flexed at the elbow. Distraction (elevation) of the arm by an assistant will open the axillary space (**Fig. 14.5**).

A transverse incision is made at the inferior margin of the hairline parallel with the skin crease (**Fig. 14.6**). Posteriorly it is limited by the latissimus dorsi muscle, and anteriorly by the pectoralis major muscle (**Fig. 14.7**).

The axillary fat pad is next encountered, and within it, passing from the second intercostal space to the inner aspect of the upper arm, is the intercostobrachial nerve (**Fig. 14.7**). This nerve provides sensation to the inner aspect of the upper arm, and if an unpleasant area of anaesthesia is to be avoided postoperatively, great care should be taken to preserve it.

Once the upper part of the chest wall is exposed, the first rib is identified. The assistant raises the arm and in doing so opens the costoclavicular recess. Periodically the arm should be lowered to reduce the pull on the neurovascular structures. The anterior and medial scalene muscles and subclavius muscle are separated from the first rib. This is easily accomplished by pulling the fibres away with a right-angled forceps (**Fig. 14.8**). Next, the periosteum over the rib is incised with the diathermy point and a periosteal elevator used to strip it, first from the inferior and then from the superior surface of the rib (**Fig. 14.9**). Great care is taken not to injure the great vessels or first thoracic nerve. Anteriorly the costoclavicular liga-

Figure 14.7

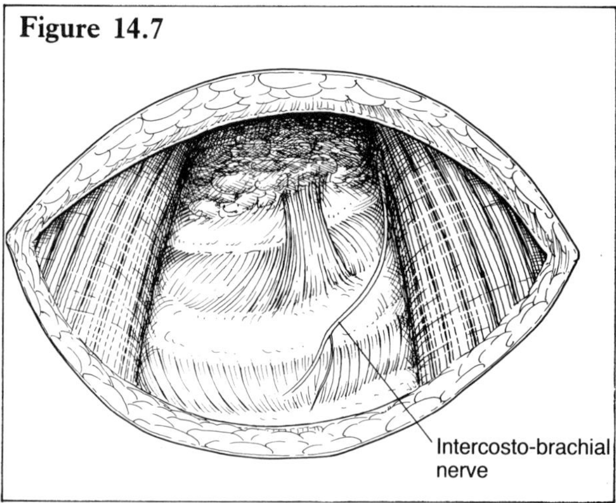


Figure 14.8

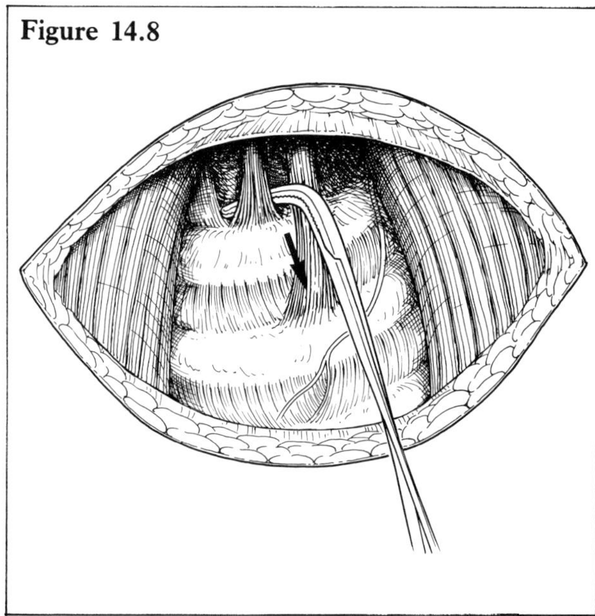

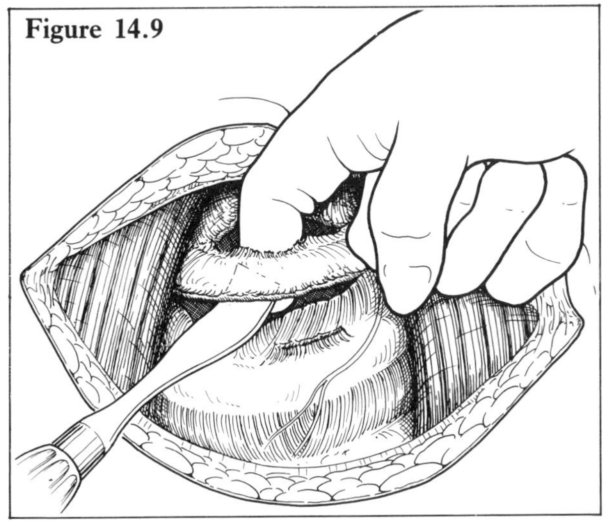

Figure 14.9

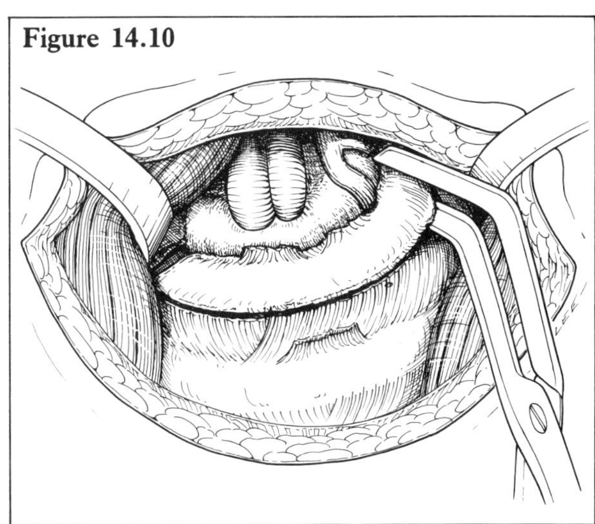

Figure 14.10

ment is sectioned and the anterior end of the rib divided with appropriately angled rib shears.

Finally the dissection is carried posteriorly beyond the tubercle of the rib, where it is sectioned with angled rib shears (**Fig. 14.10**). The whole rib is removed and any bony spicules are trimmed with bone nibblers.

If a cervical rib is present it is detached from the first rib and resected at this stage. Similarly, any cervical fibrous band is divided.

By pouring warm saline into the wound at this stage, any hole in the pleura may be identified and repaired. It is not usually necessary to use a pleural drain. If a hole is present a suction catheter can be placed in the pleural space and withdrawn when the wound has been closed.

### Closure

An absorbable suture is used to close the fat and subcutaneous layers over a vacuum drain. A subcuticular absorbable suture is used for skin closure. The drain is removed when drainage ceases. This prevents a subcutaneous haematoma or seroma forming and reduces the risk of infection.

# 15 Thoracoplasty

Thoracoplasty was once the standard surgical treatment for pulmonary tuberculosis affecting the upper lobes; it was used effectively to close tuberculous cavities. This indication is now rarely necessary. Thoracoplasty is more commonly used to obliterate a persistent pleural space, usually in the presence of chronic infection and a bronchopleural fistula.

The operation involves resection of three to seven or more ribs. This mobilization of the chest wall may result in paradoxical movement which can interfere with the patient's respiratory function. The degree of paradoxical movement depends on the rigidity of the mediastinum and the walls of the pleural cavity. Where these rigid surfaces prevent paradoxical movement the operation can be carried out in a single stage; otherwise it is carried out in two or more stages, spread over 10 to 14 days. Much more delay may result in fixation at the previous operative site and limit the final degree of collapse that can be achieved. In the first stage the upper three ribs are removed. For successful closure of a pulmonary cavity or pleural space the apex of the lung and the dome of the pleura must be lowered by an extrafascial apicolysis, otherwise the cavity or pleural space will persist in a narrow recess adjacent to the mediastinum.

**Figure 15.1**

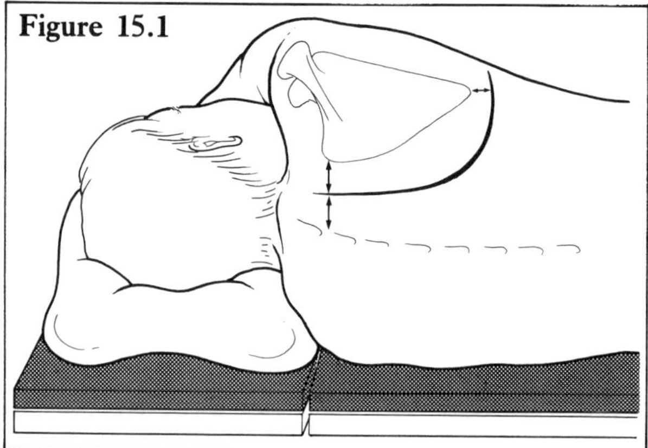

**Figure 15.2**

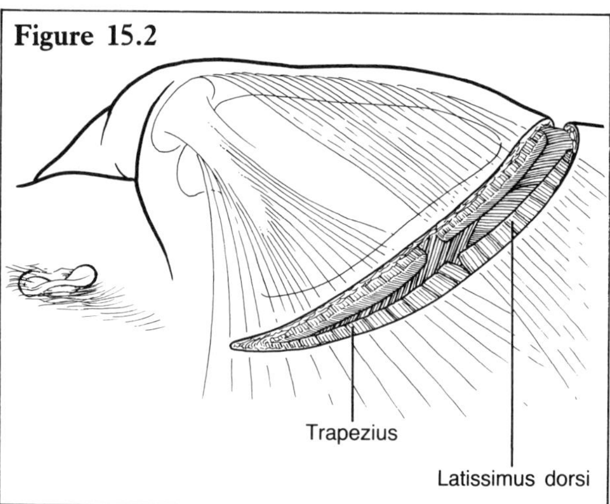


## Procedure

The patient is placed in the lateral position with the uppermost arm directed forwards over the edge of the table.

The incision begins at the level of the spine of the scapula and is carried parallel to the thoracic spinous processes, halfway between them and the medial edge of the scapula, to about the level of the seventh rib (i.e. to a point about 25 mm below the inferior angle of the scapula). Here it is carried forwards at right angles terminating about 4 cm anterior to the inferior angle of the scapula (**Fig. 15.1**). The trapezius and latissimus dorsi muscles are divided in the line of the incision and the rhomboid muscles divided in the same line (**Fig. 15.2**). The scapula is retracted forwards and upwards and the connective tissue between it and the chest wall divided, thus exposing the first three digitations of the serratus anterior muscle. A finger can then be passed into the gap between the scalenus medius and the uppermost digitation of serratus anterior, thus protecting the contents of the axilla.

The scapular retraction is increased, putting the digitations of serratus anterior attached to the first four ribs under tension. They can then be detached from the periosteum of the ribs with the diathermy point (**Fig. 15.3**). The serratus posterior superior muscle is excised. The scalenus medius and scalenus posterior muscles, attached respectively to the outer surface of the first and second ribs, are detached by tearing through their muscle fibres a few at a time with closed scissors or blunt-nosed right-angled forceps (**Fig. 15.4**). The whole outer margins of the first and second ribs are now exposed and

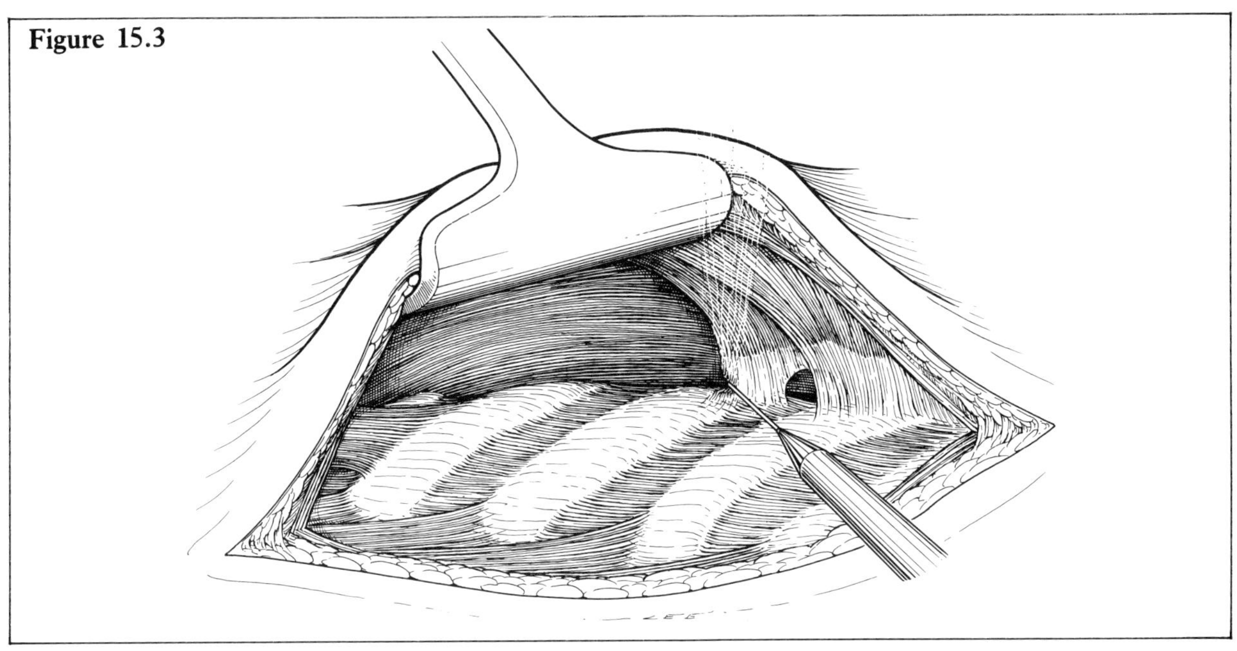
Figure 15.3

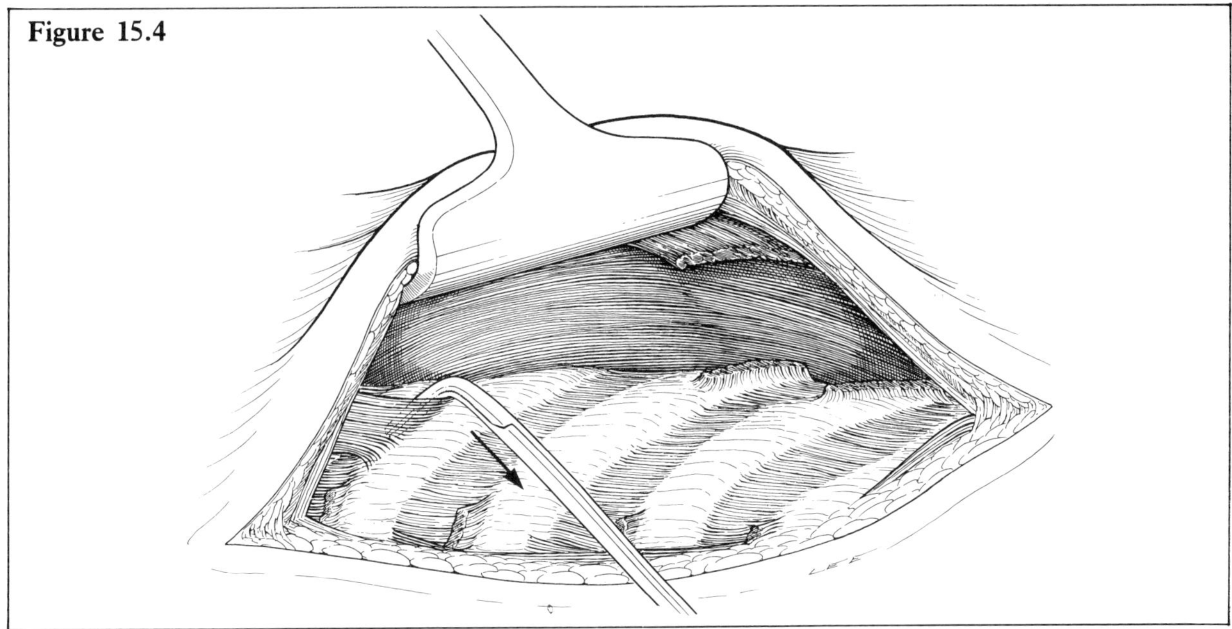
Figure 15.4

the neurovascular structures leading to the arm can be seen above the first rib. Anteriorly a collapsing area is identified as the subclavian vein. Immediately behind it the subclavian artery can be seen or felt to be pulsating, and behind it, close to the neck of the rib, is the first thoracic nerve (see **Fig. 14.10**).

A vertical incision is made with the diathermy point along the lateral border of the sacrospinalis muscle, over the necks of the ribs. The periosteum of the third rib is incised with diathermy from the vertical incision posteriorly to the anterior axillary line (**Fig. 15.5**), and the periosteum is elevated from the outer surface, and then the inner surface, of the rib. Posteriorly the periosteal elevation continues to the anterior surface of the neck of the rib. The neck of the rib is divided adjacent to (or just central to) the transverse process with right-angled rib shears. The rib is grasped and divided anteriorly with rib shears, the handles of which are curved to accommodate the curve of the chest wall.

By a similar technique the second rib, which is now more accessible, is excised. The line of excision anteriorly is through the costal cartilage.

The outer surface of the first rib can now be clearly seen. The rib is flat and wide. The periosteum is incised (**Fig. 15.6**) along the outer edge of its upper surface and also the outer edge of the lower surface. A broad, flat periosteal elevator is used to strip the periosteum gently from the inferior surface. The direction of stripping is parallel to the surface, i.e. directed towards the anterior and posterior ends of the rib. As soon as

Figure 15.5

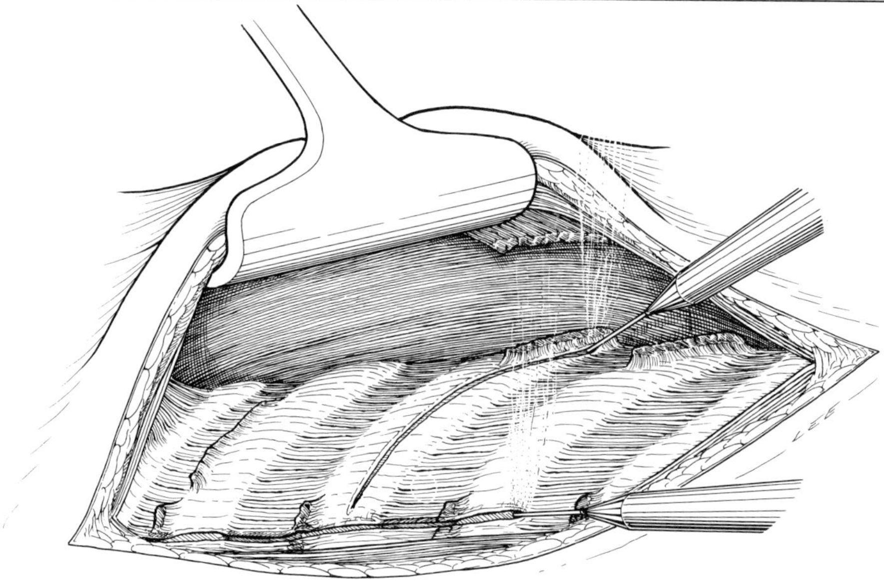

Figure 15.6

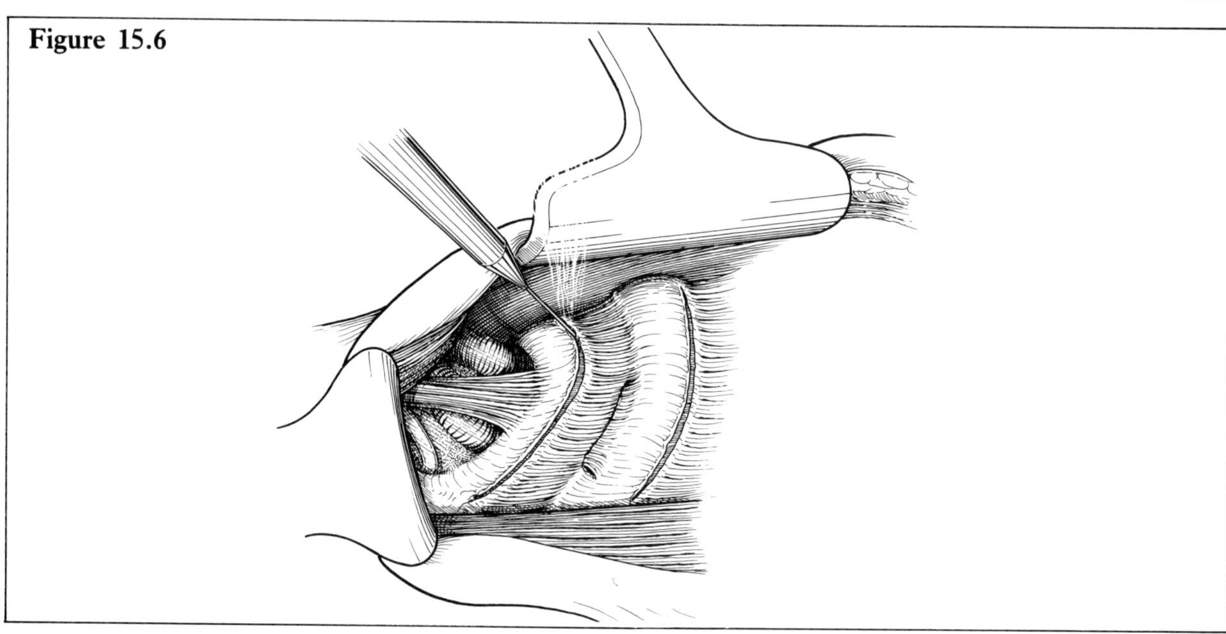

Figure 15.7

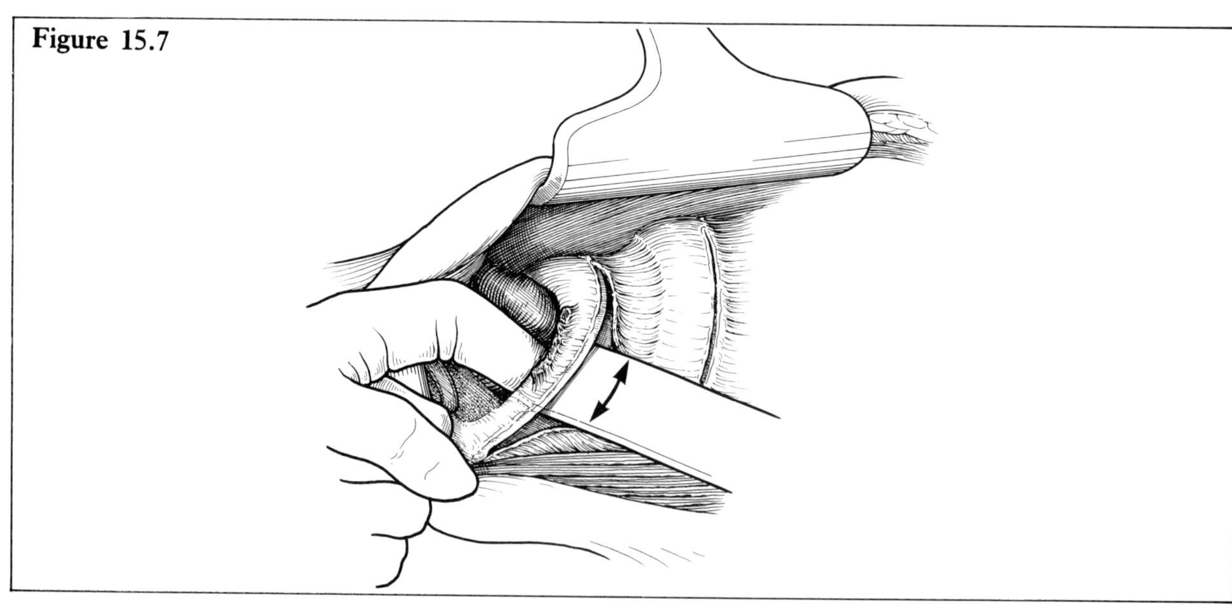

Figure 15.8

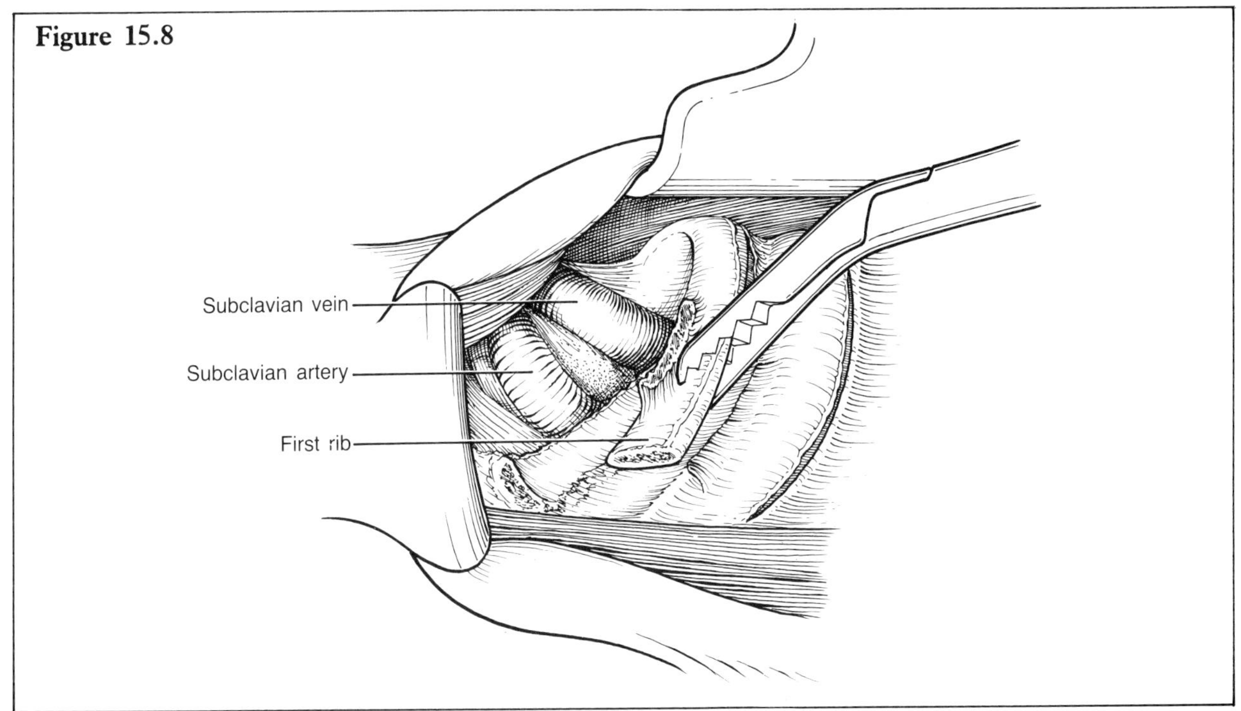


the medial margin of the rib can be recognized, a finger is hooked around it from above and a curved rugine used to free the periosteum from the medial margin. The finger can now protect the subclavian artery and vein while the medial border of the rib is freed of periosteum (**Fig. 15.7**).

Blunt dissection along the medial margin of the anterior half of the rib now reveals the scalene tubercle and the insertion of the scalenus anterior muscle. The rib is divided just behind the scalene tubercle, the index finger of the left hand still protecting the subclavian vessels. The posterior half of the rib is grasped with bone forceps and the neck cleared of periosteum with the periosteal elevator (**Fig. 15.8**). Traction on the posterior half of the rib at this stage will often result in its being avulsed completely together with the head and neck. If this manoeuvre is unsuccessful, rib shears are insinuated across the neck of the rib, taking great care to protect the first thoracic nerve. The rib shears are then gently closed, and the posterior half of the rib is removed.

By downward traction on the anterior half of the rib, the tendon of the scalenus muscle comes into view and is divided with diathermy. Further traction downwards and forwards exposes the costoclavicular ligament. The subclavian vein is continuously protected while the ligament is divided with scissors. The costochondral junction now often dislocates from the sternum, but if not the cartilage is divided and the rib removed.

### Extrafascial apicolysis

The endothoracic fascia lining the muscles of the chest wall has fibrous extensions which are attached to the transverse processes of the cervical vertebrae. These bands extend downwards between the nerves and vessels of the thoracic inlet and support the apical pleura (**Fig. 15.9**). They must therefore be divided before the apex of the lung can be lowered.

The first step in this manoeuvre is to divide the periosteum of the posterior ends of the first, second and third ribs. The endothoracic fascia is encountered immediately deep to the periosteum, and by advancing the dissection along the anterior surfaces of the transverse processes on to the sides of the bodies of the vertebrae, the apicolysis is initiated from behind.

Figure 15.9

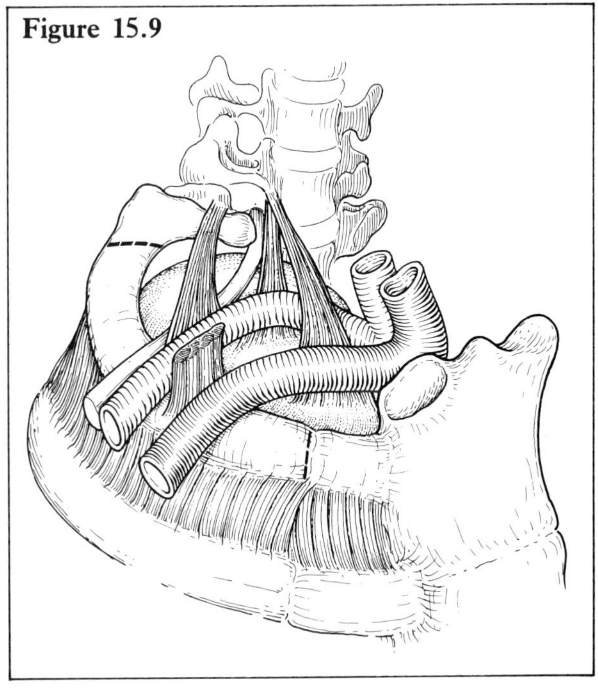

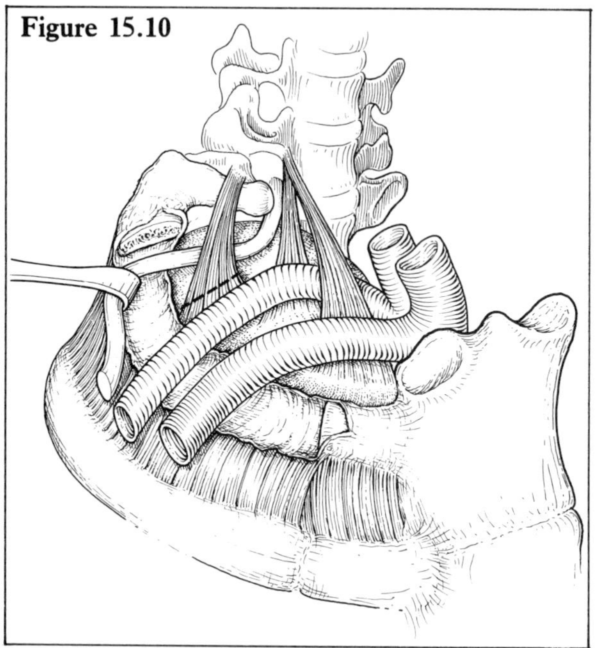

Figure 15.10

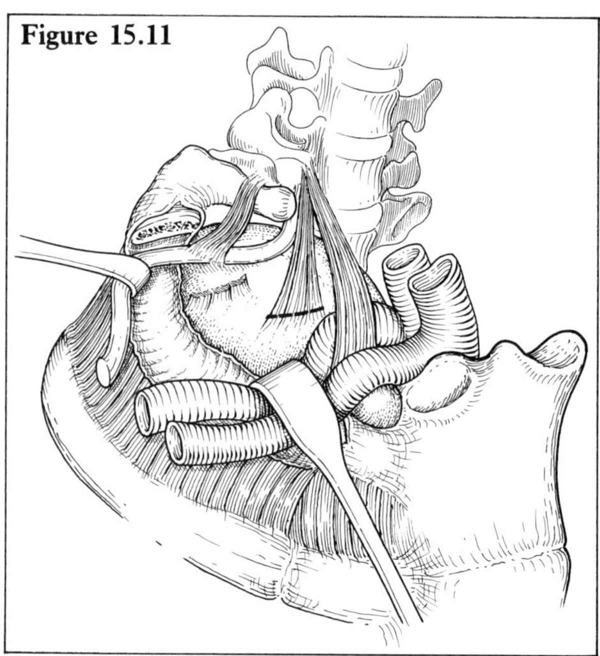

Figure 15.11

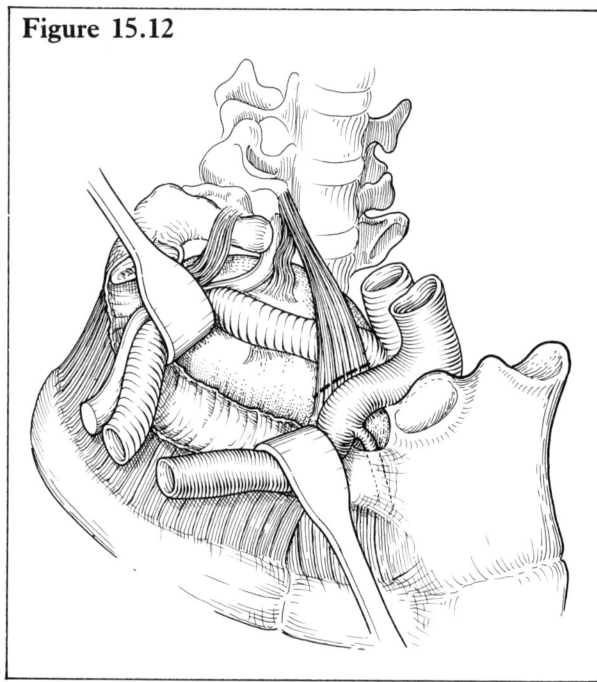

Figure 15.12

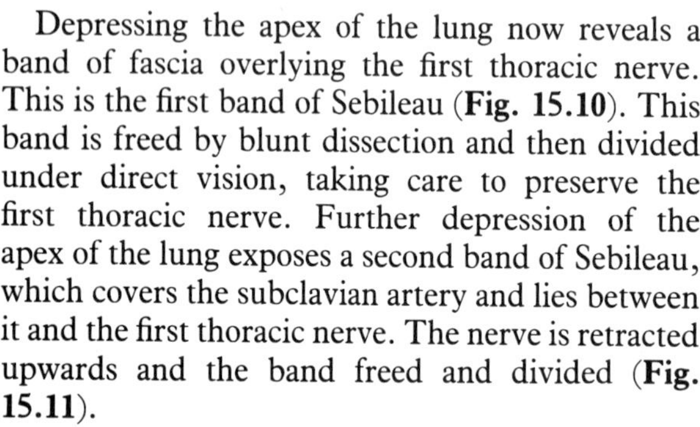

Depressing the apex of the lung now reveals a band of fascia overlying the first thoracic nerve. This is the first band of Sebileau (**Fig. 15.10**). This band is freed by blunt dissection and then divided under direct vision, taking care to preserve the first thoracic nerve. Further depression of the apex of the lung exposes a second band of Sebileau, which covers the subclavian artery and lies between it and the first thoracic nerve. The nerve is retracted upwards and the band freed and divided (**Fig. 15.11**).

The third band lies between the subclavian artery and vein (**Fig. 15.12**). The fascia around both these vessels is dissected away and the line of dissection is continued downwards and forwards to expose the internal mammary vessels. These vessels lie in the plane in which the extrafascial apicolysis is to be continued on the mediastinal aspect. The exposed periosteum at the posterior end of the second and third ribs is now divided, and the neurovascular bundles of each of the first three ribs is isolated, ligated and divided. By blunt dissection the apex of the lung is freed from the mediastinum as far down as the azygos vein on the right side, and the arch of the aorta on the left. The vagus and phrenic nerves are identified and preserved.

The freeing of the anterior part of the upper lobe can be extended by separating the perichondrium from the back of the third rib anteriorly. The divided chest wall muscles are now repaired with continuous sutures, and the skin incision closed.

The space between the ribs and scapula—the Semb space—is not drained and is allowed to fill with fluid, which aids in the compression of the apex of the lung and prevents it from rising.

### Subsequent operations

The number of subsequent operations to complete the thoracoplasty depends on the extent to which the lung is to be collapsed or chest wall allowed to cave in, and also on the degree of fixation of the mediastinum and pleura. This determines the amount of paradoxical movement which will occur after the rib resections. A seven-rib thoracoplasty usually necessitates three stages, and has the advantage that on its completion the inferior angle of the scapula beds itself inside the ribs. If only five or six ribs are removed the inferior angle of the scapula may impinge repeatedly on the rib causing discomfort.

Successive stages of the operation should be carried out at two-weekly intervals. At a second-stage operation the whole wound is reopened, the scapula mobilized and retracted, and clot and serum removed from the subscapular space. About half of the fifth rib and two-thirds of the fourth are resected. This allows access to the anterior end of the third rib which is removed completely.

Between the thoracoplasty stages the apex of the lung tends to rise up the mediastinum and it must therefore be mobilized again at subsequent stages. To do this safely, the dissection begins posteriorly by division of the periosteum of the necks of the fourth, fifth and sixth ribs and the corresponding intercostal bundles. The extrafascial plane is therefore entered at the back of the mediastinum and enlarged forwards and upwards until the apex can be freed from the mediastinum. The wound is then closed.

Resection of the posterior halves of the sixth and seventh ribs, which is carried out at the third stage, can be achieved by opening the lower half of the incision only. The intercostal bundles are divided as for the upper ribs.

## Thoracoplasty for obliteration of an empyema cavity associated with a bronchopleural fistula

The problem here is one of obliterating a rigid pleural space, usually after pneumonectomy. If viable lung remains in the pleural space the ideal operation is decortication of the lung and excision of the empyema lining the space. The bronchopleural fistula is excised and repaired at the same time and the lung can then usually be persuaded to fill the pleural space, if necessary by the induction of a pneumoperitoneum.

After pneumonectomy the problem is much more difficult. Closure of the space can only be achieved by approximation of the outer wall of the hemithorax to the mediastinum. Thus an extensive thoracoplasty is necessary.

### Procedure

There will usually be a tube track extending into the pleural cavity from a point somewhere below the inferior angle of the scapula. This track is excised and the incision extended posteriorly and anteriorly as a posterolateral thoracotomy. The pleural space is entered by a long fifth intercostal incision. The walls of the cavity are cleaned of granulation tissue partly by sharp dissection, which is appropriate to the parietal wall, and partly by a combination of sharp dissection and curettage, which is more suitable for the mediastinal aspect where the underlying structures cannot be seen. Curettage should continue on the diaphragmatic surface.

The upper ribs are then resected throughout their length over an area that encompasses the whole extent of the empyema cavity. The resection must include the first rib, otherwise a narrow space is liable to persist adjacent to the mediastinum.

If the layer of intercostal muscles, periosteum and fibrous tissue does not fall in to meet the mediastinum and diaphragm, several steps can be taken to increase its mobility. These are:

1. Excision of a wedge of fibrous tissue from the interior aspect of the region of the necks of the ribs.
2. Detachment of the intercostal muscles and periosteum anteriorly adjacent to the sternum.
3. Detachment of the lower margin of the outer layer at its attachment to the diaphragm.

The management of the bronchopleural fistula itself is dealt with on p. 147.

#### Closure

Three drains are placed in the space and brought out below the incision. They are connected via an underwater seal to a vacuum of 60 mmHg (8 kPa). The pleural space and subscapular spaces are heavily powdered with appropriate antibiotics and the muscle layers of the chest wall tightly closed. A systemic course of broad-spectrum antibiotics must also be given.

# 16 Rib resection for empyema

## Indications

1. Failure to cure by aspiration or by irrigation via an intercostal tube.
2. Decortication contraindicated by the patient's age or debilitated state.
3. The presence of a bronchopleural or oesophago-pleural fistula.

## Procedure

In order to avoid aspiration of the empyema contents into the opposite lung the operation should be performed under local anaesthesia with the patient upright, or under general anaesthesia with the aid of a double lumen tube with the patient in the lateral position. If the procedure is to be carried out in the upright position the patient is seated on a stool, feet resting on a support and elbows leaning on the operating table. A pile of pillows supports the head (**Fig. 16.1**). The rib level at the most dependent part of the empyema cavity is sought. This is identified on an over-penetrated PA and lateral chest film after contrast material has been instilled into the pleural cavity.

The chosen rib is identified by counting from above and below. The pleural cavity is aspirated

**Figure 16.1**

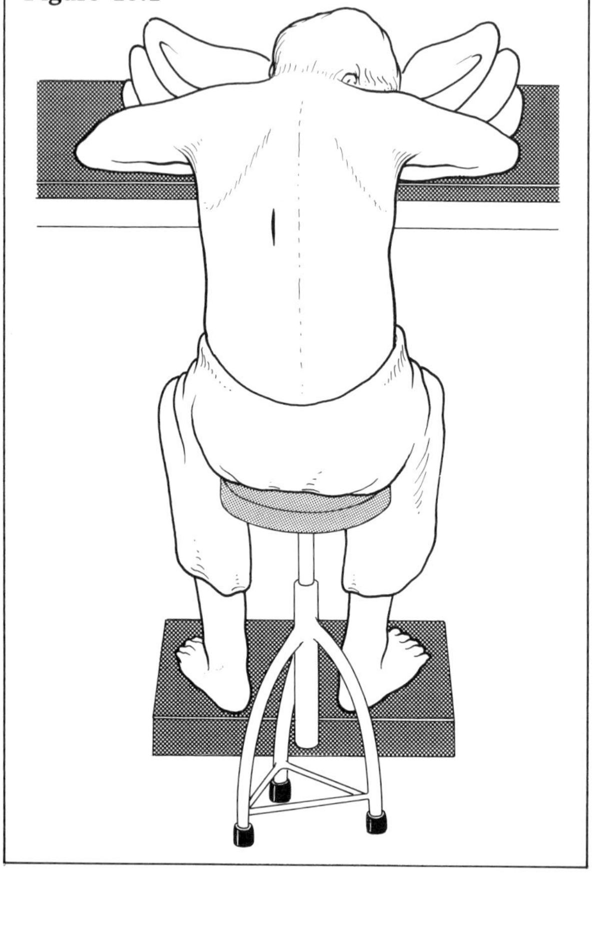

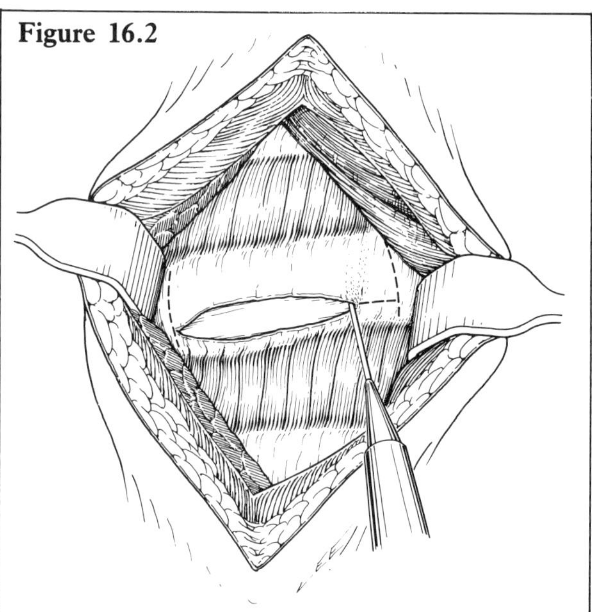

**Figure 16.2**

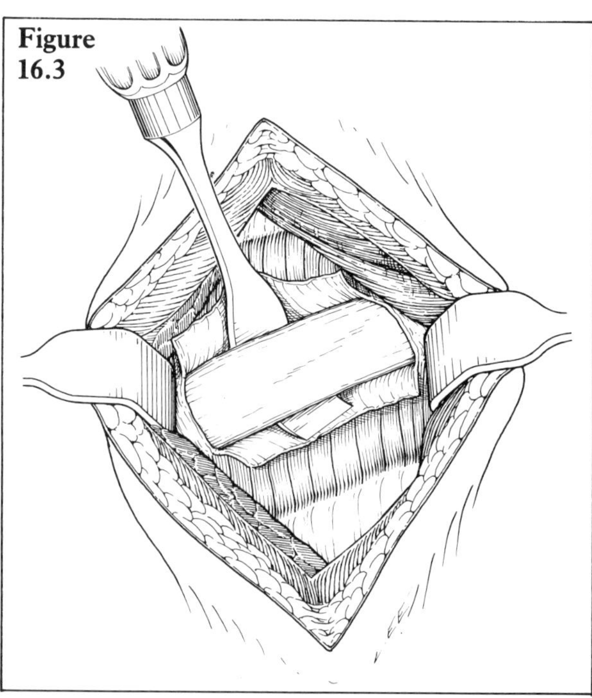

**Figure 16.3**

with a wide-bore needle which can be left *in situ*.

A vertical incision is made with diathermy down to (and centred on) the chosen rib. The muscles are retracted laterally. An incision about 8 cm long is made through the periosteum of the outer surface of the rib and a transverse incision at each end (**Fig. 16.2**). The periosteum is freed completely (**Fig. 16.3**) and the section of rib removed with a bone cutter (**Fig. 16.4**). A further aspiration is carried out through the periosteal bed of the rib to confirm the presence of pus or air (**Fig. 16.5**). The needle track can be enlarged with diathermy or opened with an artery forceps.

A large section of the outer wall of the empyema is removed with diathermy and preserved for histological examination.

Next, a finger is introduced to palpate the walls of the empyema and particularly to determine that the site of the rib resection is level with the floor of the cavity. If it is not, the opening is extended downwards (**Fig. 16.6**).

Using a fibre-optic light to illuminate the cavity, retained pus is sucked away and the walls thoroughly debrided with a gauze swab held in sponge forceps. As much as possible of the slough and fibrin is removed from the cavity.

A tube 20–30 mm in diameter is passed into the pleural cavity for about 5 cm. Its outer end is pierced with a safety pin which is used to affix adhesive strapping to hold the tube in position (**Fig. 16.7**). Suturing of the muscles and skin is often unnecessary, as they soon approximate.

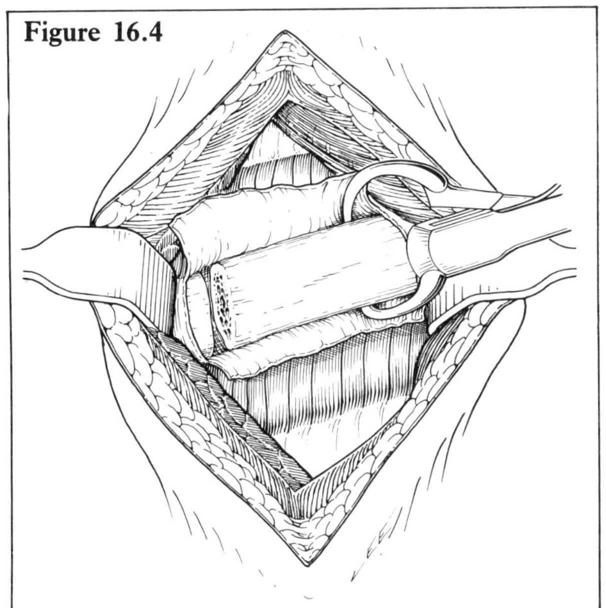
**Figure 16.4**

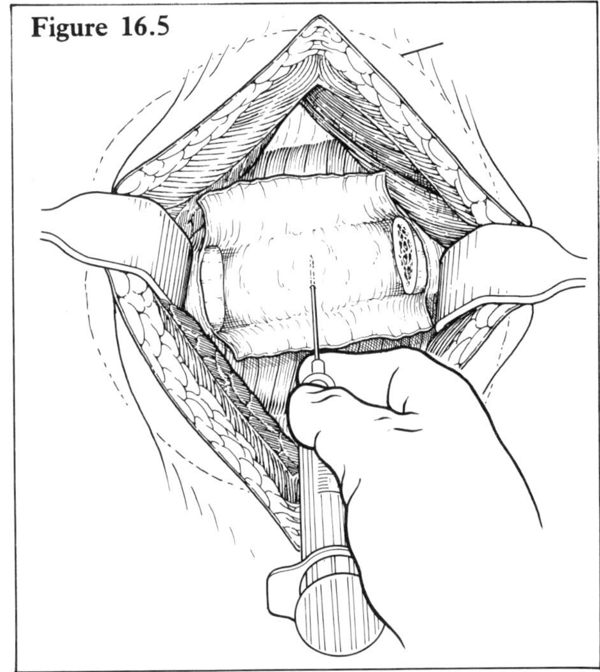
**Figure 16.5**

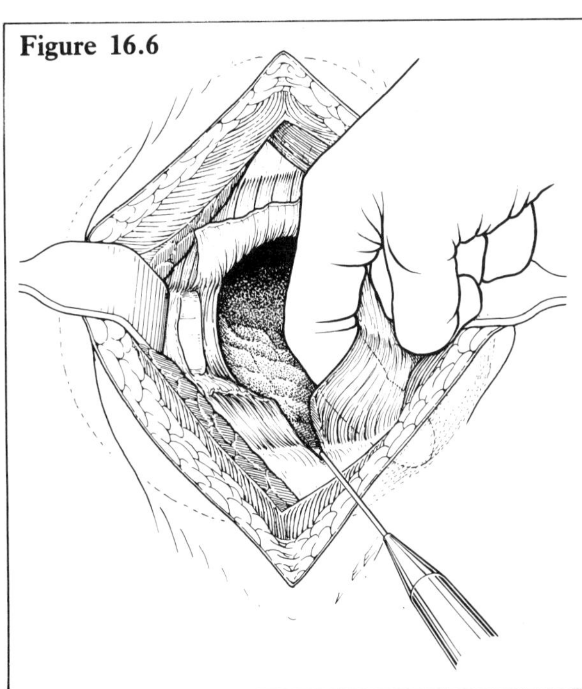
**Figure 16.6**

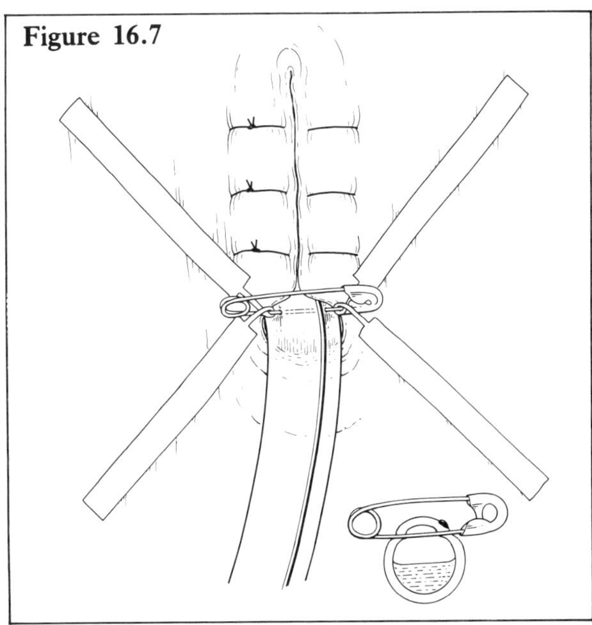
**Figure 16.7**

### Postoperative management

It is convenient to connect the tube to an underwater seal to which suction of 50–100 mmHg (7–13 kPa) is applied. This treatment continued for the first week ensures that most of the pus drains into the bottle and diminishes soiling around the wound. After this the tube can be cut short and allowed to drain into dressings.

PA and lateral chest radiographs are obtained the day after operation to ensure that the tube is correctly sited, with an appropriate length inside the chest so that fluid cannot collect below it. During healing the rise of the diaphragm may necessitate increasing the length of the tube inside the cavity.

The tube is changed at six-weekly intervals, and on these occasions a sinogram or pleurogram is carried out. When the pleural cavity has been reduced to the size of the tube track, the tube is replaced by a much smaller one, which is then gradually withdrawn over the course of some weeks.

## Treatment of empyema by cyclical irrigation

Frequently it is possible to treat an established empyema by a system of cyclical irrigation. The indication for this treatment is an empyema that has been present for at least one week and whose resolution is unlikely because the pleura is thickened.

### Procedure

Initially two intercostal tube drains are inserted under local anaesthesia. One tube is positioned at the apex of the cavity for the instillation of the irrigation fluid. The other is placed at the most dependent part of the space to act as a drain. If there are many adhesions these may be broken down with the aid of a thoracoscope. At that time the pus may be aspirated and the pleural space irrigated with normal saline. This procedure will require a general anaesthetic (see section on thoracoscopy, p. 10).

On return to the ward a solution of normal saline is instilled through the superior drain. During the inflow phase the basal drain is elevated to shoulder level to create a safety valve, thus ensuring the complete filling of the space and at the same time preventing the generation of high pressure which could result in air embolism. No benefit is achieved by using antiseptics or antibiotics for the irrigation.

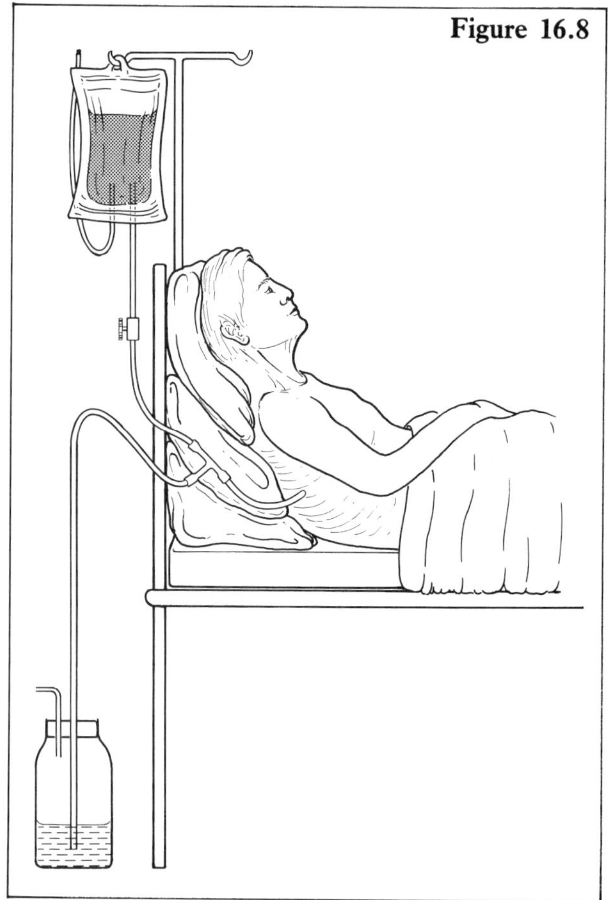

**Figure 16.8**

The system may be simplified using a single drain connected by a 'Y' connector to both the irrigation set and the drainage bottle (**Fig. 16.8**).

Irrigation is done in four-hourly cycles. The fluid (200 to 500 ml) is run into the cavity and retained for three hours. It is then allowed to drain for the remaining hour using suction. If the patient has a fever, a course of appropriate antibiotics is given.

Samples of the drain effluent are sent daily for culture. Irrigation is continued for 5 to 10 days until the draining fluid becomes clear and sterile. On completion of the irrigation period the space is filled with the appropriate volume of normal saline containing a combination of antibiotics to which the organisms are sensitive, the tubes are withdrawn and their sites sutured.

The occasional recurrence following this technique necessitates decortication (see p. 135).

# 17 Cervicothoracic sympathectomy

## Indications

Cervicothoracic sympathectomy is indicated for:

1. Hyperhidrosis of the hands.
2. Advanced cases of Raynaud's phenomenon (its value is limited with this disease because of a 50 per cent recurrence rate within one to two years).

## Procedure

The two sides may be treated by separate thoracotomies in one session, or on separate occasions.

A double lumen endotracheal tube is used so that the lung on the affected side can be deflated when the pleural cavity has been opened. The approach is via an axillary thoracotomy (p. 38) through the bed of the third or fourth rib. After a rib spreader has been inserted, the apex of the lung is depressed with the aid of a malleable spatula or a mounted swab.

The sympathetic chain is seen lying on the heads of the ribs beneath the parietal pleura. This is incised vertically over it, from the fourth rib to the apex. The sympathetic chain is picked up with a nerve hook. Most of the dissection can be carried out with this instrument (**Fig. 17.1**). The dissection should begin at the level of the head of the fourth

**Figure 17.1**

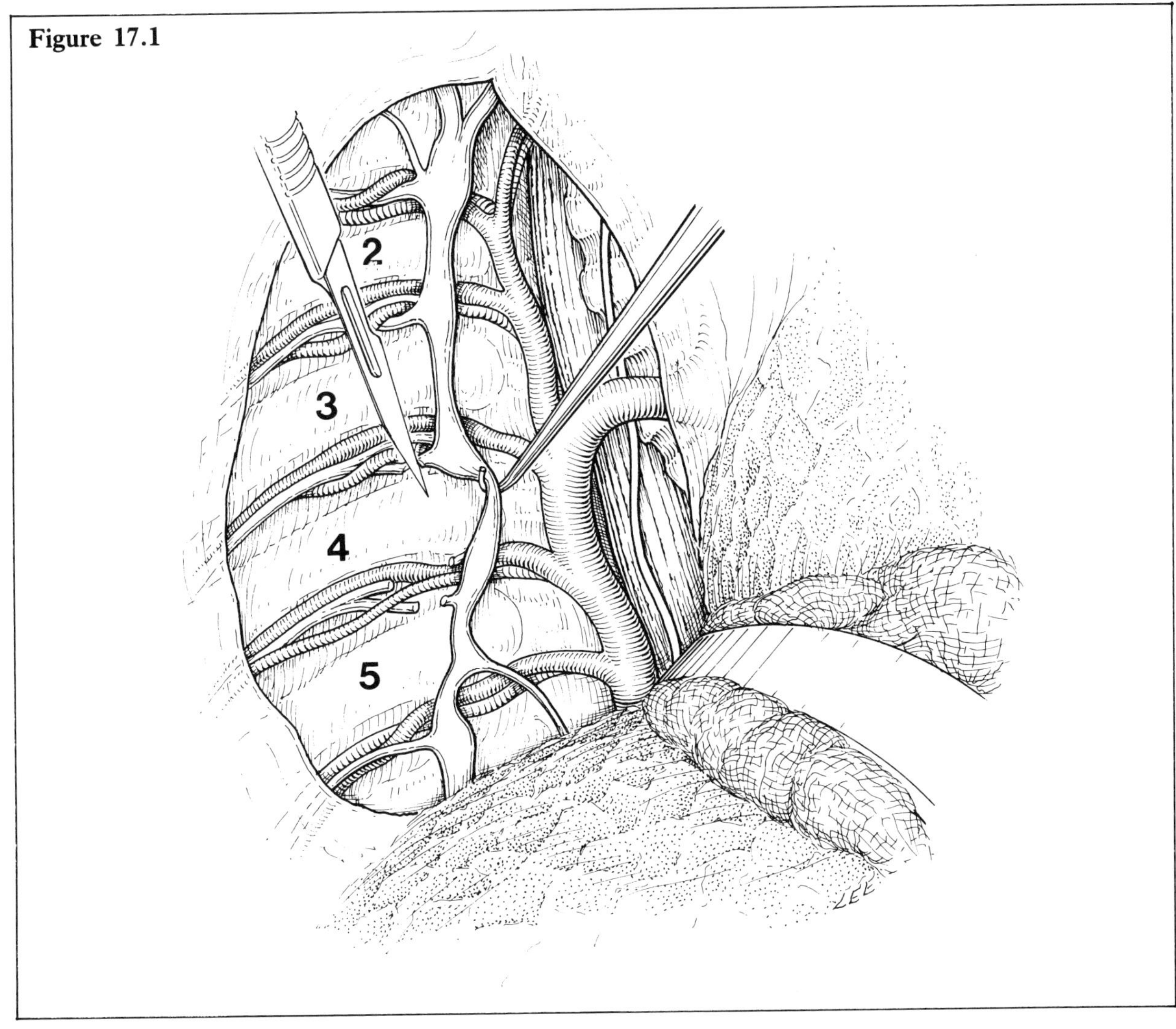

rib and proceed in a cephalad direction. The two rami communicantes connecting each ganglion to the corresponding intercostal nerve can then be seen and cut. The chain should not be divided at this stage as it is more apparent if left intact. Most of the intercostal arteries and veins lie deep to the chain, but a few branches lie in front of it. These can be secured with diathermy or the chain slipped from beneath them after it has been divided. As the dissection proceeds upwards the first rib is identified, and the stellate ganglion is seen overlying its head. The ganglion is recognized by an expansion in the chain, its sides diverging to form a 'V'.

The chain is divided at the level of the fourth rib and gentle traction exerted on it with a haemostat (**Fig. 17.2**). The upper line of division is where the expanded chain again becomes parallel, i.e. at the upper limit of the 'V' (**Fig. 17.2**, inset). This technique removes only the lower third of the stellate ganglion and obviates the risk of producing Horner's syndrome. The small amount of bleeding that occurs when the chain is divided should be controlled by pressure rather than by diathermy for the same reason.

A size 20 Argyle catheter is passed into the pleural cavity as a drain, the lung is re-expanded and the incision closed.

**Figure 17.2**

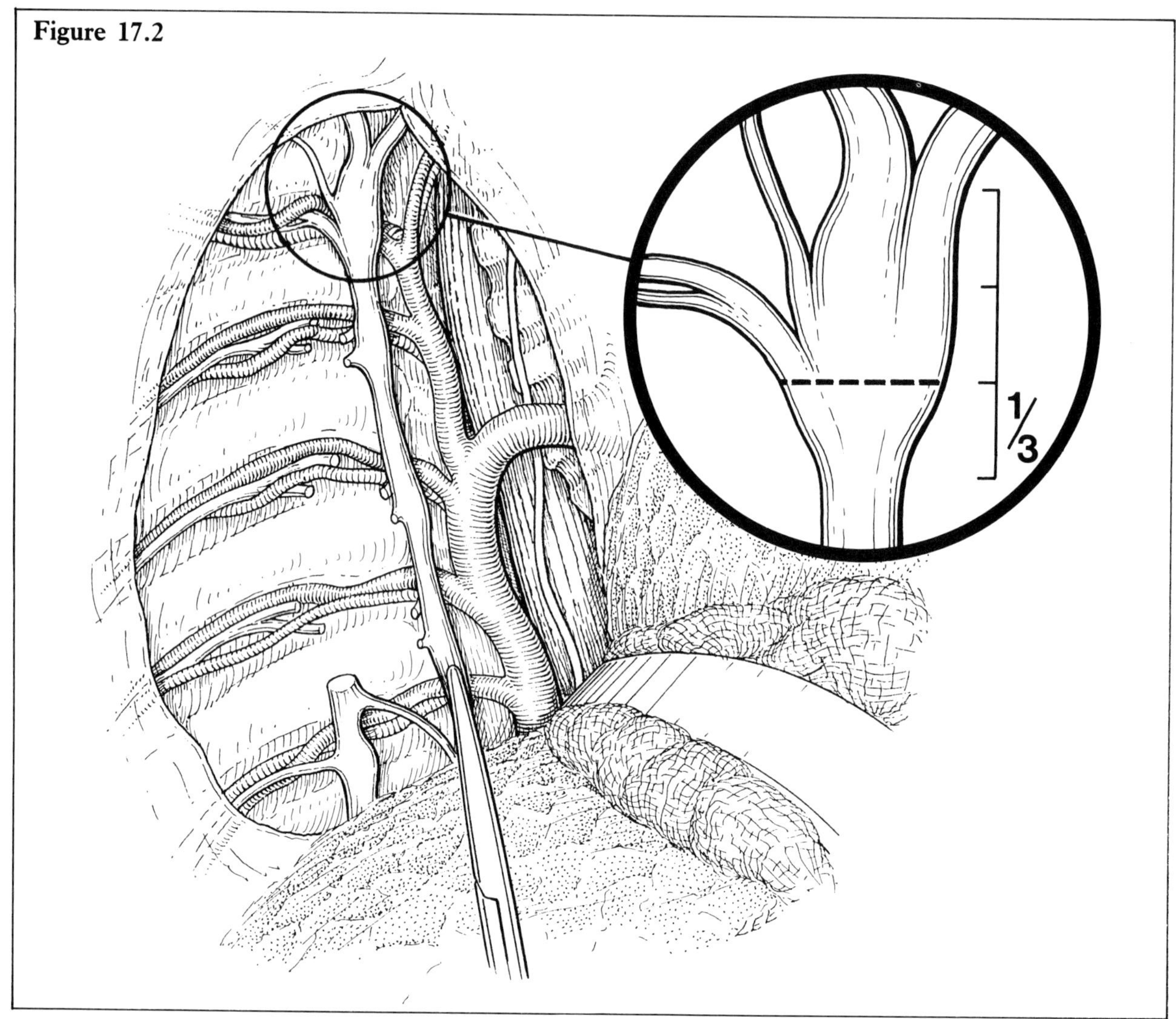

SECTION 4

# SURGERY OF THE TRACHEA

# 18 Surgical anatomy of the trachea

The trachea begins below the larynx at the level of the sixth cervical vertebra. It ends at the level of the sternal angle, where it bifurcates to form the right and left main bronchi. It is 'U'-shaped in cross-section, being supported anteriorly and laterally by the cartilaginous tracheal rings. Posteriorly it is flat; this is the membranous part. Smooth muscle fibres are found within the fibrous membrane. Contraction of the transversely orientated fibres can reduce the diameter of the trachea.

The cervical portion is quite superficial, being separated from the skin by the strap muscles of the neck and the isthmus of the thyroid gland. Lying behind the trachea and in the tracheo-oesophageal grooves are the recurrent laryngeal nerves. The right-sided nerve joins the trachea after looping around the right subclavian artery. The left-sided nerve joins the trachea after looping around the ligamentum arteriosum in the mediastinum (**Fig. 18.1**). The blood supply of the trachea is via a series of end-arteries, segmentally distributed, (**Figs. 18.2, 18.3**).

**Figure 18.1**

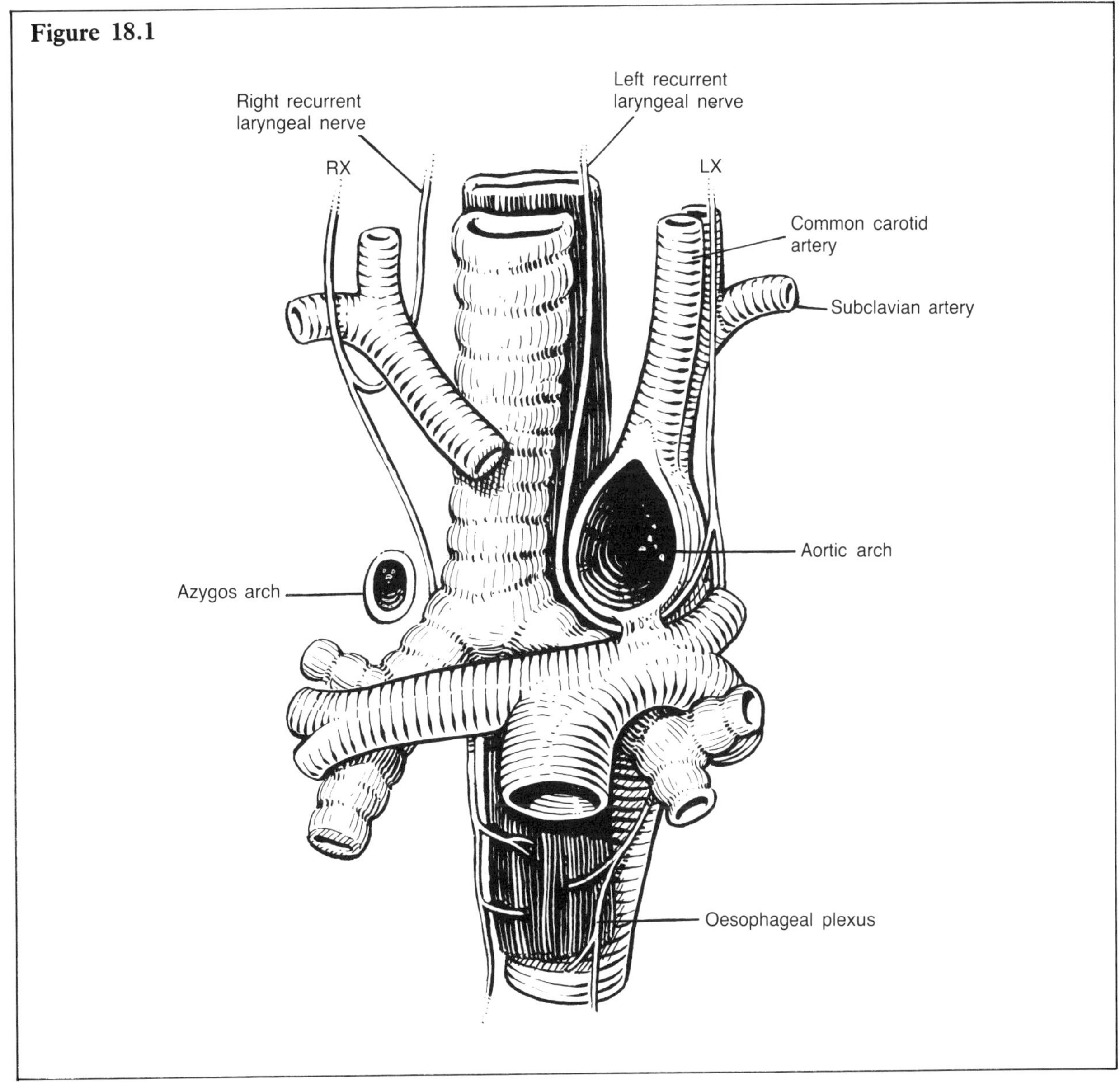

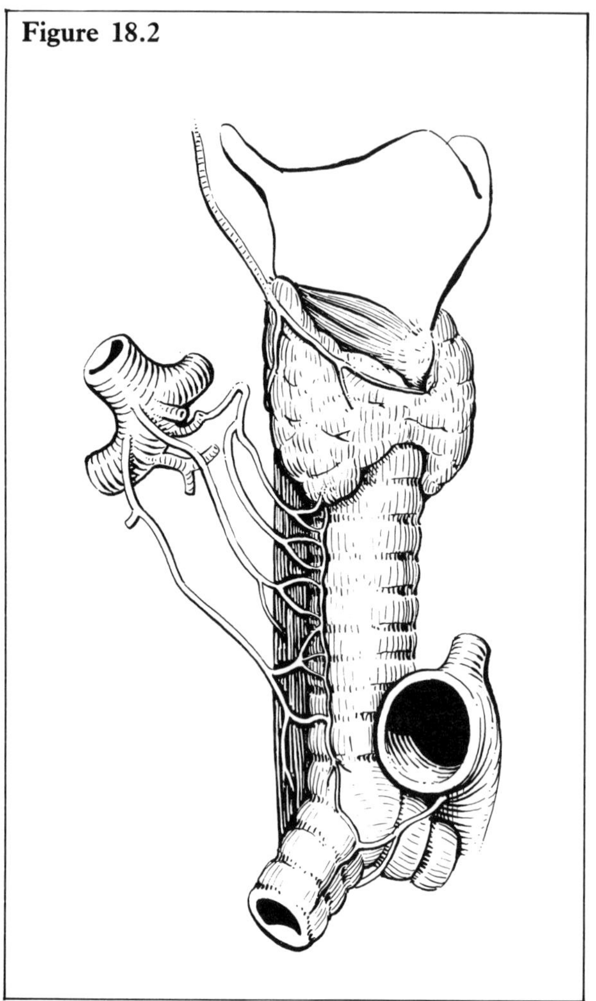
Figure 18.2

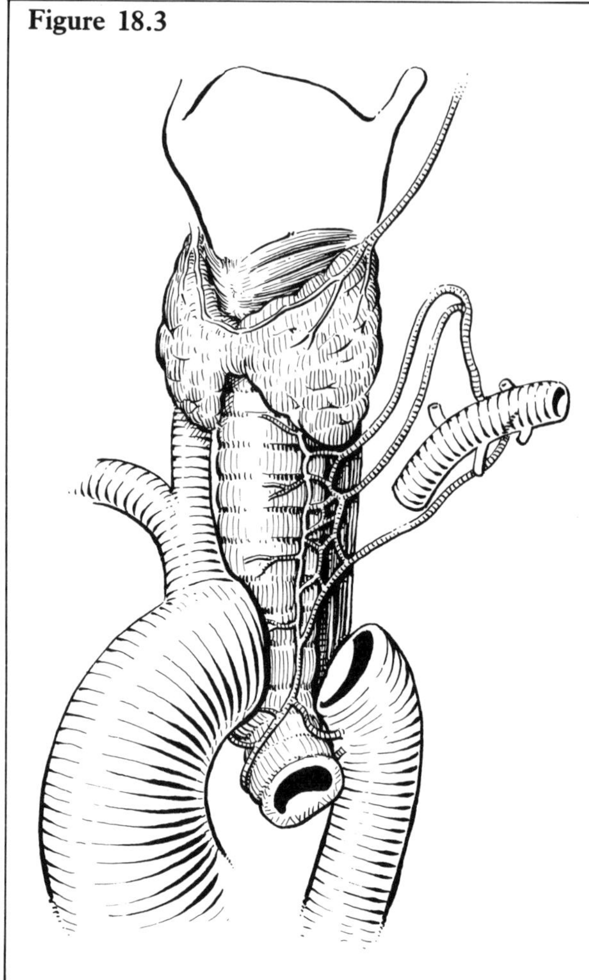
Figure 18.3

The trachea occupies a central position until it reaches the level of the aortic arch, where it is deviated to the right by that structure. Partially encircling the trachea just below the thoracic inlet are the great vessels arising from the aortic arch. Lying anteriorly and to the right of the trachea is the superior vena cava. Crossing the trachea just above the right main bronchus to join the superior vena cava is the azygos vein. On the right side the vagus nerve crosses the mid-portion of the trachea from anterior to posterior. It is both vulnerable and available for division through the mediastinoscope at this point.

Posterior to the trachea throughout its length is the oesophagus.

# 19 Tracheostomy

With improvements in endotracheal tubes, the need for early tracheostomy has diminished significantly. The low-pressure cuffed tubes currently available may be safely left *in situ* for up to two weeks.

The creation of a tracheostomy must be conducted with care and with great attention to detail. It should preferably be carried out under a general anaesthetic in an operating theatre with full aseptic precautions.

## Indications

1. Prolonged positive pressure ventilation beyond two weeks.
2. A large flail segment of chest wall following chest trauma, especially if in association with decreased lung compliance.
3. Severe head injury.

A common indication in the past was for persistent secretions that were difficult to clear, often necessitating repeated bronchoscopy for aspiration. Now it is usually possible to gain adequate control of this problem with a mini-tracheostomy tube (see p. 12).

## Procedure

The patient is anaesthetized, intubated and positioned supine on the operating table with the shoulders elevated on a pad to extend the neck; this thrusts the trachea closer to the skin in the neck. Care must be taken, however, not to over-extend the neck which might result in placing the tracheal opening too low. The head is stabilized with a rubber ring placed under the occiput.

A 25 mm transverse skin incision is made midway between the sternal notch and the cricoid cartilage between the medial borders of the sternocleidomastoid muscles (**Fig. 19.1**). This is deepened through the platysma muscle and fascial layers to the strap muscles, which are separated in the

**Figure 19.1**

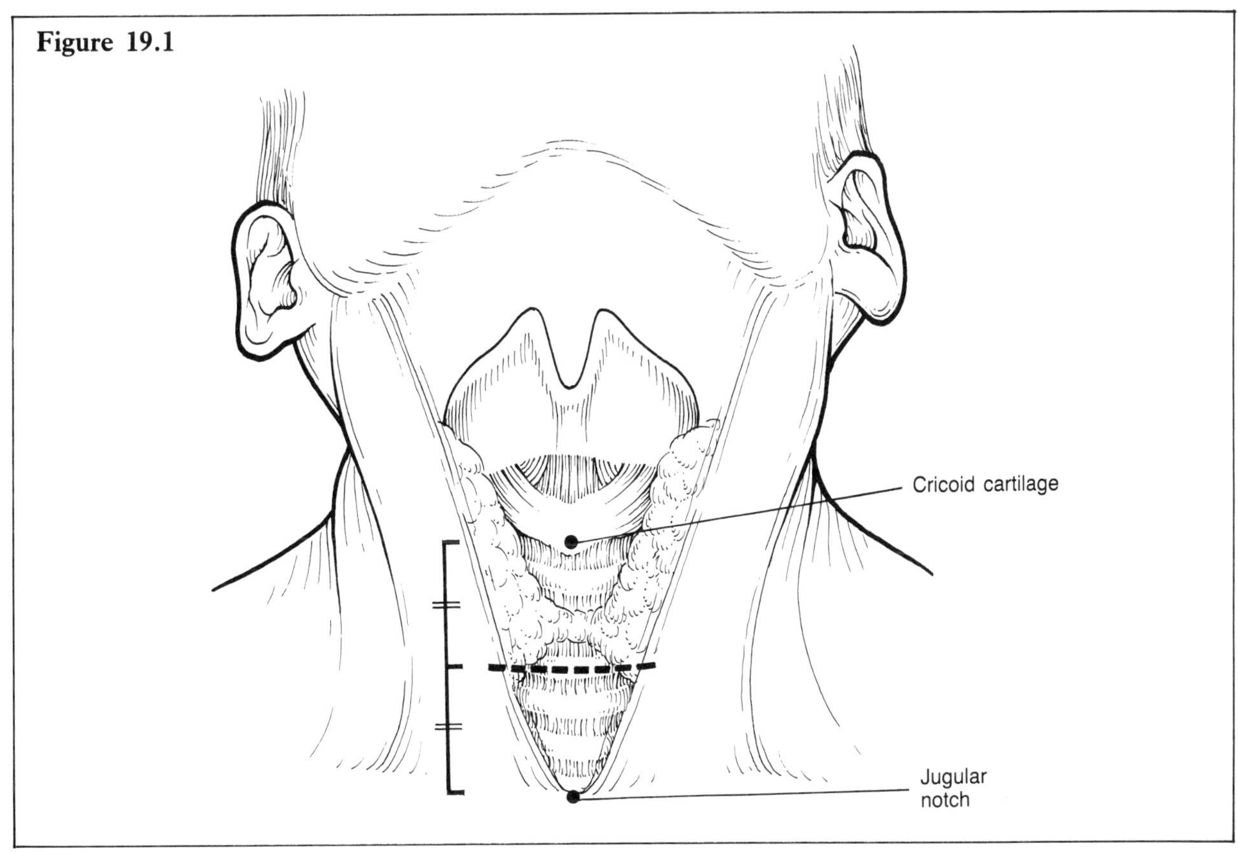

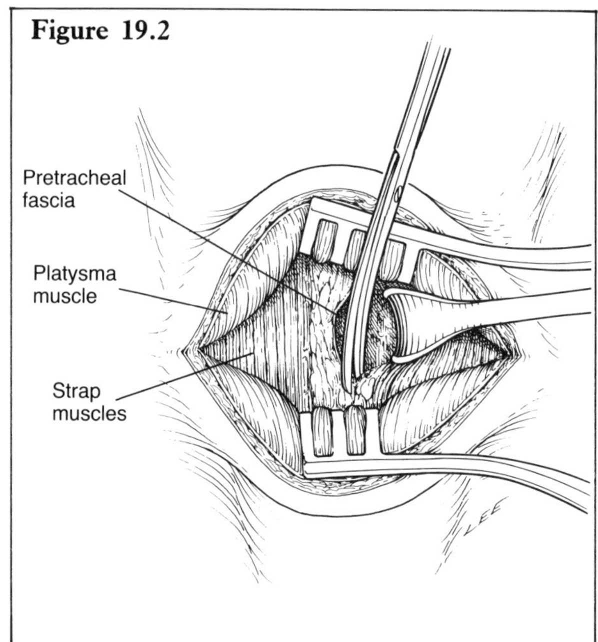


**Figure 19.2**

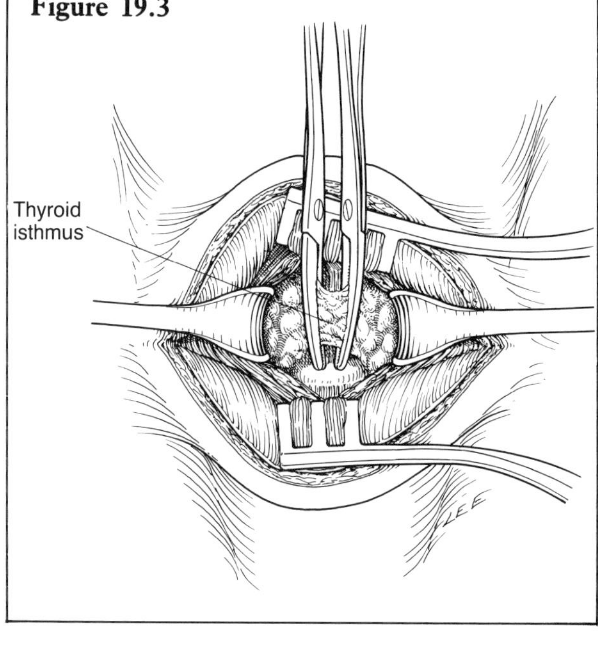


**Figure 19.3**

midline, exposing the pretracheal fascia (**Fig. 19.2**). The isthmus of the thyroid gland may be encountered at this point in some patients (**Fig. 19.3**); if this is so, it will be necessary to divide the isthmus in the midline between short artery clamps. The ends are then oversewn with an absorbable suture. The inferior thyroid veins may also need division and ligation. Before opening the trachea, complete haemostasis should be obtained.

The appropriate size of tracheostomy tube is chosen and all the connections must be checked. All the air in the tube cuff is aspirated and the outside well lubricated ready for insertion. When the surgeon is ready to open the trachea, the anaesthetist is asked to deflate the cuff on the endotracheal tube and withdraw it to a level just above the proposed incision.

**Figure 19.4**

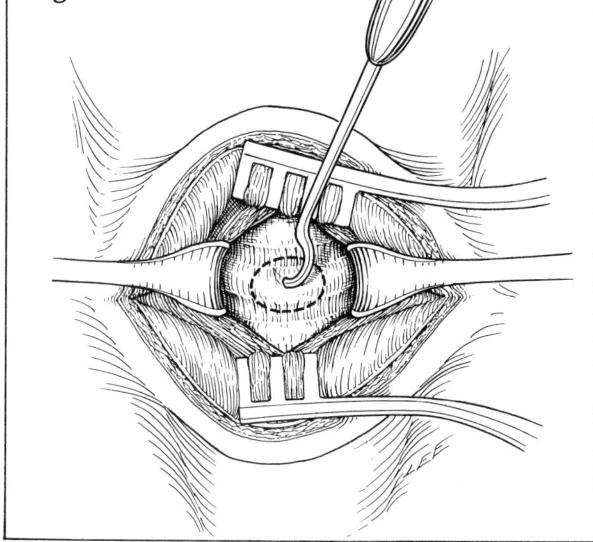

### Stoma creation in the adult

A sharp tracheal hook is inserted into the anterior surface of the trachea at the level of the second tracheal ring (**Fig. 19.4**). The first ring must never be interfered with as this may result in subglottic stenosis. An oval section of trachea large enough to allow the insertion of the tracheostomy tube is then resected using a knife (**Fig. 19.5**). The incised edges of the trachea are gently cauterized to gain haemostasis. The tracheostomy tube is then inserted (**Fig. 19.6**), the obturator removed, the cuff inflated to the minimal occluding volume, and the connections made to the ventilator tubing. The skin on either side of the tracheostoma is then closed with interrupted non-absorbable sutures. The restraining ribbons are passed through the flanges on either side of the tracheostomy tube and secured around the patient's neck, snugly but not tightly.

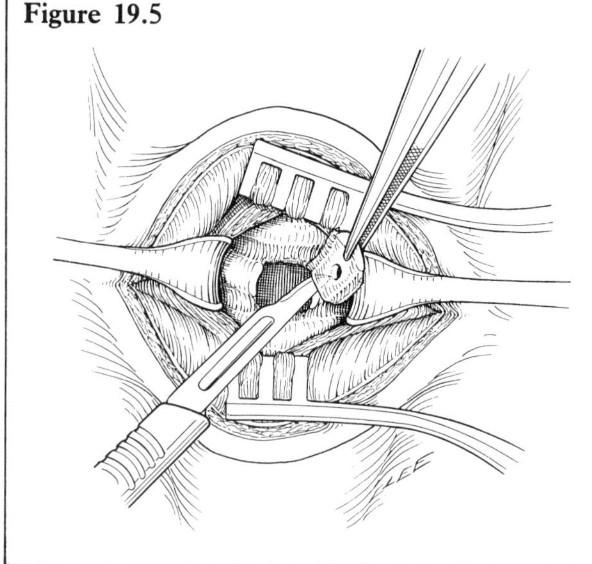

**Figure 19.5**

**Figure 19.6**

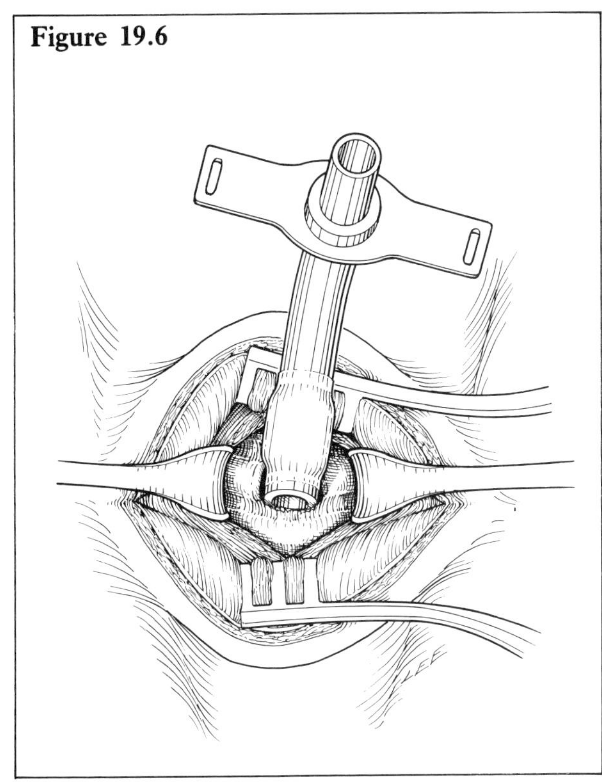

### Stoma creation in a child

In children under 12 years old the procedure is the same except that no section of the trachea is removed. All that is required is a vertical incision in the midline long enough to allow the insertion of the tracheostomy tube. To facilitate the insertion of the tube a stay suture is placed on either side of the proposed incision to allow traction.

## Postoperative care

The patient should be nursed in an intensive care unit and constantly supervised. Aspiration of bronchial secretions is performed as frequently as necessary to maintain a clear airway. Aspiration should be done by a nurse wearing disposable gloves using a sterile suction catheter. The inspired gases should be humidified to minimize the desiccation of secretions, which may block the tubing and coat the wound edge.

## Complications

### Dislodgement of the tube

If the tube is not properly secured, or if the anaesthetic tubing is allowed to drag, the tube may be dislodged. Tracheostomy retractors should be kept at the bedside constantly for speedy reinsertion should the tube fall from the trachea. Trauma to the tracheostoma and surrounding structures by constant pulling may result in catastrophic haemorrhage.

### Sepsis

The wound may become infected if the dressings surrounding it are not frequently changed and careful wound toilet carried out. Infection can result in secondary haemorrhage from the brachiocephalic artery, which is usually fatal.

### Obstruction of the tube

Obstruction may occur without dislodgement for various reasons. The tube may become blocked with hardened secretions, or the balloon cuff may prolapse over the end of the tube. Rarely, the tracheostomy tube may collapse due to overinflation of the cuff.

### Tracheal stenosis

Tracheal stenosis is a rare occurrence with the low-pressure cuffs that are now in universal use.

## Extubation

When the patient is able to support his or her own respiration, it is time to move towards extubation. As a first step the tube may be changed for another of the same size but with the cuff deflated. After one or two days this may be changed for a smaller tube for one or two more days, prior to removal of the tube altogether. The tracheostoma is then covered with a light, dry dressing. The stoma will close over the next three or four days. If the patient is making rapid progress, then the tracheostomy tube may be replaced by a silver speaking tube. This has an obturator which enables the patient to speak, while allowing endotracheal suction.

# 20 Specific tracheal resections

Tracheal resection is most commonly required for strictures following prolonged intubation or tracheostomy. These strictures may be situated at the site of a tracheostomy in the cervical trachea, or at the site of maximal compression by the cuff of an endotracheal tube in the mediastinum. The majority of them are short, from 2 to 4 cm in length, and therefore extensive mobilization of the trachea is not necessary.

A much less common indication for tracheal resection is tracheal tumour. These tumours are nearly all malignant, usually either squamous carcinomas or adenoid cystic carcinomas. As a result of local extension and lymph node involvement, squamous carcinomas are rarely suitable for surgical treatment. The adenoid cystic carcinoma is much more commonly localized and slow-growing. It may, however, be quite extensive and require resection of a considerable length of trachea, making reconstruction difficult.

### Preoperative investigation

When planning the operation and the appropriate incision, the upper and lower limits of the lesion must be identified. This can best be achieved by the study of oblique tomograms of the whole length of the trachea. When the stenosis is tight, contrast studies and endoscopy are dangerous procedures because they may worsen the degree of airway obstruction. The former should not be employed, and the latter should, if possible, be carried out only immediately prior to the operation.

Although in cases of tracheal tumour a histological diagnosis before operation is desirable, the bleeding caused by biopsy can be extremely hazardous. CT scanning of the neck and mediastinum will demonstrate any tumour extension beyond the confines of the trachea and enlargement of mediastinal lymph nodes which may be due to tumour infiltration. Squamous carcinomas that have not extended in this way should be treated by resection, so that biopsy becomes unnecessary.

When the resection is being performed for stricture, inflammation and ulceration of the tracheal mucosa make it difficult to distinguish between irreversibly damaged and viable trachea. To achieve maximal healing before the operation, it is advisable if possible to remove the tracheostomy tube and to allow the stoma to close. The airway can be maintained by intermittent dilatation of the stricture.

## Resection of the upper trachea for stricture

A cervical incision will permit adequate access to the whole of the cervical trachea and the upper two-thirds of the mediastinal trachea.

The patient lies supine, with the neck extended and a pillow between the shoulders. The incision is made in a skin crease 4 cm above the suprasternal notch from the posterior border of one sternomastoid muscle to that of the other. If there is a tracheostomy, the opening is included in the incision and excised. The platysma is divided throughout the length of the incision and skin flaps elevated upwards and downwards. The upper limit of the dissection is the thyroid cartilage; the lower limit is the suprasternal notch. The sternohyoid and sternothyroid muscles are separated in the midline and retracted laterally, exposing the thyroid gland. A right-angled forceps is passed between

**Figure 20.1**

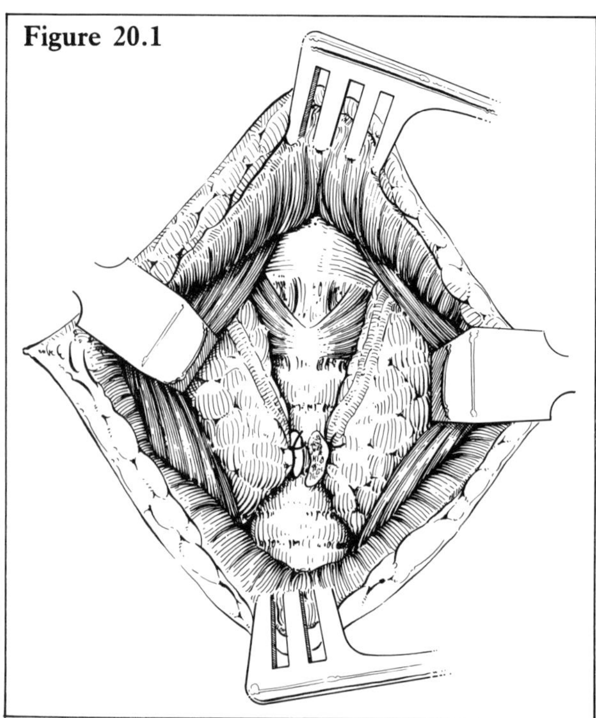

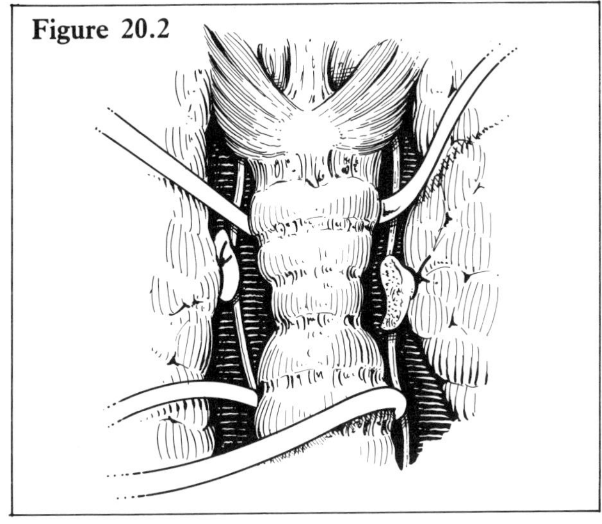
Figure 20.2

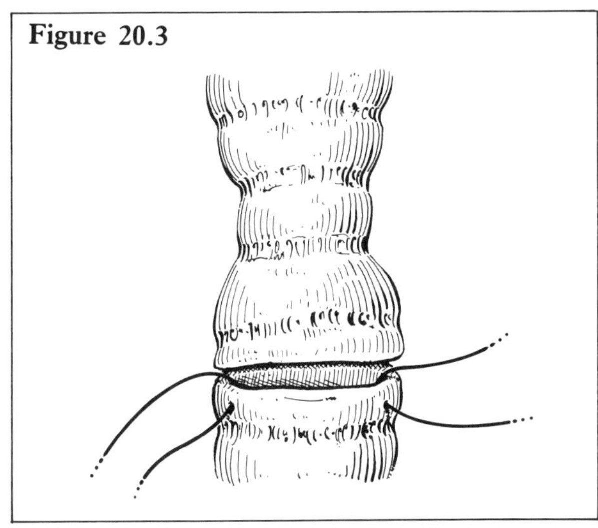
Figure 20.3

the isthmus of the thyroid gland and the trachea, and the isthmus divided between clamps (**Fig. 20.1**).

In cases of benign stricture the region of narrowing is now identified. There is usually extensive fibrosis outside the trachea in the region of the stricture. However, the dissection must keep close to the tracheal wall in order to avoid damage to the recurrent laryngeal nerves in the tracheo-oesophageal angles.

The easiest course is to mobilize the whole circumference of the trachea immediately above and below the stricture, first freeing it from the oesophagus posteriorly. This mobilization should not extend more than 1 cm beyond each end of the stricture because of the danger of damaging the tracheal blood supply, which is segmental and enters the trachea at its posterolateral angles. Tapes are passed round the trachea above and below the stricture, which can then be freed by sharp dissection (**Fig. 20.2**).

The trachea is divided immediately below the stricture. The incision must be through undamaged tracheal wall, because if there is fibrosis at this level the stricture will recur. It may be necessary to excise additional segments until healthy tracheal wall is encountered. As the division is made a series of stay sutures are placed in the cut edge of the lower trachea to prevent it from retracting (**Fig. 20.3**).

When this division has been completed, a sterile endotracheal tube is inserted into the lower trachea and connected across the operation field to the anaesthetic apparatus (**Fig. 20.4**).

The stricture is now elevated and any remaining posterior attachments to the oesophagus divided under direct vision. The trachea is divided above the stricture, again taking care to ensure that healthy tissue has been reached, and a series of stay sutures is placed in the divided upper margin (**Fig. 20.5**).

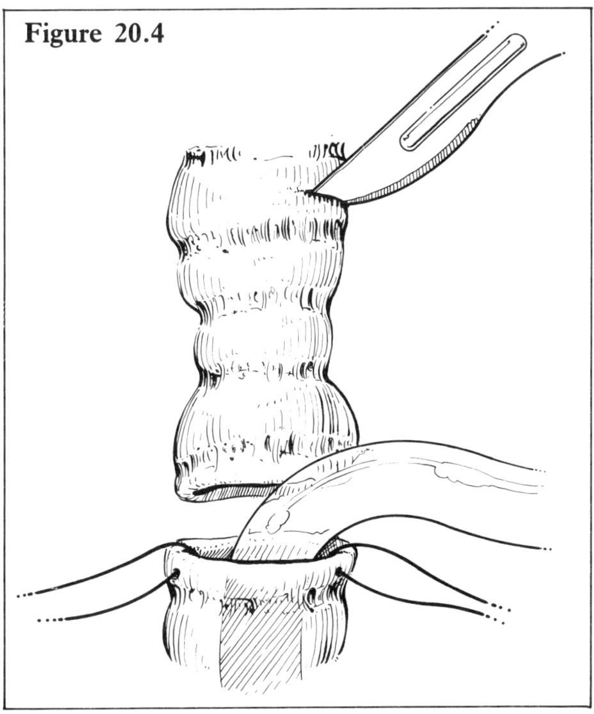
Figure 20.4

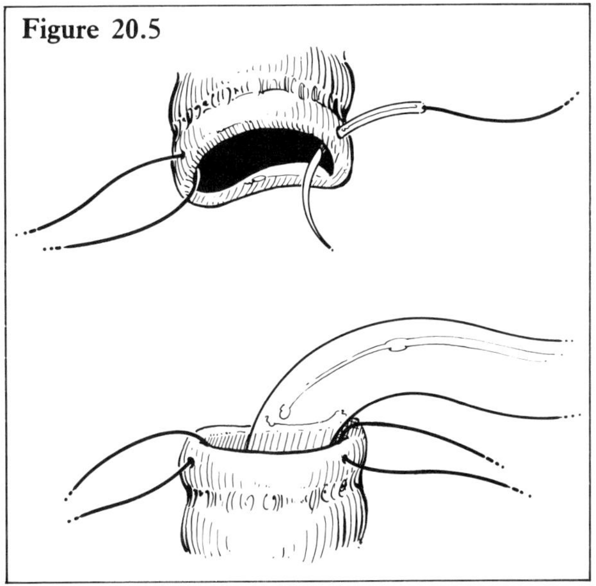
Figure 20.5

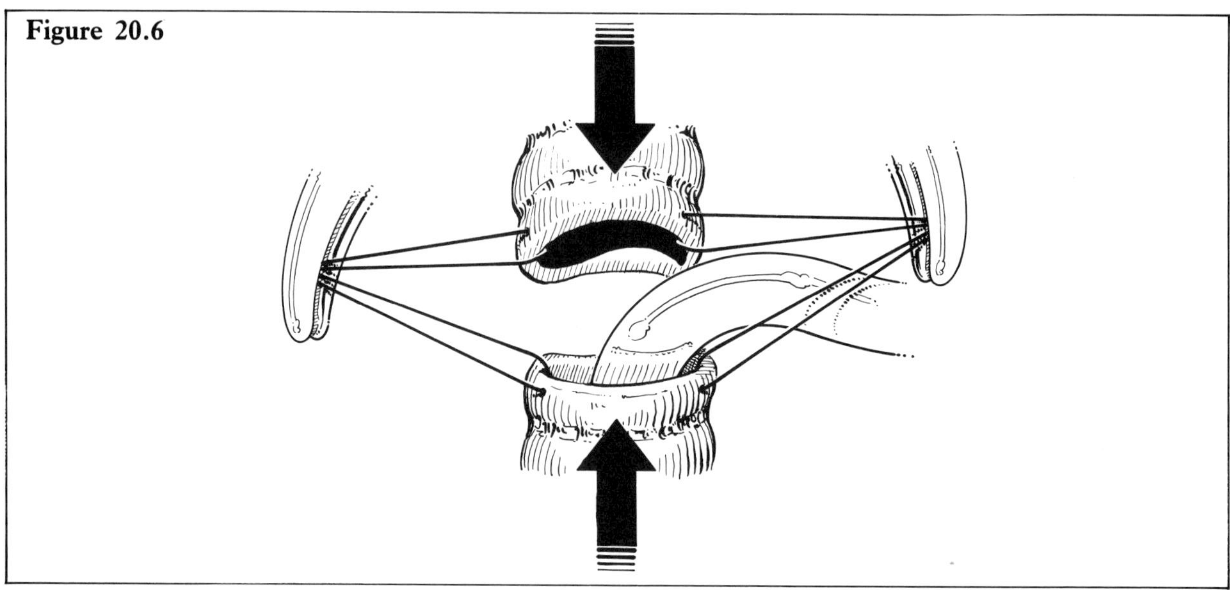
Figure 20.6

Sometimes the location of the stricture cannot be determined from external inspection. The anaesthetist should then replace the endotracheal tube by a bronchoscope, to ascertain the level of the stricture. With the theatre darkened, the bronchoscope light can be clearly seen through the tracheal wall. The proximal end of the stricture is thus identified.

The neck is now flexed and the traction sutures approximated to determine whether the ends of the trachea can be brought together without tension (**Fig. 20.6**). If so (and this can always be achieved if the segment resected is no longer than 3 cm), the anastomosis proceeds. If not, further mobilization of the trachea must be carried out. The anterior and anterolateral walls of the trachea are freed by blunt dissection from the cricoid cartilage above to the bifurcation of the trachea below. The posterior surface can also be mobilized by separating the membranous wall from the oesophagus, but the posterolateral vascular attachments must be left intact. This mobilization, together with flexion of the neck, will allow resection of 6 cm of trachea, which is adequate for almost all cases of benign stricture.

If approximation with the traction sutures shows that the anastomosis can be made without undue tension, the neck is extended a little to allow separation of the two ends of the trachea, and a row of interrupted fine sutures is placed in the membranous wall but not tied. In our opinion the best suture materials are polygalactin (Vicryl) 4/0, the knots of which may be placed on the outside of the trachea, or fine wire, which may be tied with the knots inside the trachea. Interrupted sutures of 4/0 polypropylene may also be used, but continuous non-absorbable suture material is not advisable because it may ulcerate into the lumen and cause granuloma formation and obstruction.

All the sutures of the posterior row are inserted, and then traction is applied to the stay sutures to approximate the two ends of the trachea while the sutures are tied (**Fig. 20.7**).

The endotracheal tube passed into the lower trachea is now removed and a suitably sized tube passed from the upper trachea across the gap into the lower trachea. Anaesthesia is continued via this tube. The anterior and lateral walls of the trachea

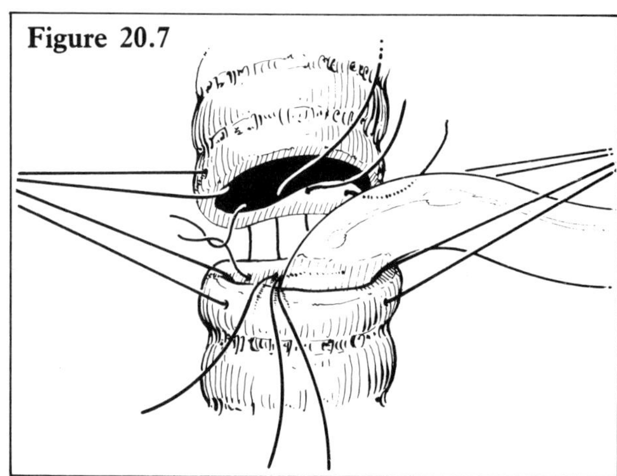
Figure 20.7

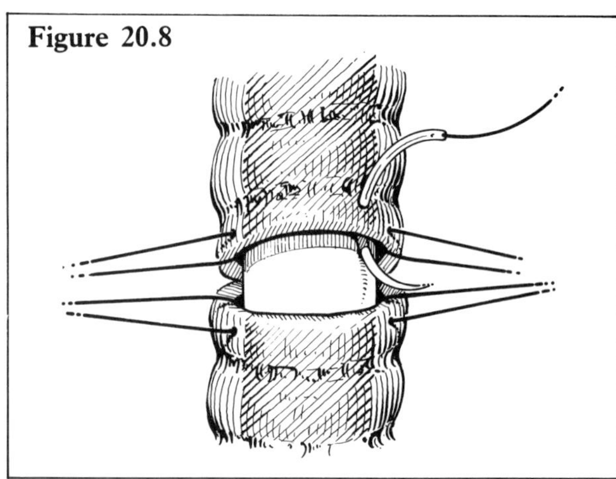
Figure 20.8

are now anastomosed with similar interrupted sutures (**Fig. 20.8**). It is usually possible to place these without difficulty with the endotracheal tube in position. However, if difficulty is encountered the tube may be withdrawn into the upper trachea and ventilation suspended for a minute or so at a time.

The remaining wire sutures are tied and the traction sutures relaxed and removed. There should be minimal tension on the anastomosis. Meticulous haemostasis must be achieved. The sternohyoid and sternothyroid muscles are sutured together in the midline and the platysma and skin closed with interrupted non-absorbable sutures (**Fig. 20.9**) or skin clips.

Tracheostomy must be avoided at all costs. Indeed the endotracheal tube should be removed at the end of the operation and the patient allowed to breathe spontaneously.

Flexion of the neck is maintained by a suture between the skin of the chin and the upper chest. This prevents extension of the neck, but it should be appreciated that it also impairs the efficiency of coughing. Where the tracheal resection has been short this step may be omitted. The suture is removed after two weeks.

## Resection of the upper trachea for tumour

The procedure is similar to that described for stricture. The collar incision can be combined with a median sternotomy, which allows a more extensive mobilization of the lower trachea and carina. The brachiocephalic vein is retracted or divided, and the brachiocephalic and left common carotid arteries and the arch of the aorta are freed from the trachea by blunt dissection.

The trachea is divided 1 cm beyond the macroscopic limit of tumour at each end. The line of division should be immediately examined by frozen section to ensure the limits of the tumour have been reached.

**Figure 20.9**

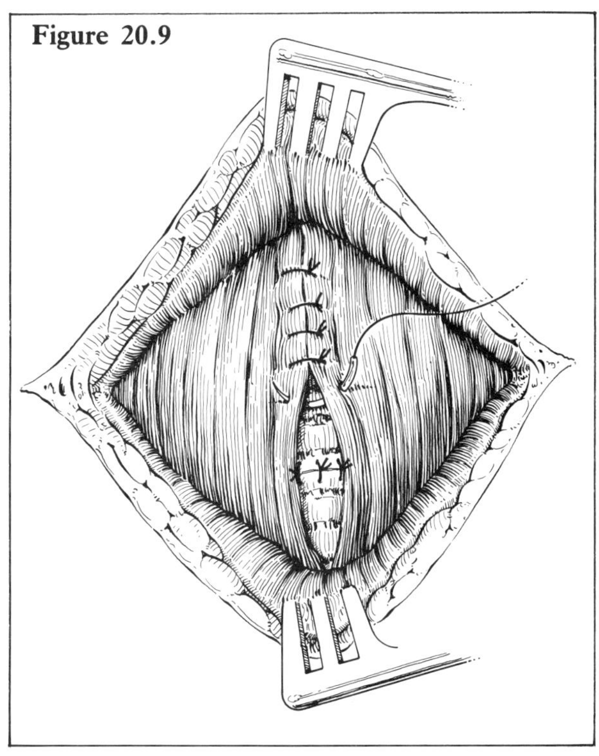

The mobilization of the trachea is completed. The neck is now flexed and the traction sutures approximated. If the two ends of the trachea cannot be united without undue tension, the suprahyoid release operation described below is to be preferred to the laryngeal drop technique, since the former is less frequently followed by dysphagia.

### Suprahyoid release procedure

The skin incision is carried to the angle of the jaw, so that a skin flap containing the platysma can be elevated above the level of the hyoid bone. The muscles attached to the upper part of the body of the hyoid bone are transected. This incision begins in the midline, but stops on either side at the point of attachment of the digastric muscle sling. Laterally the insertion of the stylohyoid is divided (**Fig. 20.10**). The muscles divided from front to

**Figure 20.10**

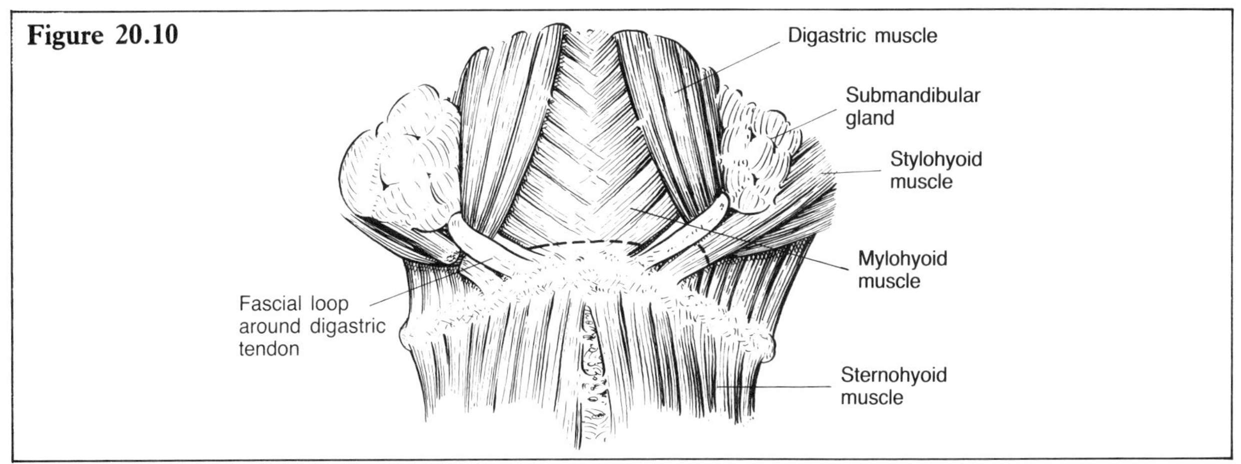

Figure 20.11

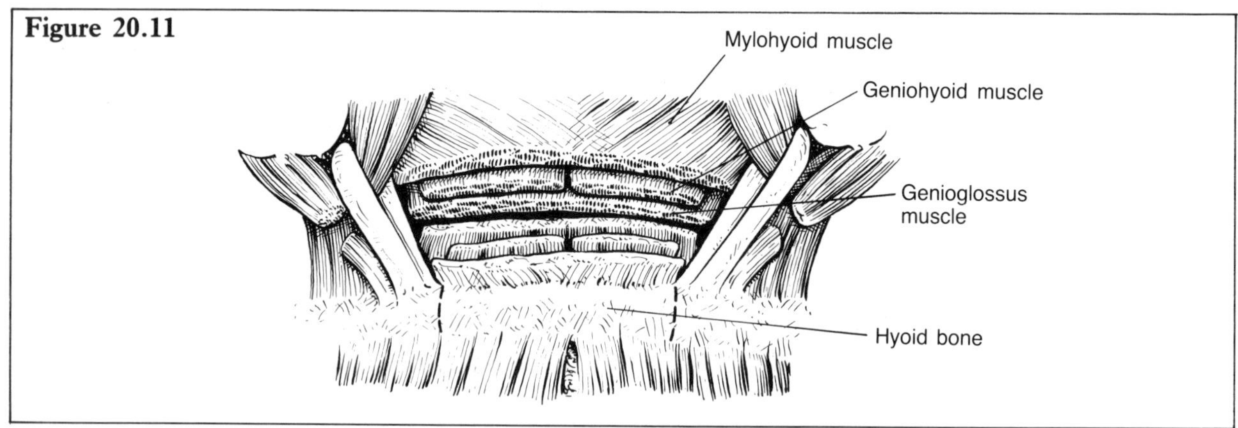


back are the mylohyoid, geniohyoid and genioglossus muscles.

Next the cornu of the hyoid bone is transected (**Fig. 20.11**). This releases the chondroglossus muscle and some of the fibres of the middle constrictor.

Finally the body of the hyoid bone is sectioned at either end, at the origin of the greater cornua, just in front of the digastric attachments (**Fig. 20.12**). This allows considerable drop of the body of the hyoid bone, and hence the hyoid cartilage.

Figure 20.12

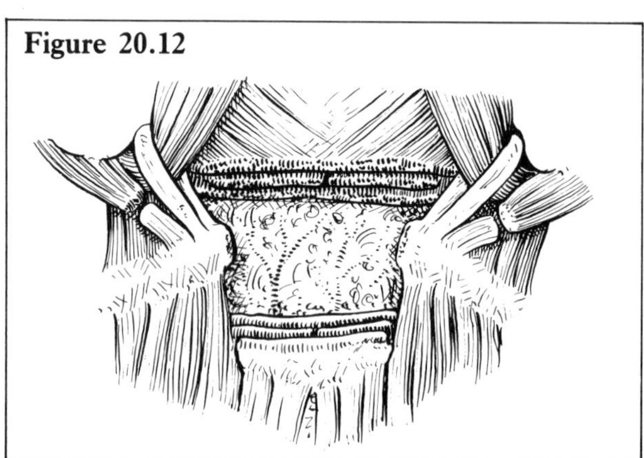

## Resection of the lower trachea

Resection of the lower trachea is usually performed for tumours.

The incision is a right posterolateral thoracotomy, stripping the lower border of the fourth or fifth rib to enter the pleural cavity. The right lung is deflated. If there is severe airway obstruction this may not be possible and then satisfactory ventilation of the left lung must be established immediately.

The right lung is retracted forward and the pleura incised immediately in front of the vagus nerve over the right main bronchus and trachea up to the apex of the chest. The azygos vein is divided between ligatures (**Fig. 20.13**). The right

Figure 20.13

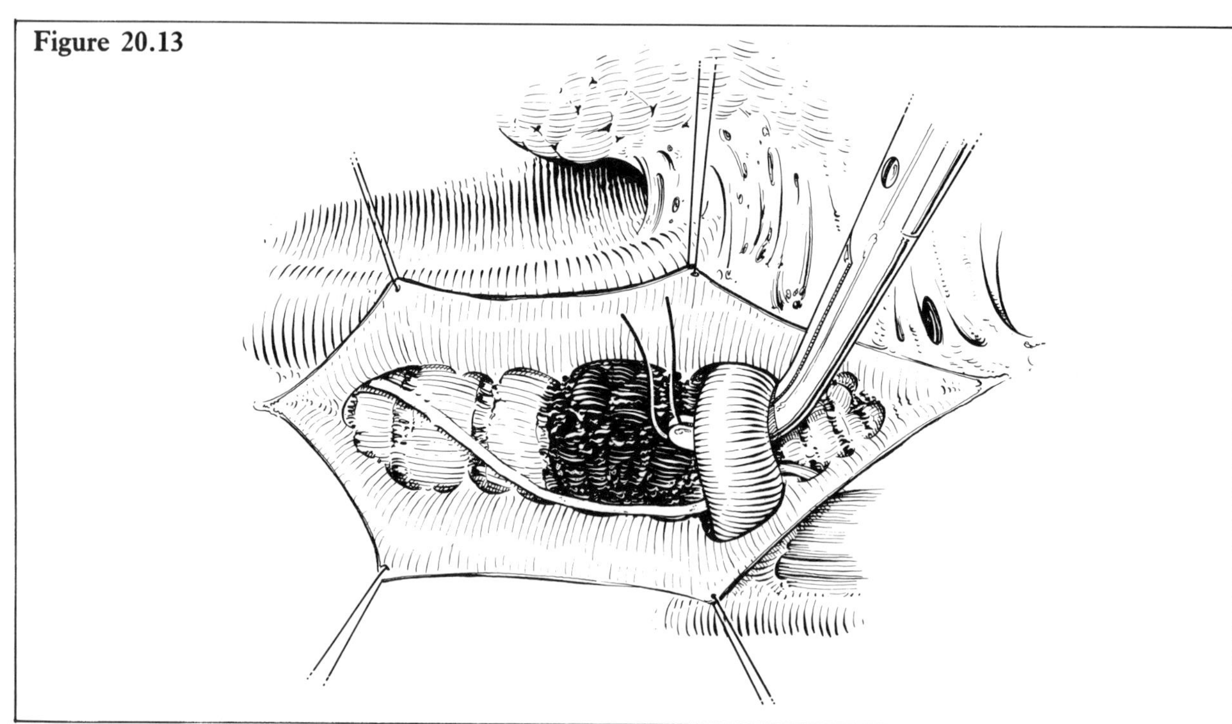

main bronchus is dissected out and a tape passed round it. The lower end of the trachea is similarly mobilized and surrounded by a tape. With traction on these two tapes the left main bronchus comes into view and can be mobilized (**Fig. 20.14**). The trachea is now divided below the tumour and ventilation continued by an endobronchial tube passed across the operation field into the left main bronchus (**Fig. 20.15**).

The trachea is mobilized throughout its length, but the lateral vascular attachments are preserved (**Fig. 20.16**). The trachea is then divided above the tumour (**Fig. 20.17**).

To obtain maximum mobilization of the carina, the right pulmonary ligament is divided, and the right and left main bronchi are mobilized as far as

**Figure 20.14**

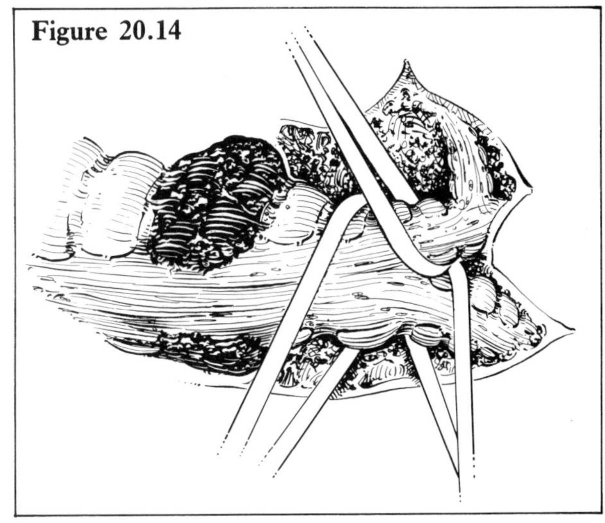

**Figure 20.15**

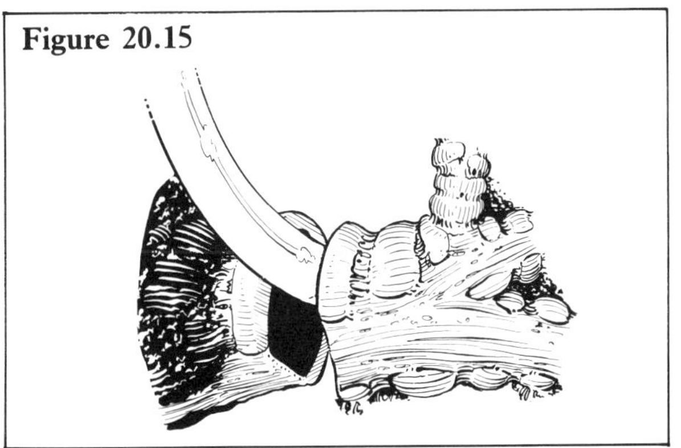

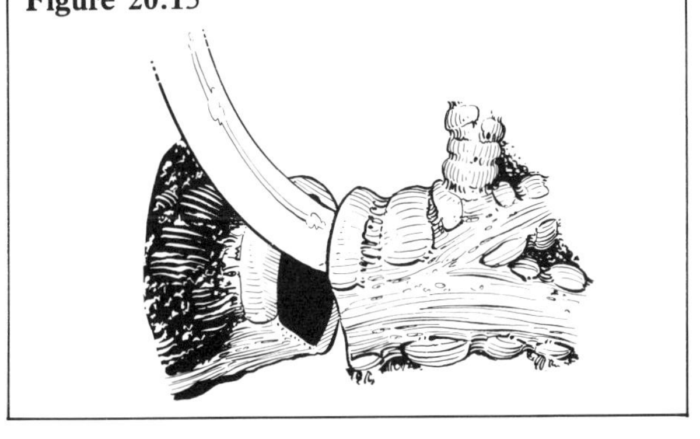

**Figure 20.16**

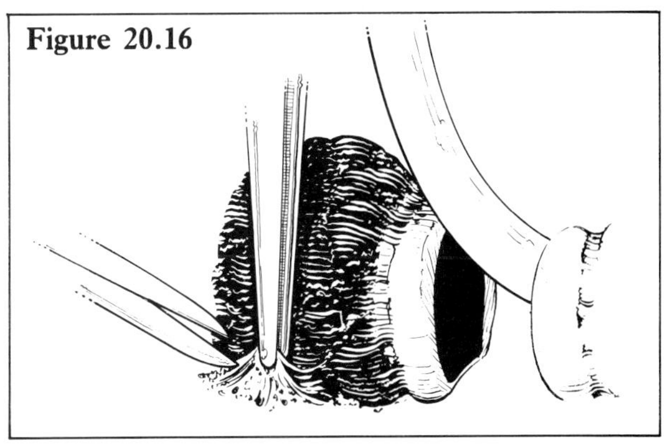

**Figure 20.17**

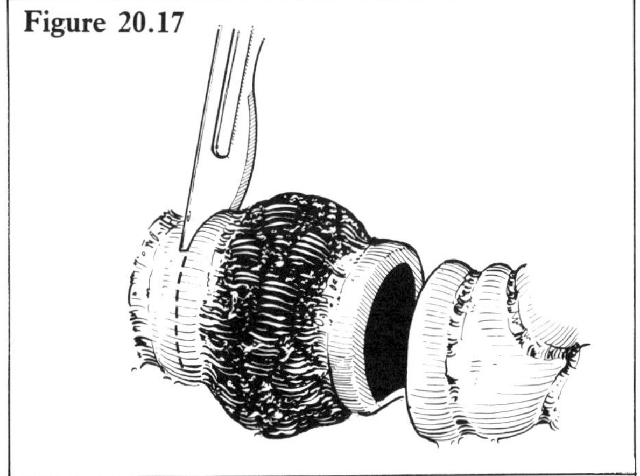

**Figure 20.18**

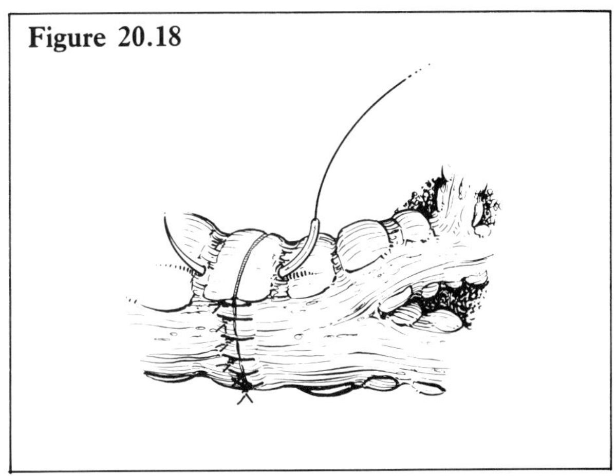

**Figure 20.19**

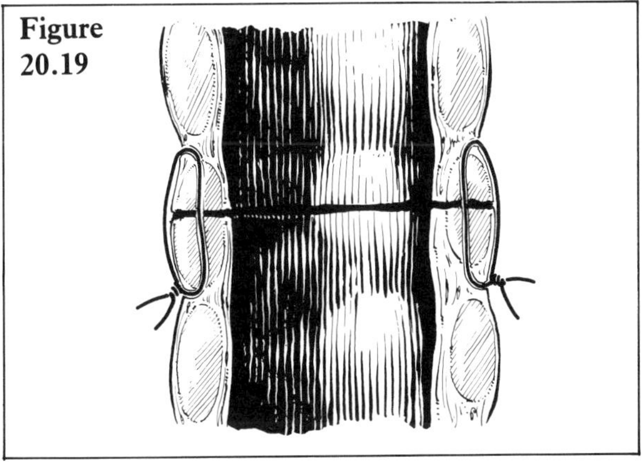

**Figure 20.20**

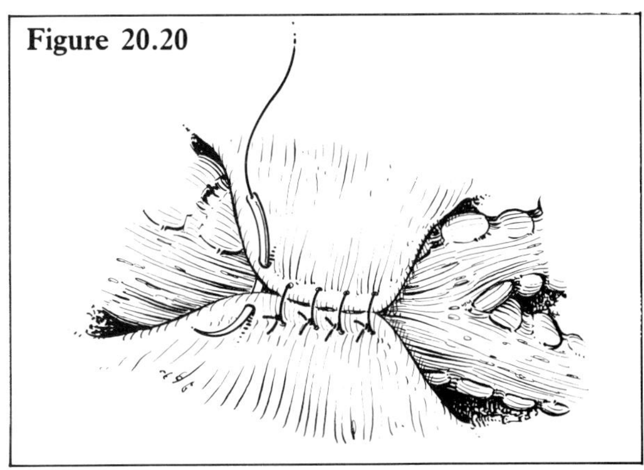

possible. The pericardium is entered just anterior to its reflection on the pulmonary veins, and the right pulmonary artery and both veins are completely freed.

If the anastomosis is still likely to be under too great a tension, consideration should be given to the cervical mobilization previously described. The anaesthetist is asked to flex the patient's neck. This should allow a gap of up to 7 cm to be closed. The anastomosis is carried out as described on p. 79 (**Figs. 20.18, 20.19**). The suture line is then protected by wrapping around it a pedicled flap obtained from the adjacent pleura or pericardium (**Fig. 20.20**).

## Resection of the carina

When the tumour involves the carina it is necessary to resect the origins of both main bronchi as well as the lower trachea. The trachea, carina and main bronchi are mobilized as described above (**Fig. 20.21**). By traction on the tapes surrounding the right main bronchus and the trachea the whole length of the left main bronchus is mobilized beneath the arch of the aorta, taking care to preserve the bronchial blood supply and the left recurrent laryngeal nerve (**Fig. 20.22**). The right main bronchus is incised 1 cm beyond the macroscopic limit of the tumour and traction sutures are placed 5 mm from the cut edge as the incision proceeds (**Fig. 20.23**). The left main bronchus is

**Figure 20.21**

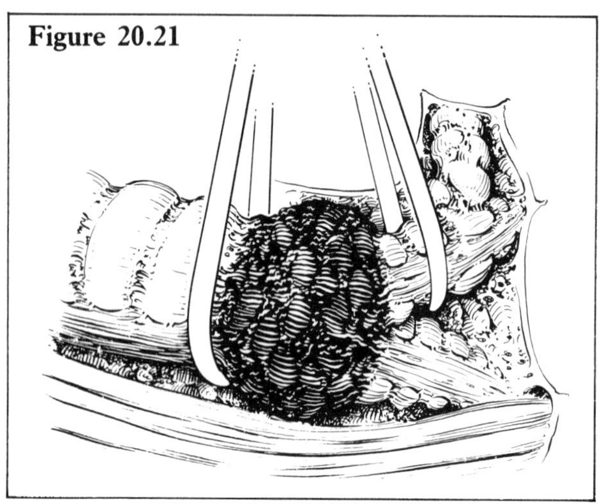

**Figure 20.22**

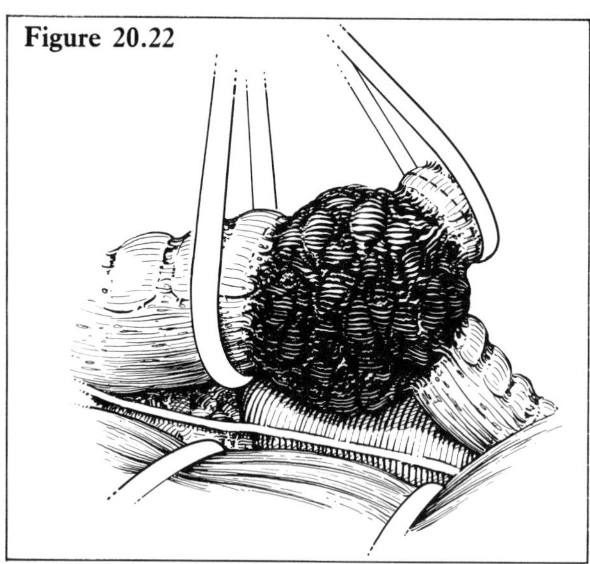

**Figure 20.23**

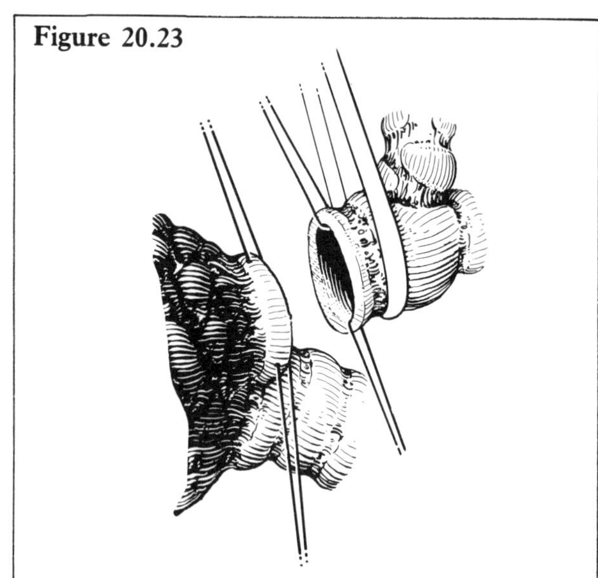

**Figure 20.24**

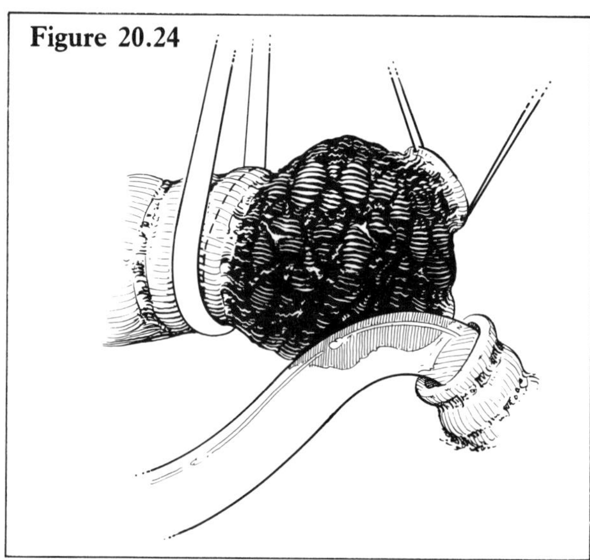

**Figure 20.25**

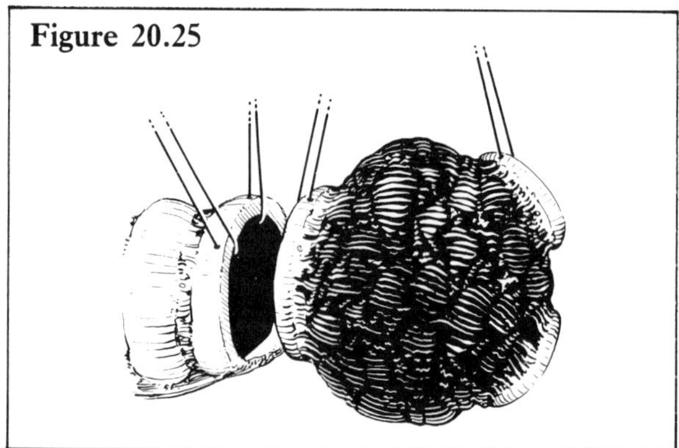

similarly incised; when it has been divided, a cuffed endotracheal tube is passed into it and anaesthesia continued through this (**Fig. 20.24**). The trachea is then divided above the tumour and traction sutures again inserted (**Fig. 20.25**).

## Reconstruction

Reconstruction has two stages: first, the right main bronchus is anastomosed end-to-end to the trachea, and then the left main bronchus is anastomosed end-to-side to the right main bronchus.

The neck is flexed, and with traction on the sutures in the trachea and the right main bronchus the approximation of the two is tested. A wedge is now removed from the cartilaginous trachea and the margins approximated with interrupted polypropylene sutures to reduce the size of the tracheal orifice to that of the right main bronchus (**Figs. 20.26–20.30**).

The suturing starts in the depths of the wound, i.e. on the left side of the trachea, using 3/0 polypropylene interrupted sutures. One row of sutures is placed in the cartilaginous trachea and the other in the membranous part. The sutures are left untied until all have been inserted (**Fig. 20.31**). They are then tied, starting in the depths of the incision and working towards the surface. The ventilation is now transferred to the right lung by connecting the anaesthetic machine to the endotracheal tube. The suture line should be tested for leaks by pouring a small amount of saline into the pleural cavity and, if necessary, additional sutures inserted.

**Figure 20.26**

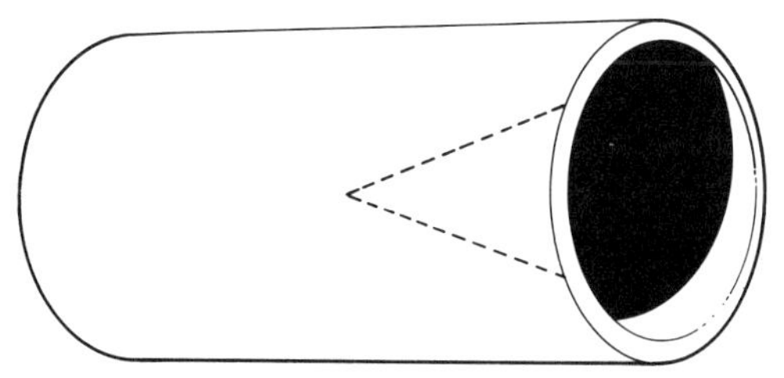

**Figure 20.27**

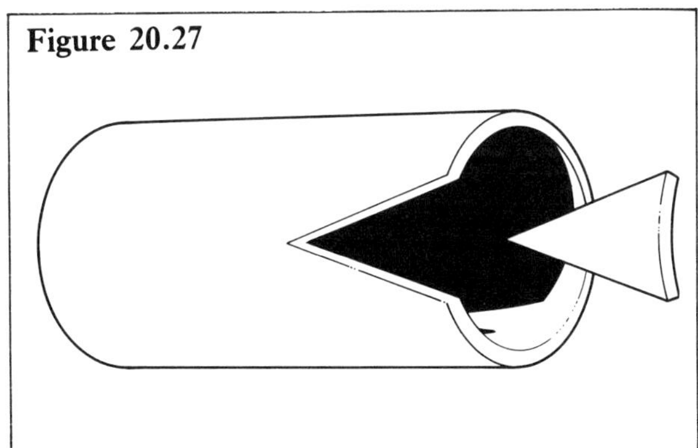

**Figure 20.28**

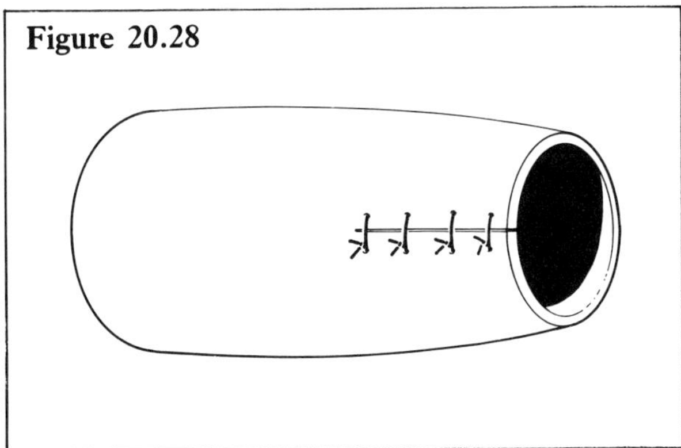

**Figure 20.29**

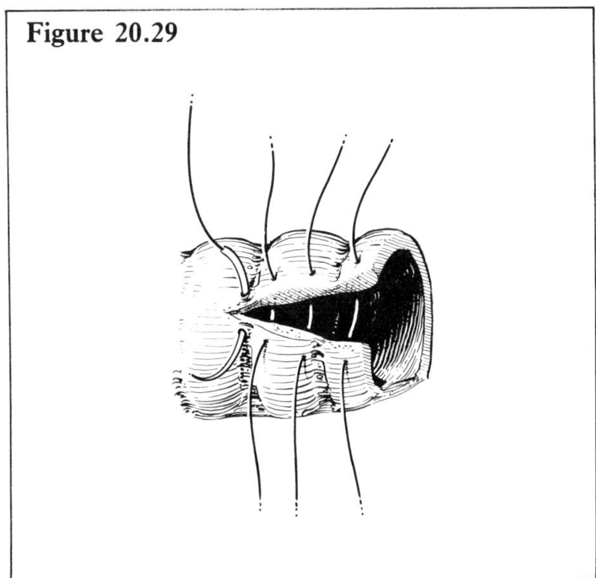

**Figure 20.30**

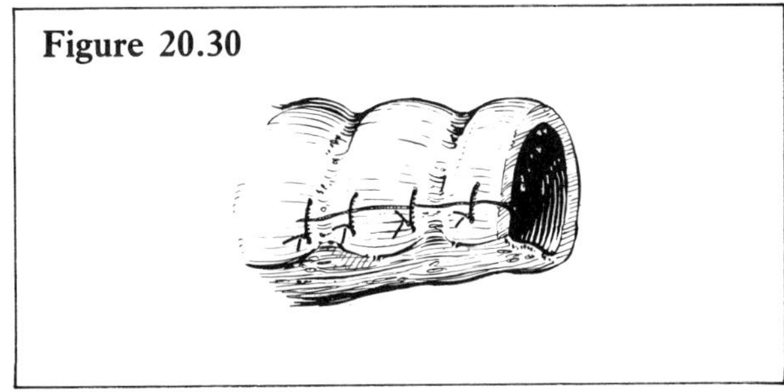

**Figure 20.31**

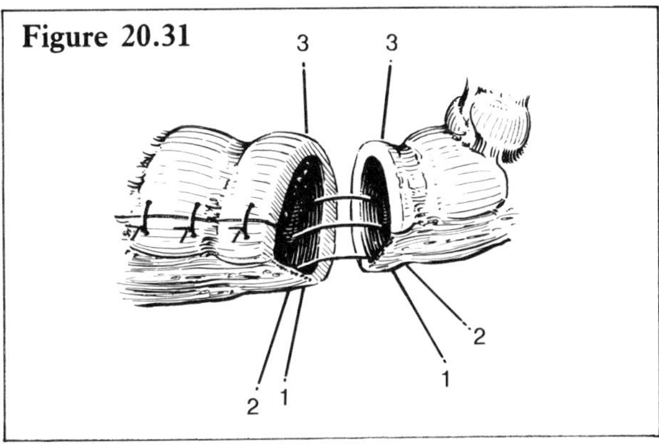

## End-to-side anastomosis of left main bronchus

The right lung is retracted forward and the left main bronchus held up beneath it with the aid of stay sutures (**Fig. 20.32**). An incision about 2 cm long is made at the junction of the cartilaginous and membranous portion of the intermediate bronchus opposite the opening in the left main bronchus, and the two openings are united by a series of interrupted 3/0 polypropylene sutures. The first suture is placed in the centre of the incision, and by holding this up, insertion of sutures on either side is facilitated (**Fig. 20.33**). The whole posterior row is placed before any of the sutures is tied (**Fig. 20.34**). Between the insertion of each suture the opening in the intermediate bronchus is temporarily occluded with a mounted swab to permit ventilation to continue. When this row of sutures has been completed all are tied and cut, leaving the knots on the inside of the lumen. The row of sutures joining the membranous portion of the bronchi is then inserted in a similar manner (**Fig. 20.35**). This suture line is also tested for leakage and adequate inflation of the left lung is confirmed. Two drains are placed in the right pleural space and the chest is closed in the usual way.

**Figure 20.32**

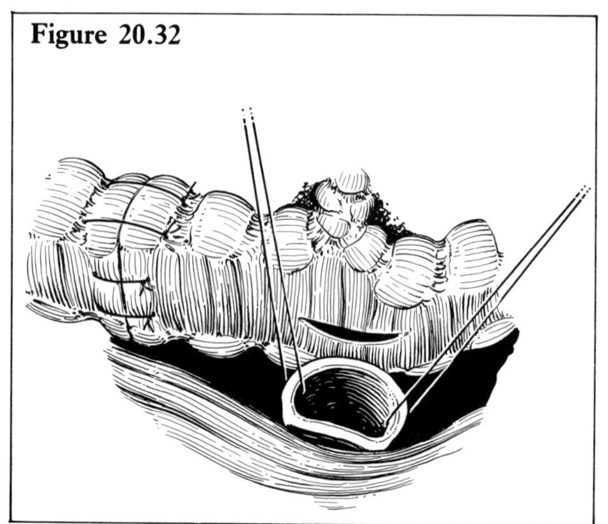

**Figure 20.33**

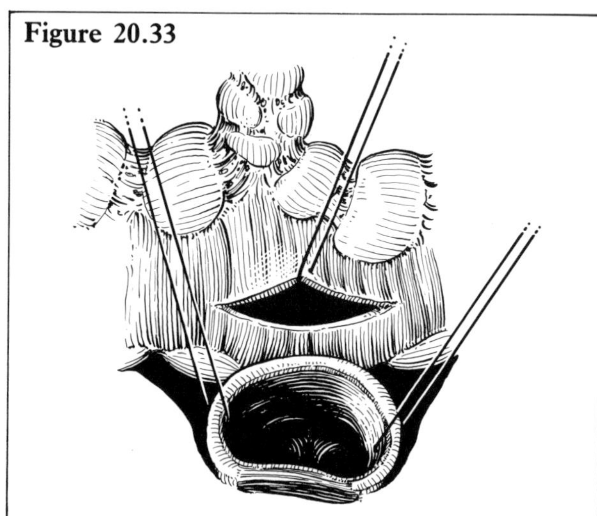

**Figure 20.34**

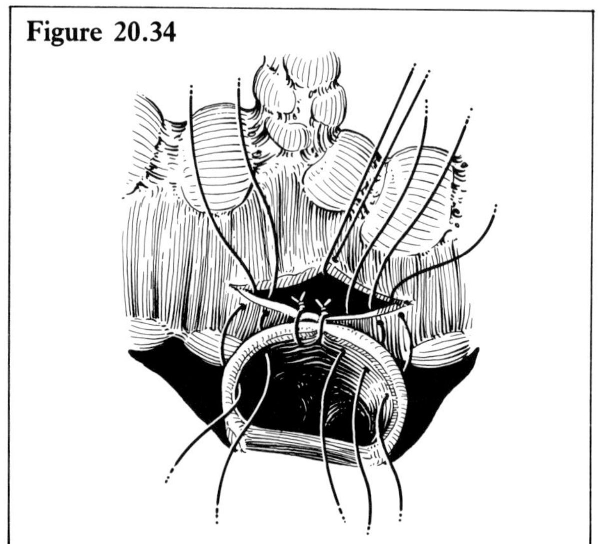

**Figure 20.35**

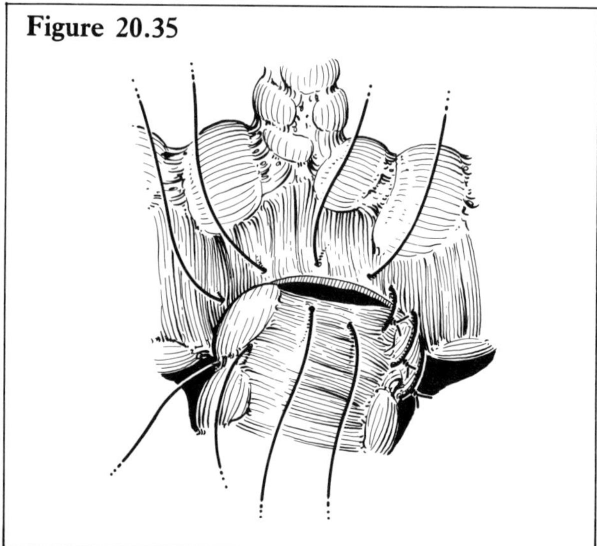

SECTION 5

# SURGERY OF THE LUNG AND PLEURAL SPACE

# 21 Open lung biopsy

An open lung biopsy is indicated when transbronchial or needle biopsies are unlikely to yield sufficient tissue for a pathological diagnosis. This is usually the case when there are diffuse lung changes. Open excision biopsy is also indicated when tissue samples obtained by needle or drill biopsy are inadequate.

The tip of the inferior segment of the lingula should be avoided as the changes in it tend to be atypical. If the chest radiographs or CT scan do not point to a specific area for biopsy, as is often the case, an anterior thoracotomy through a submammary incision is the best approach. This provides access to the middle and lower lobes on the right, and to the lower lobe on the left, and the incision heals with little discomfort to the patient (see p. 34 for the details of this part of the procedure). Provided that the thorax is entered through the fifth intercostal space, good access is assured.

Care should be taken to avoid crush damage to the piece of lung to be removed, and it is preferable to grasp it only with the fingers. If the line of resection is to be sutured rather than stapled, a clamp is placed across the base of this portion of lung, excluding a piece about 4 cm × 4 cm which is excised close to the clamp leaving a margin of 3–4 mm (**Fig. 21.1**). The cut edge is oversewn underneath the clamp with a continuous horizontal mattress suture of 3/0 polypropylene in one direction (**Fig. 21.2**), and an over-and-over suture with the same material in the opposite direction (**Fig. 21.3**). This gives an airtight suture line.

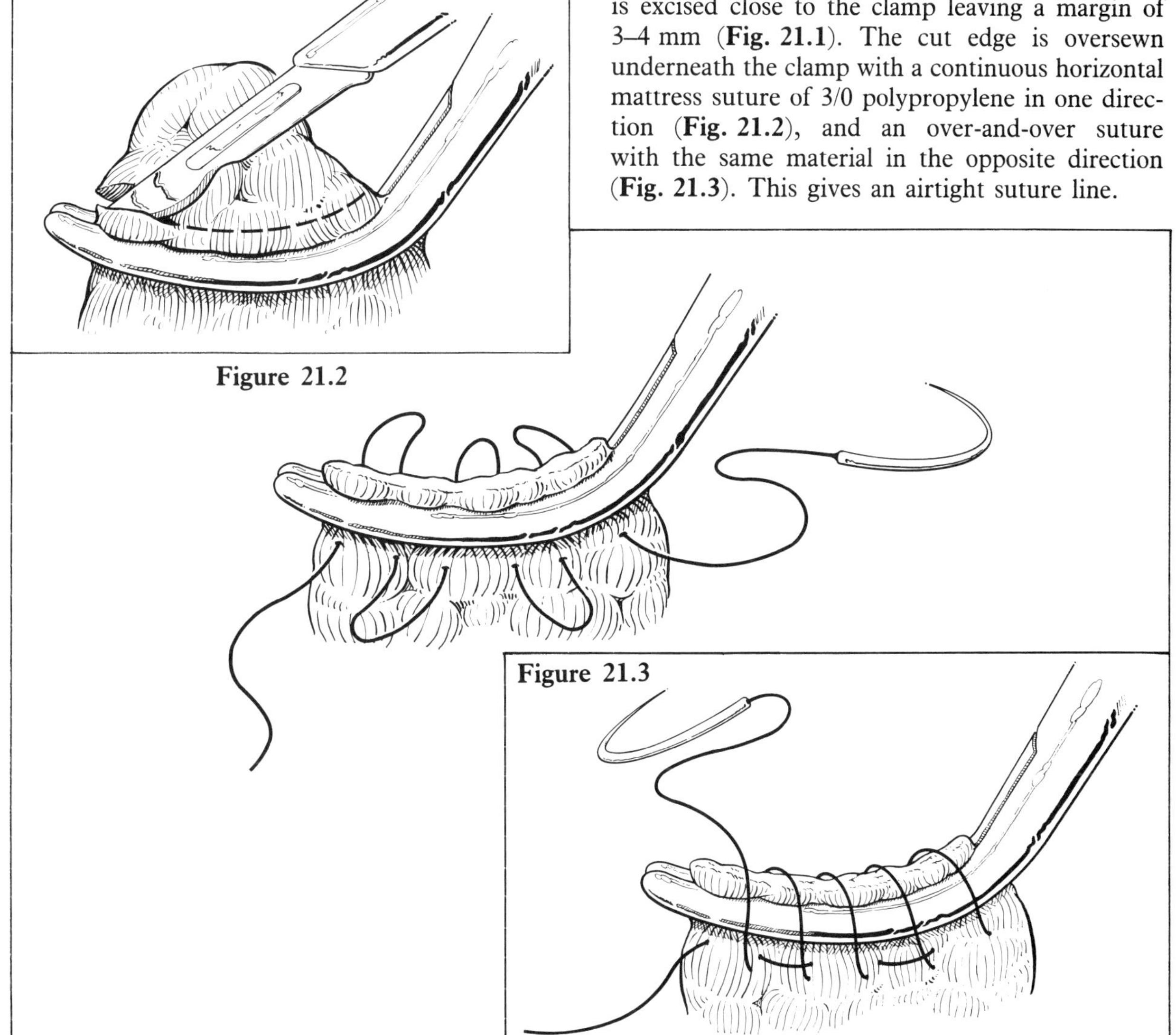

**Figure 21.1**

**Figure 21.2**

**Figure 21.3**

An alternative is to use a staple gun. The blade of the 55-mm instrument is easily introduced into the pleural cavity through this incision. With the piece of lung to be removed held in the fingers, the stapler loaded with 3.5 mm staples is placed across its base and fired. The lung is transected with a knife close to the stapler (**Figs. 21.4, 21.5**).

There should be no air leak after this operation. However, despite this the chest should be closed over a 10-mm chest drain, as the compliance of diseased lung is usually impaired and this may give rise to an unexpected air leak.

When closing the chest it is not necessary to suture the whole length of the intercostal layer. Three or four bites of nylon suture taken around the rib above and the intercostal muscle below in the accessible anterior portion of the incision are usually sufficient to approximate the whole length.

**Figure 21.4**

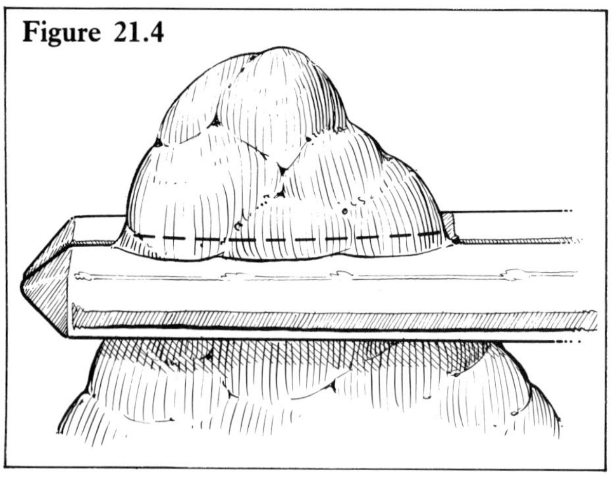

**Figure 21.5**

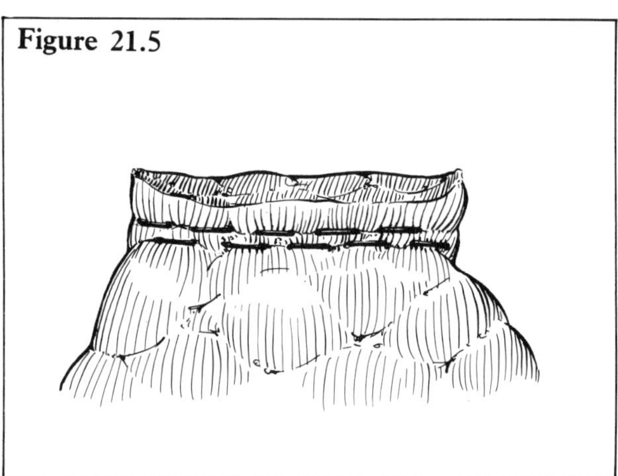

# 22 Operations for spontaneous pneumothorax

These procedures are required for the management of chronic or recurrent pneumothoraces. A chronic pneumothorax may be defined arbitrarily as one that has persisted for five days or more. Recurrent pneumothorax is an indication for surgical treatment when a third one has occurred on the same side or a second one has occurred after a pneumothorax has developed on the opposite side.

The procedures available are pleurodesis, pleurectomy, and an apical pleurectomy with abrasive pleurodesis of the remainder of the hemithorax. Pleurectomy may make a subsequent thoracotomy very difficult, therefore it is most important to deter any patients who are smokers from this habit at the time of treatment. A more immediate and serious potential complication of pleurectomy is haemorrhage. For this reason extra care should be taken to ensure that the raw surface is not bleeding prior to closing the chest. We advocate the use of pleurodesis by abrasion for most patients. On completion of the pleurodesis it is most important to deal with any pulmonary bullae or blebs that are present.

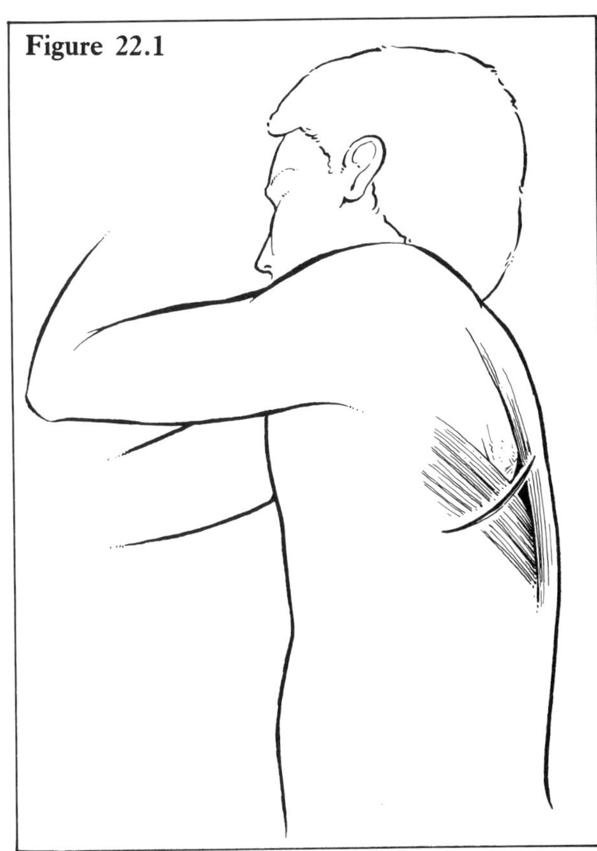

**Figure 22.1**

## Procedure

The operation is performed through a lateral thoracotomy. The skin incision should be quite small—no more than 15 cm in length (**Fig. 22.1**). The operation can be performed through an axillary thoracotomy; this limited approach may be useful in frail patients in whom only an apical pleurodesis is necessary. This is not routinely recommended because a complete inspection of the lung is not possible, and thus success cannot be guaranteed.

If a pleurodesis is to be done, the pleural space is entered as the chest is opened and the whole of the parietal pleura abraded with a gauze sponge mounted on a sponge-holding forceps (**Fig. 22.2**). These swabs should be changed as soon as they become moist as the friction then ceases to be adequate to abrade the pleura. The abrasion is carried out vigorously until the pleural surface is inflamed and bleeding.

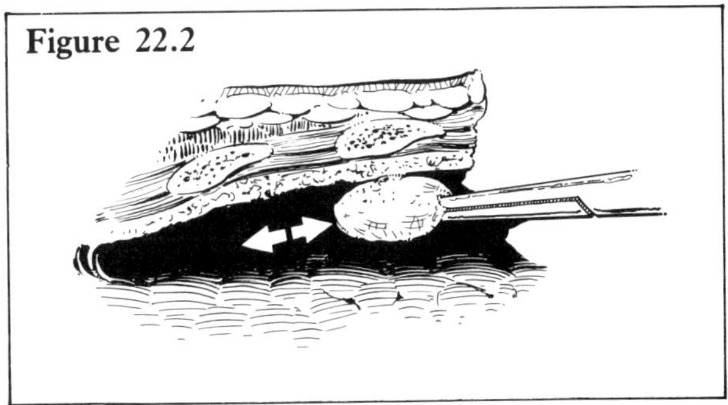

**Figure 22.2**

Once this has been completed the whole of the lung is inspected. There may be multiple bullae of sizes varying from 5 mm to 100 mm or more. In younger patients, however, the most common abnormality is a group of small bullae, often incorporated in some thickened pleura at the apex. These are isolated from the underlying lung with a stout ligature, or a row of 3.5 mm staples fired from a TA30 or a TA55 staple gun. It is not necessary to resect the excluded portion of lung. If there are multiple bullae, these should all be picked up in a similar way and stapled at the base. Multiple staple cartridges are expensive and so we use multiple ligatures which are equally effective.

Figure 22.3

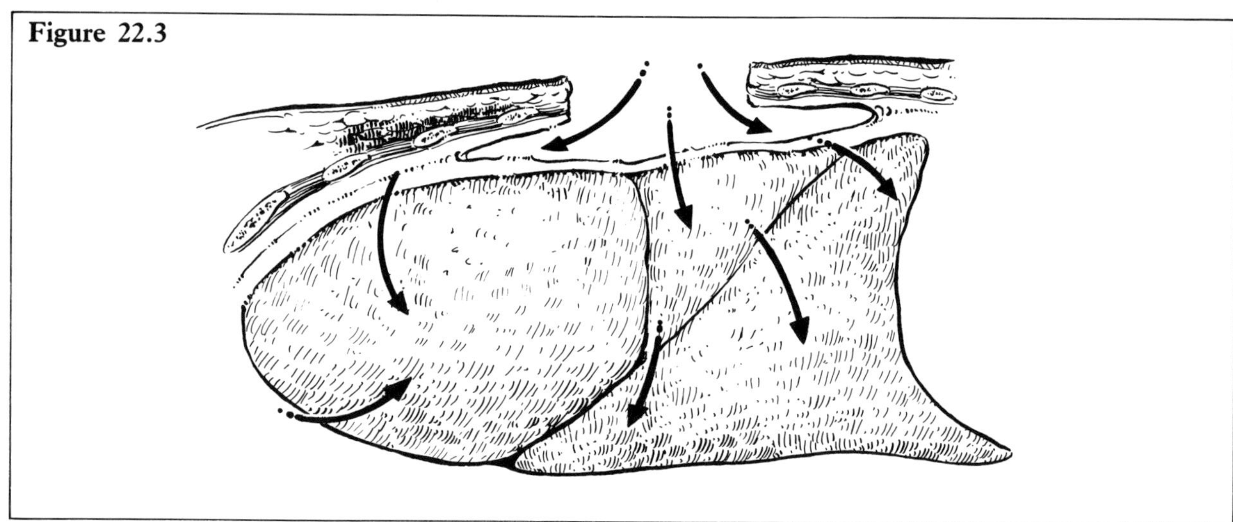

Here also the portions of lung beyond the ligatures should not be excised. These procedures are carried out with the lung partly inflated so that the bullae can be easily identified.

If a pleurectomy is to be performed, the pleural strip is begun before the pleural space is opened (**Fig. 22.3**). This makes the procedure very much easier. The pleura is stripped from the whole of the chest wall and the mediastinum down to the azygos vein and around the hilum of the lung. The pleural strip is not continued past the costophrenic recess because the diaphragm may be detached in the process. It is important, however, to abrade the pleural surface of the diaphragm to prevent the formation of a subpulmonary pneumothorax.

Prior to closing the chest a very careful inspection for bleeding from the chest wall is made and any significant bleeding points cauterized. The lung is reinflated to a pressure of 40 $cmH_2O$ (3.9 kPa) after filling the chest cavity with warm saline to test for air leaks. If any are found they are repaired either with a polypropylene stitch or a further ligature. The chest is closed with two drains in the pleural space, inserted through an intercostal space two ribs below the incision. The reason for inserting two drains is that not only may there be some air leak, but also that the only serious complication of this operation is the formation of a haemothorax. The tubes can be removed after 24 to 48 hours, and the patient is usually fit to go home at the end of five days.

# 23 Surgical treatment of bullous disease of the lung

Most patients with large cysts of the lung have generalized emphysema. However, when a cyst or group of cysts compresses the surrounding lung parenchyma, considerable improvement in the dyspnoea experienced by the patient can be achieved by their removal. The condition may be bilateral; if so, operations should be staged. High kV chest radiographs give valuable information about the size and position of the cysts. Crowding of the vessels at the hilum identified on a plain chest radiograph indicates compressed lung parenchyma, and is as good a way as any other of deciding whether removal of the space-occupying lesion (the bulla) will improve the patient's dyspnoea.

Lung function tests performed at rest, and if possible after exercise, should be obtained before embarking on surgical treatment, and a ventilation–perfusion scan will give information about non-functioning areas of lung.

## Preoperative preparation

This is aimed at eliminating bronchial infection as far as possible. The patient should not be operated on within four weeks of an upper respiratory tract infection. If the sputum is purulent it should be cultured and a five-day course of the appropriate antibiotic given.

## Anaesthesia

The application of positive pressure to the lungs before the chest has been opened can result in the development of a tension cyst with the same manifestations as a tension pneumothorax. The trachea should therefore be intubated under local anaesthesia and the patient allowed to breathe spontaneously until the chest has been opened. Ventilation can be controlled even better by the use of a jet ventilator.

## Procedure

As access to the whole of the lung may be necessary, a full posterolateral thoracotomy stripping the lower border of the fifth rib is the best approach. The largest cystic area under tension should be punctured as soon as the pleura has been opened.

The procedure varies according to the position and nature of the cysts. As the whole of the lung parenchyma is usually involved in the disease process, resection of lung tissue should be a last resort. It is almost always possible to exclude the bullae from the rest of the lung without resection, thus removing the space-occupying lesion and retaining all the functioning lung tissue. It is always surprising how much functioning lung tissue remains even around some of the most emphysematous areas.

Large cysts may be dealt with in the following way. The cyst is held with forceps and opened (**Fig. 23.1**). The base may be closed with a mechanical stapler (**Fig. 23.2**), or with a full-

**Figure 23.1**

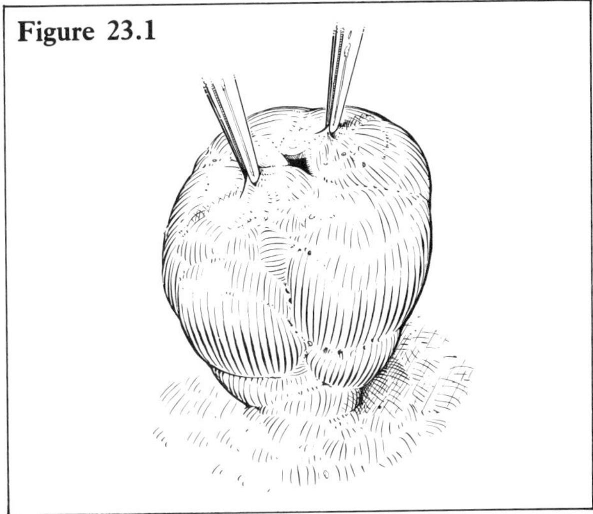

**Figure 23.2**

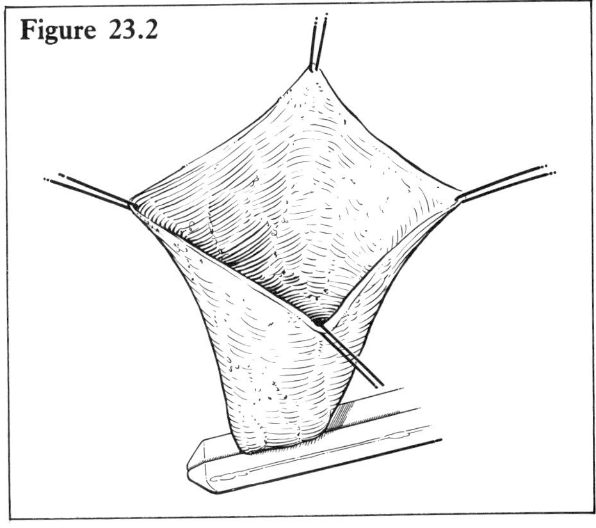

thickness purse-string suture (**Fig. 23.3**). The redundant tissue is then resected, leaving enough for a suture line of 3/0 polypropylene to reinforce the repair (**Fig. 23.4**). Small cysts may be held up and the pedicle ligated without opening the bulla. It is not necessary to excise that part of the cyst beyond the ligature.

In some cases a row of cysts may be seen along one margin of the lung. It may be possible to exclude these with the use of the stapler or otherwise to incorporate them all in a running suture.

The parietal pleural surfaces are now abraded as in a standard pleurodesis.

Because a persistent air leak is the major complication of this procedure, two or three drains should be placed in the pleural cavity. They are connected to an underwater seal and suction at 100 mmHg (13 kPa) is applied.

Pain relief is of more importance than usual following this operation to allow full ventilation by the patient early after surgery. The appropriate intercostal nerves may be frozen with the cryoprobe before the chest is closed.

## Postoperative management

The patient is initially given 28% oxygen to breathe as the respiratory centre may be insensitive to $CO_2$, making anoxic respiratory drive all-important. High oxygen concentrations may lead to increasing hypercapnia. Blood gases should therefore be estimated frequently in the early postoperative period. Spontaneous respiration should be established as early as possible; this is facilitated by the use of a short-acting muscle relaxant during the operation. In the presence of a large air leak, obstruction of a chest tube may lead to a tension pneumothorax or to massive surgical emphysema. Therefore the patency of the drainage tubes must be ensured at all times.

**Figure 23.3**

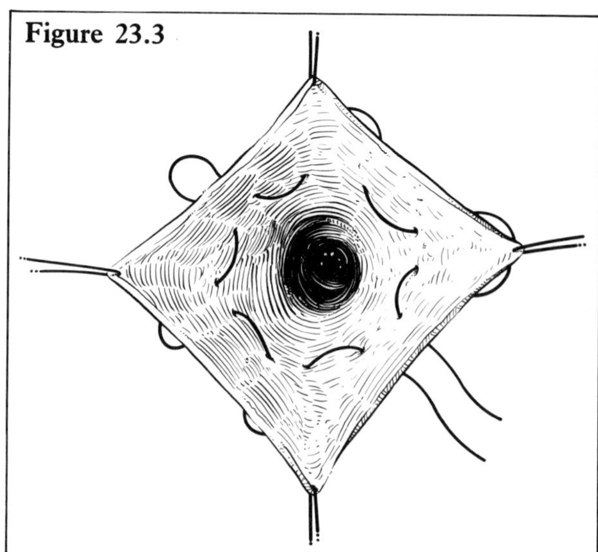

**Figure 23.4**

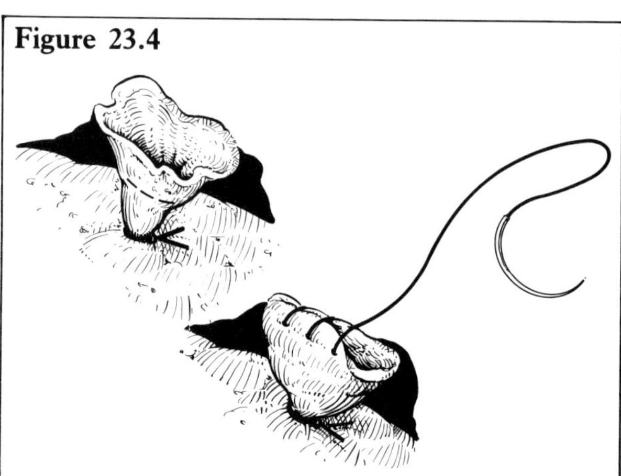

# 24 Right pneumonectomy

The approach is via a right posterolateral thoracotomy through the bed of the fifth rib (p. 24). The lung is fully mobilized and any adhesions to the chest wall are divided. The location and extent of the tumour and the involvement of lymph nodes are identified. If the tumour is centrally placed, before proceeding to a pneumonectomy, the operator should expose in turn the pulmonary artery, both pulmonary veins and the main bronchus, although not in any particular order, so as to ensure that each can be safely divided.

Individual surgeons will have their own preference for the order in which they identify and divide the major pulmonary structures. We describe the approach that has evolved in our practice and that we have found safe and effective.

The lung is retracted backwards and downwards to expose the azygos vein crossing the right main bronchus to join the superior vena cava. The phrenic nerve lies on the superior vena cava immediately over the area of the dissection. The mediastinal pleura is incised just behind it so that the nerve can be displaced forward. It is convenient to begin the operation by the division of the superior pulmonary vein which can be seen overlying the right pulmonary artery (**Fig. 24.1**). After this has been done the pulmonary artery can be seen more clearly. The vein is short but it must be dissected close to its point of emergence from the pericardium; distal dissection may result in damage to the posterior segmental vein which arises from the posterior aspect. The posterior surface of the superior pulmonary vein is closely applied to the inferior division of the pulmonary artery, and is separated from it by a tongue of pericardium. The separation of these two structures must be carried out under direct vision by lifting the upper and lower margins of the vein in turn and incising the fascial plane which is closely applied to it (**Fig. 24.2**). When this is done the underlying artery wall will be seen very clearly. It will then be found possible to pass a right-angled forceps safely beneath the vein (**Fig. 24.3**). As the vein is too short to be divided between two ligatures, separate ligatures must be placed on each of the individual tributaries distally. A clamp is placed across the vein centrally and the vessel divided. A

**Figure 24.1**

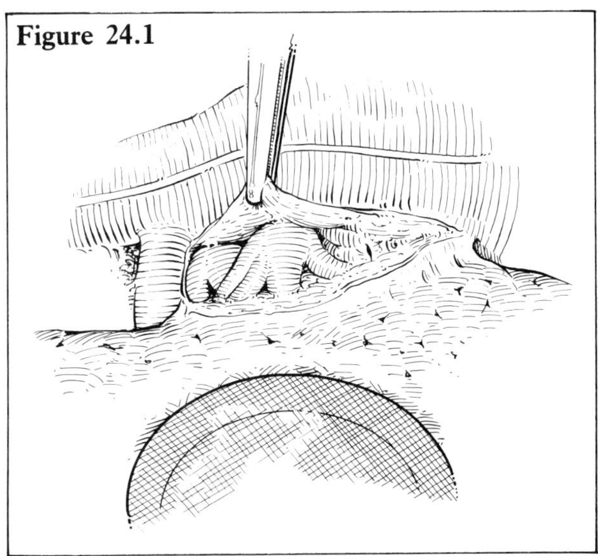

**Figure 24.2**

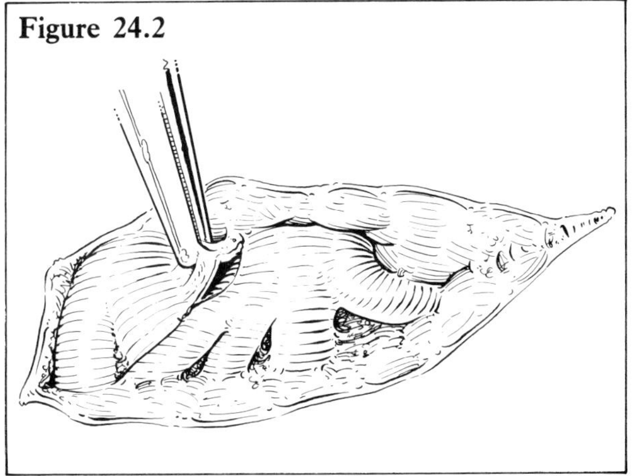

**Figure 24.3**

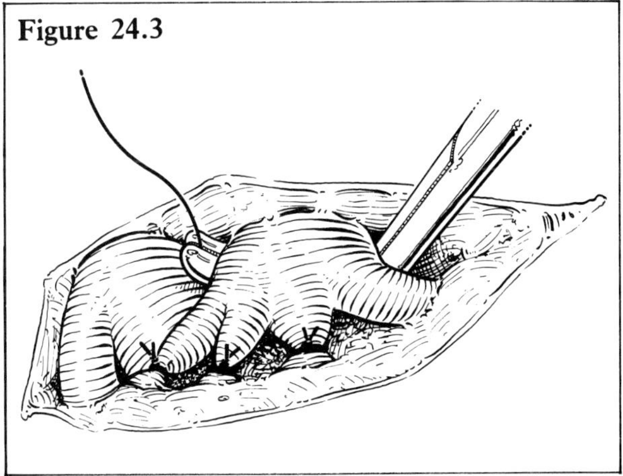

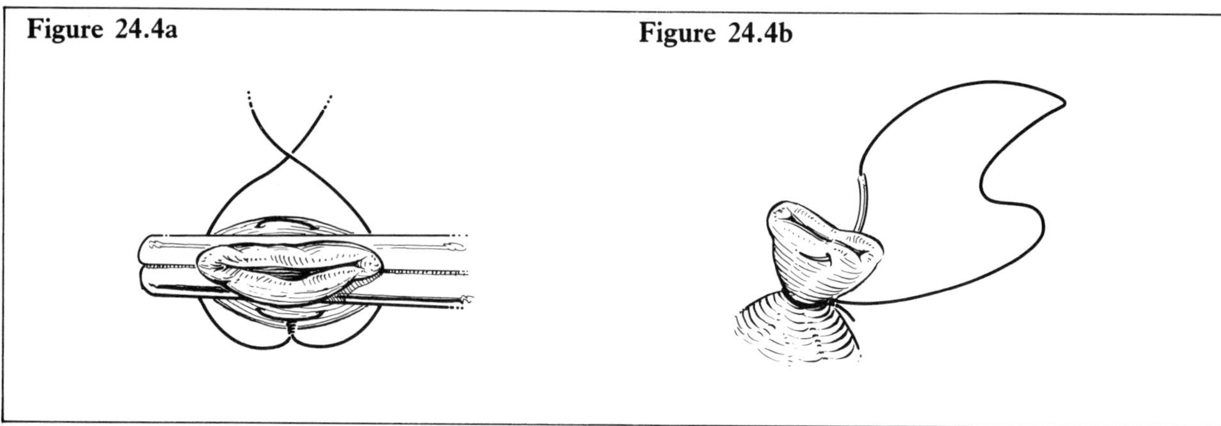
Figure 24.4a

Figure 24.4b

3/0 polypropylene stitch is then passed through the vein as a horizontal mattress stitch beneath the clamp, and a single knot thrown before passing the suture back around the vein, under the clamp (**Fig. 24.4a**). As the clamp is removed the knot is tightened around the vein, and four further knots thrown securely. The suture is then carried over and over the vein and tied again to give a very secure closure (**Fig. 24.4b**).

When the vein is divided, the line of incision should be at the junction of the central two-thirds and the distal third of the distance between the ligatures. The reason is to ensure that the major cuff is on the central side so that the ligature cannot slip off.

Attention is now turned to the pulmonary artery. The mediastinal pleural incision is continued over the top of the hilum following the lower border of the azygos vein, which is divided between strong ties. This will expose the first division of the pulmonary artery and the right main bronchus and vagus nerve (**Fig. 24.5**).

The pericardium overlying the main pulmonary artery is lifted up and retracted forwards. The fibrous extension of the pericardium from the upper margin of the main pulmonary artery to the superior vena cava can now been seen and divided. The fascia surrounding the artery is incised along both the upper and lower margins (**Fig. 24.6**). It should now be possible to pass a finger around the artery close to its origin behind the superior vena cava (**Fig. 24.7**). This permits any remaining firm bands of fascia to be put on the stretch and divided with scissors. In this way an opening is made behind the artery through which a Semb pneumonectomy forceps can be passed. With this a heavy linen thread ligature is drawn behind the artery and tied with three knots. Distally the ligatures are placed around the right upper lobe artery and intermediate artery and, again, a very wide cuff is left centrally to obviate any possibility of the ligature slipping. Sometimes, as a result of encroachment of a tumour on the branches of the right pulmonary artery, there is insufficient length to permit a division

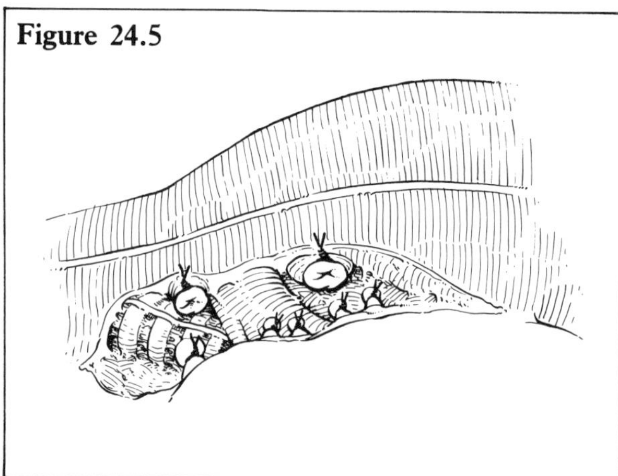
Figure 24.5

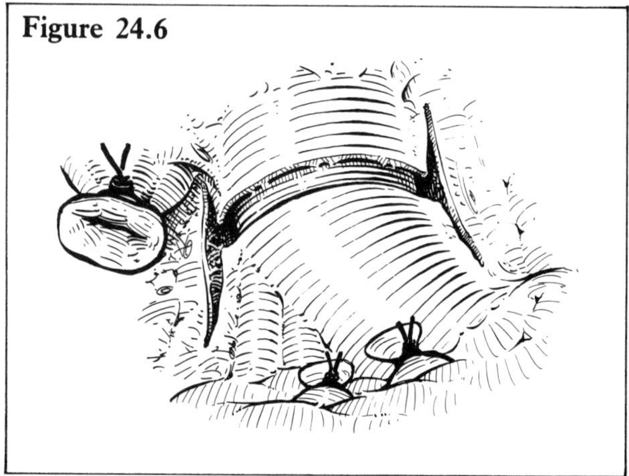
Figure 24.6

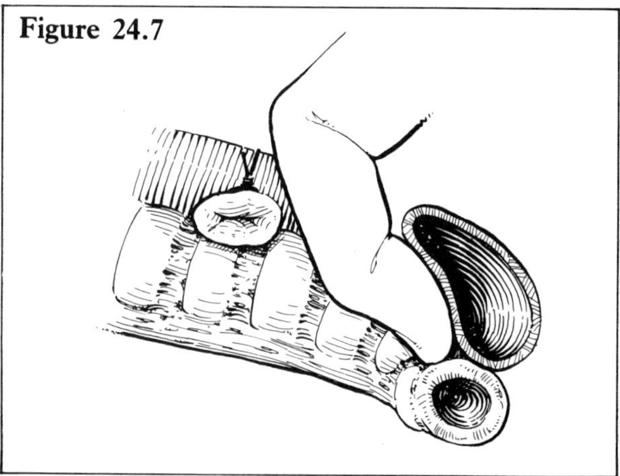
Figure 24.7

between ligatures. In these cases the central end of the artery is occluded with an angled vascular clamp. The artery is divided leaving a cuff of at least 2 mm beyond the clamp. The cut edge is closed with a continuous suture of 4/0 or 5/0 polypropylene, which can be run conveniently from one end of the cuff to the other and then back again so that the two ends can be tied together. The clamp should be opened before the suture is cut. In this way one can see whether the suture line is blood-tight. If it is not, a little traction on the end of the suture makes clamping of the divided artery much easier.

In some cases the extent of a tumour makes it impossible to pass ligatures round the distal branches of the artery. The artery can be divided after its central end has been secured and distal bleeding controlled by suturing the distal cut ends with the accompanying tumour.

Attention is now turned to the posterior aspect of the hilum. The mediastinal pleura is incised along the anterior margin of the vagus nerve. The lower lobe of the lung is lifted up, exposing the pulmonary ligament which should be divided close to the oesophagus (**Fig. 24.8**). There are several arteries in this ligament, in particular one at the lower end and one just below the lower margin of the inferior pulmonary vein. The latter always has a lymph node in association with it.

The inferior pulmonary vein can now be clearly seen. Its sheath is incised along the upper and lower margins, and dissection is continued distally to expose its two branches. This is often best accomplished with a small dental swab sweeping the sheath proximally and distally (**Fig. 24.9**). The main trunk and its two branches are then ligated and divided as for the superior pulmonary vein (**Fig. 24.10**).

As the dissection proceeds upwards, the carinal lymph nodes are encountered lying on the posterior aspect of the pericardium over the left atrium between the two main bronchi (**Fig. 24.11**). The lower margins of both main bronchi are carefully dissected to allow this group of glands to be removed *en bloc*. Bleeding from small bronchial arteries is controlled with diathermy.

Attention is now turned to the right main bronchus. The sheath of the bronchus is entered by sharp and blunt dissection with scissors at the lower right side of the trachea extending to the tracheobronchial angle. By lifting the bronchus and working from both above and below it is possible to free it by blunt dissection.

The anaesthetist must now be warned that the bronchus is about to be clamped, in case an endotracheal or endobronchial tube is projecting beyond the carina, and the anaesthetist must be given time to withdraw the tube into the trachea.

**Figure 24.8**

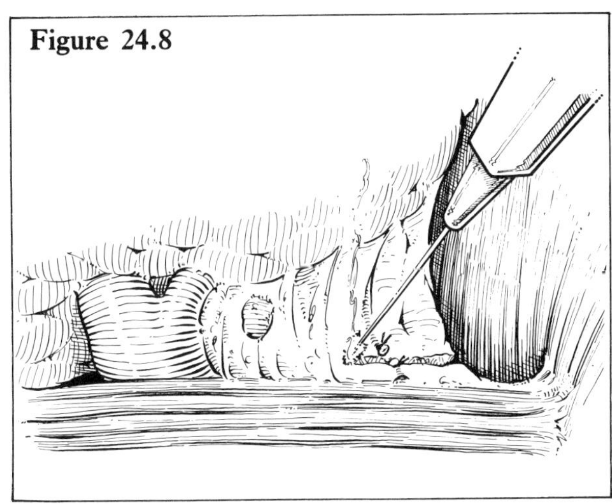

**Figure 24.9**

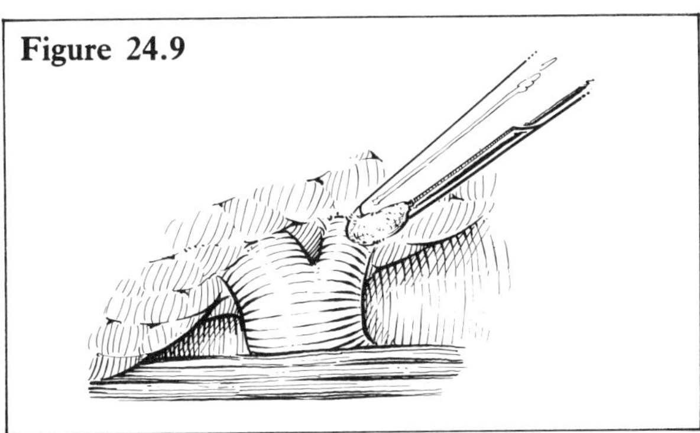

**Figure 24.10**

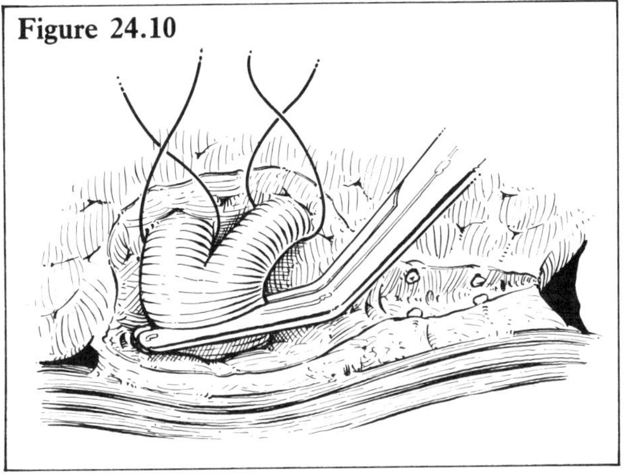

**Figure 24.11**

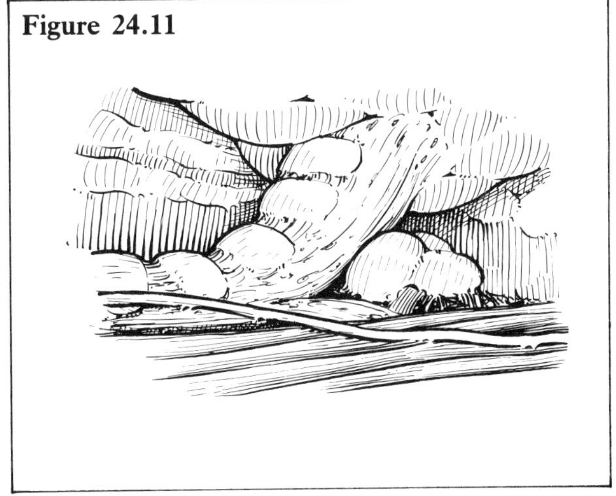

The right main bronchus is clamped exactly at its origin; if the clamp is not placed exactly parallel with the trachea, a sump may be left which may act as a focus for sepsis (**Fig. 24.12**). A second clamp is placed more distally. The bronchus is then divided using a scalpel with a large blade. The division should leave at least 5 mm of bronchial wall projecting beyond the clamp on the proximal side. Our own preference is for a continuous horizontal mattress suture proximal to the clamp, continued as an over-and-over stitch around the clamp back to the origin of the suture where it is securely tied. The clamp is removed before the suture is tied over the cut end of the bronchus. As it is being tied the anaesthetist should be asked to stop ventilating the lung, to avoid tension on the bronchus at that moment; this prevents tearing, especially of the membranous portion.

The lung is now removed. The next task is to remove the right paratracheal lymph nodes which are situated between the trachea and the superior vena cava (**Fig. 24.13**). Blunt dissection along the right margin of the trachea and the posterior margin of the superior vena cava isolates these lymph nodes in a mass of fatty tissue which extends from the pulmonary artery sheath below to the scalene nodes above, and is related on its left side to the pericardium, ascending aorta and aortic arch. This mass of lymph nodes and fatty tissue can be removed *en bloc*. Care must be taken when approaching the apex of the chest to identify the right brachiocephalic artery and then the recurrent laryngeal nerve as it arises from the vagus and passes upwards behind the pulmonary artery.

The fascia surrounding the oesophagus is now sutured over the bronchial suture line on to the anterior wall of the bronchus with a continuous suture or several interrupted sutures (**Fig. 24.13**). When these are tied the fascia covers the bronchial suture line, so excluding it from the pleural cavity.

**Figure 24.12**

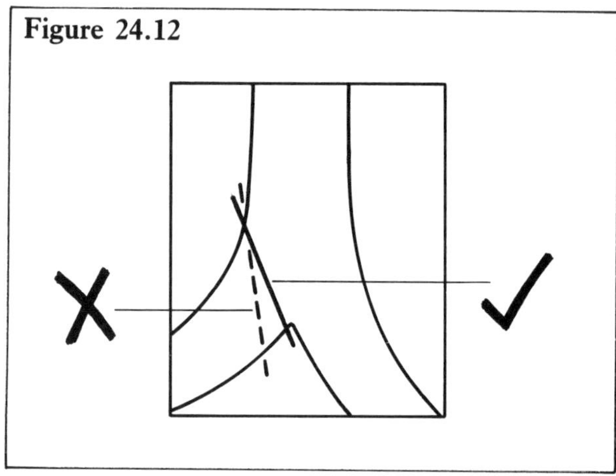

**Figure 24.13**

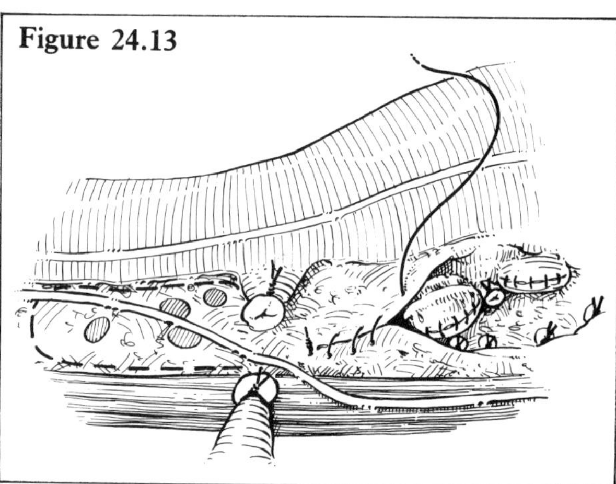

The chest is closed as described on p. 27, over a single chest drain. The drain should reach no higher than the hilum, nor be lower than the level of the divided inferior pulmonary vein. This prevents the chest either overfilling or underfilling with fluid, which could cause excessive mediastinal shift. The drain is kept clamped and released for one minute each hour to allow neutralization of the mediastinal position, and is removed the day after the operation.

# 25 Right intrapericardial pneumonectomy

Intrapericardial pneumonectomy is necessary when the tumour is at the hilum and has encroached upon the pulmonary artery or pulmonary veins.

**Figure 25.1a**

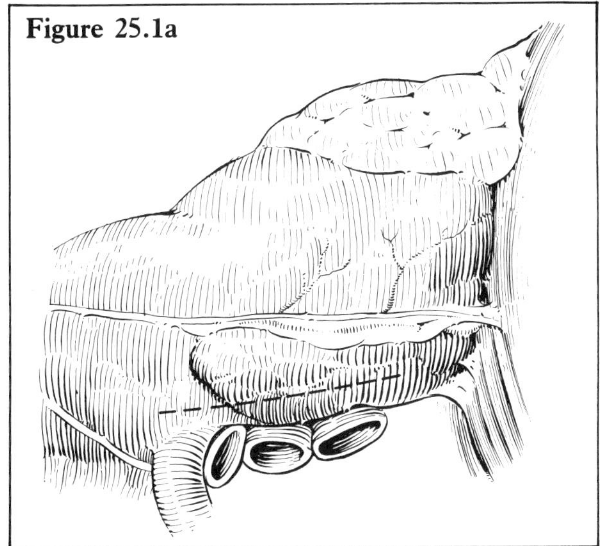

## Procedure

The azygos vein is divided. A vertical incision is made in the pericardium behind the phrenic nerve and anterior to the hilum of the lung, as close as possible to the point where the right pulmonary veins can be seen emerging from the pericardium (**Fig. 25.1**). If any tumour can be seen here the incision should be made 1 cm medially to it if possible. The incision is continued upwards on to the superior vena cava to the limit of the pericardial reflection, and downwards to the lower margin of the inferior pulmonary vein. The pericardial fluid obscures the view and should be sucked away as soon as the opening has been made. The extension of the incision is facilitated if the cut edges are grasped with long haemostats so that they can be held away from the underlying thin-walled right atrium.

At the lower margin of the inferior pulmonary vein there is a double pericardial fold which attaches it to the inferior vena cava (**Fig. 25.2**).

**Figure 25.1b**

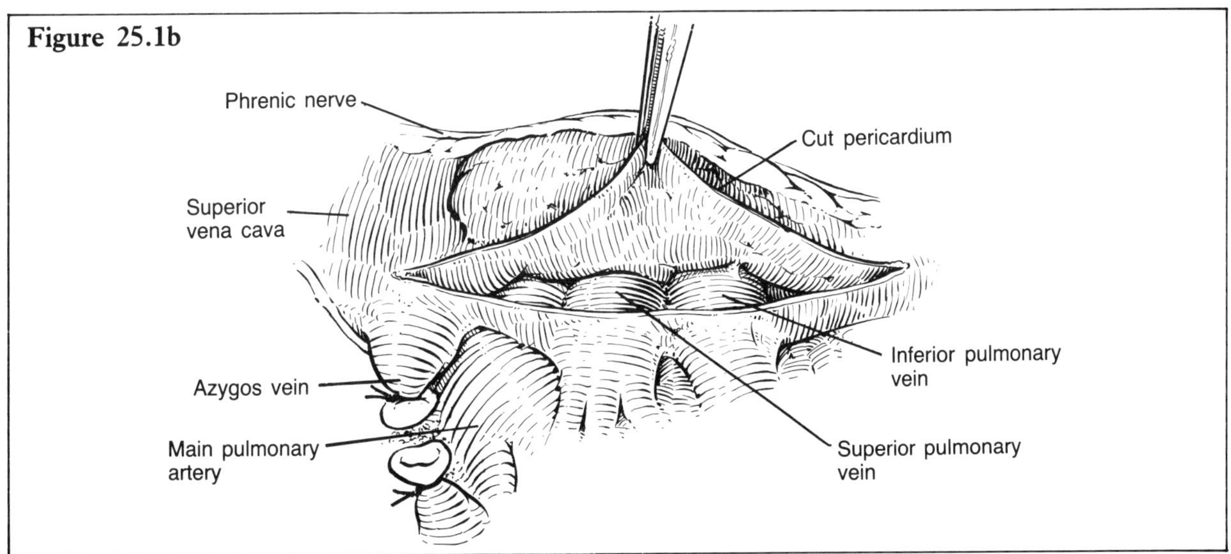


**Figure 25.2**

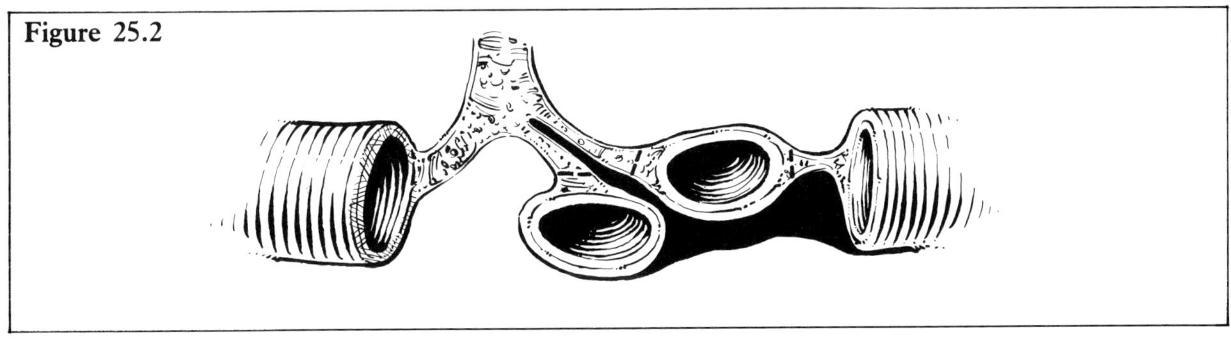

This fold should be divided close to the pulmonary vein, taking great care not to injure it or the inferior vena cava. The oblique sinus of the pericardium is thus entered. The incision can now be carried vertically upwards for a short distance along the posterior surface of the inferior pulmonary vein. The superior vena cava and the right atrium are retracted medially with a retractor or a swab to expose the pulmonary veins (**Fig. 25.3**). The retraction should be intermittent so as not to impede the venous return to the right atrium for too long. Undue pressure may also initiate atrial dysrhythmias. The pericardial reflections around each of the pulmonary veins are divided right up to the wall of the left atrium, and an instrument is passed beneath the veins (**Fig. 25.4**). A clamp is now placed across the wall of the left atrium (**Fig. 25.5**). The two veins are each ligated distally, and divided. The veins may be divided outside the pericardium in order to retain a greater length within the pericardium for safety. The line of division may go through the wall of the left atrium. The resection margin in the clamp is secured with a continuous suture of 3/0 polypropylene. The clamp is then cautiously released to make sure there is no bleeding between the stitches.

The right pulmonary artery can be secured as in a conventional pneumonectomy, or it can be located as it passes behind the ascending aorta and the superior vena cava. If the latter technique is used, the superior vena cava is elevated and retracted laterally with a pair of forceps and the ascending aorta pulled medially by the assistant. The pulmonary artery can then be seen running transversely beneath the pericardial recess. The pericardium is picked up and incised along the upper and lower margins of the pulmonary artery, which is mobilized by a combination of blunt and sharp dissection (**Fig. 25.6**).

A useful tip to remember is that if the main pulmonary artery has been injured outside the pericardium lateral to the superior vena cava during any operation on the right lung, pressure on it in this pericardial recess will stop the bleeding. It is then usually possible to dissect out the pulmonary artery while compression is maintained by the assistant, so that the artery can be clamped and the bleeding controlled. The artery can then be ligated or sutured, when it has been dissected completely in the aortocaval recess.

When both veins and the artery have been

**Figure 25.3**

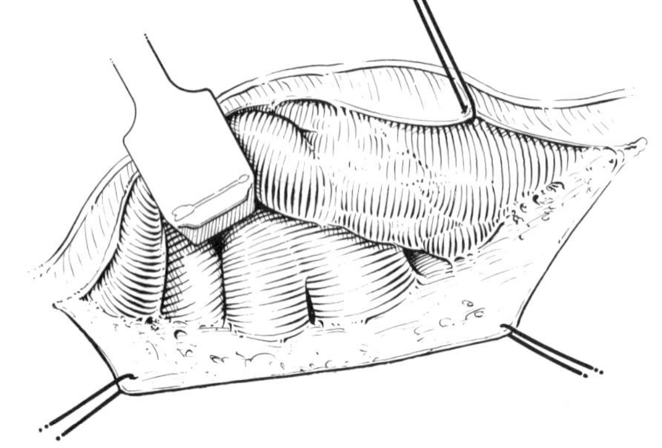

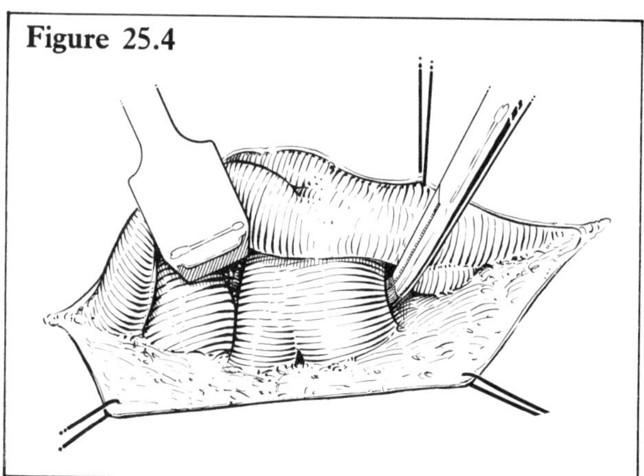

**Figure 25.4**

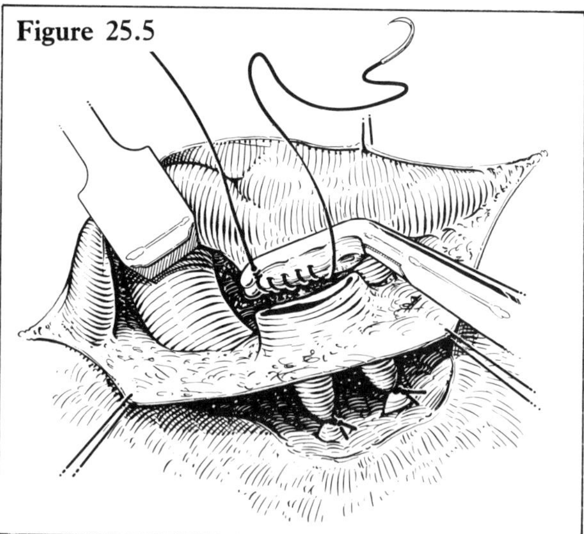

**Figure 25.5**

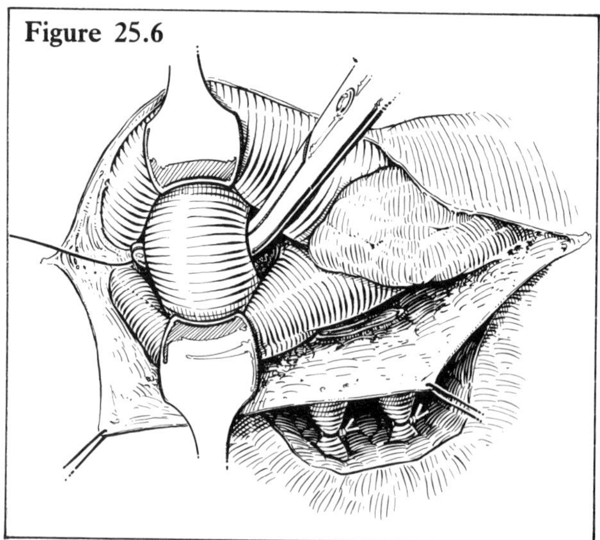

**Figure 25.6**

divided, the posterior layer of the pericardium is exposed. This is divided upwards as far as the pulmonary artery, thus exposing the anterior wall of the right main bronchus, which is secured as previously described and the lung is removed. The lymph nodes from the carinal and para-oesophageal regions are removed as described on p. 95.

The remaining defect in the pericardium may measure from 3 to 10 cm in diameter. Herniation of the heart can occur through this defect and therefore it must be closed. This can sometimes be achieved by approximation of the anterior and posterior cut edges, working from both ends with interrupted or continuous sutures. During this procedure a close watch must be kept on the systemic arterial and central venous pressures. A fall in arterial pressure or a rise in venous pressure indicates that the pericardial closure is causing cardiac compression, and an alternative method of closure must be used. Our preferred method is to use a piece of fine Marlex mesh cut to the appropriate size and shape, and sutured to the free edges of the pericardium with a 3/0 polypropylene suture (**Fig. 25.7**).

**Figure 25.7**

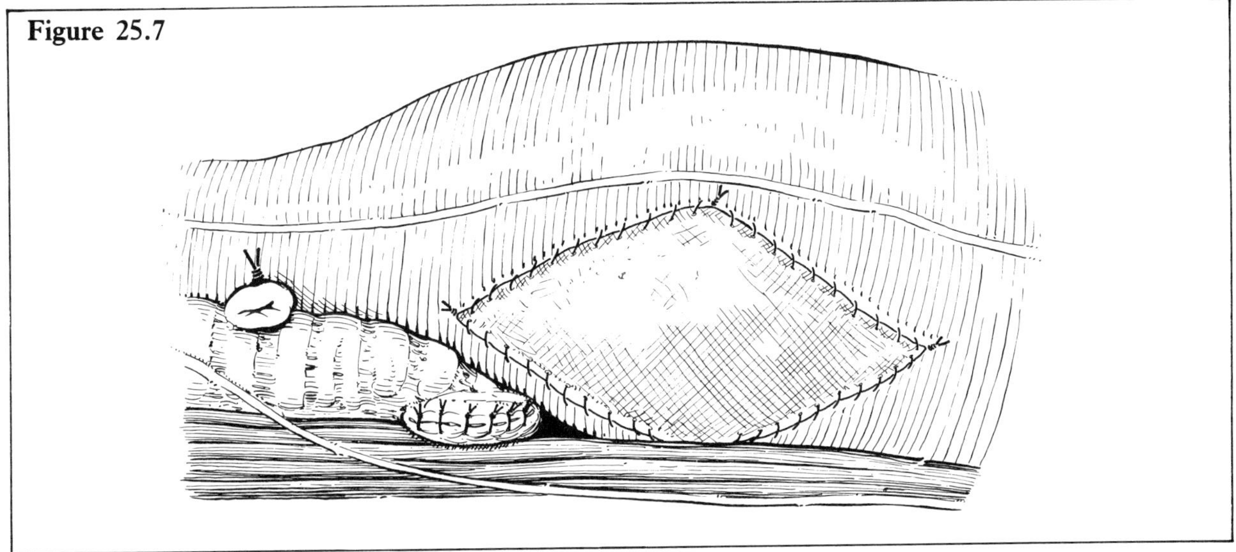

# 26 Left pneumonectomy

The patient lies on his or her right side. The incision is a left posterolateral thoracotomy (p. 24), and the pleural cavity is entered through the bed of the fifth rib. Any adhesions between the chest wall and the lung are divided, and the primary tumour in the lung is palpated to determine its size and extent. The pulmonary veins and bronchus are inspected in turn to determine whether they can be safely divided. If any one of these structures looks difficult to mobilize because of the extension of the tumour or its lymph nodes, it should be dissected first so that the patient is not subjected to an extensive dissection only to find that the lung cannot be removed. If tumour encroaches upon the vessels at the hilum the pericardium should be opened in preparation for an intrapericardial resection as described on p. 98.

The apex of the lung is grasped in Duval forceps and retracted downwards and backwards (**Fig. 26.1**). This exposes the phrenic nerve running down to the diaphragm anteriorly, and behind it the vagus nerve situated between the left common carotid and left subclavian arteries. The mediastinal pleura is incised over the left main pulmonary artery and the superior pulmonary vein immediately posterior to the left phrenic nerve. The left superior intercostal vein is ligated at the point where it reaches the descending thoracic aorta from the chest wall, and again where it enters the left innominate vein to prevent tearing a hole in the left innominate vein during retraction (**Fig. 26.2**).

The fatty tissue and accompanying lymph nodes in the superior mediastinum are dissected downwards towards the aortic arch and then over it as far down as the left pulmonary artery. The vagus and phrenic nerves must be carefully preserved. The left pulmonary artery and left superior pulmonary vein now come into view. As the vein lies anterior to the artery and obscures its lower margin, it is usually better to divide it first. The technique is the same as that described for the right lung (p. 95). A single proximal ligature together with individual ligatures for the peripheral branches are usually satisfactory, but a proximal clamp underrun with a 3/0 polypropylene suture gives greater security. Note that the lowest of the tributaries enters the main venous trunk at right angles and runs downwards on the anterior aspect of the upper lobe to reach the lingula (**Fig. 26.3**).

The left pulmonary artery is exposed. It should be dissected as far centrally as possible, to avoid the fragile branches which emerge from its inferior aspect. Once the pleural reflection has been opened it may be swept away from the artery with a dental swab mounted on a Roberts clamp (**Fig. 26.4**). A heavy thread ligature is passed around the artery centrally with the aid of a Semb forceps (**Fig. 26.5**).

**Figure 26.1**

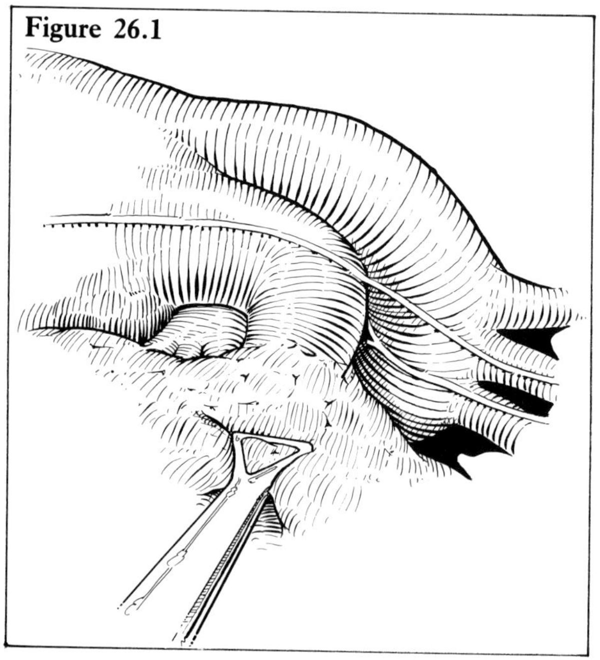

**Figure 26.2**

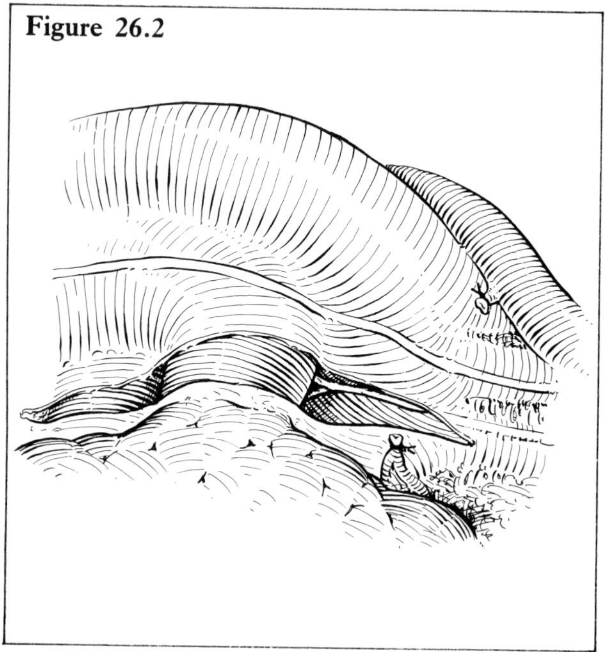

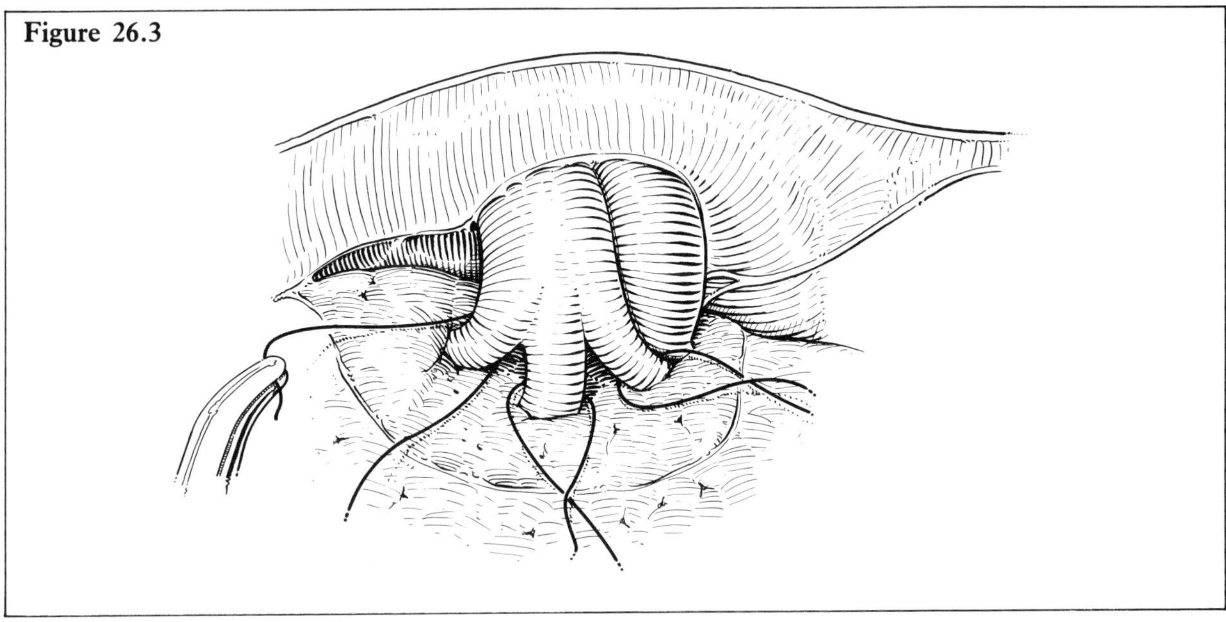

Figure 26.3

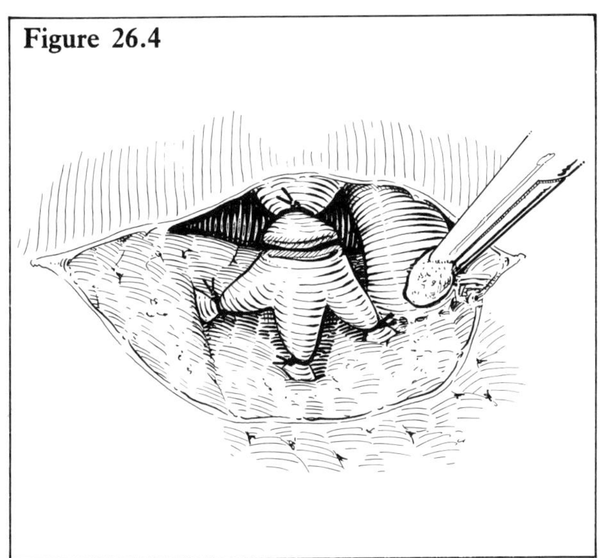

Figure 26.4

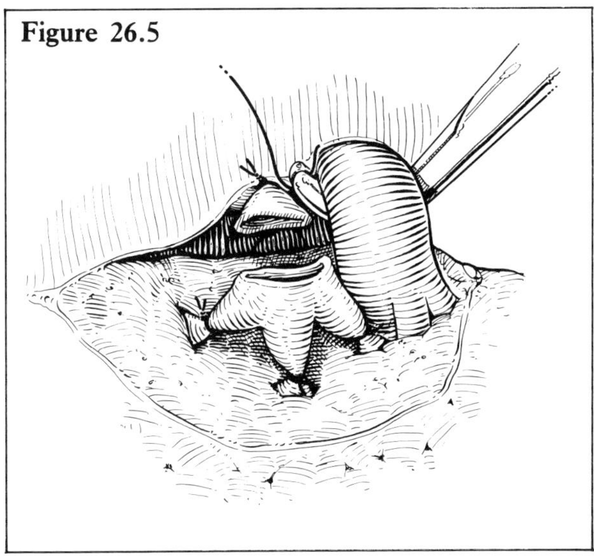

Figure 26.5

It is wise to dissect the distal end of the artery before the proximal ligature is tied; the reason for this is that tying the proximal ligatures puts the adjacent part of the artery under tension. An excessive amount of traction on the distal end is then likely to cause tearing where the ligature has been tied.

It may be necessary to expose and divide one or two of the upper lobe branches in order to obtain enough length of artery to permit a distal ligature to encircle it. The two ligatures are then tied as far apart as possible and the artery divided between them. This exposes the anterior aspect of the left main bronchus.

The inferior pulmonary vein is approached from the posterior aspect of the hilum. The lung is held up and the pulmonary ligament divided. Forward traction on the lung then exposes the inferior pulmonary vein and its two divisions. The oesophagus lies immediately behind it. The vein may be dissected with sharp instruments or encircled by a finger. The common basal and apical lower tributaries are isolated distally, and then the main trunk and branches are ligated with heavy linen thread (**Fig. 26.6**).

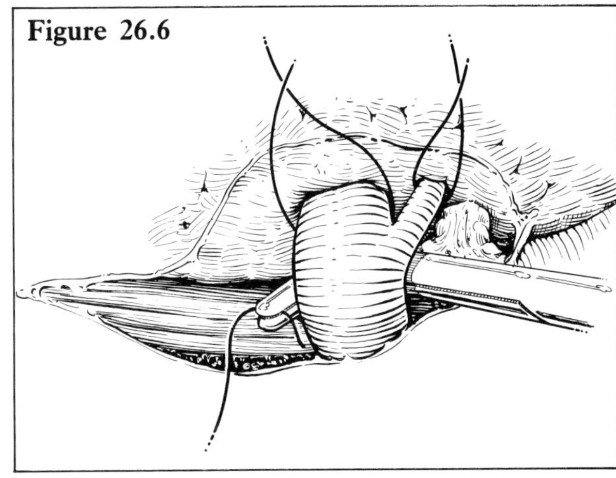

Figure 26.6

By pulling the lung posteroinferiorly the left main bronchus is exposed immediately above the vein. Its fascial sheath is picked up and opened. Blunt dissection inside this layer frees the bronchus from all surrounding tissue. A finger can then be passed around the bronchus and the lung elevated away from the mediastinal structures to allow the application of a bronchus clamp. To improve access to the carina the junction of the aortic arch and descending thoracic aorta is retracted backwards using Cummings' retractor (**Fig. 26.7**).

The anaesthetist is warned that the bronchus is to be clamped, and must be given time to withdraw the tube into the trachea. When the anaesthetist is ready the bronchus is clamped at its origin as close to the carina as possible. A second clamp is then placed distally on the bronchus 1 cm away from the first. The bronchus is divided with a knife 5 mm distal to the proximal clamp. Any secretions that emerge from the bronchus are immediately sucked away. The lung is removed, and the central end of the bronchus is closed with a 3/0 polypropylene suture as described on p. 96.

Finally, the lymph nodes of the subaortic fossa (i.e. those situated along the upper margin of the left main bronchus and in the left tracheobronchial angle) become accessible and can be removed by blunt dissection. Great care must be taken to identify the recurrent laryngeal nerve, which courses between these lymph nodes. It must be held out of the way with a dissecting swab while the lymph nodes are being removed. Bleeding arising from the small bronchial arteries that supply these lymph nodes should *not* be controlled with diathermy, as the recurrent laryngeal nerve is easily damaged. If the fossa is packed for five minutes this bleeding will usually cease. If it does not, then the vessel should be held in a haemostat and tied with a ligature.

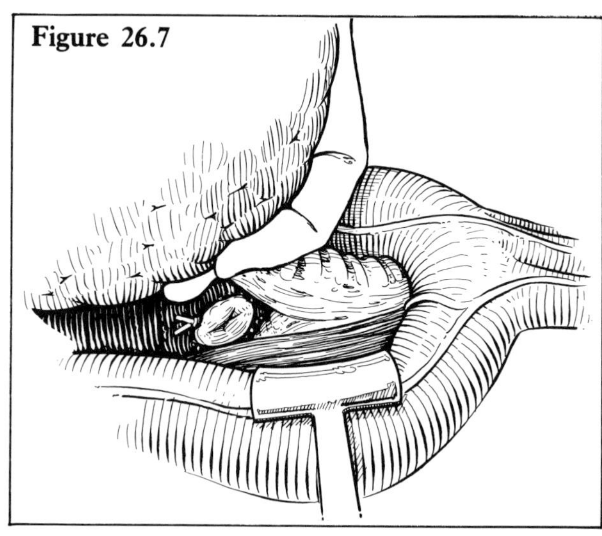
**Figure 26.7**

The aortic retractor is now shifted to a point just below the left main bronchus. This exposes the carinal lymph nodes lying behind the pericardium that overlies the back of the left atrium. These lymph nodes should be removed as far to the right as the origin of the right pulmonary veins, thus leaving a clear view of the medial wall of the right main bronchus.

Next, 500 ml of sterile water is placed in the pleural cavity and the anaesthetist is asked to raise the inflation pressure to 50 mmHg (7 kPa) for a short time. This test will reveal any leak from the bronchus or the stitch holes in it. Such leaks can be dealt with by the insertion of an additional suture, or by tamponading with adjacent tissue such as pericardium or oesophageal fascia.

The chest is now ready for closure as described for the right lung (p. 27).

# 27 Left intrapericardial pneumonectomy

The pericardium is opened by an incision posterior to and parallel with the left phrenic nerve. Superiorly, this incision continues to the limit of the pericardial reflection on the aortic arch overlying the ligamentum arteriosum. Inferiorly, it extends well below the inferior pulmonary vein. The left pulmonary artery is seen in the cranial part of the incision (**Fig. 27.1**).

To improve the mobility of the left pulmonary artery, the ligamentum arteriosum should be divided between ligatures. The fascia on either side of it (fibrous pericardium) is picked up and divided with scissors. Great care should be taken to preserve the vagus and recurrent laryngeal nerves. As dissection proceeds the ligamentum becomes well defined as a cord which is transected close to its aortic end. The fibrous tissue behind the upper border of the pulmonary artery is then picked up and divided (**Fig. 27.2**). This opens up the serous pericardial space on the deep surface of the artery.

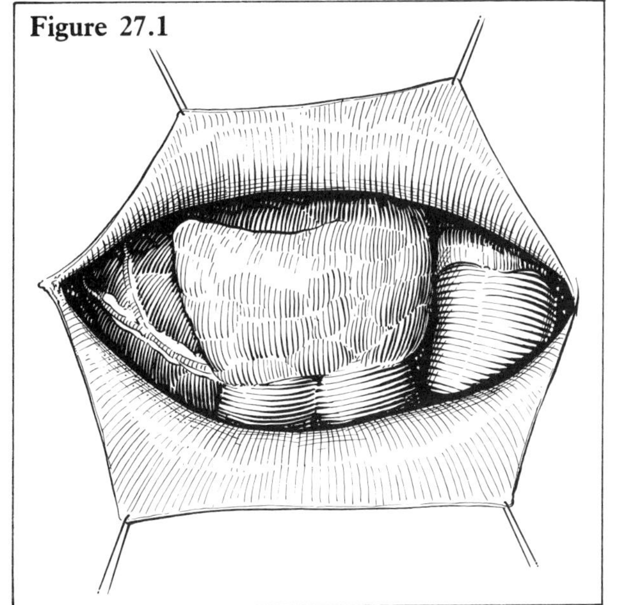

**Figure 27.1**

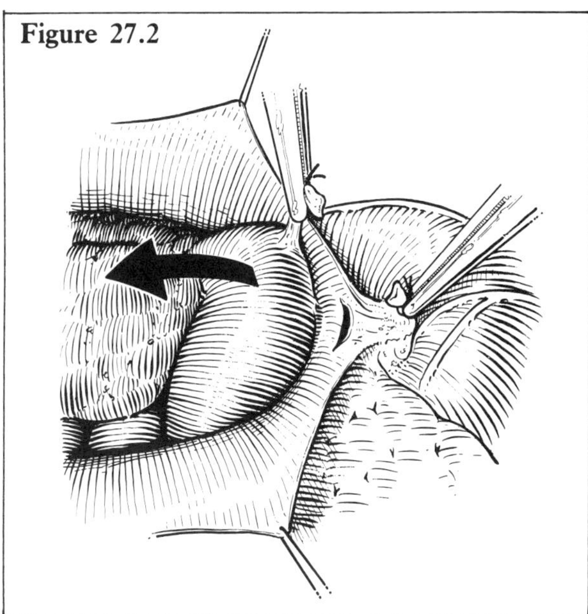

**Figure 27.2**

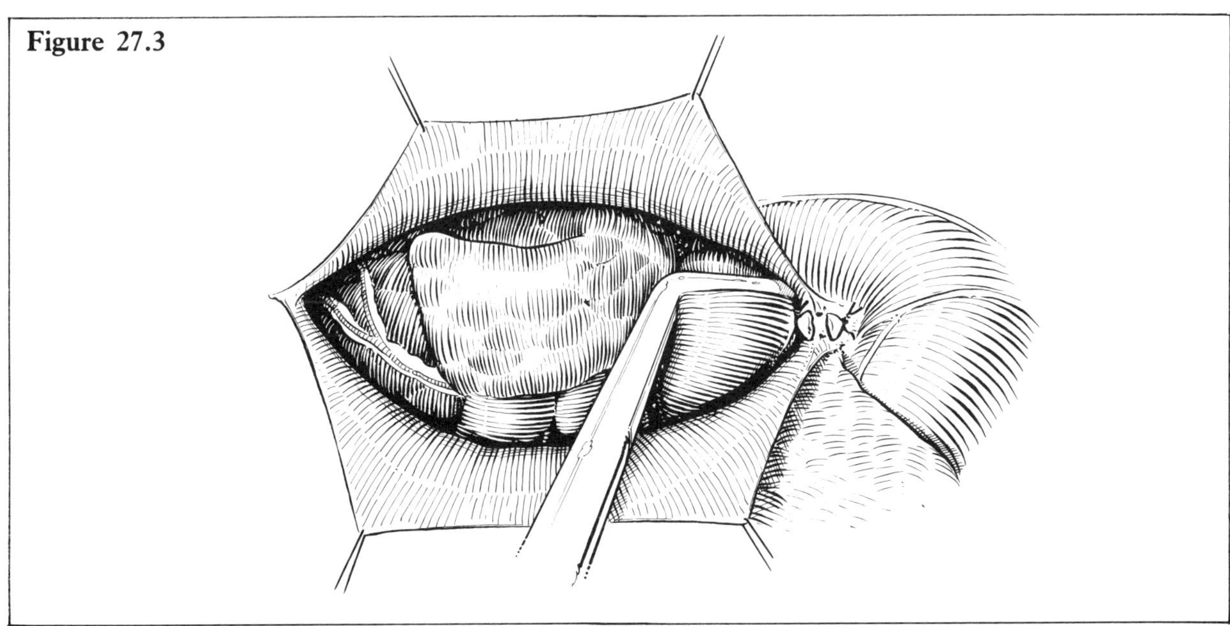

**Figure 27.3**

A finger is passed into it to emerge between the lower margin of the artery and the upper border of the superior pulmonary vein. It may be necessary to divide the fold of Marshall, which stretches from the junction of the superior pulmonary vein and the left atrium to the undersurface of the pulmonary artery. The pulmonary artery has then been fully mobilized.

The left pulmonary artery is occluded with two arterial clamps (**Fig. 27.3**), divided between them, and oversewn. The distal cut end is closed with a continuous suture of 4/0 polypropylene. When the clamp is removed the remaining stump of the artery retracts, so that the main pulmonary artery appears to continue into the right pulmonary artery.

There is no pericardial fold attaching the lower margin of the left inferior pulmonary vein to the parietal pericardium, so an instrument can be passed from below, close to the left atrium, to emerge above the upper margin of the left superior pulmonary vein. Both veins are then ligated distally. Centrally a clamp is applied to the wall of the left atrium, the veins divided and the central end closed with a continuous suture of 3/0 polypropylene as described on p. 95.

The posterior parietal pericardium is now incised behind the left atrium and the pulmonary veins. This will expose the left main bronchus, the trachea above it and the carina and oesophagus beneath it. The carinal lymph nodes may then be dissected out. The left main bronchus is divided at its origin between bronchus clamps. The lung can then be removed, and the central cut end of the bronchus closed with a continuous 3/0 polypropylene suture as described on p. 96.

For a description of how to close the opening in the pericardium, see p. 99.

# 28 Right upper lobectomy

This operation is carried out through a postero-lateral thoracotomy stripping the lower border of the fifth rib. The pleural cavity is opened, and the diagnosis and the site and extent of the disease confirmed. The pulmonary veins, pulmonary artery and upper lobe bronchus are palpated to ensure that they can be divided clear of the disease.

The lung is retracted backwards to expose the anterior surface of the hilum. The right superior pulmonary vein overlies the right pulmonary artery (**Fig. 28.1**). The vein is dissected along its upper and lower margins until the upper and middle lobe tributaries have been clearly identified. The middle lobe vein is the lowest tributary and runs downwards at almost 90 degrees to the main trunk (**Fig. 28.1**). An interlobar vein usually drains into the junction between the upper and middle lobes. This vein may be safely divided, as it has no effect on venous drainage from the middle lobe. The dissection should be carried out at a little distance from the pericardium to avoid opening it. It must be remembered that the posterior segmental vein enters the deep surface of the upper lobe vein and can be injured when passing an instrument behind the latter. Immediately behind the upper lobe vein lies the descending limb of the right pulmonary artery. An instrument passed beneath the vein must therefore stay closely applied to it to avoid injury to the artery. This is ensured by dissecting within the fascial sheath around the vein. A vascular clamp is applied centrally to the superior pulmonary vein and then each of the tributaries are tied separately. This is necessary because the vein is short and its tributaries diverge so rapidly that a distal ligature is liable to slip off. The vein is divided with scissors and closed with a 3/0 polypropylene suture. A stapling device may be used to close the vein prior to division.

Immediately beneath the divided superior pulmonary vein, the pulmonary artery runs down to enter the greater fissure. Its first branch arises from the upper border of the main artery behind the superior vena cava. It divides into two branches, one for the anterior segment and one for the apical segment of the upper lobe. The upper lobe artery is ligated centrally close to its origin. Each of the two segmental branches is ligated separately and divided (**Fig. 28.1**).

The anterior margin of the descending limb of the right pulmonary artery sometimes gives off one or two small, additional branches which enter the right upper lobe. These are thin-walled and tear easily if they are stretched. They are best controlled with a fine suture.

The posterior segmental artery arises from the main pulmonary artery as it crosses the lesser

**Figure 28.1**

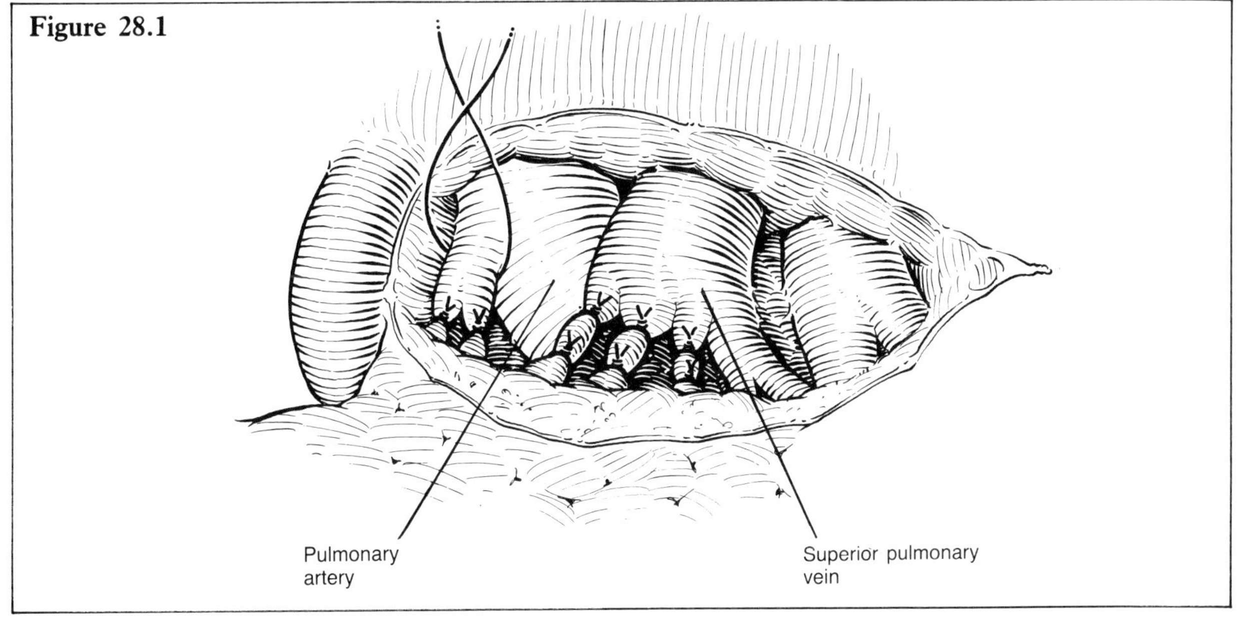

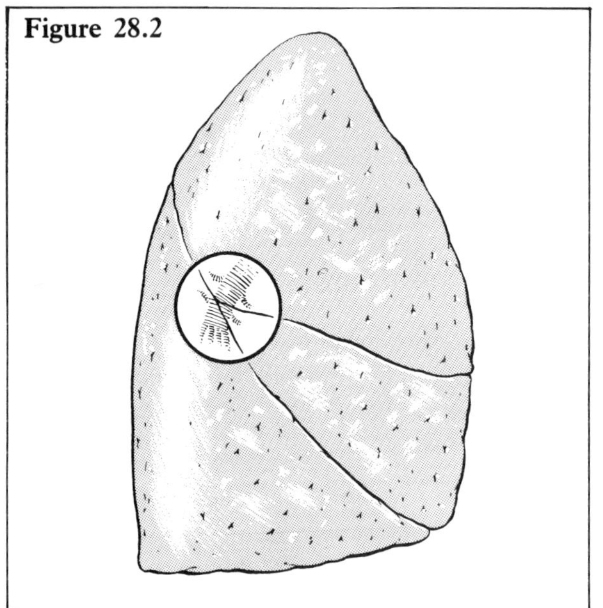
Figure 28.2

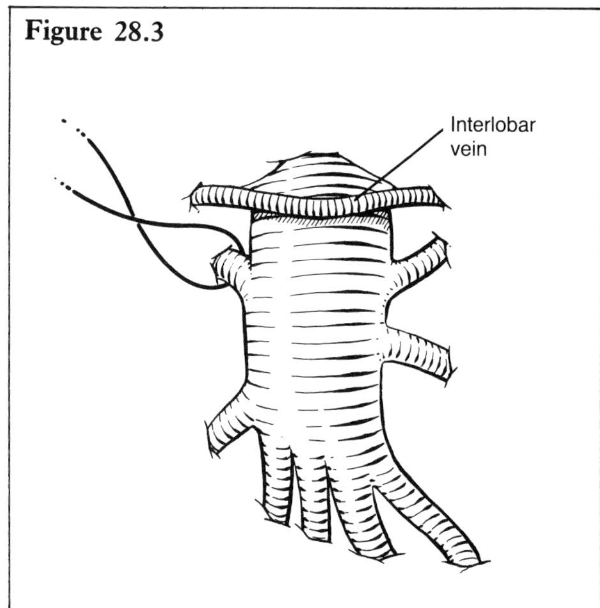

Figure 28.3

fissure, and is found by opening the junction of the greater and lesser fissures (**Fig. 28.2**). It runs upwards and backwards from this point to lie posterior to the upper lobe bronchus. To locate it, the sheath of the pulmonary artery must be opened and dissection continued within the sheath. If the fissure is well developed the artery can be secured here. However, it must be dissected for some distance distally, since it is not unusual to find a common origin of the posterior segmental artery and the artery to the apical segment of the right lower lobe (**Figs. 28.3–28.5**). Unless care is taken to determine the distal distribution of the artery arising from the fissure, there is a danger of occluding the lower lobe apical segmental artery.

If the fissure is absent or incomplete, dissection within it to search for the posterior segmental artery is best avoided. The artery can be secured after division of the upper lobe bronchus.

In order to identify the upper lobe bronchus clearly, the lung should be retracted forwards and the pleura over the posterior surface of the main bronchus incised. The vagal branches and the accompanying bronchial artery to the upper lobe are divided. The upper margin of the upper lobe bronchus may then be easily identified by following the lateral border of the trachea and upper margin of the right main bronchus. The lower margin can be found by identifying the lymph node that lies between the lower margin of the upper lobe bronchus and the intermediate bronchus (**Fig. 28.6**). The accompanying bronchial artery (omitted from the figure for clarity) is secured with diathermy. Blunt dissection in the angle between the intermediate bronchus and the upper lobe bronchus allows a plane to be entered close to the bronchial cartilage. It is now possible to pass an instrument round the upper lobe bronchus. The bronchus can

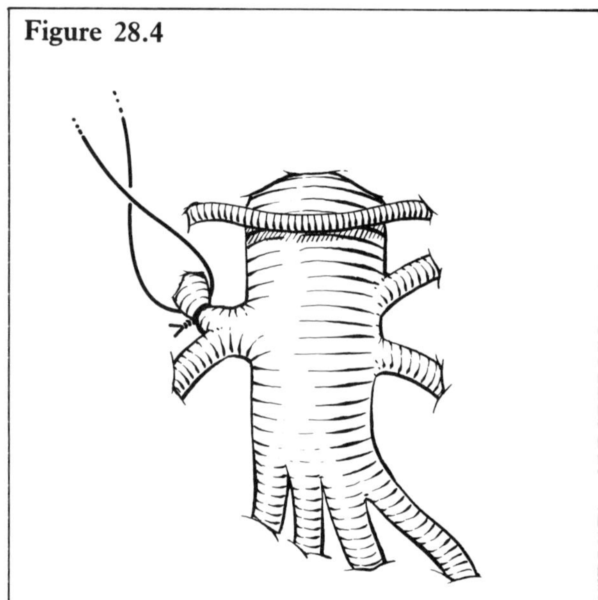
Figure 28.4

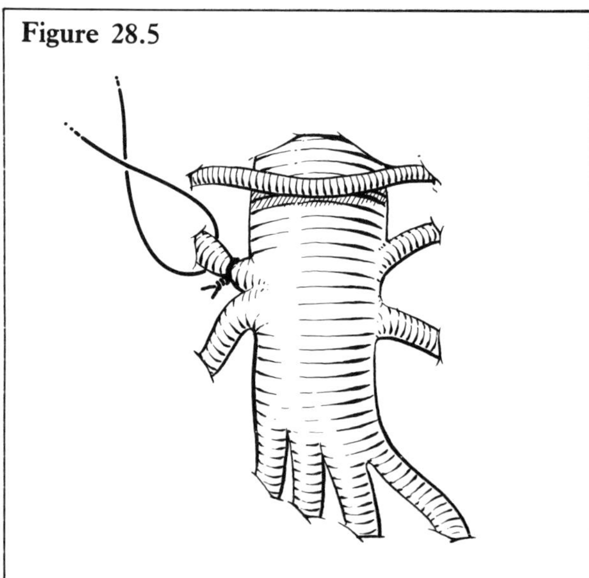
Figure 28.5

**Figure 28.6**

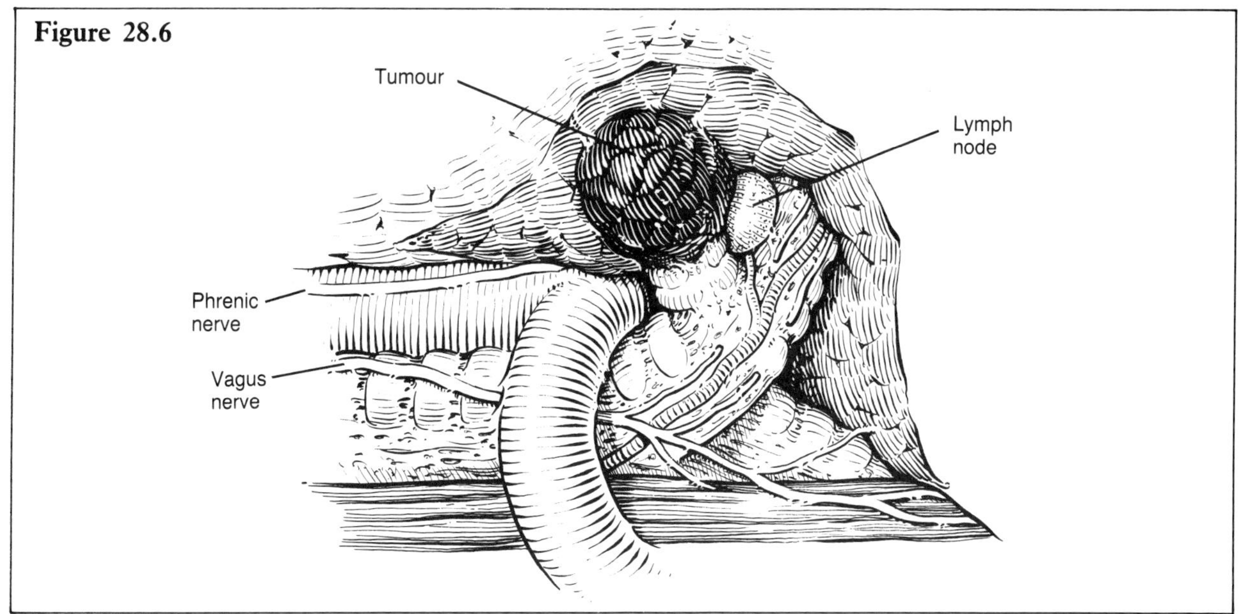


be divided after stapling it closed, or it may simply be cut across after clamping distally; in this case a cuff of about 7–10 mm should be left. Secretions within the bronchus are sucked out. The bronchus can be closed with any non-absorbable suture material. Monofilament material such as stainless steel wire or polypropylene is preferable. A continuous horizontal mattress suture in one direction with an over-and-over stitch in the opposite direction gives a very secure closure.

If the posterior segmental artery has not been divided by this stage, traction on the clamped distal end of the bronchus will reveal it arising from the posterolateral aspect of the pulmonary artery as it descends to the lower lobe. A little dissection here will soon reveal whether the apical lower artery arises from this trunk; very often the origin of the apical lower artery, immediately below this point, is now obvious. The assistant must be warned not to exert too much traction on the bronchial clamp as it is quite easy to tear the artery. The posterior segmental artery is then ligated and divided.

The bronchus clamp is lifted further forward and the medial aspect of the pulmonary artery scanned for any other small branches entering the upper lobe, which are then divided. If the fissures are complete there are now no attachments to the lobe other than the visceral pleura which can be cut. However, the fissure is usually incomplete and may even be completely absent. The lobe must then be separated by traction.

Unless there is fibrosis in the interlobar plane, the upper and middle lobes will separate very easily. Initially the venous branches and strands of fibrous tissue adjacent to the upper lobe bronchus should be divided with scissors. The plane of incision should be immediately adjacent to the wall of the bronchus. The bronchus clamp holding the distal bronchus is then drawn upwards, while pressure is applied with a swab to the region of the apical segment of the lower lobe. It is important that the movement is much more one of pressure downwards than of traction upwards. (It is difficult to teach this manoeuvre and it has to be learned by experience.) It may also be advantageous to move the index finger along the edge of the upper lobe into the plane between it and the adjacent lobes. This, without tearing into the lung, will easily separate the interdigitated alveoli.

Great care must be exercised as the plane of dissection moves from the lower lobe (i.e. from the posterior end of the greater fissure) to the middle lobe (i.e. into the lesser fissure). There is a danger here that adherent lymph nodes may cause the traction to be transmitted to the middle lobe arteries and these may be torn out of the pulmonary artery. Scissors should be used to snip away the attachments of these lymph nodes, taking them with the specimen, so that they cannot exert traction on the pulmonary artery, and pressure should be downwards on to the pulmonary artery and the middle lobe, so that the middle lobe arteries are never under tension.

As separation reaches the outer limits of the lobe, it is convenient to spread the upper lobe over the margin of the wound so that the interlobar surfaces of the middle and lower lobes are stretched out. In this way bleeding interlobar venous branches, which will be seen spreading in a fan-like pattern on the interlobar surfaces, can be secured with diathermy, and any torn small bronchi suture-ligated. When the raw surfaces are quite dry, the remaining pleural attachment of the upper lobe is divided.

It may be helpful to carry out this separation with the remaining lung inflated, so as to define the interlobar plane, although this is not always effective because of the phenomenon of collateral air drift. However, once the lobe has been removed the remaining lobes should be inflated for two reasons. First, inflation results in a considerable diminution of bleeding from the raw surface, and second, it enables identification of any small torn bronchi which can then be sutured.

As in all cases where a large bronchus has been divided, 500 ml of warm saline should be placed in the pleural cavity and the lung inflated to a pressure of about 50 mmHg (7 kPa) while the bronchial suture line is observed to ensure that it is watertight.

Prior to closure, it is customary to divide the pulmonary ligament from the diaphragm up to the inferior pulmonary vein. It is said that this allows the lower lobe to rise up in the chest and fill the remaining pleural space.

If the fissure between the middle and lower lobes is complete, the middle lobe can now be seen to be suspended on a narrow pedicle; the lobe may therefore rotate, causing torsion and obstruction of the vascular pedicle which may lead to venous thrombosis. This can be prevented by securing the middle lobe to the lower lobe at two or three points along the outer margin of the greater fissure (**Fig. 28.7**). We prefer to do this by placing apposed artery forceps at these points and then tying together the minute portions of lung held in the tips of the forceps, a technique less likely to cause an air leak than the penetration of a suture.

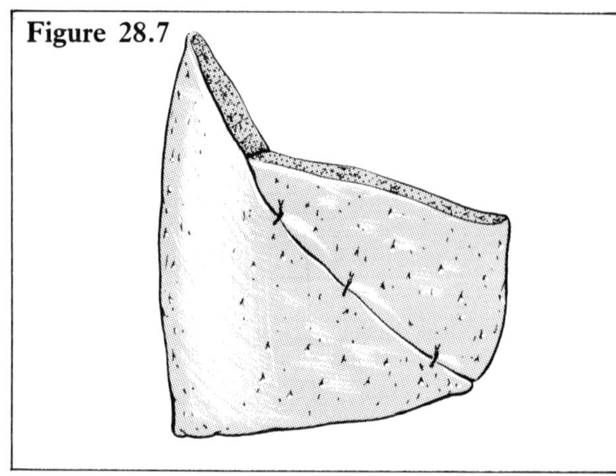

**Figure 28.7**

Two drains are placed in the pleural space. It is probably worth while ensuring that one of these is located in the area in which a space is most likely to be found in the postoperative period, namely towards the apex anteriorly. If one of the tubes does not sit comfortably in this position it should be fixed there by a suture through the parietal pleura. The chest is then closed as described on p.27.

# 29 Middle lobectomy

Middle lobectomy is performed through a right, fifth intercostal space, posterolateral thoracotomy. An anterolateral approach might seem to be attractive, but the pathological conditions involving the middle lobe that necessitate its removal are likely to make this a difficult and dangerous procedure. Adequate access to the main pulmonary artery is therefore imperative.

The lung is retracted backwards and the lower part of the superior pulmonary vein exposed. The middle lobe vein is isolated and traced distally into the lobe (**Fig. 29.1**). Immediately above it the small interlobar vein is identified. The middle lobe vein is divided between ligatures. The central ligature should not be tied so far proximally as to allow the possibility of narrowing of the upper division of the vein; this can lead to thrombosis of the vein and infarction of the upper lobe.

Immediately beneath the vein, the middle lobe bronchus is identified. Enlarged lymph nodes are usually found between the lower margin of the middle lobe bronchus and the anterolateral aspect of the lower lobe bronchus. These should be removed by sharp dissection, the numerous bronchial arteries in the region being coagulated with diathermy. When the lower edge of the bronchus has been cleared in this way, attention should be directed towards the upper edge of the middle lobe bronchus. The dissection here should keep very close to the wall of the bronchus because the middle lobe artery or arteries lie immediately above it.

A right-angled clamp is passed round the middle lobe bronchus, and the dissection carried centrally to the origin of the bronchus from the intermediate bronchus. The distal end is clamped and the bronchus divided about 5 mm from its origin. To prevent retraction of the bronchus it is often convenient to divide it halfway across and then insert the first bronchial suture. This should be of soft material such as Mersilene (or an absorbable suture such as polygalactin) and not wire or polypropylene, the projecting ends of which could penetrate the adjacent lower lobe pulmonary artery. When tied, the suture may be left long for traction at this stage.

There may be one or two separate middle lobe arteries. These are clearly seen when the bronchus has been divided, and they are carefully isolated and divided. Distally it is usually necessary to ligate the two branches separately. This technique avoids the difficulty of having to expose the pulmonary artery in the depths of a fused fissure, which can be a bloody, time-consuming and even dangerous procedure.

If the greater fissure is more or less complete,

**Figure 29.1**

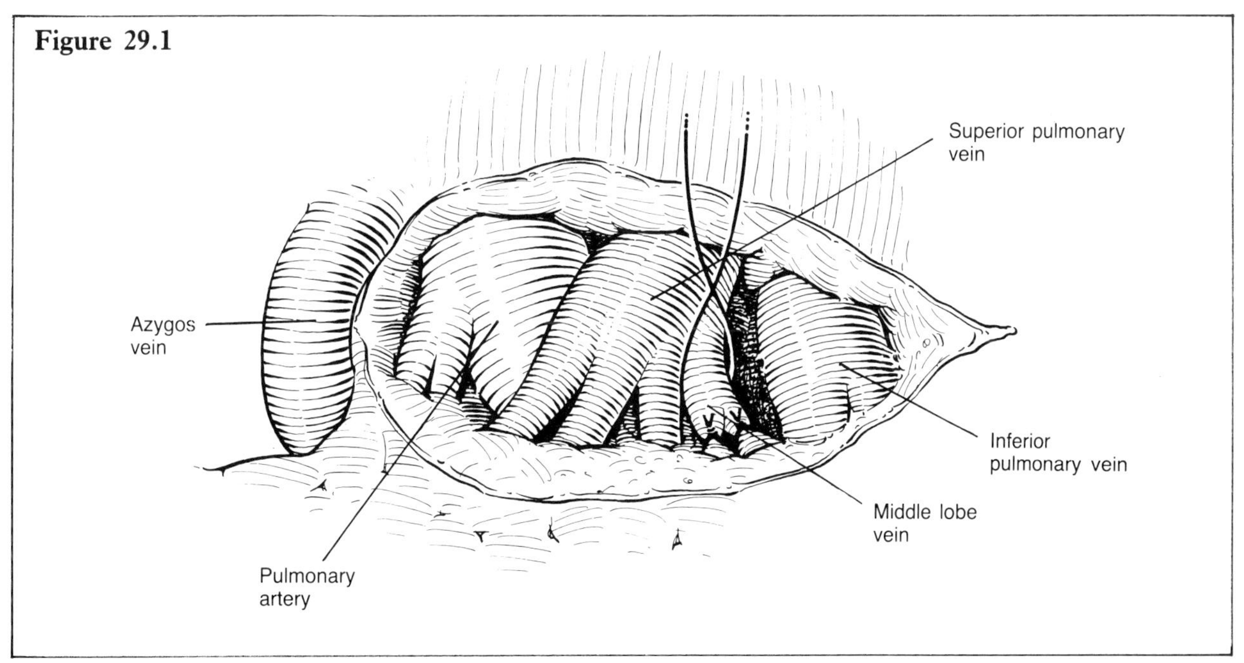

the middle lobe artery can be identified by incising the pleura and then the sheath of the pulmonary artery at the posterior angle of the middle lobe. Here the origins of the posterior segmental, apical lower and middle lobe arteries are found together, the middle lobe arteries being directed anteriorly. They are dissected out, ligated and divided. The bronchus is found immediately below them (**Fig. 29.2**).

Because of the partial fusion of one or other fissure, the removal of the middle lobe is usually achieved by traction. The clamp holding the distal end of the middle lobe bronchus is elevated, and veins and bands of fibrous tissue closely attached to the bronchus are divided with scissors. Pressure on the upper and lower lobes, and steady traction on the middle lobe, will gradually free it, until finally only the visceral pleura remains to be divided.

In some cases of non-malignant middle lobe disease, fibrosis extends beyond the fissures. It may then be necessary to divide bands of fibrous tissue and small bronchi by sharp dissection, securing the cut ends with artery forceps and subsequently ligating or suture-ligating them.

The upper and lower lobes are inflated and any visible cut bronchi are suture-ligated. Haemostasis on the cut surfaces is achieved with diathermy. The bleeding usually stops when the lobes have been inflated.

**Figure 29.2**

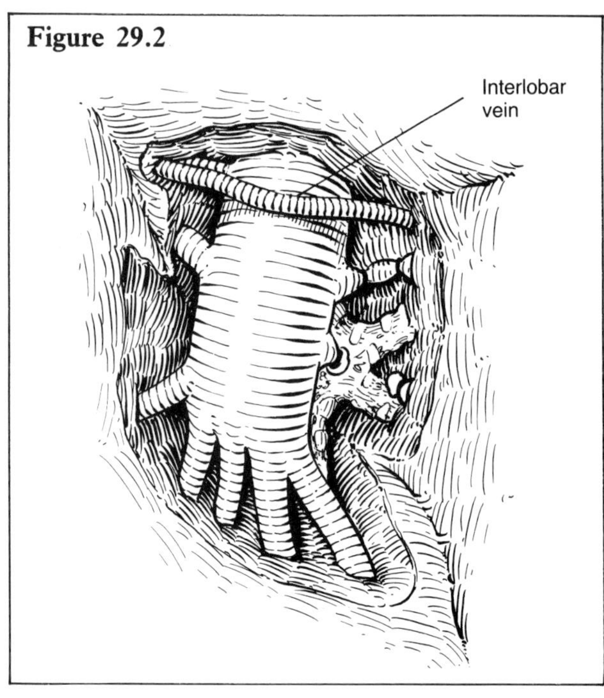

# 30 Middle and right lower lobectomy

The chest is entered through a right, fifth intercostal space posterolateral thoracotomy.

If the greater fissure is more or less complete, the dissection should begin by exposing the pulmonary artery. A lymph node in the depths of the fissure marks the site of the pulmonary artery. The sheath of the artery is picked up and incised, revealing the strikingly white wall of the vessel. The opening in the sheath is extended both proximally and distally to display the arterial branches. The middle lobe arterial branches arise anteriorly, almost at a right angle to the main artery. The apical lower segmental artery emerges from the posterior aspect of the main trunk, and runs at first parallel to the artery that supplies the basal segments. More proximally the posterior segmental artery arises from the lateral aspect of the pulmonary artery and disappears beneath the superior pulmonary vein. In order to leave an adequate cuff on the pulmonary artery, it is usually necessary to ligate the common basal, apical lower and middle lobe arteries separately (**Fig. 30.1**).

If the fissure is obliterated, the dissection begins with the inferior pulmonary vein, accessible from the anterior or the posterior aspect of the lung. To identify the inferior pulmonary vein the pulmonary ligament is divided and its vessels secured with diathermy (see **Fig. 24.8** on p. 95). This incision is continued up to the lower margin of the inferior pulmonary vein. The lung is then held forward and the inferior pulmonary vein dissected out, together with its apical lower and common basal branches. The vein is divided using heavy ligatures or a stapler. Its exposure from an anterior approach is shown in **Fig. 30.2**.

**Figure 30.1**

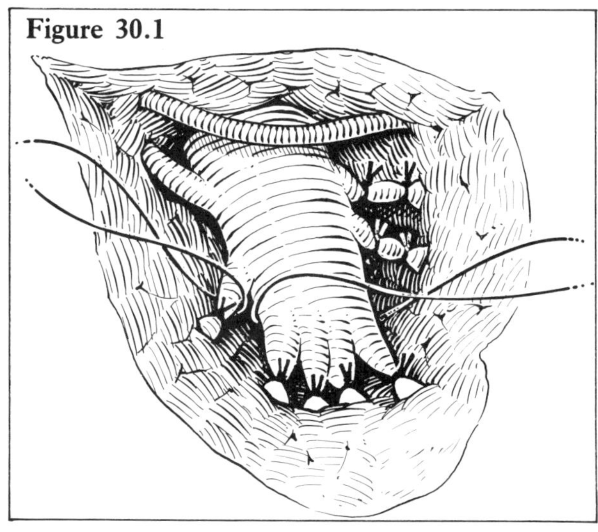

The middle lobe vein is identified next and divided at its origin. This is the lowest branch of the superior pulmonary vein, arising anteriorly in conjunction with the interlobar vein between right upper and middle lobes (**Fig. 30.2**).

**Figure 30.2**

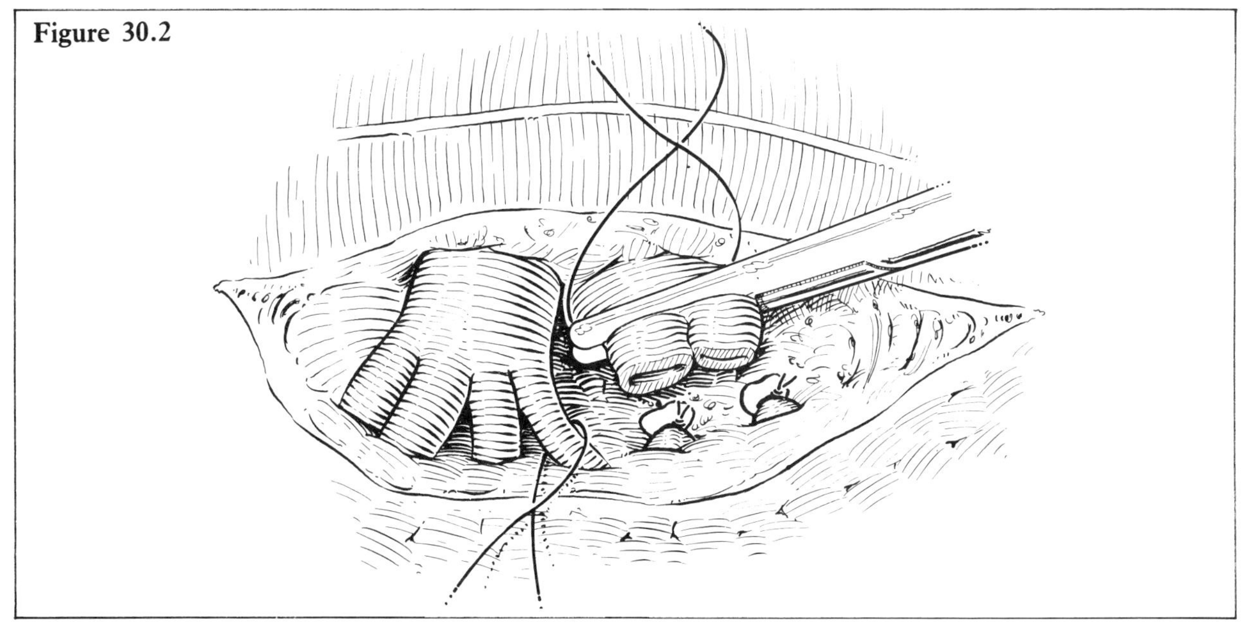

It is often convenient at this stage to separate the apical segment of the lower lobe from the posterior segment of the upper lobe. This is done by introducing an artery forceps through the fissure below the point where the pulmonary artery has been divided, and allowing it to emerge posteriorly between the upper lobe bronchus and the intermediate bronchus. There is only some loose areolar tissue in this region. A finger is then passed along this track and, with the aid of a little sharp dissection with scissors, the two lobes can be separated quite easily. If a small portion of lung resists separation, it can be divided between clamps and the two portions ligated, or sealed with a stapling gun.

The lower lobe is held forward and the vagal nerve branches and bronchial arteries supplying the lobe identified and divided as they pass over the back of the bronchus. The intermediate bronchus is now visible and the lymph node between it and the lower margin of the upper lobe bronchus can be identified (**Fig. 30.3**). This lymph node is dissected away from both bronchi. Its bed exposes the plane in which an instrument can be passed round the intermediate bronchus, which is then divided 7 mm beyond the lower margin of the upper lobe bronchus after applying a clamp distally (**Fig. 30.4**).

A suction catheter is then passed into the right upper lobe and right main bronchi through the open intermediate bronchus to remove secretions. The bronchial stump is closed as described on p. 96. Alternatively, the intermediate bronchus may be closed by stapling.

The middle and lower lobes are now removed. Traction is exerted on the clamp on the intermediate bronchus, while pressure is applied to the upper lobe. The middle lobe now separates easily from the anterior segment of the right upper lobe. Before the separation is completed all bleeding vessels are secured by diathermy, and small bronchi leaking air are ligated. The carinal lymph nodes and right paratracheal nodes are dissected out, mainly for staging purposes.

The integrity of the bronchial suture line is tested by inflation to 50 mmHg (7 kPa) after placing 500 ml of warm saline in the pleural cavity. Two drains are placed in the pleural space, one of these being fixed in the paravertebral gutter (where any residual space is likely to persist).

**Figure 30.3**

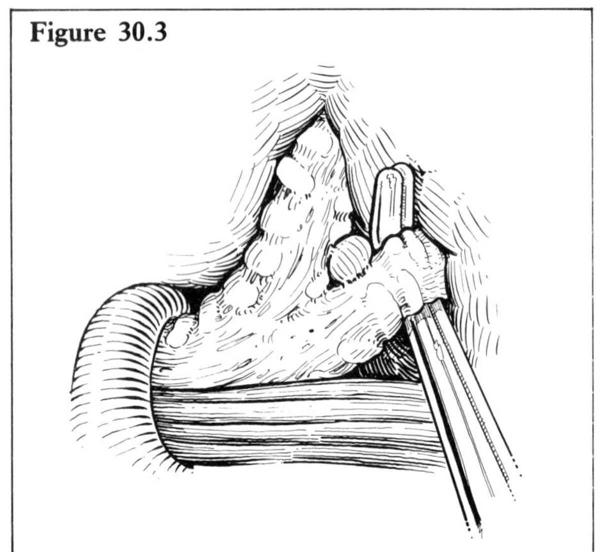

**Figure 30.4**

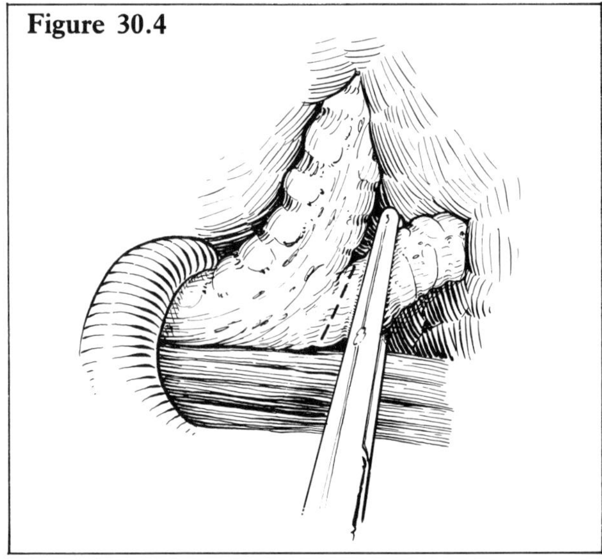

# 31 Right lower lobectomy

The chest is entered through a posterolateral thoracotomy above the sixth rib. To help to spread the ribs without injuring them, a short segment of the posterior end of the sixth rib may be excised with rib shears.

The pulmonary ligament is divided and the vessels within it are ligated and divided. The pleural reflections at the hilum are divided on either side of the inferior pulmonary vein. The superior margin of the vein is identified and after a little dissection a curved forceps can be insinuated beneath it. Ligatures are passed around it and tied, and the vein divided (**Fig. 31.1**). The proximal end is oversewn with a 3/0 polypropylene suture. The vein can also be approached from in front and below (**Fig. 31.2**).

Next, the confluence of the greater and lesser fissures is opened to reveal the pulmonary artery

**Figure 31.1**

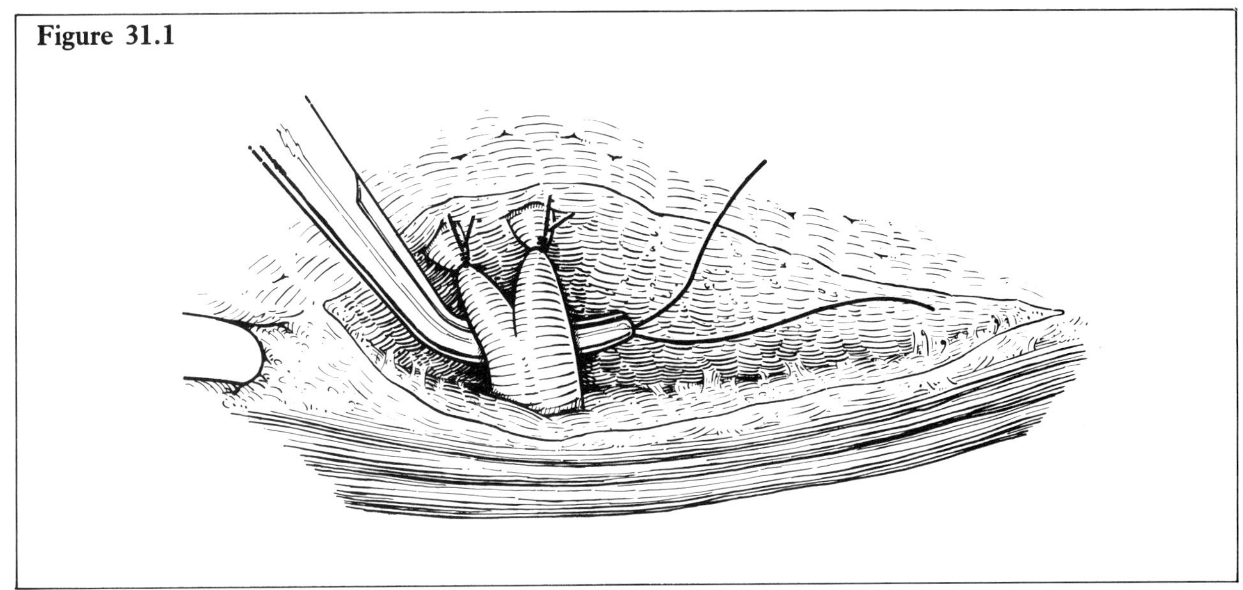

**Figure 31.2**

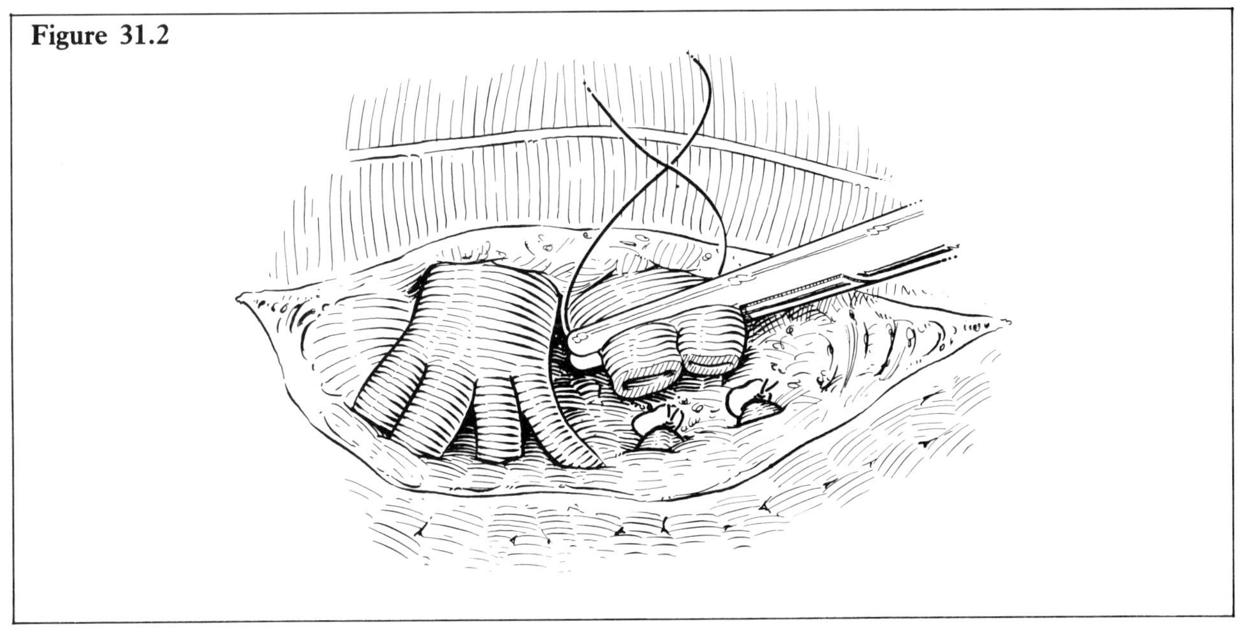

in its depths (see **Fig. 29.2** on p. 110). The branches to the middle lobe can be seen running medially (**Fig. 31.3**). These vessels must be preserved. The branches to the basal segments are dissected free from the pulmonary parenchyma by sharp dissection. Ligatures are passed around the segmental arteries and tied, and the vessels divided. The apical lower segmental artery often arises more posteriorly in the greater fissure. This vessel may be missed in the initial dissection. If this is so, care should be taken not to tear it when the lobe is finally being separated from the remaining lung. The common anomalies of this vessel are described on p. 106.

The lower lobe bronchus can now be identified in the depths of the fissure. It is usually possible to secure the common basal bronchus with a single bronchial clamp (**Fig. 31.3**). If the basal bronchi arise early it may be necessary to deal with each segmental bronchus individually. The apical segmental bronchus of the right lower lobe must be divided individually, as it usually arises from the main bronchial stem opposite the middle lobe orifice (**Fig. 31.4**). If it is possible to secure the lower lobe bronchus with one clamp, it must be placed obliquely to avoid narrowing the middle lobe bronchus (**Fig. 31.5**). The divided bronchus is then oversewn with a 3/0 polygalactin suture.

**Figure 31.3**

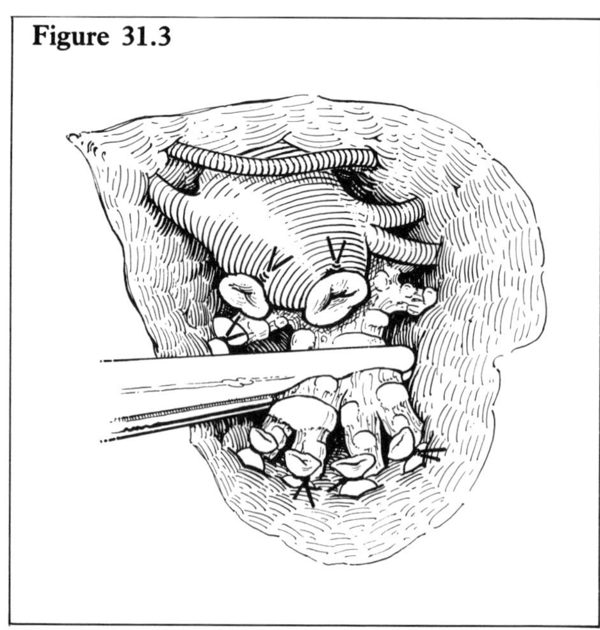

The bronchial stump is tested by asking the anaesthetist to inflate the lungs at a pressure of 50 $cmH_2O$ (4.9 kPa) after filling the pleural space with sterile saline.

All subcarinal and paratracheal lymph nodes are removed for histological examination for staging purposes.

The chest is closed as described on p. 27.

**Figure 31.4**

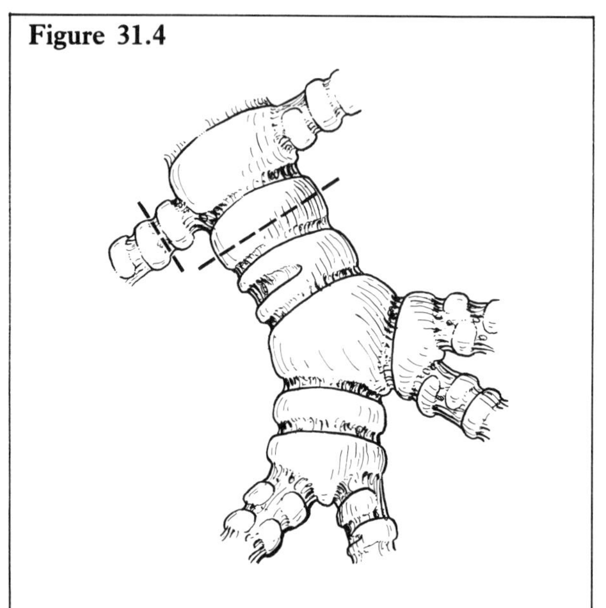

**Figure 31.5**

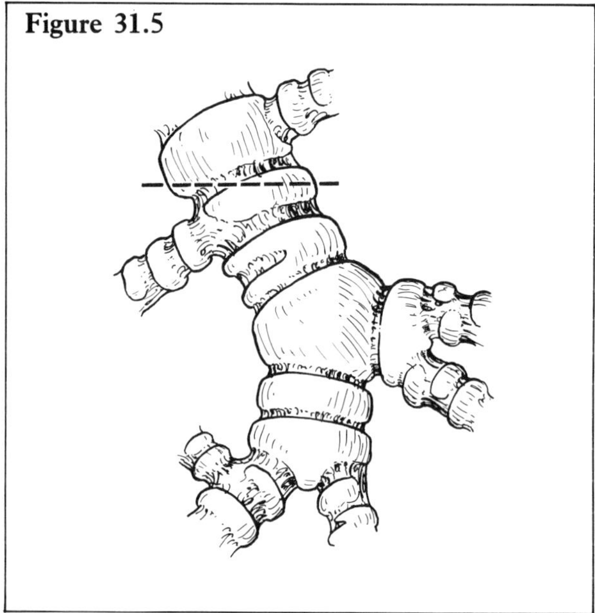

# 32 Left upper lobectomy

The pleural cavity is entered through a left posterolateral thoracotomy, stripping the periosteum from the lower border of the fifth rib. Adhesions between the lung and the parietal pleura are divided and the apex of the lung is retracted downwards and laterally. The mediastinal pleura is incised behind the phrenic nerve and over the pulmonary artery, which is the highest structure in the hilum of the lung.

As the superior pulmonary vein lies anteriorly, it is often easier to divide it before dealing with the branches of the pulmonary artery to the upper lobe. The central end of the vein is covered by a recess of pericardium; this should be opened first (**Fig. 32.1**) to reveal the segmental tributaries, as the main vessel is quite short. The lowest branch runs downwards at right angles to the main trunk and drains the lingula. The dissection of the vein is begun distally (**Fig. 32.2**). Each tributary is mobilized and a ligature placed around it, so that

**Figure 32.1**

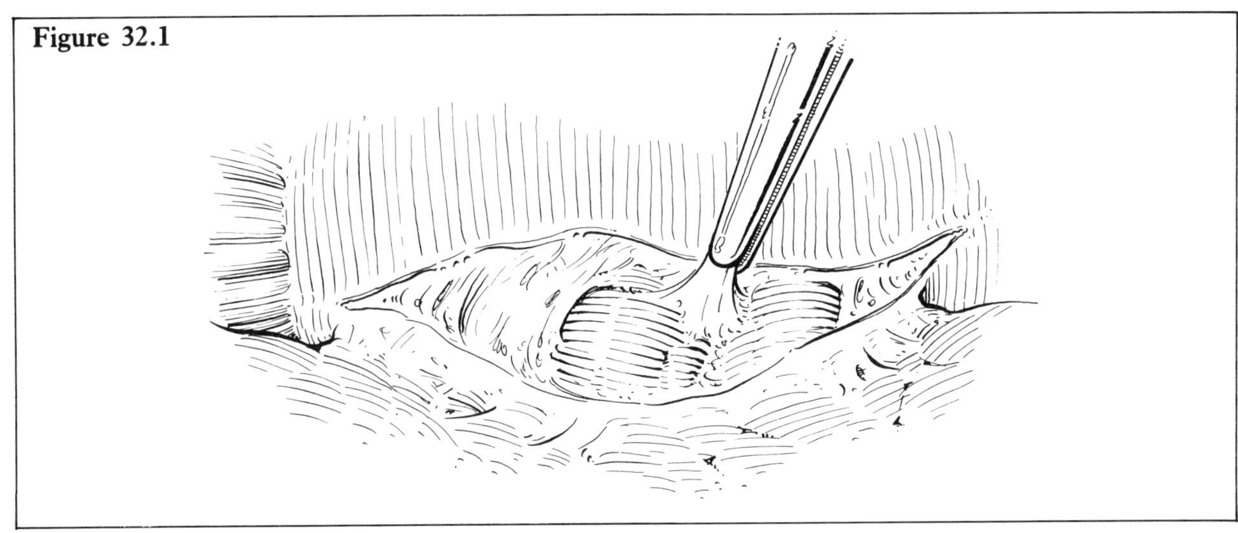

**Figure 32.2**

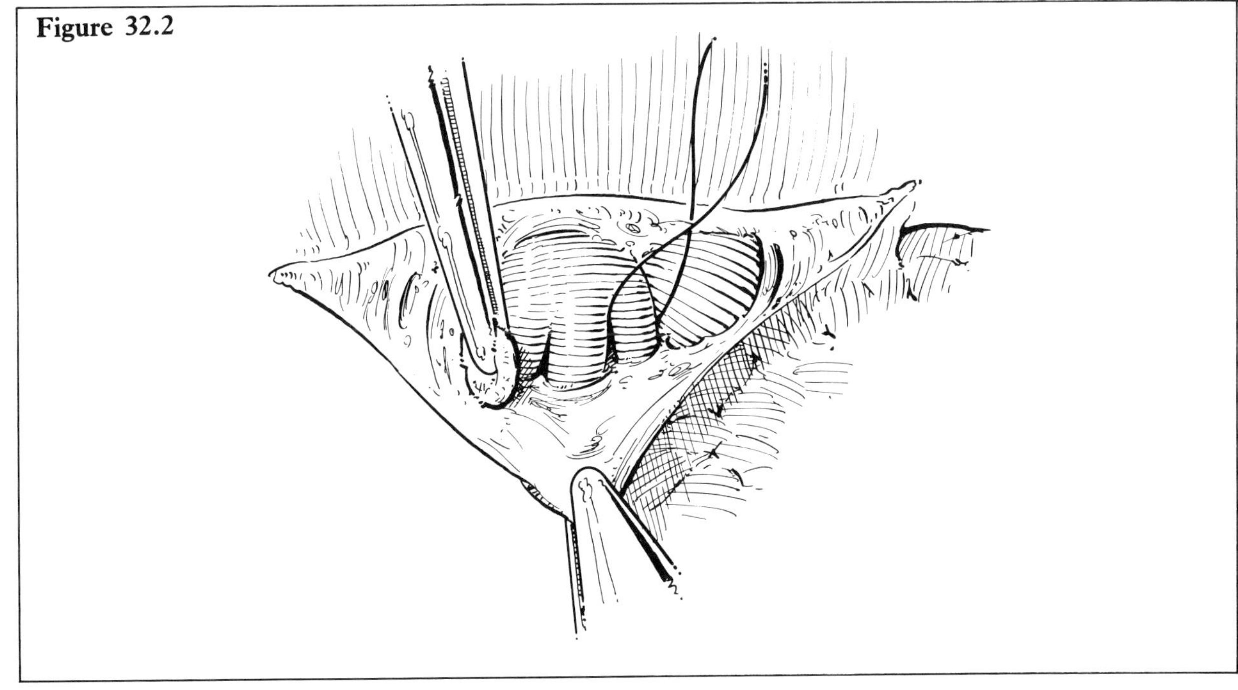

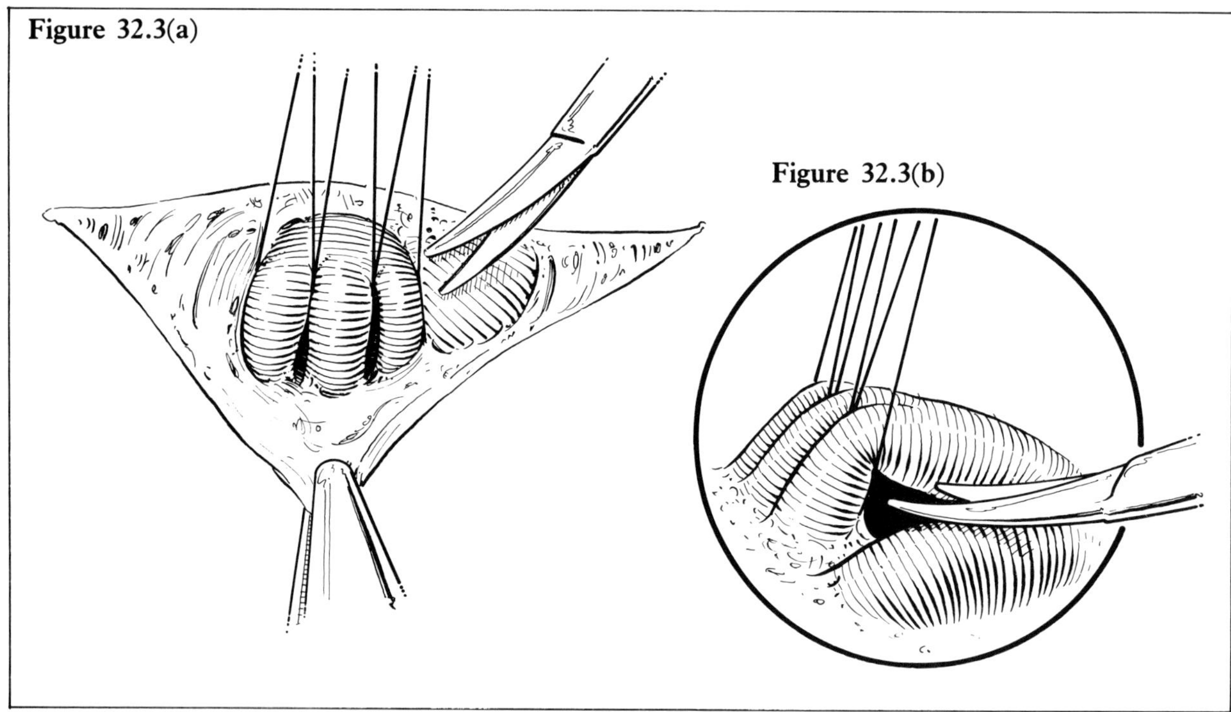
Figure 32.3(a)

Figure 32.3(b)

by holding the ligatures up it is possible to see beneath the vein (**Fig. 32.3**) and to dissect a sufficient length of it medially to allow for the application of a central ligature or of a stapler. The distal ligatures are then tied and the veins divided.

The number of branches from the left main pulmonary artery supplying the upper lobe varies from two to seven. The earliest of these arises as the pulmonary artery passes over the left main bronchus where it enters the hilum of the lung. The main artery then passes into the fissure and runs between the upper and lower lobes, behind the left upper lobe bronchus, giving branches to both lobes. Usually the last branch running forward to the upper lobe is one (or occasionally two) supplying the lingula. Rarely, the lingular artery is the first branch of the pulmonary artery and runs downwards anterior to the hilum to supply it.

The pulmonary artery is best exposed before it enters the main fissure as it emerges from beneath the arch of the aorta. By opening the fascia overlying the artery as it enters the fissure, it becomes very simple to dissect and ligate each branch in turn (**Fig. 32.4**). Although this part of the dissection is not difficult, great care is needed for two reasons. First, the arteries may be densely adherent to adjacent lymph nodes or the underlying bronchus; and second, a pulmonary artery branch may bifurcate immediately after its origin, with one branch (hidden from the operator) running away at right angles from the main trunk. A right-angled clamp passed around the origin of the branch may then penetrate the thin-walled bifurcation.

The dissection proceeds distally, well into the lung, so that an adequate length of the arterial branch is obtained, thus permitting division between ligatures. The dissection then continues down along the anterolateral aspect of the artery and into the fissure. The last branch to be divided will usually be the lingular artery.

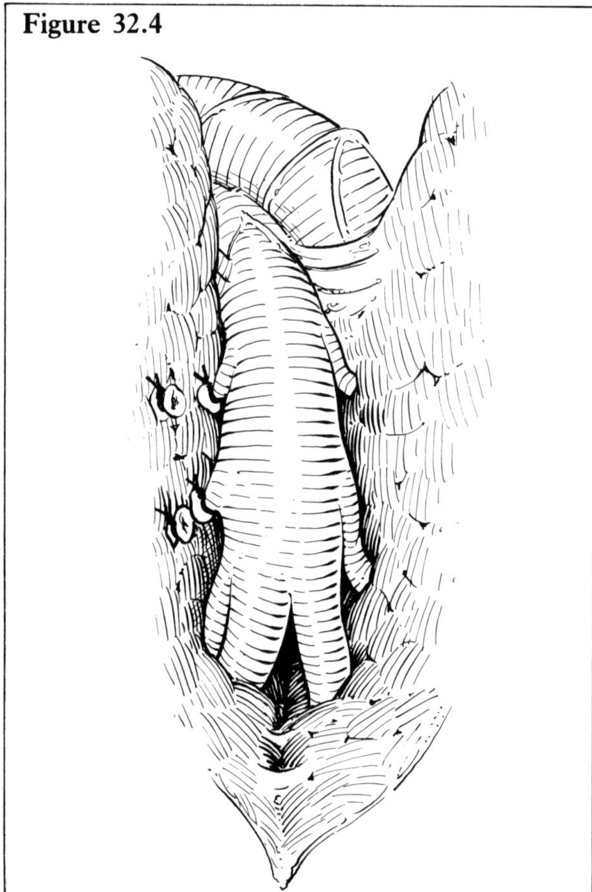
Figure 32.4

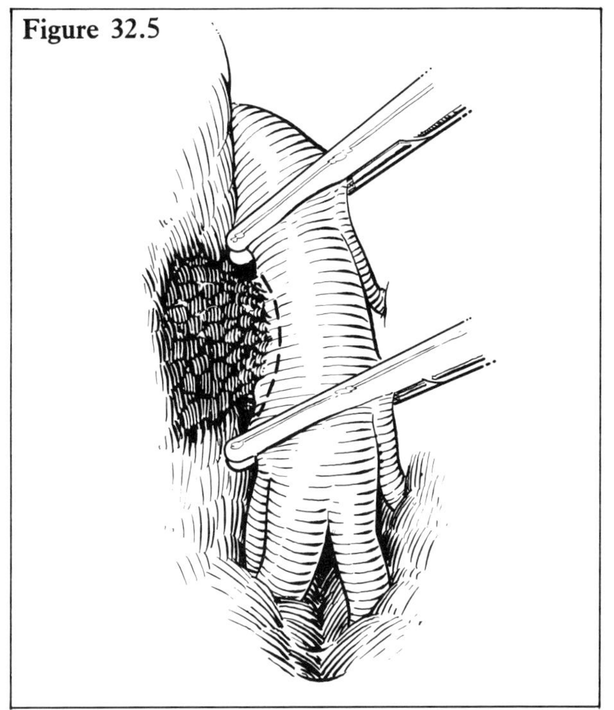

Figure 32.5

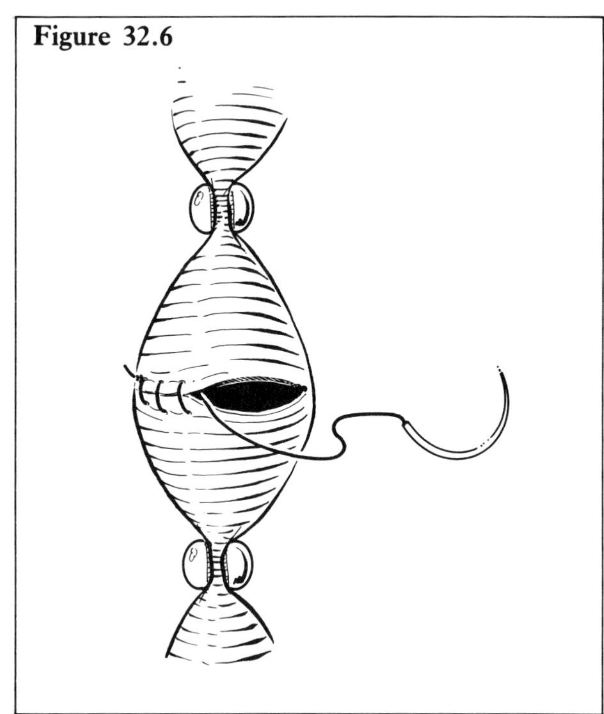

Figure 32.6

Occasionally the tissue surrounding the artery is very dense and adherent, or tumour may be very closely applied to it, rendering the dissection difficult. If this is so, then the main pulmonary artery should be dissected out immediately beyond the ligamentum arteriosum and a tape passed around it. This will make it possible to apply a clamp without delay if a branch is torn. In some cases it may be safer to divide the branch between clamps and to close each end with an arterial suture. In others it may be advisable to clamp the main pulmonary artery proximal and distal to the branch, excise a small portion of the wall of the main artery containing the branch or branches, and repair the artery with a transverse suture line that will avoid narrowing it (**Figs. 32.5, 32.6**). In yet other cases it may be necessary to excise a complete segment of the left pulmonary artery bearing a number of branches, and then to perform an end-to-end anastomosis. This procedure is sometimes referred to as a sleeve resection of the pulmonary artery (**Figs. 32.7, 32.8**).

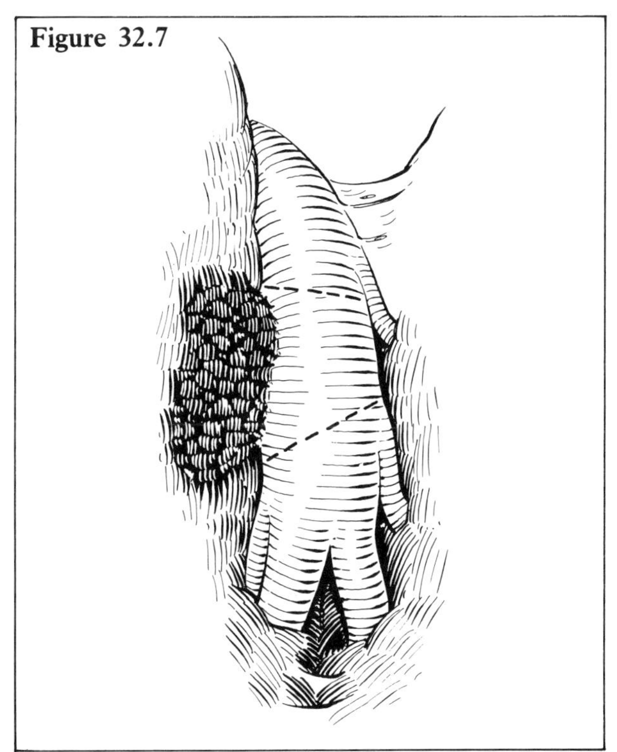

Figure 32.7

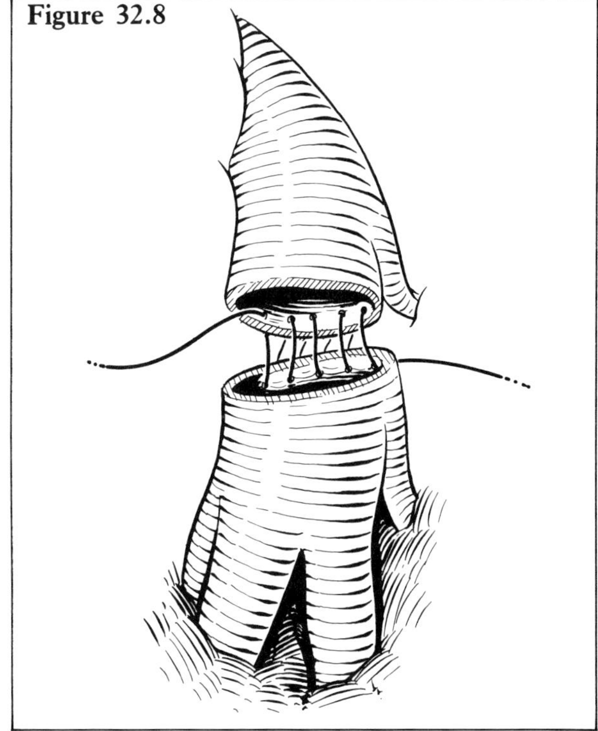

Figure 32.8

When all the arterial branches to the upper lobe have been divided, the artery is retracted backwards with a mounted swab. This exposes the left upper lobe bronchus. The lower margin of the bronchus is now dissected out as it enters the lung and the dissection is carried towards its origin. Thus the carina between the left upper lobe and left lower lobe bronchi is exposed. Any lymph nodes at that point are removed. Any bronchial arteries that are cut are coagulated with diathermy.

The upper margin of the left upper lobe bronchus and adjacent main bronchus is now dissected. An instrument is passed round the upper lobe bronchus, which is clamped distally and divided about 7 mm from the lower lobe carina (**Fig. 32.9**). The proximal end is closed with the stapler, or with a continuous 3/0 polypropylene suture as a horizontal mattress in one direction and an over-and-over stitch in the opposite direction. The lobe is now removed. Some fusion between the upper and lower lobes may be separated by traction or by division between clamps or stapling devices.

The left lower lobe is inflated, and the bronchus tested for leaks.

After removal of the upper lobe the residual space lies anterosuperiorly, and one of the drainage tubes should be placed there. A stitch passed through the pleura of the anterior chest wall will hold the tube in place. A second drain should be placed between the lateral aspect of the lower lobe and the lateral chest wall, with the tip 25 mm below the apex of the thorax.

**Figure 32.9**

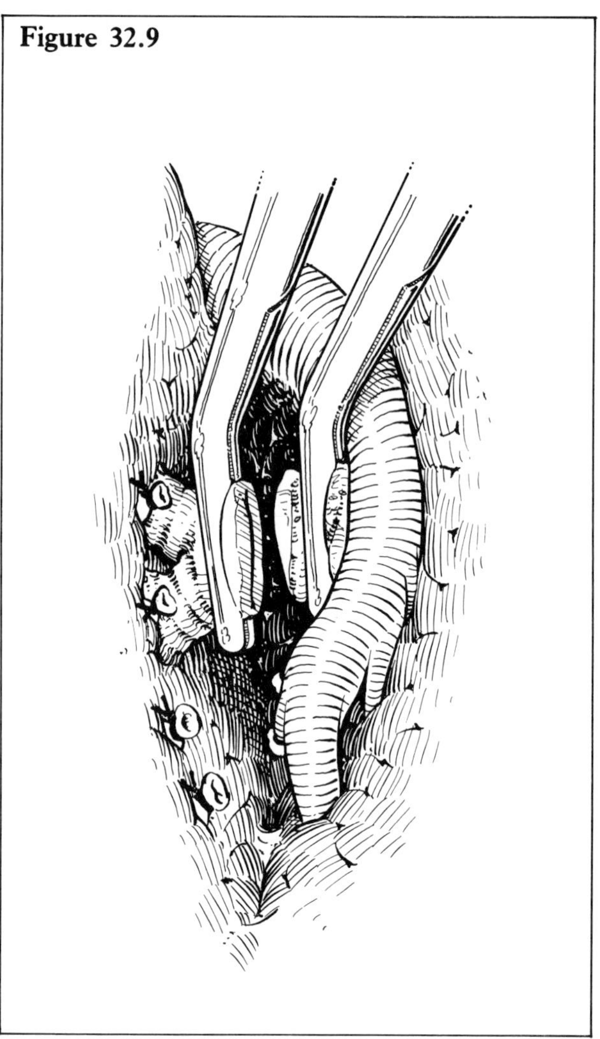

# 33 Left lower lobectomy

This procedure is carried out through a postero-lateral thoracotomy stripping the upper border of the sixth rib.

After any adhesions have been separated, the lower lobe is elevated and the pulmonary ligament divided (**Fig. 33.1**). The inferior pulmonary vein is dissected free of the surrounding tissue and a ligature passed around it centrally. By stroking the divided pleural reflection distally on the vessel with a dental swab mounted on a Roberts clamp the lower lobe vein segmental tributaries will be exposed. Ligatures can then be passed around each in turn (**Fig. 33.2**), and the vein is then divided.

Next, the pulmonary artery is dissected out within the greater fissure. The upper lobe is retracted anteriorly and the pleural reflection over the pulmonary artery divided. The periarterial fascia is opened and this plane followed into the greater fissure. The segmental branches are then identified. The pulmonary artery branches to the lower lobe are divided between ligatures (**Fig. 33.3**). Care must be taken distally, as the

**Figure 33.1**

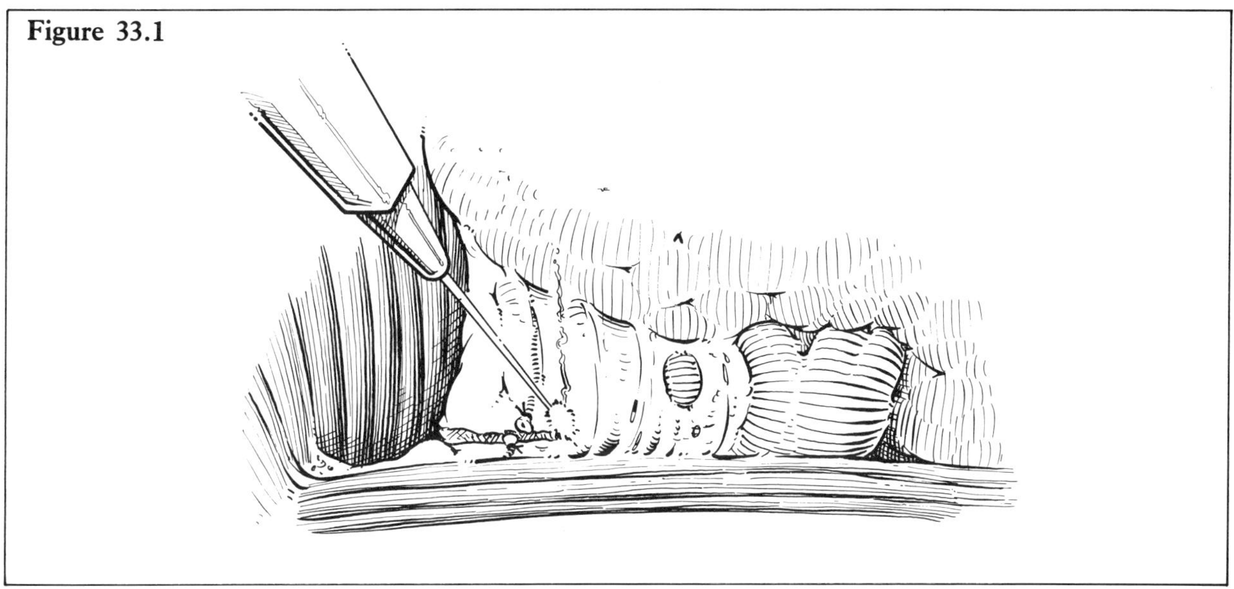

**Figure 33.2**

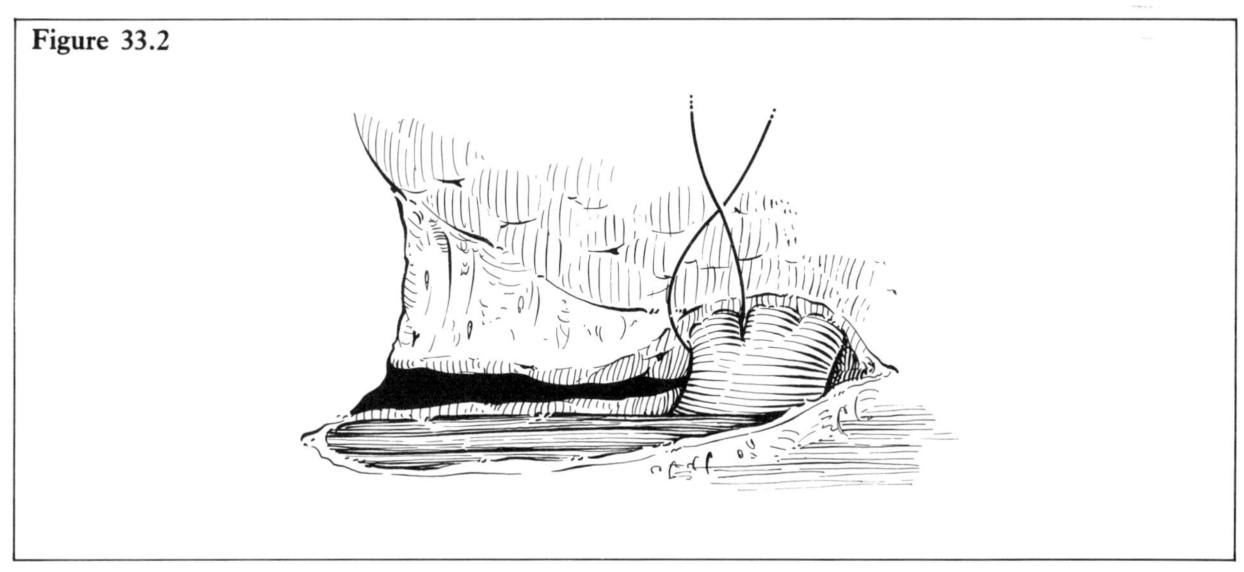

Figure 33.3

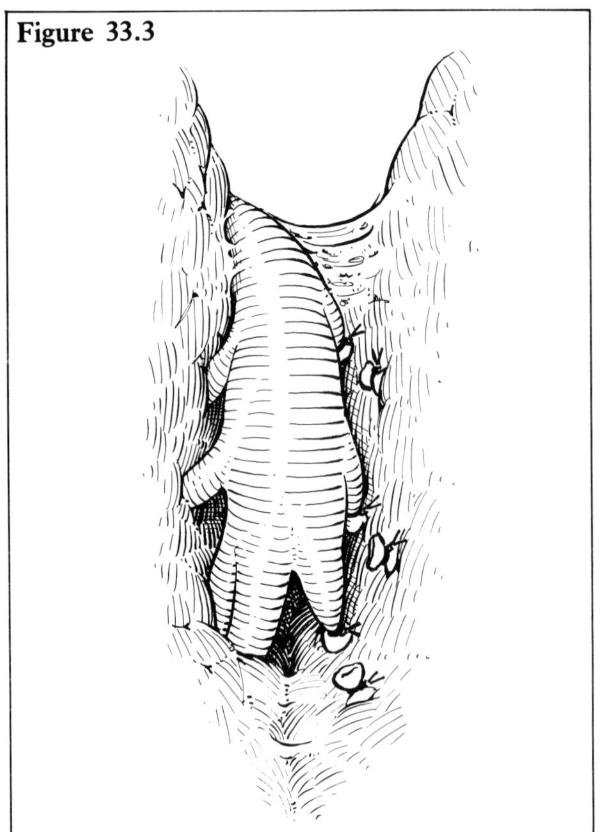

Figure 33.4

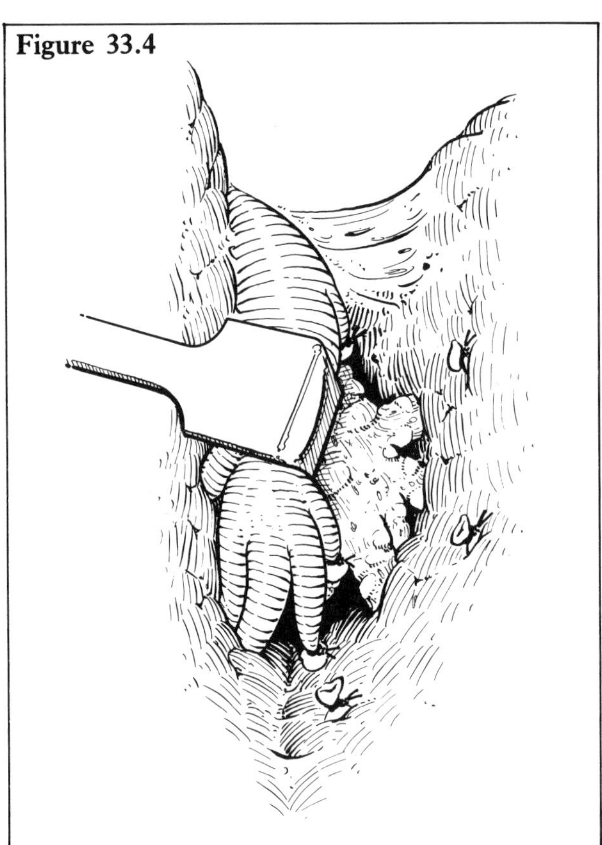

lingular branches usually arise opposite the basal segmental arteries, making it difficult or impossible to incorporate the basal segmental trunk in one ligature. If this is the case the branches should be ligated and divided individually.

The divided lower lobe pulmonary artery can then be retracted superomedially to expose the lower lobe segmental bronchi beneath (**Fig. 33.4**). Dissection from the carina between the upper and lower lobe bronchi will expose enough of the latter to allow a clamp to be placed distally prior to transecting the bronchus and removing the lower lobe. It is important to transect the bronchus so that when sutured the bronchial stump is flush with the upper lobe bronchus. This is to avoid the creation of a bronchial sump in which secretions may collect and become infected, predisposing to breakdown of the bronchial suture line and fistula formation.

At this stage of the dissection only the remaining areas where the fissure is incomplete, usually at the anteroinferior end, prevent the removal of the lobe. If this is the case it may be teased apart by traction on the lower lobe. Alternatively, the remaining parenchyma may be divided using a stapling device or simply between clamps and the resection margin oversewn with a 3/0 polypropylene suture.

Once the lobe has been removed the bronchial stump is tested by inflating the lung to 50 mmHg (7 kPa) under warm saline. Finally, the subcarinal and tracheobronchial lymph nodes are removed for staging purposes.

One chest drain is placed posterolaterally in the basal space vacated by the lower lobe, fixed with a suture if necessary. A second drain is placed anteriorly to the apex of the thorax. The chest is closed in layers as described on p. 27.

# 34 Upper lobectomy with sleeve resection of the main bronchus

This procedure is used to conserve functioning lung tissue when tumour extends into the junction of the upper lobe bronchus with the main and intermediate bronchus (**Fig. 34.1**). The procedure is most suited for the right upper lobe because the intermediate bronchus has sufficient length and circumference to allow a satisfactory anastomosis to the main bronchus. This is not the case on the left side, and although it is occasionally possible, the early origin of the lower lobe segmental bronchi and the rapid tapering of the main bronchus render it difficult.

After dissection and division of the lobar arteries and veins, the bronchus is freed from the remaining structures. A sleeve of main and distal bronchus with the upper lobe bronchus attached is resected (**Fig. 34.1**). The main bronchus is transected just proximal to the upper lobe bronchus. The line of division is angled so that it is more proximal on the side of the origin of the upper lobe bronchus and more distal on the opposite side. Distally the lower lobe or intermediate bronchus is divided. This line of division is made more distal on its lateral side and more proximal on the medial side, but care is needed not to encroach on the origin of the apical lower and middle lobe bronchi. The object is to ensure that the line of resection is well away from the encroaching tumour.

The cut ends of the main and intermediate bronchus on the right, and the main and the lower lobe bronchus on the left, are reanastomosed (**Fig. 34.2**). As mentioned above, this anastomosis is more difficult on the left side, because of the position of the aorta and the more rapid tapering of the left lower lobe bronchus compared with the intermediate bronchus on the right. If the pulmonary artery is involved a sleeve of it can also be resected and the ends anastomosed (see **Figs. 32.7, 32.8** on p. 117).

If there is a large discrepancy in size between the resected ends of the bronchi, the main bronchus can be reduced in diameter as shown in **Figs. 20.27–20.30** on p. 83: a wedge of bronchial wall is resected and the margins are closed with interrupted polygalactin sutures. Alternatively, if the discrepancy is not too great, compatibility in size may be achieved by cutting the distal bronchus obliquely and the proximal main bronchus at right angles to its axis: this will give the smallest possible circumference for the main bronchus and a larger

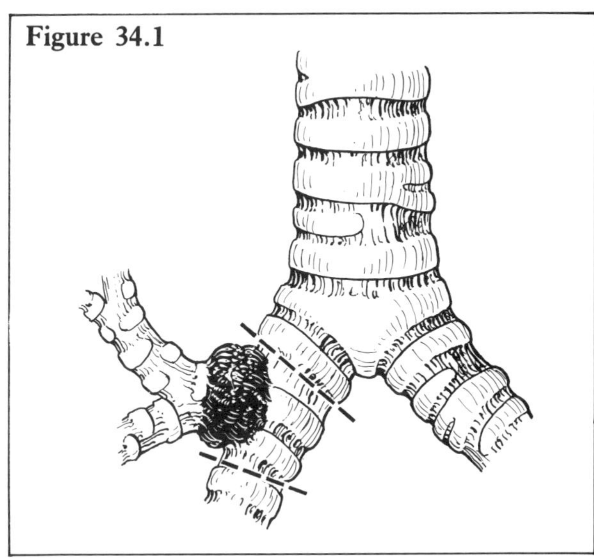

Figure 34.1

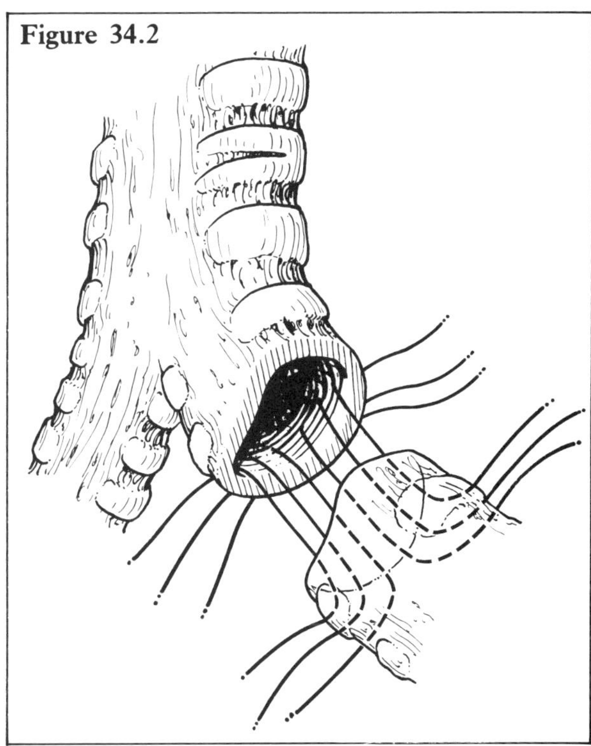

Figure 34.2

than normal circumference for the distal bronchus. The obliquity of the distal resection line should not be too great, however, as it may distort the subsequent anastomosis and lead to bronchial stenosis.

The anastomosis is constructed with interrupted 3/0 polygalactin sutures. All the sutures are inserted and held in individual artery forceps placed in order around the wound. It is helpful to slide one of the finger rings of the artery forceps holding each stitch over a Roberts clamp to keep them in order. The sutures are placed from the outside to the inside of the main bronchus, and in the reverse direction through the lower lobe or intermediate bronchus so that the knots will be on the outside. The suture line is begun at the furthest point away, which is the junction of the medial wall of the bronchus with the membranous wall. The subsequent sutures are inserted in the same way, progressing towards the anterior surface and ending at the posterolateral junction with the membranous part again. An elegant modification of the suture technique is to pass the stitches as described, but in such a way that they do not pass through the mucosa (**Fig. 34.3**). This results in no suture material being visible within the bronchus when the ends are drawn together and the sutures are tied.

By traction on the sutures the medial end of the membranous wall is brought into view, and sutures are then placed in the membranous portion starting at the furthest point (i.e. the medial end) and working towards the surface (i.e. the lateral end). The sutures securing the medial wall of the bronchus (furthest from the operator), should be tied first, followed by those of the anterior wall, then the lateral wall (closest to the operator), and finally those securing the membranous portion of the bronchus which lies posteriorly (**Fig. 34.4**). This is to reduce the chance of these sutures tearing out if the tension on them is too great.

The remainder of the operation is completed in the same way as for any other lobectomy.

## Reversed sleeve resection

For tumours arising in the intermediate bronchus and encroaching upon the upper lobe orifice, it may be possible to carry out the procedure sometimes referred to as a 'reversed sleeve' resection. The principle of the procedure is the same, in that the aim is to remove the tumour with clear resection margins of bronchus, but at the same time retaining as much functioning lung tissue as possible. In this case the right upper lobe is preserved, whilst the middle and lower lobes are removed (**Fig. 34.5**).

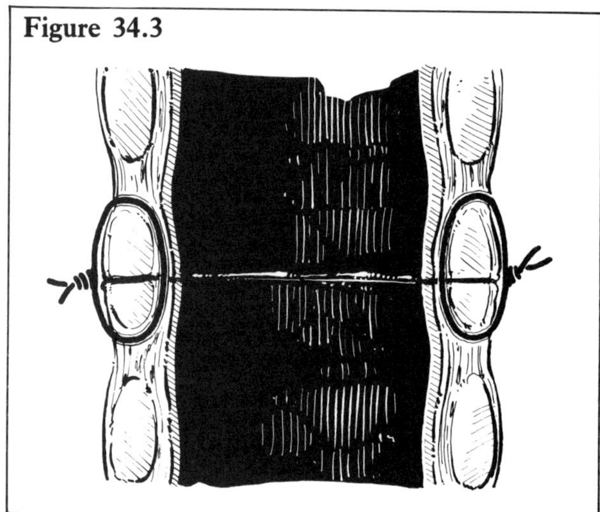
Figure 34.3

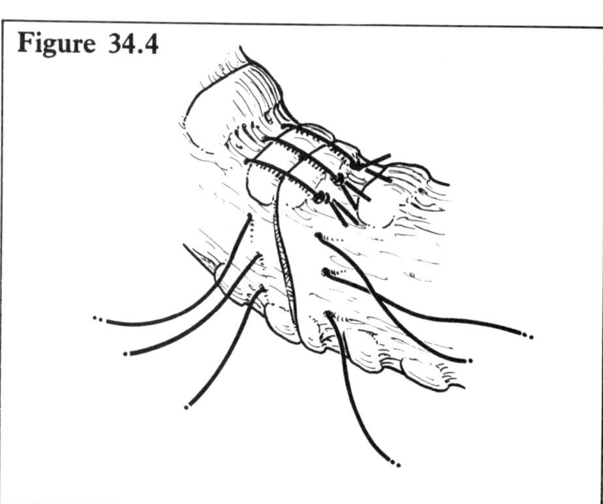
Figure 34.4

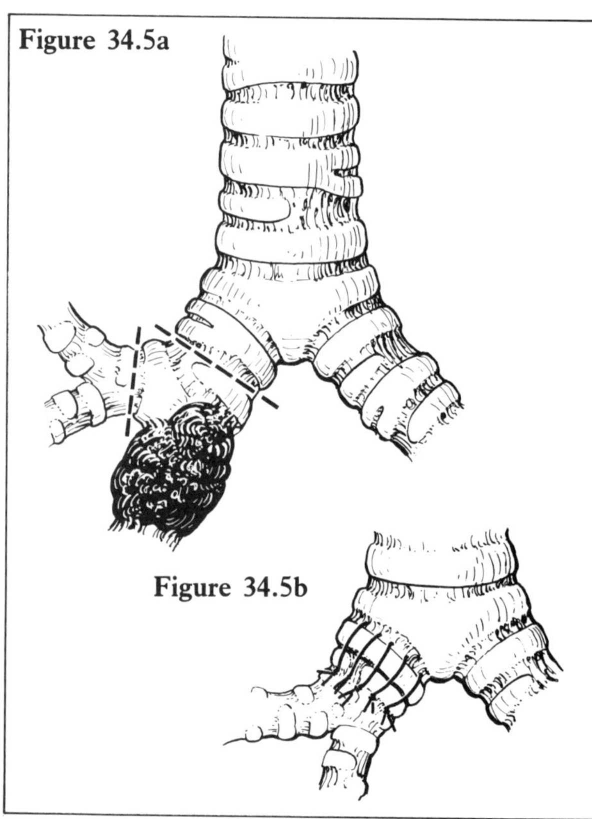
Figure 34.5a

Figure 34.5b

# 35 Chest wall excision in combination with pulmonary resection

In cases where a tumour of the lung is found to have invaded the chest wall, but the invasion is limited, it is possible to resect a portion of the chest wall together with the tumour. Although this is clearly a more advanced stage of disease than that confined within the lung, good five-year survival rates can be expected provided there is no mediastinal lymph node involvement.

## Procedure

The pleural cavity is entered through an intercostal space outside the involved area, either above or below it (**Fig. 35.1**). A small retractor is used to open the intercostal space sufficiently wide for an exploring finger to define the limits of the attachment of the tumour to the chest wall. The area of chest wall to be resected should extend at least one rib and one intercostal space above and below the tumour, and 4–5 cm beyond its anterior and posterior limits.

Diathermy is used to incise the periosteum of the ribs above and below the intercostal space that is to be entered. If the area of chest wall to be resected lies under the scapula it will be necessary to retract the scapula away from it. This is done by opening the chest at the lower level of the proposed chest wall resection, and placing the lower blade of the chest retractor over the ribs and the upper blade under the scapula. On opening the retractor, the scapula is lifted away from the chest wall giving excellent exposure (**Fig. 35.2**).

The intercostal bundle is freed from the rib above and below with a rugine. The whole bundle can then be divided between clamps and the ends ligated. This procedure is continued for each space that is to be entered. The ribs are then divided

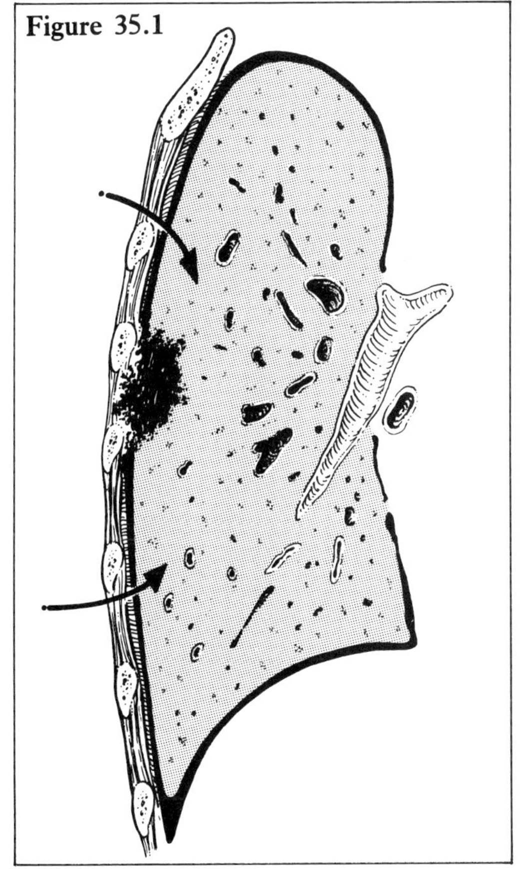

**Figure 35.1**

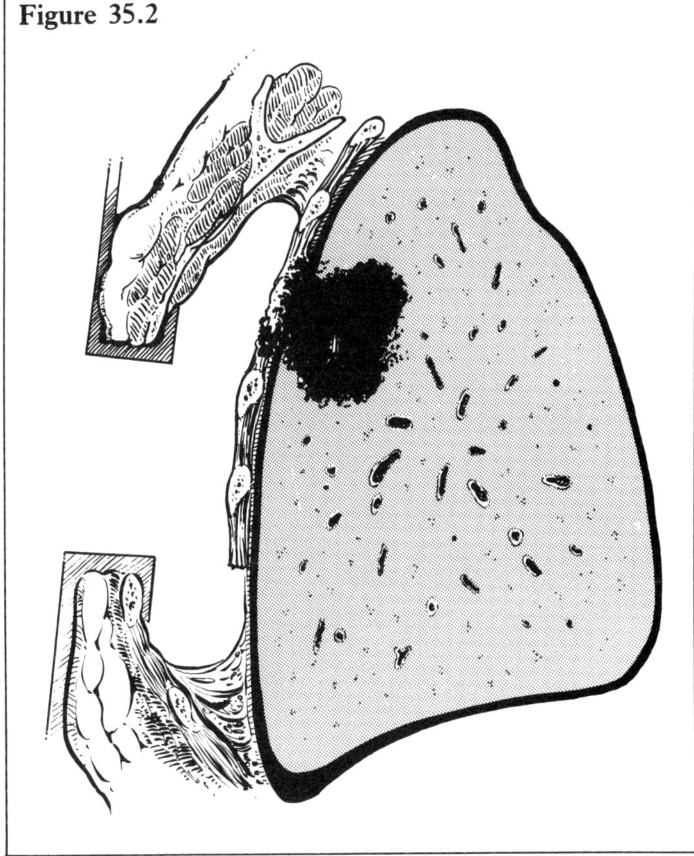

**Figure 35.2**

**Figure 35.3**

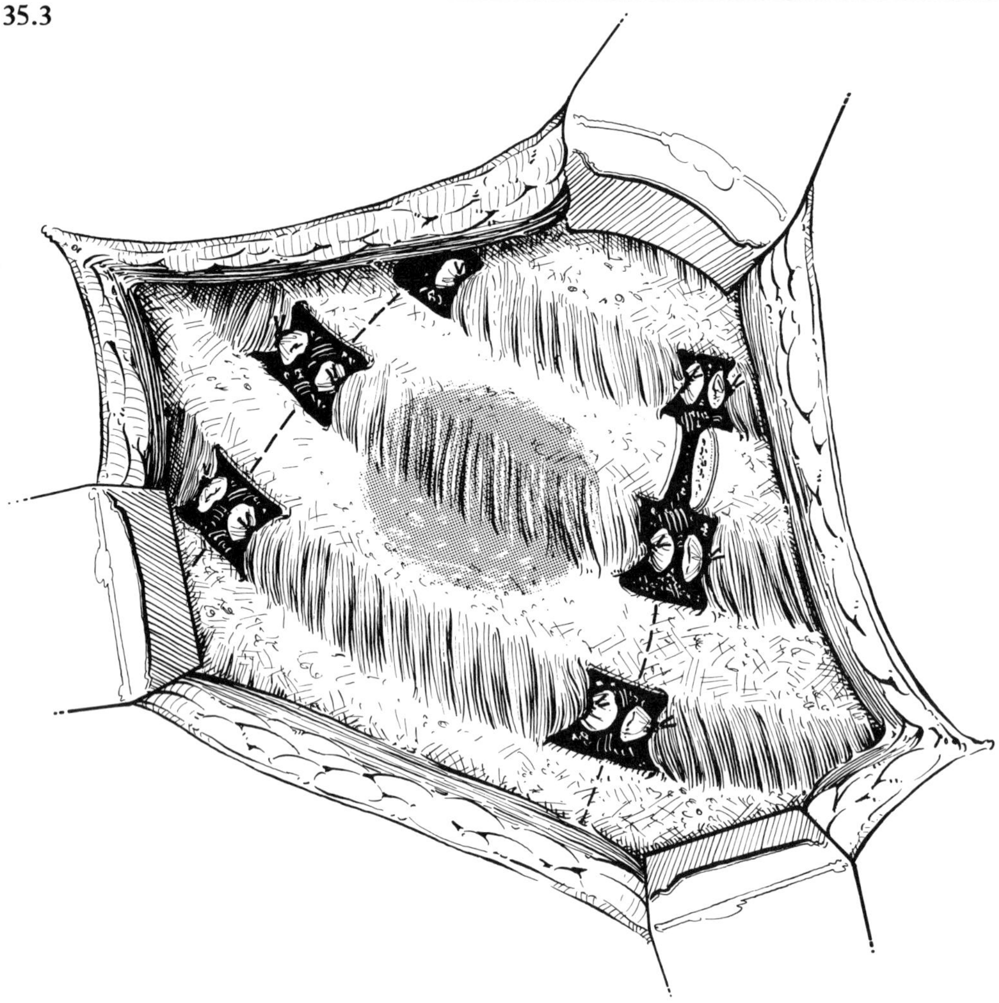

with a costotome (**Fig. 35.3**). Once the area of chest wall that is involved has been freed, it is allowed to fall into the pleural cavity after the anaesthetist has deflated the lung. The pulmonary resection can then be carried out in the usual way.

In the past it has been the general opinion that where the defect in the chest wall is posterior, particularly if it is covered by the scapula, repair is unnecessary. However, more recently it has become apparent that a large, unsupported chest-wall defect in the presence of a pneumonectomy space (wherever it is situated) interferes with the mechanical function of the chest wall, and gives rise to great difficulty in coughing and in clearing secretions from the contralateral lung. It is therefore our opinion that after pneumonectomy all these defects should be closed. In the case of small defects this can often be achieved by approximating adjacent tissues.

For defects larger than about 8 × 8 cm, we have found that a Marlex mesh patch which is both strong and flexible will give the support that is required. It should be cut to a size about 2 cm greater than the measured defect. The edge is then folded over and fixed to the inside of the pleural

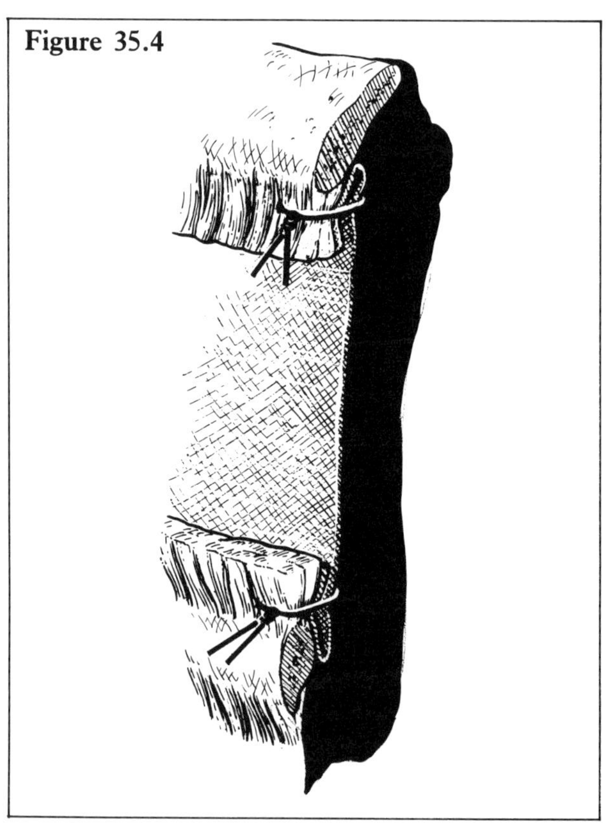

**Figure 35.4**

cavity by a series of mattress sutures, which are made more secure by passing them through a double fold at the edges of the material (**Fig. 35.4**). The sutures are tied as they are inserted along three sides of the defect. Along the fourth side, for adequate access, the whole row of sutures is inserted before any are tied. Before the final row of sutures is tied, one drain is placed within the pleural cavity and brought out through the skin below the incision. A vacuum drain may be placed outside the ribs beneath the scapula (or pectoral muscles as the case may be) to ensure the adherence of tissue at that point and to prevent the formation of an effusion outside the chest wall. The remainder of the chest wall closure is as described on p. 27.

For very large defects that lie within the areas of the chest wall where the curvature is at its greatest, the use of a stretched Marlex patch will distort the normal shape of the chest. In this situation a ‘sandwich’ of methyl methacrylate between two pieces of Marlex can be moulded to the shape of the chest wall before insertion. The Marlex patches should be appreciably larger than the methyl methacrylate, so that when the latter has hardened there is a sufficient rim of Marlex for suturing (see p. 50). The desired shape may be moulded over an upturned basin or the surgeon’s hand, as the material is malleable while hardening.

# 36 Segmental resections

Segmental resections were commonly performed for tuberculosis. Since the advent of effective antituberculous therapy this is no longer the case; however, these procedures are still useful. Basal segments are commonly affected by bronchiectasis and a resection that preserves functioning lung is to be recommended. Upper lobe segmental resections, the most common for TB, are now very rarely performed, although some surgeons recommend segmentectomy for a well-circumscribed intrapulmonary tumour when a more extensive resection would not be tolerated by the patient.

Each lung is subdivided into bronchopulmonary segments (**Fig. 36.1**). Each segment has its own bronchus and arterial supply. Although they are anatomically distinct in this regard, there is considerable variation in venous drainage. Because intersegmental and subpleural veins drain neighbouring segments, the veins associated with each segment should not be ligated until all other dissection has been completed.

Although there is considerable anatomical variation between segments, there is an underlying system which should be applied in each resection.

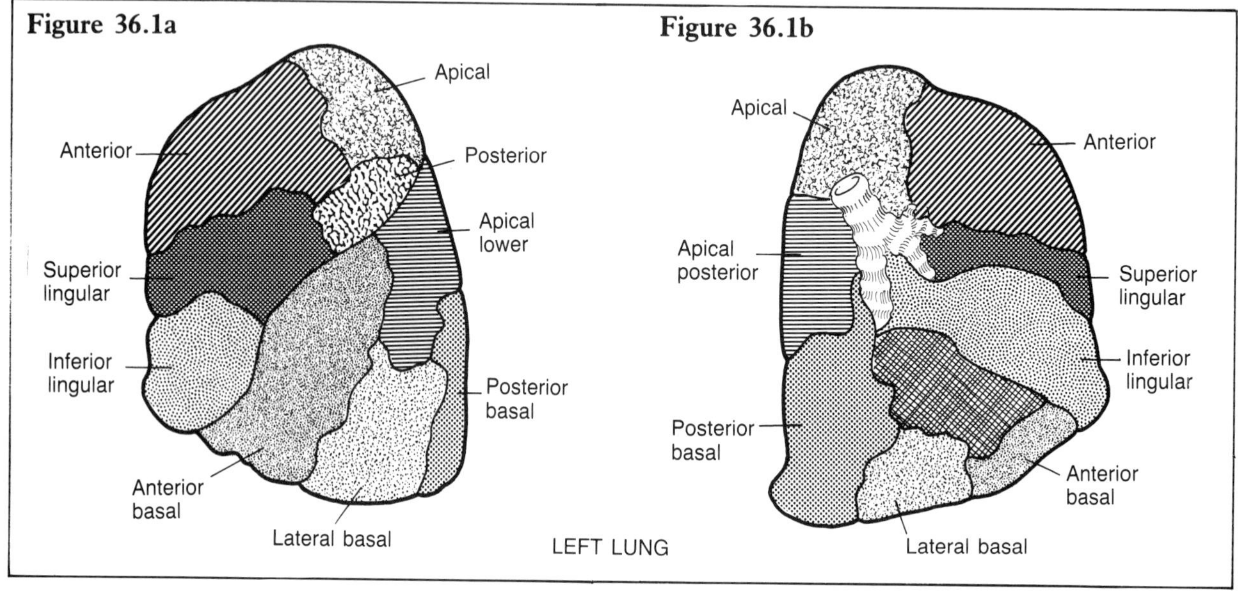


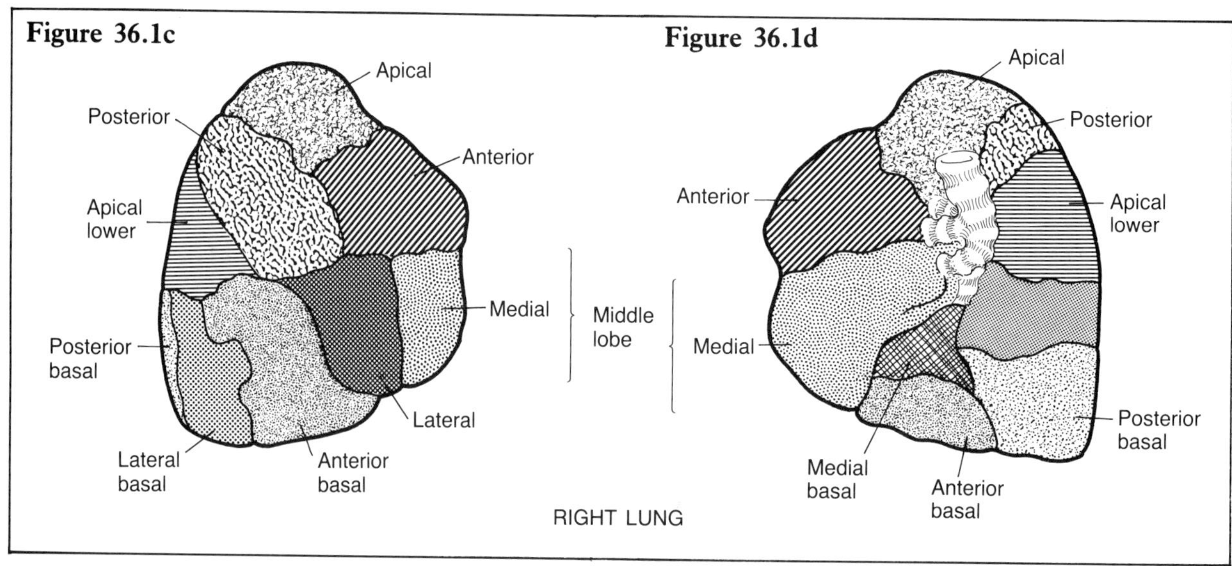

The most reliable anatomy is that of the bronchus, and for that reason it should be the first structure to be isolated. When it has been divided, gentle traction on it will reveal the appropriate segmental artery. If the bronchus cannot be seen, it may be identified by rolling the lung between a finger and thumb (**Fig. 36.2**). More often, however, it is possible to identify the appropriate bronchus by first exposing the lobar bronchus and extending the dissection back into the parenchyma of the lung from the hilum (**Fig. 36.3**). The bronchus is then clamped and the anaesthetist asked to ventilate the lung; it may then be possible to delineate the segment from the surrounding lung. Because of cross-ventilation between segments, however, the segment to be removed may also inflate. If this is the case, on stopping ventilation the segment in question is usually slow to deflate and can thus be identified. It is then safe to divide the bronchus proximal to the clamp and to oversew the stump with a polygalactin suture.

**Figure 36.2**

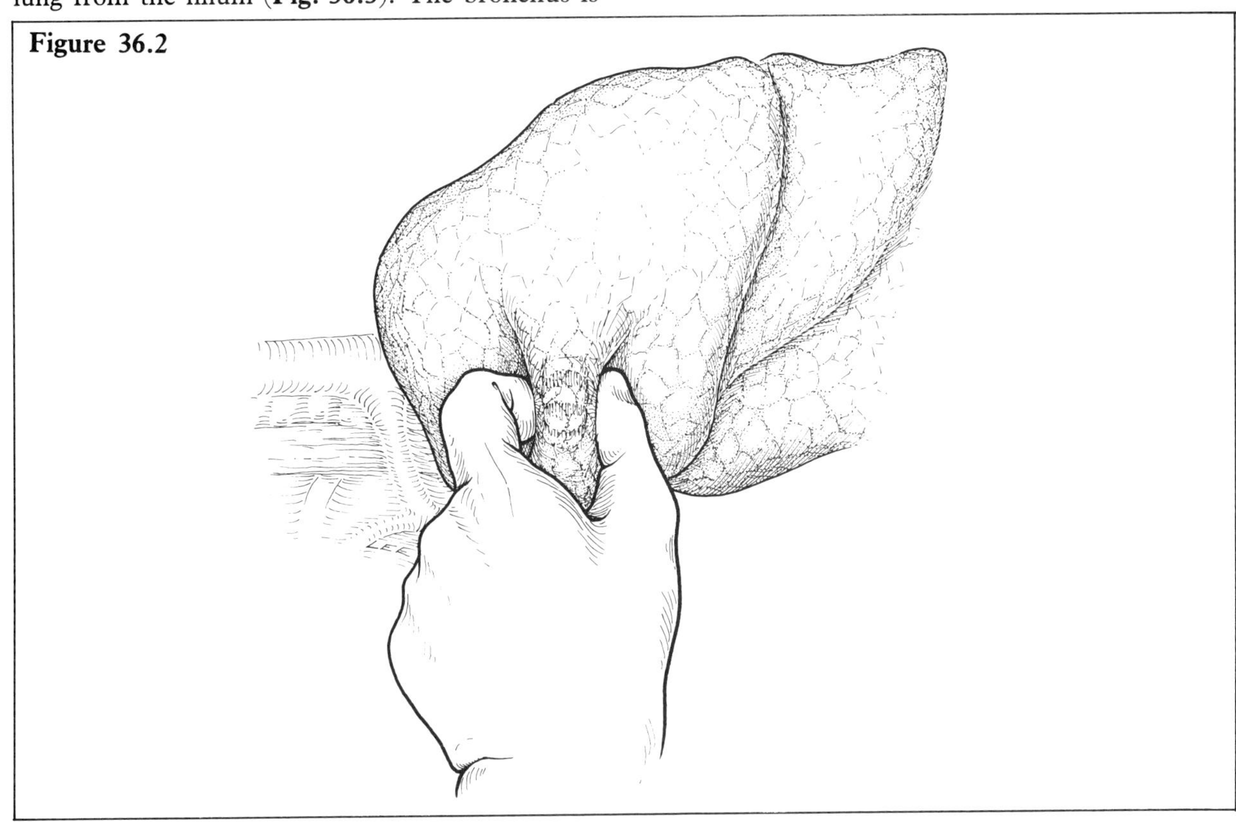

**Figure 36.3**

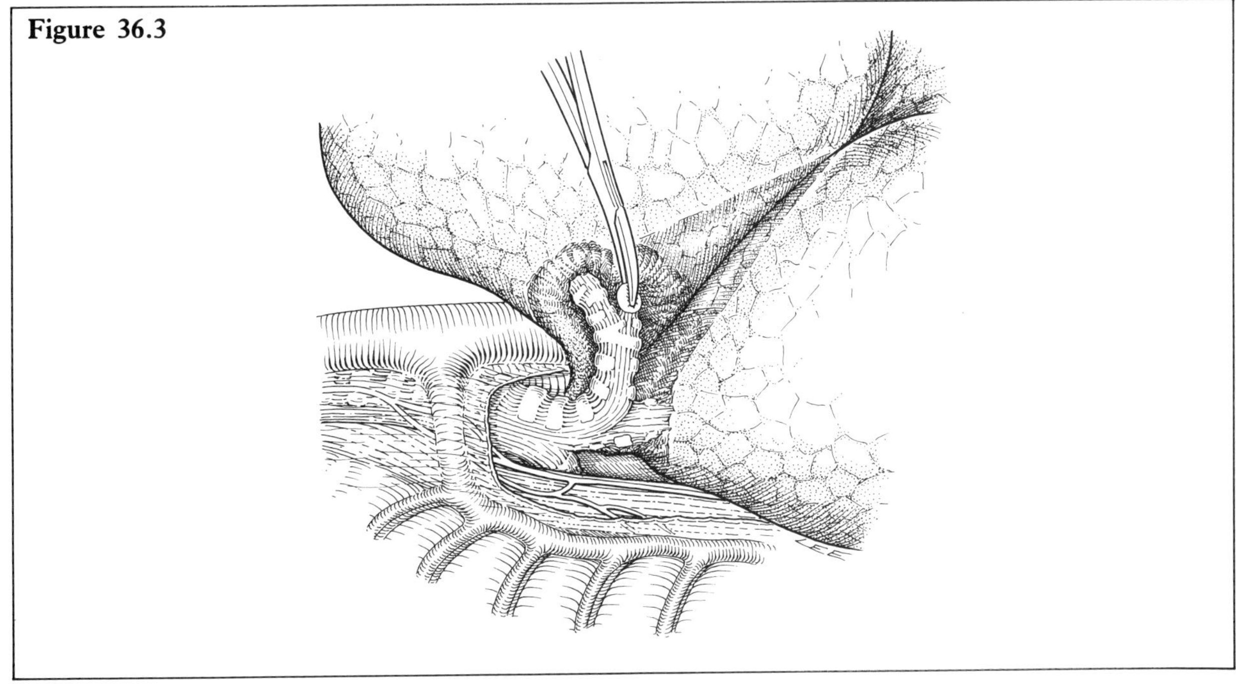

Figure 36.4

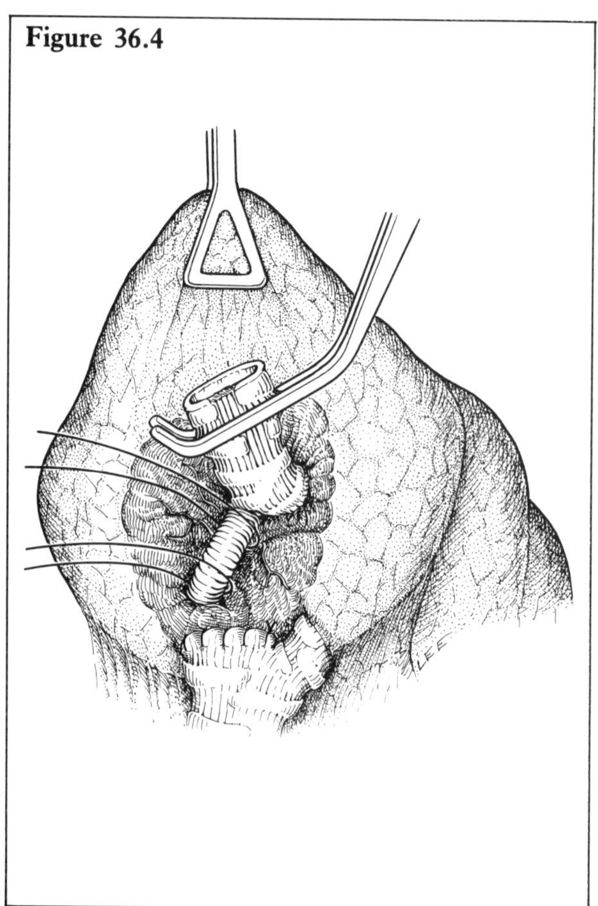

Figure 36.5

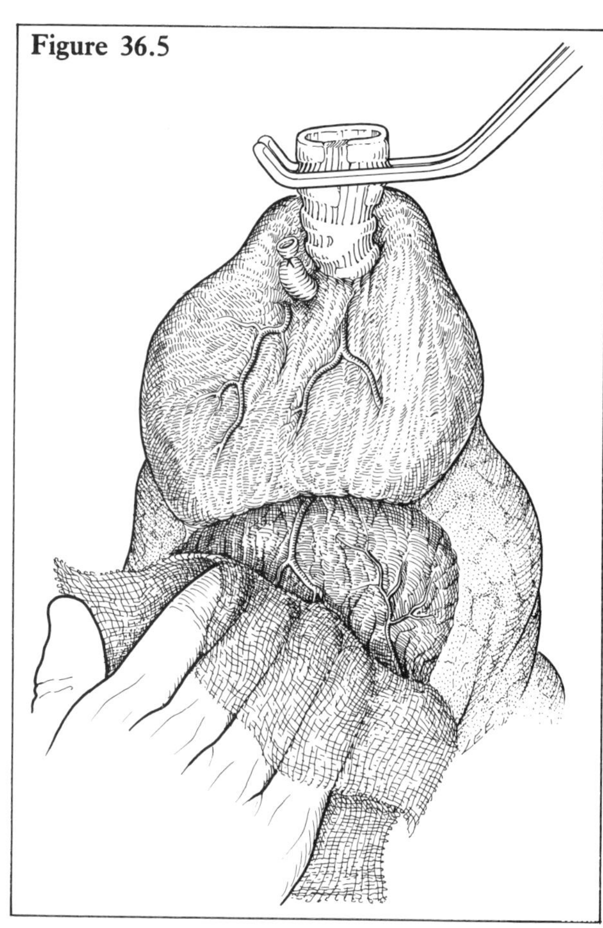

Figure 36.6

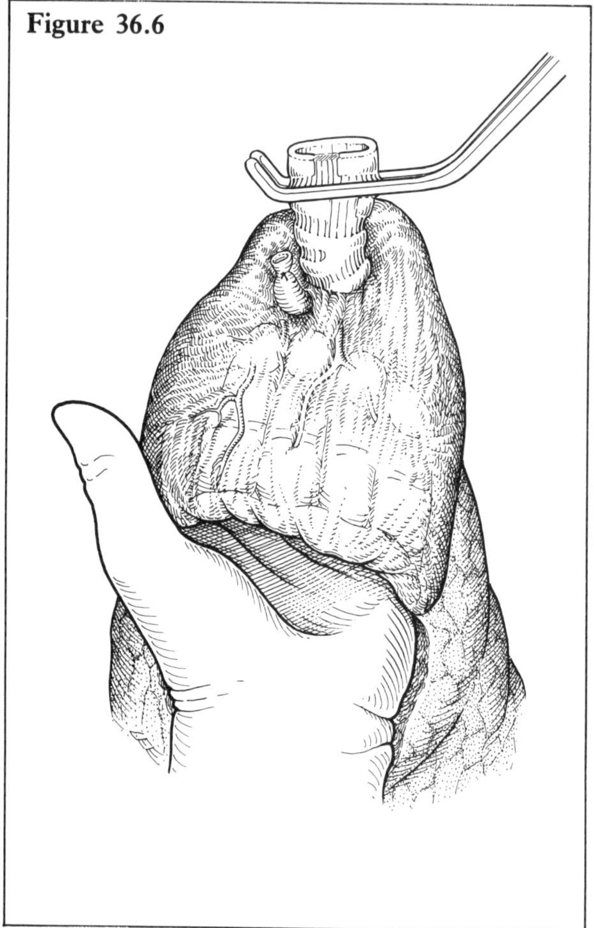

Figure 36.7

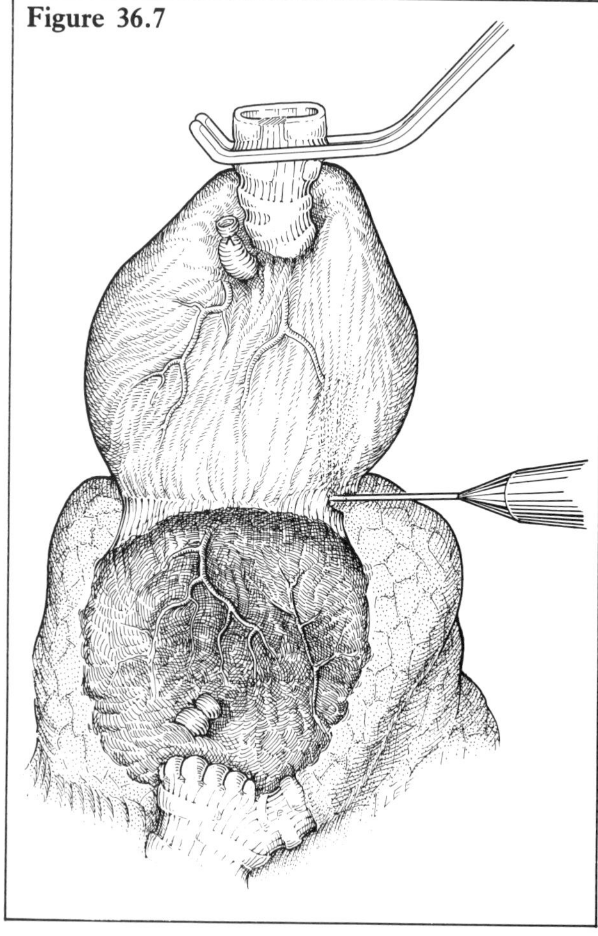

Traction on the divided bronchus will expose the segmental artery (**Fig. 36.4**); this can be ligated and divided. As the bronchus is further elevated the plane of cleavage between the segments will begin to appear. Gentle counterpressure on the remaining lung will allow separation of the segment from it (**Fig. 36.5**). As this plane develops the intersegmental veins will appear. The majority of these will remain behind. Some, however, will need to be divided and cauterized as the dissection proceeds. Further dissection is restricted by the overlying pleura, which is divided. As dissection proceeds further the intersegmental veins are divided. The operator's fingers can then be insinuated in the plane of cleavage and gently used to work towards the outer edge of the segment, when they will become visible underneath the visceral pleura (**Fig. 36.6**). The pleura is incised with either scissors or diathermy (**Fig. 36.7**). Any bleeding from the raw area should be controlled with diathermy.

The area is then tested under saline for any air leak. If there is a brisk air leak from any small intersegmental bronchus it should be underrun with a stitch. To reduce postoperative air leak the opposing edges of the area exposed may be sutured together, provided that this does not compromise lung expansion.

Postoperatively it is most important to maintain constant suction to encourage the lung to attain maximum expansion and thus to obliterate the pleural space.

## Segmental resections of the right upper lobe

The upper lobe is approached through a posterolateral thoracotomy, entering the chest through the bed of the fifth rib. The resection of the posterior or apical segment is begun by exposing the back of the right upper lobe bronchus. There is always a bronchial artery running along this part of the bronchus, and it should be divided. Along the course of this vessel also is a constant lymph node, which marks the entrance to the greater fissure and the lower margin of the upper lobe bronchus (**Fig. 36.8**).

The peribronchial tissue is opened with scissors and then cleared distally with a dental swab until the trifurcation of the bronchus is reached (**Fig. 36.8**, inset). Further dissection along the upper lobe bronchus will reveal the origins of the apical and posterior segmental bronchi. Not until this has been achieved should any vessels be divided. These bronchi should not be divided too close to their origin, for fear of injuring the anterior segmental bronchus which lies out of sight, in front of them (**Fig. 36.8**, inset).

The posterior segmental artery lies anterior to the corresponding bronchus, and when the bronchus has been divided and its distal end elevated, the artery comes into view where it enters the segment (**Fig. 36.4**). Excessive traction on the divided bronchus must be avoided, because the artery could be avulsed from the main trunk. The artery is ligated; if the available length is

**Figure 36.8**

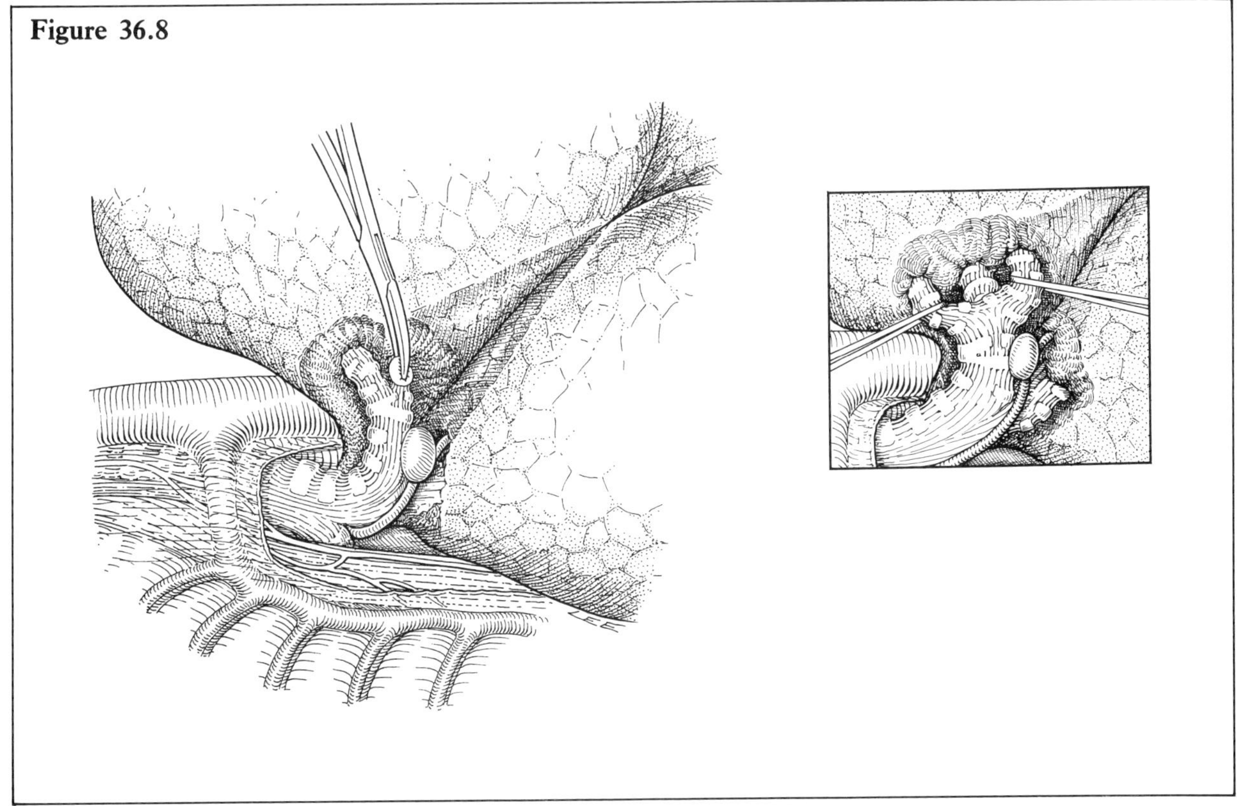

inadequate, it is underrun centrally with an arterial suture, and clamped distally before transection.

If there is difficulty in exposing the arterial branches to these segments, dissection of the superior aspect of the hilum will reveal them. To do this the pleural reflection over the pulmonary artery is divided and the arterial sheath entered (**Fig. 36.9**). The sheath may then be swept off the vessel distally, exposing the first branch of the artery which divides into the apical and anterior segmental arteries—the first passing upwards, and the second anteriorly (**Fig. 36.10**).

The anterior segment is much more difficult to remove, as the bronchus lies beneath the other two bronchi and must be approached from the front (**Fig. 36.8**, inset). It is in turn concealed by the upper lobe vessels anteriorly. Each of these vessels needs to be exposed without damage. The apical segmental vein is retracted to expose the underlying first branch of the pulmonary artery (**Fig. 36.9**). The anterior segmental artery is the anterior of the two branches of the superior arterial trunk (**Fig. 36.10**); it is ligated and divided. The anterior segmental vein is to be found between the middle lobe vein (the lowest of the tributaries of the superior pulmonary vein) and the apical venous trunk, into which empties the posterior segmental vein. The horizontal fissure has to be opened to expose the undersurface of the anterior segment. If the fissure is fused or absent it can best be approached by identifying its origin in the depths of the greater fissure. Otherwise the anterior segment must be freed from the middle lobe by careful traction on the divided bronchus and finger separation of the pulmonary parenchyma.

**Figure 36.9**

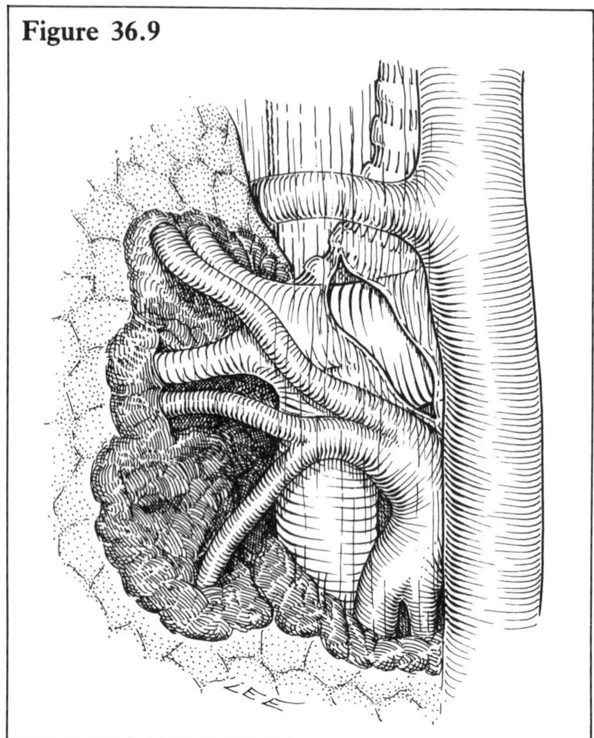

**Figure 36.10**

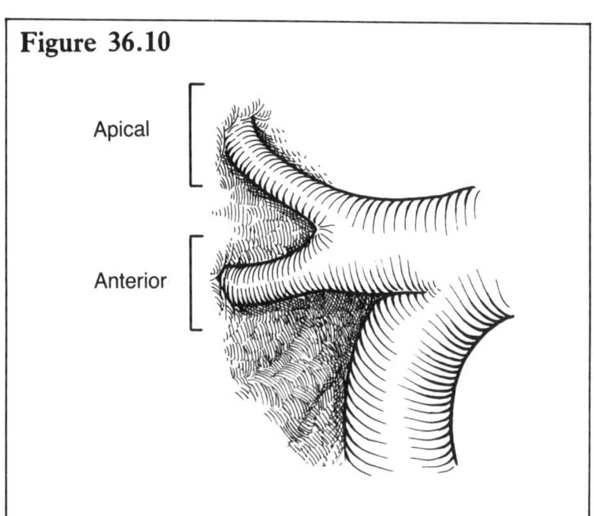


## Segmental resection of the right lower lobe

### Apical segment

The apical segment was commonly affected by tuberculosis and resected for that reason. This is now an exceedingly rare indication, but cavitation within this segment with secondary infection by bacteria or fungi is an infrequent indication for this procedure.

The upper part of the greater fissure is opened (**Fig. 36.11**) and the lymph nodes lying on the

**Figure 36.11**

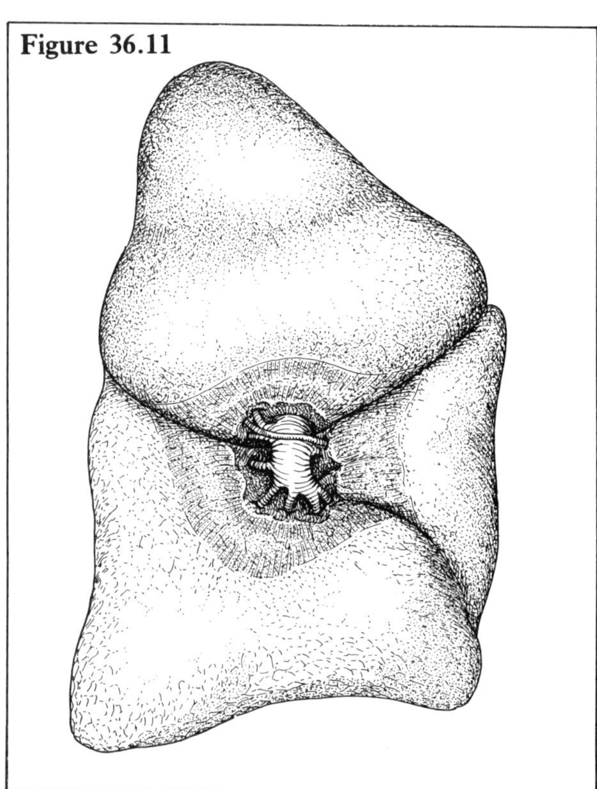

pulmonary artery are removed. The pulmonary artery sheath is incised immediately below the crossing of the posterior segmental vein (**Fig. 36.12**). Further dissection of the artery at this point reveals the middle lobe arteries running anteriorly, the apical lower artery opposite them passing posteriorly, and the posterior segmental artery of the upper lobe coursing laterally (i.e. upwards) to disappear beneath the posterior segmental vein (**Fig. 36.13**). The latter two arteries may arise in common, and therefore each must be clearly identified. The common anatomical variants are shown in **Figs. 36.13–36.15**.

The apical lower artery is ligated and divided. The segmental bronchus is seen immediately beneath it and is exposed by dividing the peribronchial fascia (**Fig. 36.16**). The bronchus arises just opposite the middle lobe bronchus (**Fig. 36.17**).

**Figure 36.12**

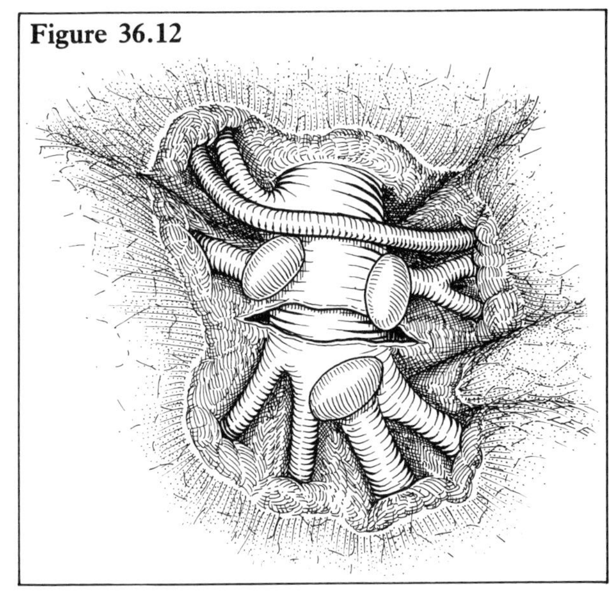

**Figure 36.13**

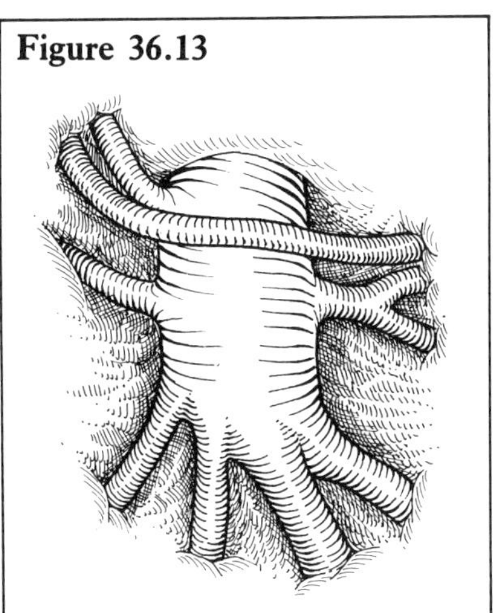

**Figure 36.14**

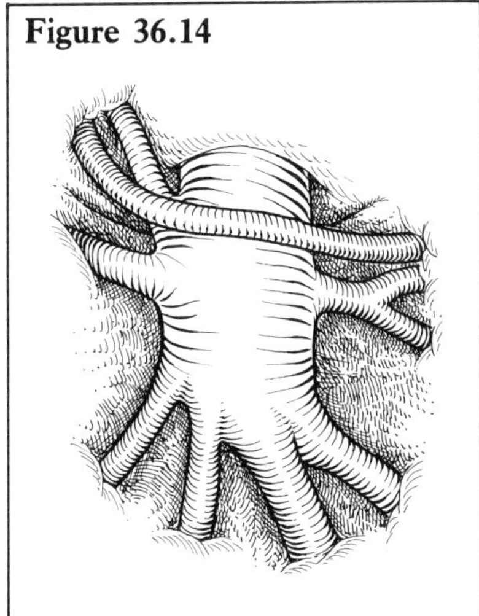

**Figure 36.15**

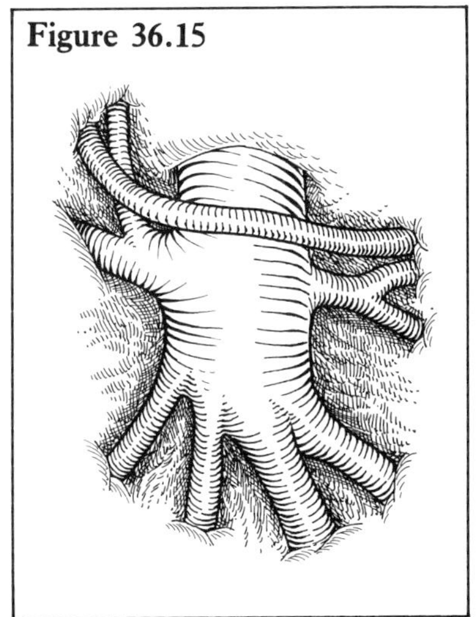

**Figure 36.16**

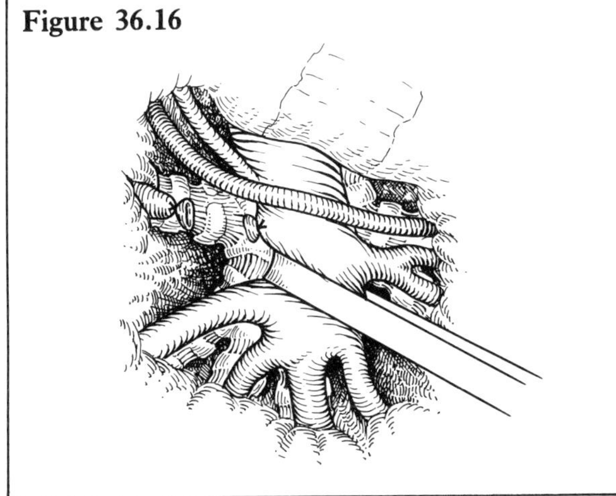

**Figure 36.17**

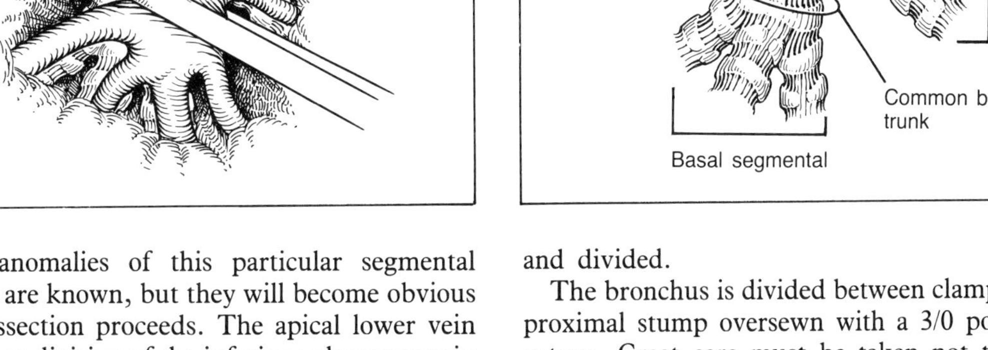


Various anomalies of this particular segmental bronchus are known, but they will become obvious as the dissection proceeds. The apical lower vein is the upper division of the inferior pulmonary vein and can be most easily identified from the posterior aspect of the lung (**Fig. 36.18**). The vein is ligated and divided.

The bronchus is divided between clamps and the proximal stump oversewn with a 3/0 polygalactin suture. Great care must be taken not to damage the middle lobe orifice which lies opposite. The clamp on the distal end can be used to retract the

**Figure 36.18**

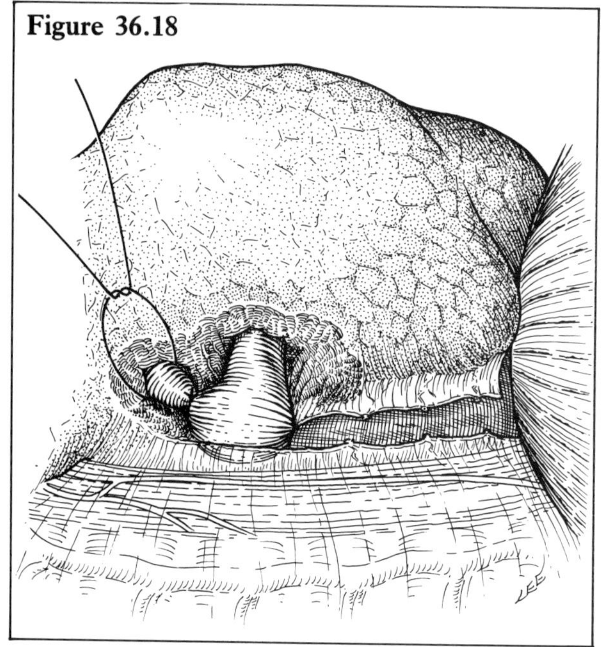

bronchus to separate it from the underlying lung. As the dissection proceeds, the pleural reflection from the segment is divided.

There is often difficulty in identifying the pulmonary artery in the greater fissure, because the fissure may be obliterated by inflammatory disease or it may be congenitally deficient. Moreover, dense fibrosis of the lymph nodes overlying the pulmonary artery may render dissection of them difficult, bloody and hazardous. If this is the case the whole dissection is carried out from the posterior aspect of the lung. The inferior pulmonary vein is dissected out, and its upper branch divided. The bronchus to the apical lower segment, now lying on the common basal bronchus, is dissected, mobilized and divided. When the bronchus is elevated the apical lower artery comes into view and is divided. An instrument is passed from behind towards the fissure, and its point can be felt and advanced into the fissure. This starts the process of traction–separation by which the segment is removed. Where the lung is unyielding along the borders of the segment the resistant area is incised between clamps.

The raw surface is then inspected for any air leak or bleeding. Any small accessory bronchi must be suture-ligated to avoid residual air leak. The chest is closed over two drains as described on p. 27.

## Basal segments

The most common indication for resection of these segments was, and is, bronchiectasis. The operation is now less frequently indicated because of the effectiveness of medical treatment.

The chest is entered through the bed of the sixth rib, and the pulmonary ligament is divided. The confluence of the greater and the lesser fissures is opened and the pulmonary artery exposed as for a lower lobectomy. The first segmental branch that the operator will come across is that of the anterior

**Figure 36.19**

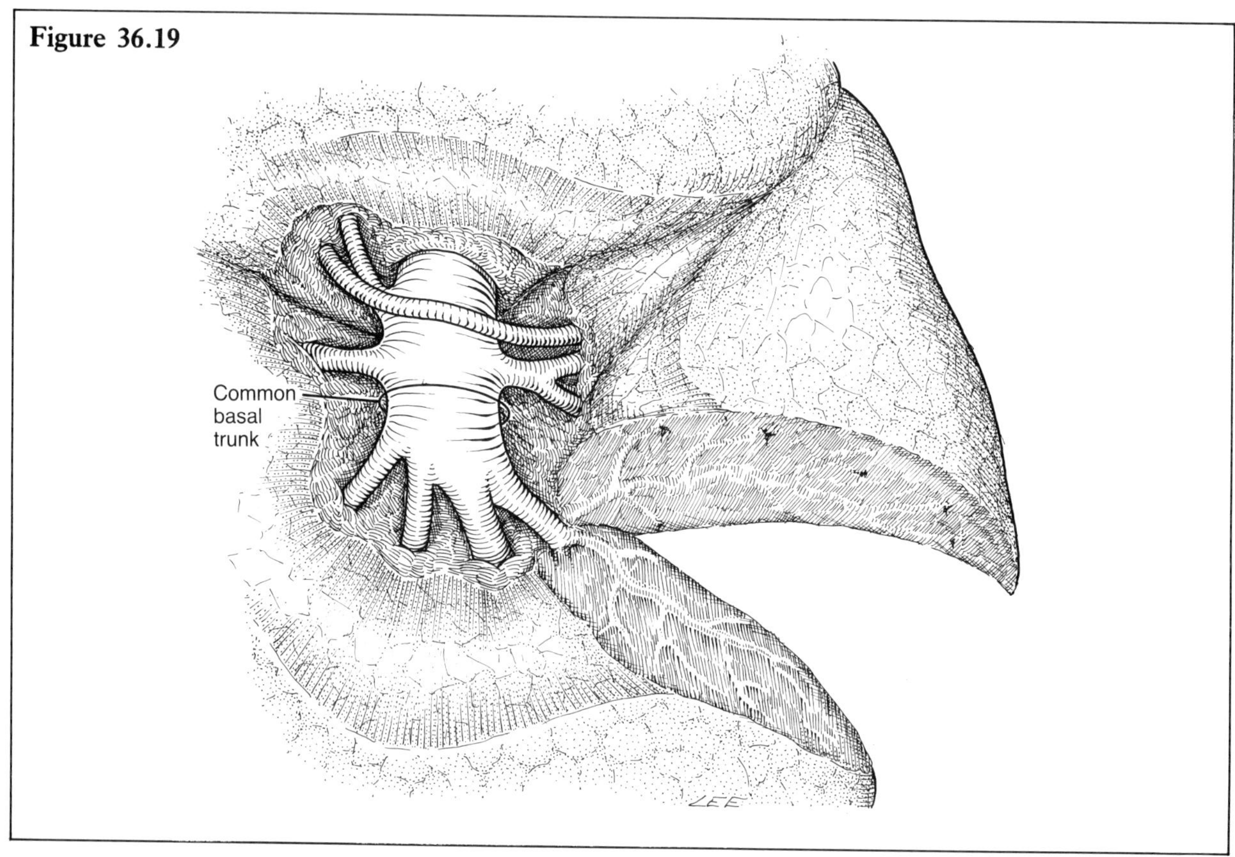

basal segment. This lies just under the pleura on the surface of the fissure. Dissection proximally will reveal the common basal trunk (**Fig. 36.19**). The apical lower artery arises separately and more proximally, opposite the middle lobe artery. Each of the basal segmental arteries can usually be exposed quite easily.

If all the basal segments are to be resected, a ligature is passed around the common basal trunk and proximally and distally round each of the segmental arteries and tied (**Fig. 36.20**). The segmental arteries are divided between the two ligatures on them, giving a secure proximal closure. Next, the common basal vein is identified from behind by retracting the lung forwards (**Fig. 36.18**). The posterior pleural reflection is divided and the pleura gently pushed off the inferior pulmonary vein and its tributaries. The inferior pulmonary vein is formed by the junction of the common basal vein and the apical lower vein; the common basal tributary is thus easily identifiable, and is divided between ligatures.

The common basal bronchus is identified via the fissure anteriorly. In the presence of bronchiectasis there are numerous, large bronchial arteries which must be ligated individually, as they are too large to be cauterized. Inflamed lymph nodes surround the bronchus and must be patiently dissected away, with meticulous control of bleeding; otherwise the field of operation rapidly becomes obscured. The operator must clearly identify the middle lobe

**Figure 36.20**

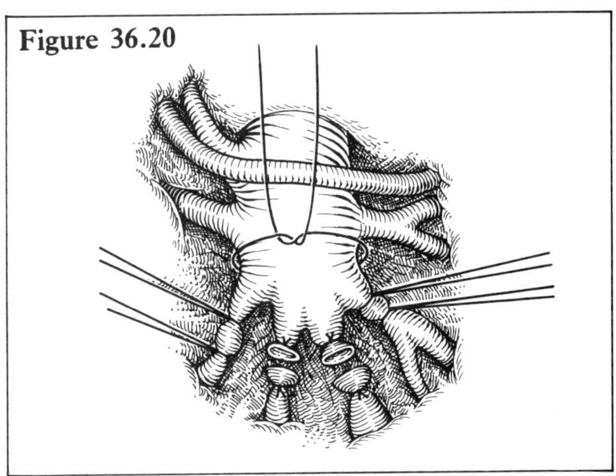

bronchus (running anteriorly) and the apical lower bronchus (running posteriorly) as they leave the lower lobe bronchus before it becomes the common basal bronchus (**Fig. 36.17**).

A bronchus clamp is applied to the bronchus distally, leaving enough length proximally to allow division and closure without interfering with the middle lobe bronchus or the apical lower bronchus. The cut bronchus is then repaired with a 3/0 polygalactin suture.

## Left lung segmentectomy

The key to left lung segmentectomies is exposure of the main left pulmonary artery and its branches in the major fissure (**Fig. 36.21**). The individual

**Figure 36.21**

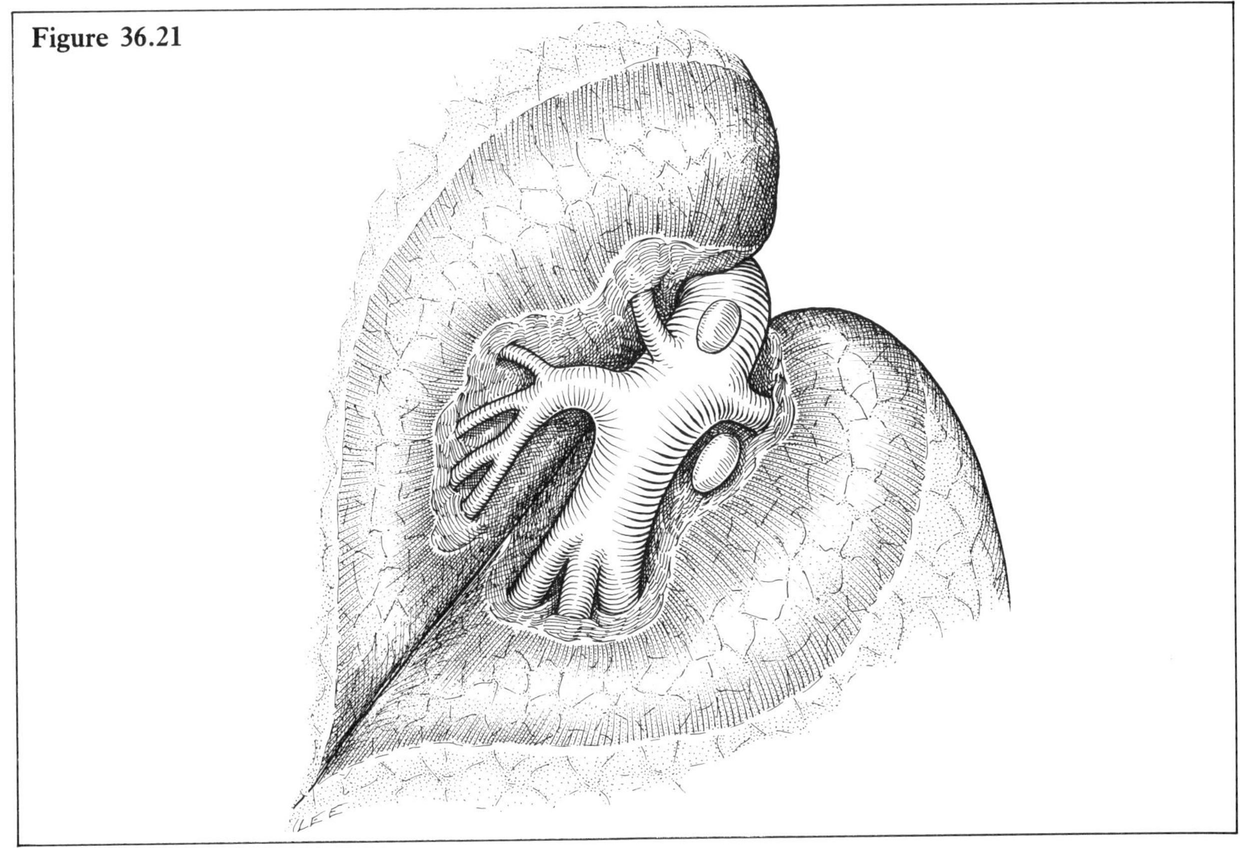

segmental arteries are very variable and therefore demand careful dissection. Sometimes the arteries to two adjacent segments have a common origin: for example, the anterior and lingular segmental arteries may arise from a common trunk (**Fig. 36.22**). Each artery must therefore be followed to the segment to be removed prior to ligation.

In the upper lobe the segmental bronchi are found beneath the appropriate arteries. By lifting the divided distal end of the segmental artery the segmental bronchus comes into view. It is dissected free from the adjacent segmental bronchi and can then be divided. Care must be taken if the apicoposterior segment is to be removed, because the anterior segmental bronchus runs horizontally at this point and may be injured. The segmental veins lie anteriorly and should be divided last. The segment is then separated as described for right upper lobectomy (p. 107). Segmental resections of the left lower lobe are almost identical to those on the right side.

**Figure 36.22**

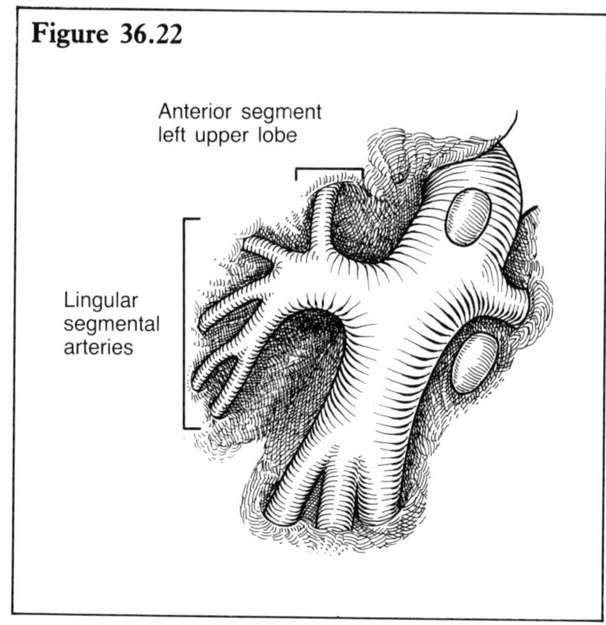

# 37 Excision of empyema and decortication of the lung

Pleural infection may result from sepsis within the lung or the chest wall, from penetrating wounds or transdiaphragmatic spread from the abdomen (liver abscess). Early acute infections may resolve with systemic antibiotics and simple tube drainage. Chronic empyemas, however, need surgical attention if conservative methods fail. An empyema is commonly referred to as chronic after being present for six weeks. A tuberculous empyema is unusual nowadays, however, and pneumonia is now the most common cause.

Decortication of the lung may be necessary for chronic empyema or for an organized and unresolved haemothorax. Decortication is contraindicated in the very elderly and infirm or in the presence of severe systemic sepsis, as it may be severely traumatic with significant blood loss.

Preoperative investigations include bronchoscopy to exclude an impacted endobronchial foreign body, bronchograms to identify and map out any areas of bronchiectasis and computed axial tomography, if available, to delineate the anatomy of the abscess and its surrounding structures. CT scanning is also very effective at defining bronchiectatic areas. Any haematological or biochemical abnormalities should be corrected.

During the procedure, the patient's arterial and venous blood pressure should be continuously monitored. Moderate pharmacological reduction of the blood pressure will help to reduce the perioperative blood loss; this may be achieved by a continuous infusion of sodium nitroprusside.

## Procedure

A posterolateral thoracotomy through the bed of the fifth rib is best for empyemas that reach the apex, and through the bed of the sixth or seventh rib where the empyema extends to the diaphragm. In chronic empyemas the ribs become triangular in cross-section and crowded together so that they overlap; a rib must therefore be removed to obtain access (**Fig. 37.1**). The deep surface of the rib is the outer surface of the parietal layer of the empyema. Along the upper and lower margins of

**Figure 37.1**

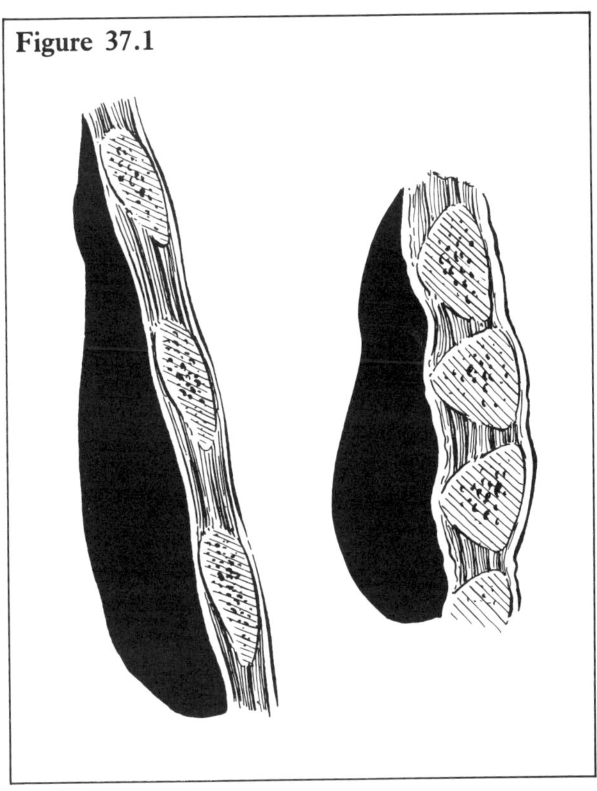

this strip of periosteum are seen the pale violet-coloured fibres of the intercostalis intimus muscle, which are divided with closed scissors. The tips of the fingers are now pressed in the angle between this layer and that formed by the ribs and intercostal muscles externally. The layer will then begin to separate from the chest wall. This separation must be continued along the upper and lower margins of the incision and round its two extremities where the sac extends over the lung. As each area is freed, the diffuse bleeding from the separated surfaces is controlled by the insertion of a hot, moist gauze pack. Attention is then turned to a different area. A small rib spreader is initially inserted, but once an adequate extrapleural space has been obtained a larger instrument is inserted which can be opened more widely as the dissection proceeds. The opening can be further increased in size by division of the posterior end of a rib above or below the excised rib, or both (**Fig. 37.2**).

**Figure 37.2**

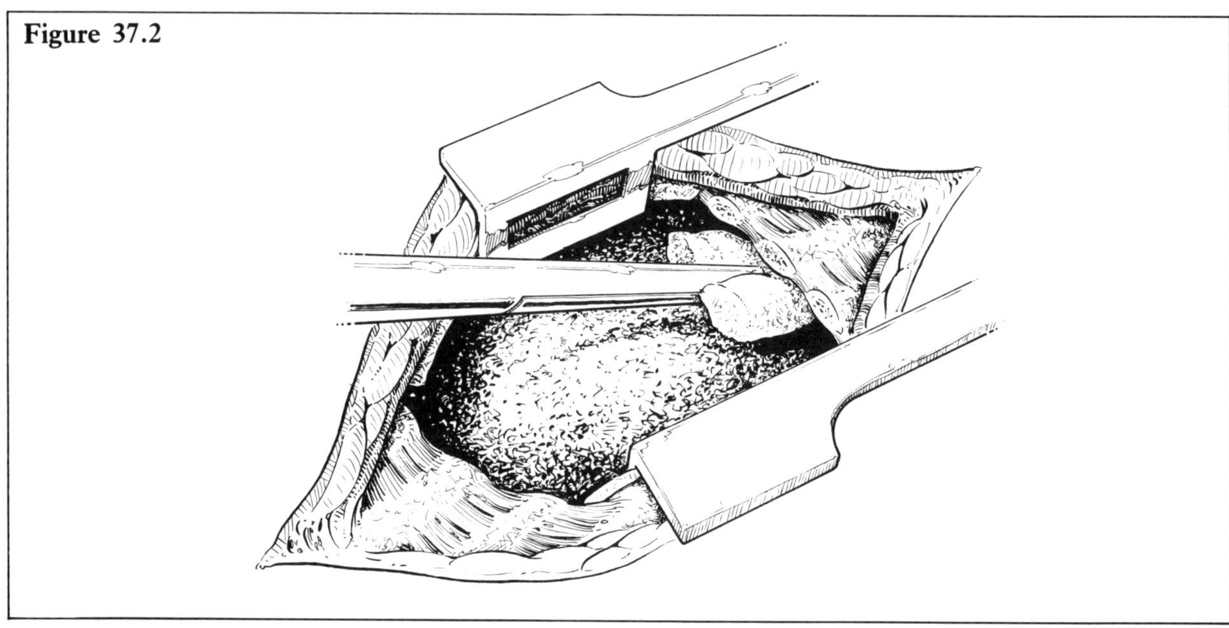

Principles of mobilization

The areas where adhesions between the pleural layers are the most dense are:

1. The costophrenic recess.
2. The diaphragm.
3. The apex.
4. The sites where intercostal tubes have previously been inserted.

The fibrosis is usually least over the mediastinum, and less over the anterior margin of the lung than over the posterior. The object is to free the least fibrosed areas first and work towards the areas of dense fibrosis. If the parietal pleural layer is very thick and the empyema cavity tense, the dissection is made easier if the sac is kept intact at this stage (**Figs. 37.3, 37.4**). In the absence of these features, or if the sac is inadvertently opened, an extensive cruciate incision is made in the outer wall and the whole of the contents sucked out (**Fig. 37.5**). The limits of the empyema cavity can then be seen from within, which is helpful in determining the line of extrapleural dissection.

Separation of the parietal cortex from the chest wall proceeds in the following sequence (**Figs. 37.6, 37.7**).

**Figure 37.3**

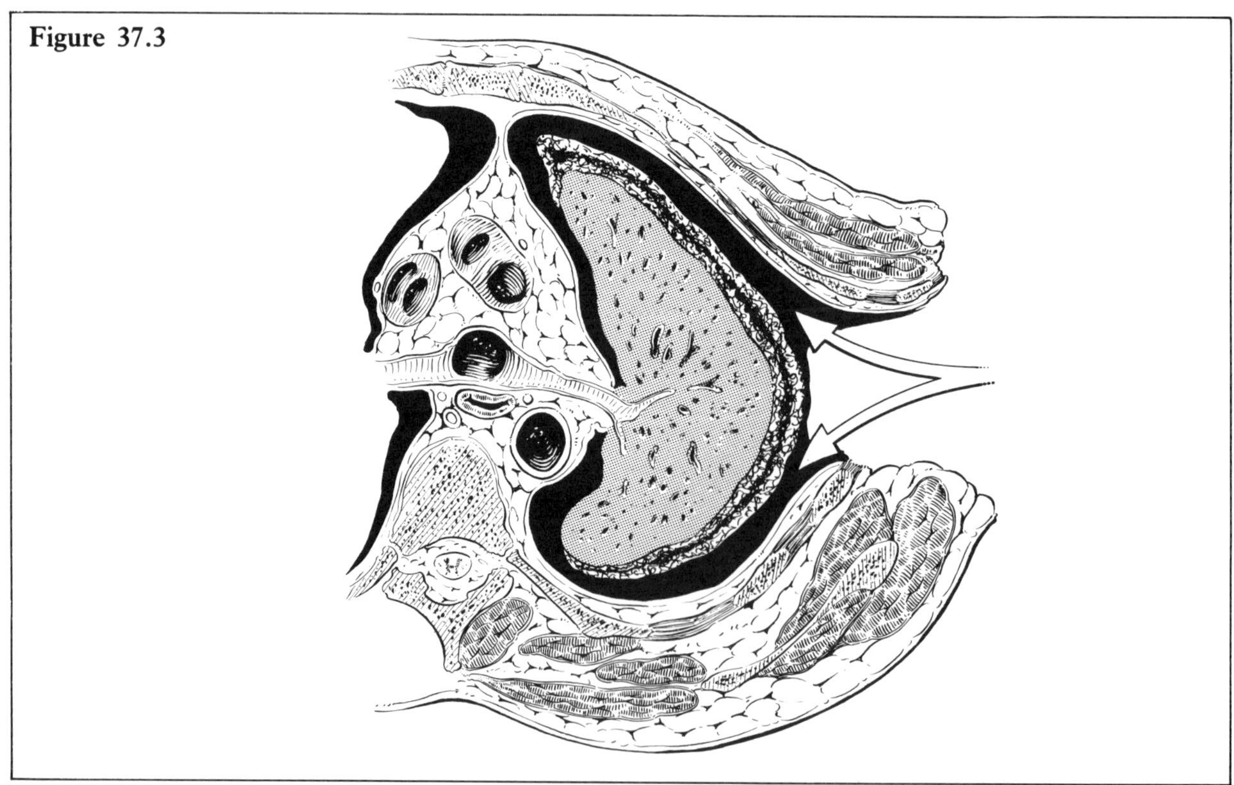

Figure 37.4

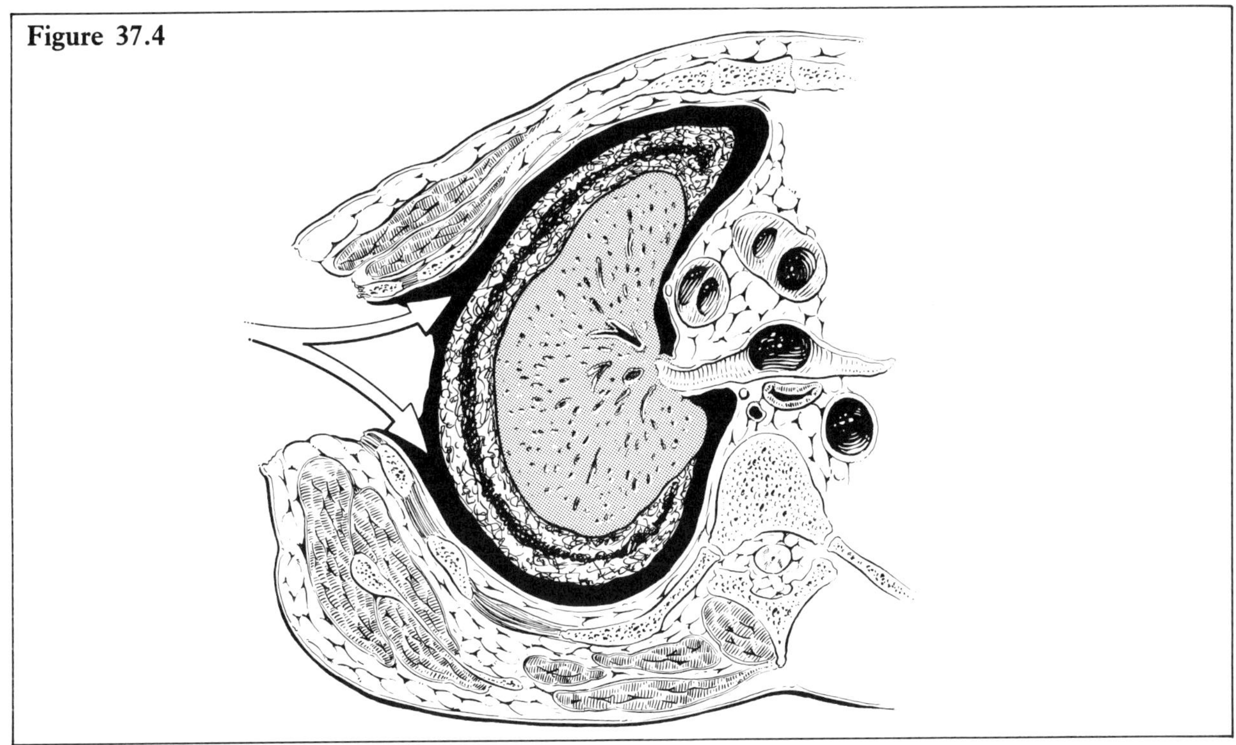

Figure 37.5

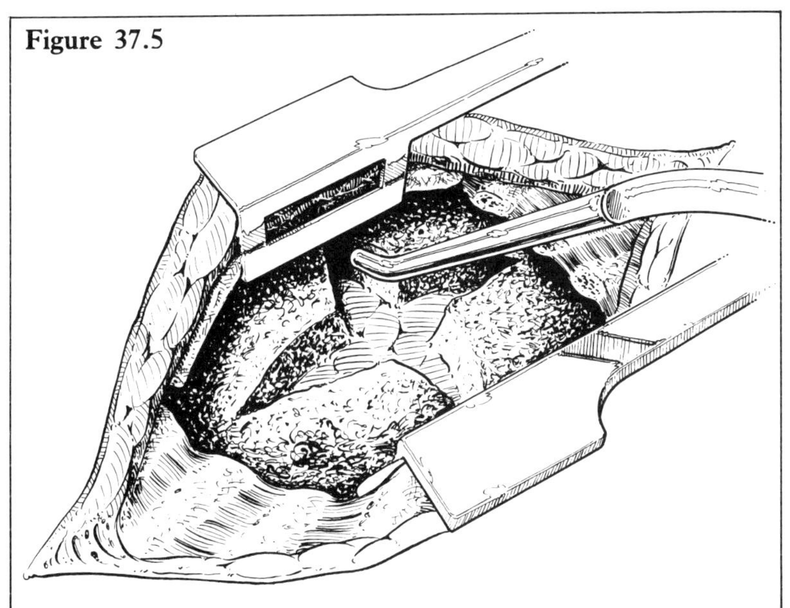

Figure 37.6

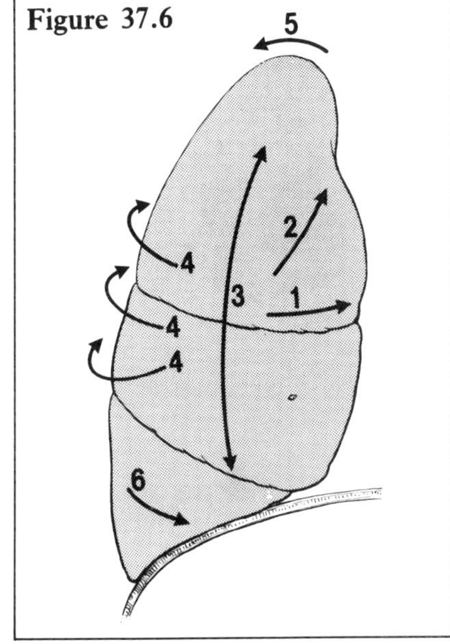


Anterior dissection

This should be the initial approach (1 and 2 in **Fig. 37.6**). Much of the separation can be done by pressing with the fingers on the empyema sac in the angle between it and the chest wall. It is essential to keep to the correct plane, and if muscle fibres are seen to have come away from the chest wall with the empyema sac the plane is too superficial. The muscle fibres must be swept off the sac with closed scissors or cut off with diathermy, and the correct plane found deep to them. As the dissection approaches the midline, the internal mammary vessels are encountered running vertically. They are identified at the plane

Figure 37.7

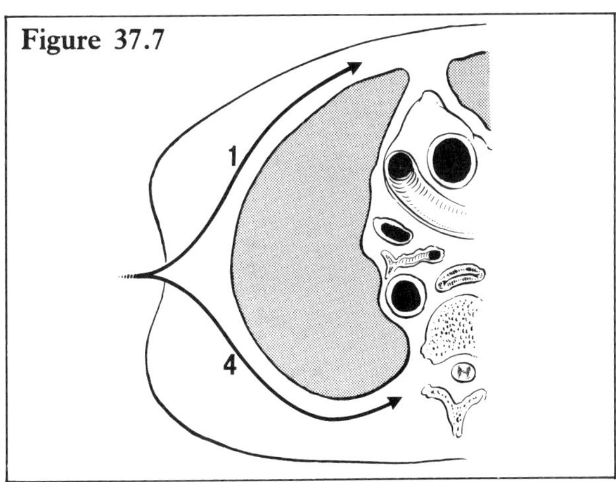

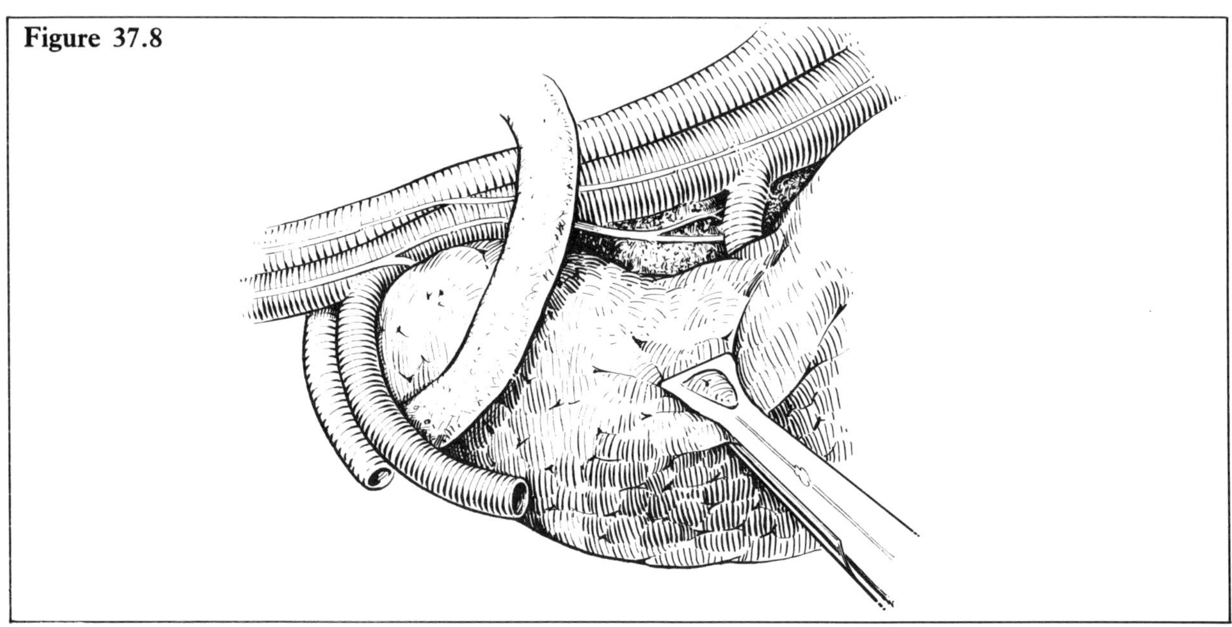
**Figure 37.8**

of separation anteriorly and can be followed upwards and downwards. If they or their branches are inadvertently torn, they are ligated. At about this position the anterior limit of the empyema cavity is encountered; medial to it lie the lung and the pericardium. With gentle movements of the fingers the lung can now be separated from the pericardium. The anterior tip of the middle lobe or of the lingula is usually firmly adherent to the parapericardial fat pad by vascular adhesions, which are divided with diathermy. Separation of the lung from the pericardium now continues in a backwards direction. When the phrenic nerve is encountered running downwards over the pericardium, it must be dissected off the lung; otherwise there is a risk of its subsequent division.

Adhesions between the lung and pericardium in this region are usually light, and by continued finger dissection backwards the hilum of the lung (in particular the superior pulmonary vein) is exposed.

The upper part of the anterior dissection is now continued in the plane of the phrenic nerve and the internal mammary vessels (2 in **Fig. 37.6**). On the right side at the upper limit of the pericardium, the superior vena cava is encountered; by following the phrenic nerve, the dissection may reach almost to the apex of the chest (**Figs. 37.8, 37.9**).

The upper dissection should not proceed further anteriorly; in front of the ascending aorta and behind the sternum the two pleural sacs are almost in contact, and there is a danger of opening the opposite pleura.

### Lateral dissection

It is now possible to extend the space beneath the ribs both above and below the level of the resected rib (3 in **Fig. 37.6**), mostly by blunt dissection

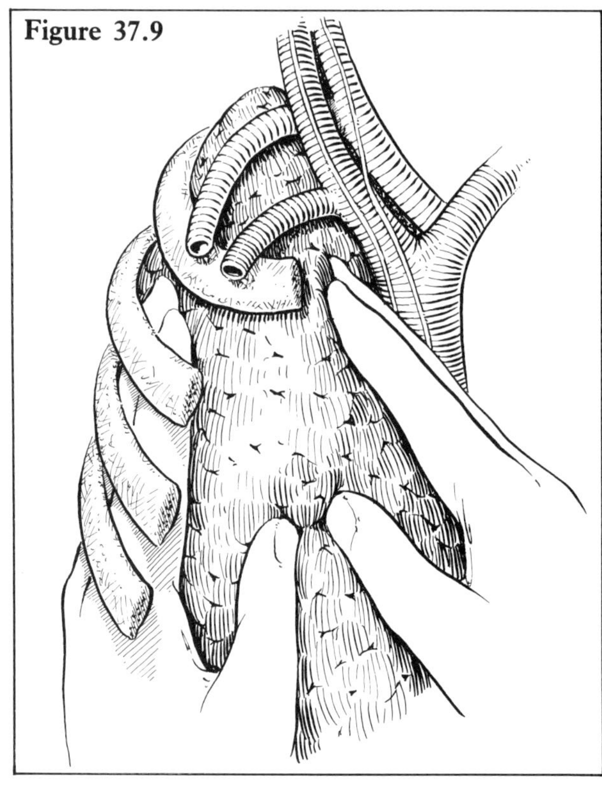
**Figure 37.9**

with the fingers. Over the lateral surface of the upper lobe, the intercostal muscle fibres tend to come away from the chest wall with the sac and must be dissected off as previously described. Working downwards over the lower lobe, areas of very dense fusion are often encountered, which may need to be levered off with a broad, flat instrument such as the Semb first rib rugine. At this stage the inferior dissection should not proceed further caudally than a line drawn through the posterior end of the ninth rib and the xiphisternum, to avoid the real danger of detachment of the margins of the diaphram from the chest wall.

### Posterior dissection

Beginning at the posterior end of the incision, the fingers are used to extend the space upwards, downwards and medially (4 in **Fig. 37.6**), pressing always in the angle between the sac and the chest wall. The correct plane is identified by the appearance of the sympathetic chain on the heads of the ribs; this structure should be followed both upwards and downwards.

On the right side, as the dissection extends round the posterior limit of the sac and proceeds anteriorly, the azygos vein is encountered. The dissection must proceed lateral to it, otherwise its intercostal branches will be torn, causing considerable bleeding. If this occurs the main trunk of the vein may itself require ligation above the diaphragm, and again where it turns forwards on to the mediastinum. In front of the azygos vein the posterior limit of the sac will be encountered, and beyond this, the lung is only lightly adherent to the mediastinum. Nevertheless, care must be taken to avoid injuring the oesophagus lying anterior to the azygos vein.

Proceeding a little higher, the finger is used to tunnel along the course of the azygos vein, across the mediastinum towards the superior vena cava. At the same time the right index finger tunnels backwards from the superior vena cava along the termination of the azygos vein immediately above the hilum (**Fig. 37.10**). The two tunnels are readily united, and the space thus formed can be extended upwards, freeing the lung and mediastinal pleura from the upper part of the superior vena cava, the side of the trachea and the upper oesophagus.

On the left side the posterior limit of the sac overlies the descending thoracic aorta. It is a common mistake to continue this dissection too far back before turning anteriorly to free the posterior limit of the sac and the lung from the mediastinum.

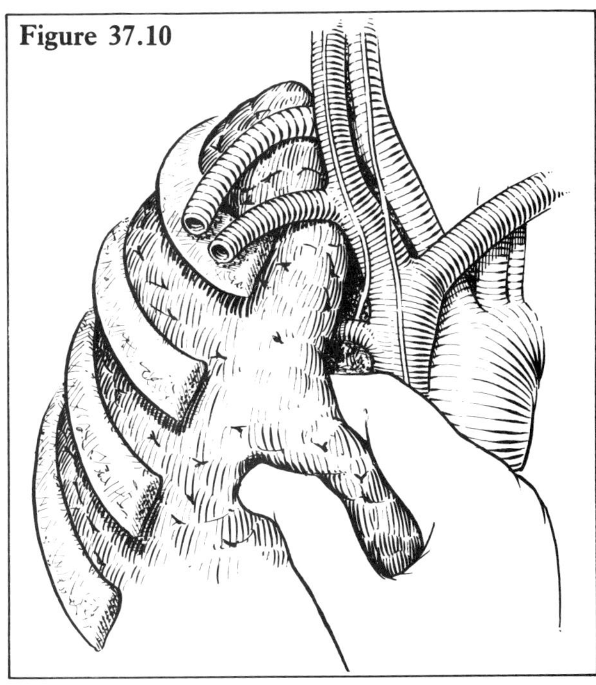
**Figure 37.10**

The intercostal arteries may then be avulsed from the aorta, and this too can be a source of serious haemorrhage. The error can be avoided by feeling the aortic pulsation and ensuring that the dissection continues on its left side. Anterior to the aorta, the oesophagus is exposed and then the hilum of the lung is reached. The inferior pulmonary vein is exposed by blunt dissection below, with the left main bronchus above it. A similar tunnelling procedure to that adopted on the right side can now be carried out along the arch of the aorta beneath the mediastinal pleura to link up with the upper anterior dissection, which has exposed the intrapericardial ascending aorta. Expansion of the dissected space upwards frees the oesophagus and left subclavian artery posteriorly, and the phrenic and vagus nerves anteriorly (**Fig. 37.11**).

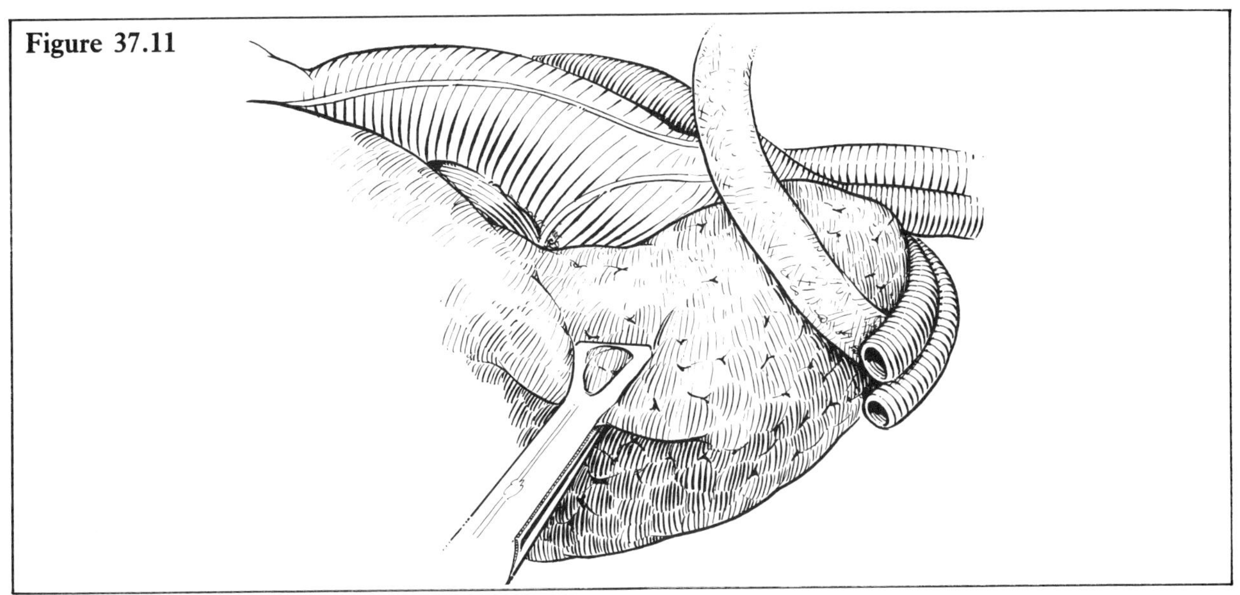
**Figure 37.11**

The thoracic duct overlies this portion of the oesophagus, and it may be torn during the dissection. The area must be inspected for evidence of persistent leakage of a little clear fluid. If this is seen, the ends of the duct should be sought and ligated to prevent the development of a chylothorax.

### Apical dissection

The upper part of the sac has now been freed all round except for the apex, which is now dissected (5 in **Fig. 37.6**). Here there may be dense fibrosis extending from the upper part of the sac, or from disease such as healed tuberculosis in the apex of the upper lobe, in the form of fibrous bands extending into the neck around the subclavian artery and vein and the first thoracic nerve. There may also be dense fusion around the upper intervertebral foramina. The sac and upper lobe are grasped with the left hand and drawn down. By a combination of traction and careful blunt dissection the apex can often be freed sufficiently for the vessels and nerve to be identified, so that the remaining strands of fibrous tissue can be divided. The first thoracic nerve may remain adherent to the fibrous tissue at the apex of the lung so that a loop of it is drawn down with the apex. The whole length of the nerve must be clearly visible in the apex of the pleural cavity before any 'fibrous tissue' bands are divided.

### Inferior dissection

This is the final stage of dissection (6 in **Fig. 37.6**). The first aim is to identify the diaphragm. This can best be done either from the anterior or the mediastinal aspect. The pleura is freed from the lowest part of the pericardium, and the dissection then extended laterally. On the right side the phrenic nerve is followed from the pericardium over the inferior vena cava and on to the diaphragm. The inferior vena cava is thin here and it must not be injured. With a similar bimanual technique to that described for dissection above the hilum, the anterior and posterior mediastinal dissections are united after division of the pulmonary ligament. The two or three small arteries in the pulmonary ligament should be coagulated with diathermy after identification of the oesophagus (necrosis of the oesophageal wall caused by diathermy may result in a perforation).

It should now be possible to identify on the diaphragm the anterior and mediastinal edges of the base of the lower lobe. Initial sharp dissection followed by blunt dissection with the fingers frees the lung without difficulty up to the point where the empyema and the diaphragm are in contact. Here the fusion is dense and sharp dissection must be used. The plane to follow is in the most superficial layer of the muscle fibres of the diaphragm. The lung is drawn upwards and the diaphragm held downwards with a mounted swab by an assistant. Bleeding from the diaphragm, which is often profuse, can be avoided by effecting this separation with the diathermy. It must be emphasized again that the plane is exactly on the surface of the diaphragmatic muscle.

As the dissection proceeds the line of section recedes continuously. Access is improved if the operator now works from the position of the patient's shoulder, facing the feet, or from a corresponding position on the opposite side of the operating table. Traction on the sac and the lower lobe will sometimes draw the diaphragm upwards and improve the visibility. If the costophrenic recess still cannot be reached, the sac is opened widely and the contents sucked out. The operator can then see the lower limit of the empyema from within and detach it by sharp dissection. It is not necessary to remove all the fibrous tissue so long as all the granulation tissue is excised.

### Completion of the operation

The operation is completed by one of three procedures.

1. If no lung resection is necessary: decortication of the lung (p. 141).
2. If a part of the lung requires excision: the appropriate lobectomy combined with decortication of the remainder of the lung.
3. When there is an indication for pneumonectomy: the hilar structures are divided and the lung and empyema are removed together.

If a portion of the diaphragm has been detached from the chest wall, it must be reattached once the empyema has been removed. This is done with a series of strong mattress sutures which are placed

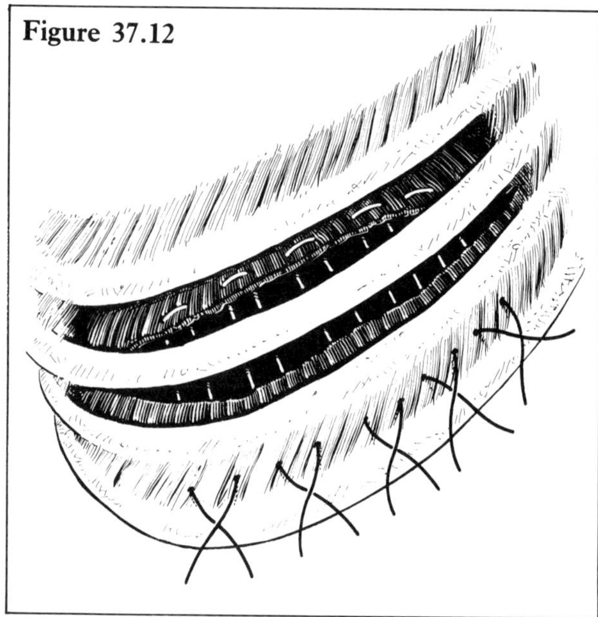

**Figure 37.12**

circumferentially in the edge of the diaphragm, passed through the chest wall through the intercostal spaces, and tied outside the rib cage (**Fig. 37.12**). If the intercostal muscle is atrophied the sutures are tied round the ribs.

## Decortication of the lung

This procedure should always be carried out in surgery for empyema when expansion of the lung is prevented by thickened, organized fibrous tissue that has formed on the surface of the visceral pleura. Such a condition may also be part of a chronic haemothorax. A restricting cortex may also form over the remaining lung when full expansion does not occur after a lung resection, and occasionally in cases of chronic pneumothorax. In empyema and organized haemothorax, excision of the parietal pleura will be necessary as well. In all other cases the excision is limited to the visceral pleura.

If the parietal pleura has been removed, the cavity walls will have been widely opened and the contents removed. Dissection of the visceral pleura is begun in a region where the thickening is minimal. The slightly thickened pleura is picked up with forceps and cut lightly with a broad-bladed knife (**Figs. 37.13, 37.14**). It should be possible to enter a plane between this redundant tissue and a shiny and intact true visceral pleural layer beneath it. Much of this separation can be done with a finger. The opening in the redundant layer of pleura is enlarged and held up with several pairs of forceps as a progressively larger space develops and a greater surface of lung is exposed (**Fig. 37.15**).

**Figure 37.13**

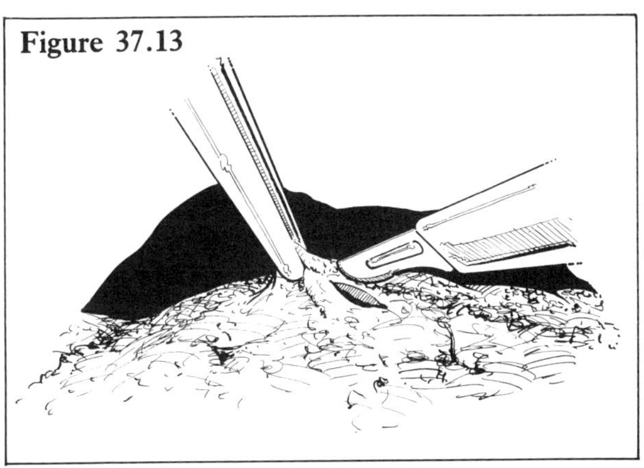

**Figure 37.14**

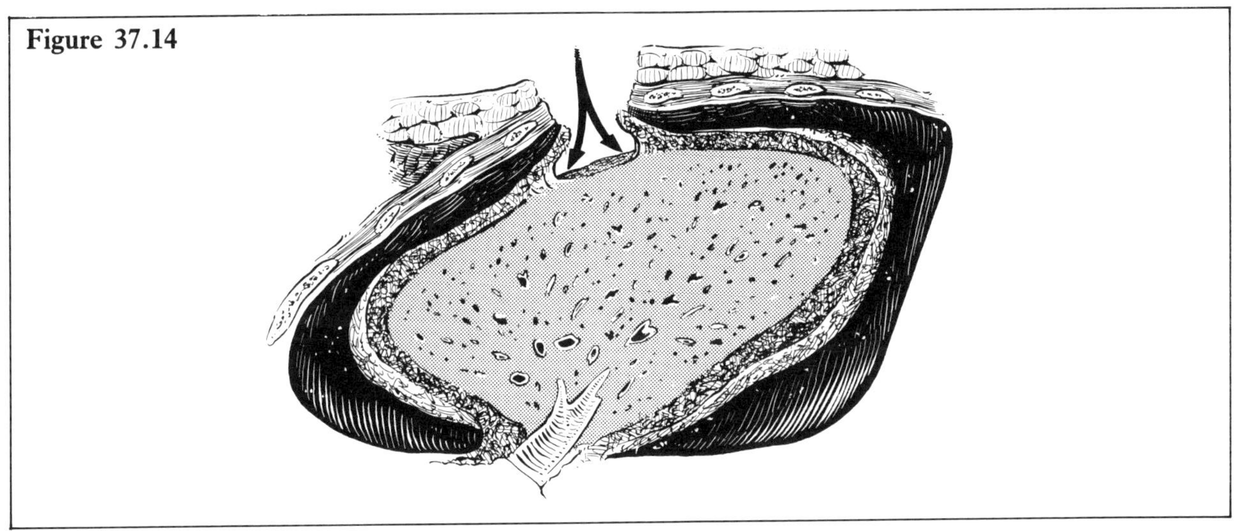

**Figure 37.15**

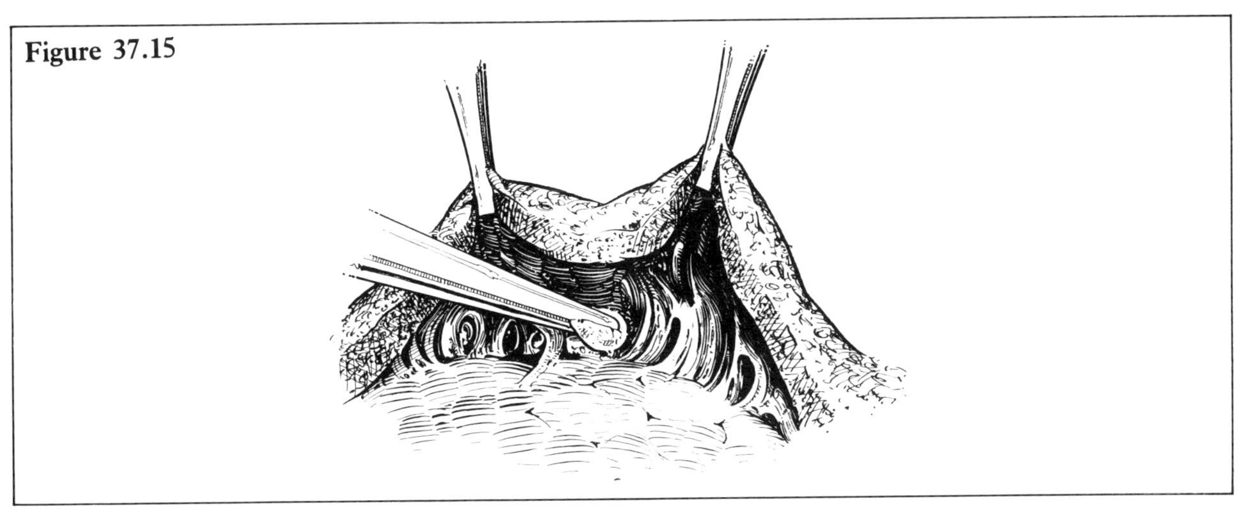

The procedure is best carried out with the lung moderately inflated. When a denser area of fibrosis is encountered, finger dissection is no longer effective and sharp dissection is used. Much of this can be done effectively with scissors cutting slightly more towards the cortex that is being removed, than into the angle between the cortex and the visceral pleura. In other areas the fibrosis may involve the visceral pleura, and here a scalpel is necessary, used with a very light touch, and cutting parallel to the inflated lung surface.

When there is no possibility of finding a plane between cortex and lung because of underlying disease or fibrosis, then the best procedure is to dissect around the fibrotic area, leaving a plaque of cortex on the surface of the lung.

The layer of thickened cortex should be followed into the lung fissures and removed, and the separation continued over the costal, mediastinal and diaphragmatic aspects of the lung until all the lobes are free. Inflation of the lung is then increased so that any constricting bands of thickened pleura left can be found and divided. Remaining restricted areas can be released by a series of cruciate incisions (**Fig. 37.16**).

## Decortication after empyema excision

In completing the operation of excision of empyema or a chronic haemothorax, the procedure to be followed is much the same, starting from the area where the fibrosis is least, which is usually the mediastinal aspect. When the edge of the empyema cavity is encountered the fibrosis becomes denser but the appropriate plane for dissection can usually be found. The operator must always be prepared to abandon one particular approach and proceed from a different direction. The operation is slow and tedious, but hurrying is likely to result in extensive damage to the surface of the lung. The empyema has often resulted from spread of infection from the lung and in the area where this has occurred, it may be necessary to leave part of the visceral wall of the sac and its granulation tissue intact. If a bronchopleural fistula is known to be present, the site of perforation of the lung should be sought and closed with fine polypropylene sutures.

**Figure 37.16**

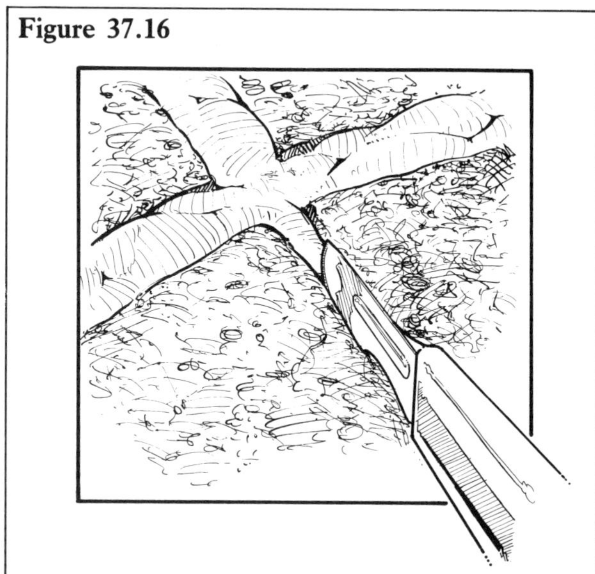

When decortication is complete the surface of the lung is carefully inspected for bleeding and for tears. Air leaks from superficial abrasion of the visceral pleura are best left alone, but accidental tears or incisions should be repaired with fine polypropylene sutures.

If induced hypotension has been used to control bleeding during excision of an empyema, the blood pressure should now be returned to normal. The packs that compressed the raw areas of the chest wall throughout the operation are removed, and all areas inspected for bleeding. All bleeding points in the chest wall should be coagulated with diathermy. A dental mirror is very helpful in visualizing the apical and basal lateral areas of the chest wall. When this technique has been adopted, control of the bleeding after restoration of the blood pressure is not usually a problem.

## Drainage

After simple decortication two pleural drains will suffice. When the operation has been combined with excision of an empyema or a chronic haemothorax, at least three drains should be used, placed anteriorly, laterally and posteriorly. Suction of 50–100 mmHg (7–13 kPa) should be continued until the lung is fully expanded and all air leak has ceased.

# 38 Early post-pneumonectomy bronchopleural fistula

Bronchopleural fistula is one of the most serious complications after lung resection. The pleural cavity inevitably becomes infected so that every case is accompanied by an empyema. The condition is less serious after lobectomy because it can be treated by excision of the empyema, decortication of the lung and closure of the reamputated bronchus. The expanded remaining lung can then obliterate the pleural space and in so doing isolate and seal the bronchial stump. If the volume of the remaining lung is inadequate to fill the pleural cavity completely a thoracoplasty can be performed at the same time, although this is very rarely necessary. An alternative is brief freezing of the phrenic nerve with the cryoprobe, producing temporary diaphragm paralysis.

The bronchopleural fistula that follows a pneumonectomy represents a much more difficult problem. The fistula may occur either early or late after the original pneumonectomy. 'Early' in this case refers to the first week following operation.

## Management of early bronchopleural fistula after pneumonectomy

One of the earliest manifestations of a bronchopleural fistula is the coughing up of watery brown fluid from the pleural space. This fluid may be aspirated into the contralateral lung.

The emergency treatment is the insertion of a basal intercostal tube to drain all the fluid from the pleural cavity and so prevent further aspiration. If some aspiration has already occurred it may be necessary to delay any operative procedure until the remaining lung has recovered fully.

Special care is necessary when inducing anaesthesia in these patients. There is a danger of aspiration of pleural contents into the opposite side (although this should be minimized by tube drainage). There is also a risk of inadequate ventilation where the fistula is large so that most of the anaesthetic gases escape through the fistula, which may result in mediastinal displacement. The patient is therefore anaesthetized sitting up at 45 degrees with an inhalation method such as nitrous oxide and halothane. An endobronchial double lumen tube is then passed so that the opposite bronchus can be excluded, before moving the patient to a supine position and beginning positive pressure ventilation.

The aim of this operation is to reamputate the bronchus and to isolate it from the infected pleural space. If the repair is carried out through a thoracotomy, an intercostal muscle bundle may be used to cover the new bronchial stump. To construct the intercostal muscle bundle it is necessary to enter the pleural cavity through a different intercostal space from the one that was used for the original operation. Thus if the original operation was carried out through the fifth intercostal space, the fourth or sixth should be utilized on this occasion.

The periosteum is incised along the middle of the outer surface of the appropriate rib and then stripped as previously described from the lower half and undersurface of the rib. A similar incision is made along the rib below and the periosteum stripped from the upper and deep surface (**Fig. 38.1**). This process must be continued anteriorly as far as the costal cartilage, where the intercostal muscle bundle and its accompanying vessels are divided (**Fig. 38.2**). Posteriorly, the

**Figure 38.1**

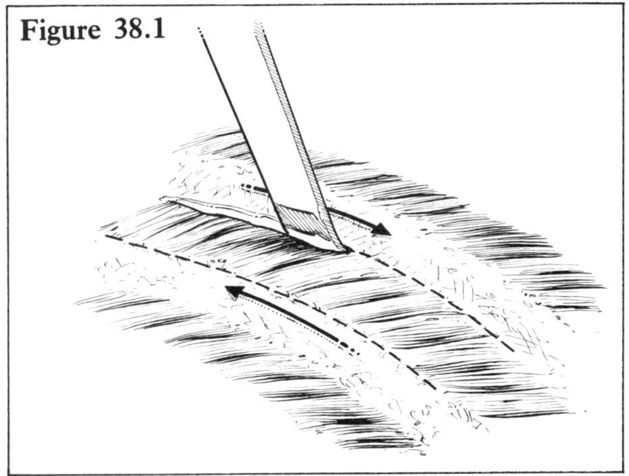

**Figure 38.2**

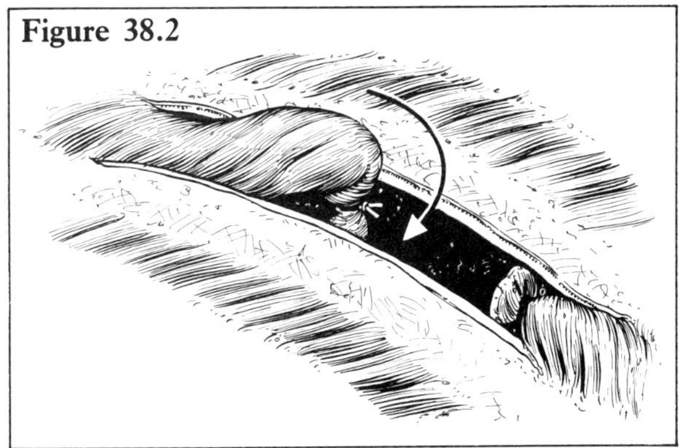

bundle is freed up to the neck of the rib, but the intercostal artery and its collateral artery are carefully preserved. The intercostal muscle flap is allowed to fall into the pleural cavity and the rib spreader is now inserted. It may be necessary to remove one of the denuded ribs to obtain adequate access. The insertion of the rib spreader is delayed to this point so that there is no danger of crushing the intercostal muscle and vessels of the prepared bundle.

Blood and fibrin in the pleural cavity are removed and the empyema cavity walls excised or curetted. If the exploration is carried out early after the original operation the fistula can usually be seen in the depths of the mediastinum. If not, the anaesthetist should be asked to deflate the bronchial cuff and inflate the tracheal cuff of the endotracheal tube. Air may then be seen emerging from the site of the fistula; if there is still doubt about its location, a small amount of saline can be introduced, through which bubbles will be seen emerging when the anaesthetist raises the ventilation pressure.

The end of the bronchus must now be dissected out. *On the right side* the main hazard is presented by the stump of the right pulmonary artery, which lies immediately anterior to the origin of the right main bronchus (**Fig. 38.3**). The dissection should therefore start along the anterior or posterior wall of the trachea *above* the level of the fistula. The lower half of the trachea is first separated from the oesophagus behind, taking great care to avoid penetrating the oesophageal wall or the membranous trachea. Anteriorly the lower half of the trachea may be fused to the posterior wall of the superior vena cava, especially if the right paratracheal nodes have been removed. By retracting the oesophagus backwards the origin of the left main bronchus is exposed. This facilitates the exposure of the carina (**Fig. 38.4**).

Keeping the dissection close to the wall of the lower end of the trachea and working distally, the operator can now free the amputated bronchus. The dissection can be facilitated by passing slings of tape or fine rubber tubes round the lower end of the trachea and the origin of the left main bronchus. The suture line and the adjacent traumatized bronchial wall are now excised and the bronchus closed with a series of four or five interrupted monofilament stainless steel wires or 3/0 polypropylene sutures. The sutures should all be placed before any of them is tied. If the bronchial stump is short these sutures will encroach on the trachea, but this is of no importance so long as the lumen of the left main bronchus is not compromised.

The intercostal muscle flap is now placed in position so that its long axis lies parallel to the suture line and with the periosteum in contact with the membranous wall of the bronchus. One edge of the flap is attached to the membranous wall of the bronchus behind the suture line, using three or four interrupted 4/0 polypropylene sutures. One more suture is inserted just beyond the ends of the bronchial suture line but not tied at this stage. The periosteum is then drawn over the bronchial suture line to its anterior aspect and similarly fixed here with three or four polypropylene sutures. The two end sutures can now be tied, thus completely covering the bronchial stump. The pleural cavity is completely filled with saline containing 150 mg of gentamicin and 5 megaunits of penicillin. Every effort is made to close the intercostal layer completely by approximating the separated ribs with pericostal tension sutures, followed by a continuous nylon suture approximating the muscles. This sealing of the space is facilitated if a rib has been removed. The chest is closed without drainage.

*On the left side*, visualizing the bronchial stump is more difficult because after amputation it retracts deeply beneath the arch of the aorta. Access to it is obtained by mobilizing the aortic arch and turning it forwards.

**Figure 38.3**

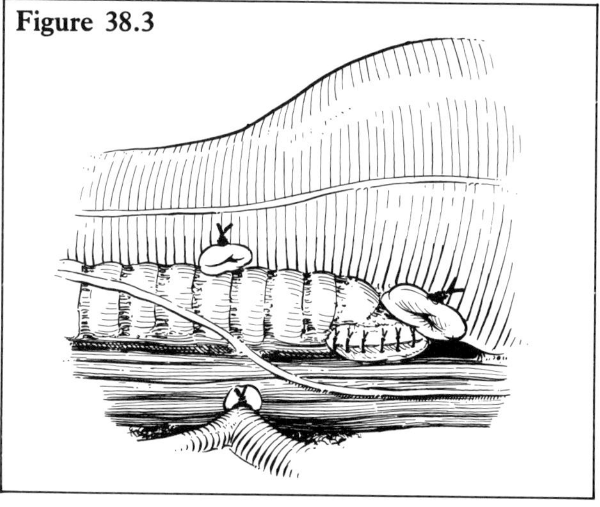

**Figure 38.4**

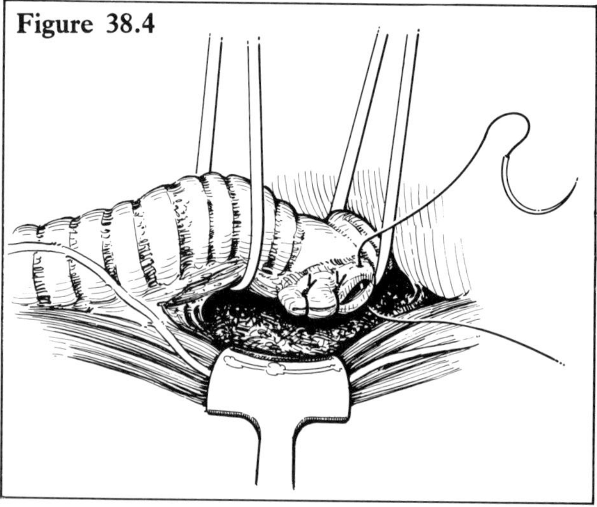

**Figure 38.5**

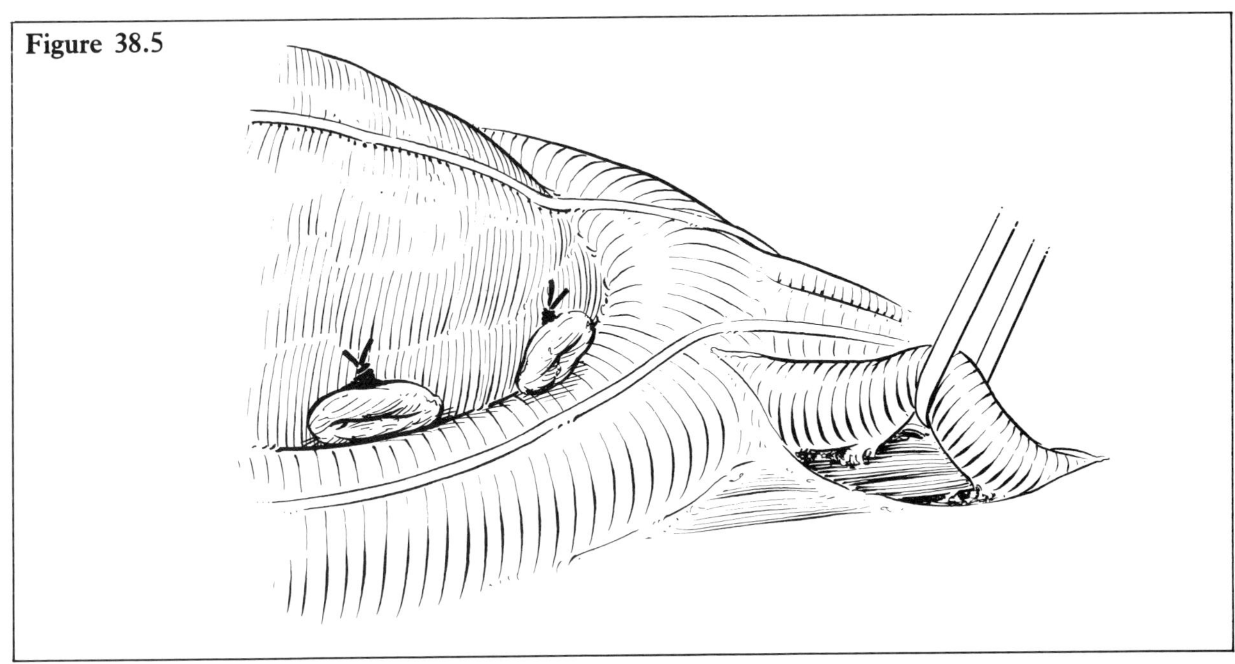

After debridement of the pleural cavity, the subclavian artery is dissected out and a tape passed around it (**Fig. 38.5**). The thoracic duct lies immediately behind the subclavian artery overlying the oesophagus in this region, and is at risk of injury. The duct may be difficult to see, but if it is divided the persistence of a small pool of clear lymph in the region indicates that it has been damaged. In such a case the two ends should be found and ligated.

Following the plane of the subclavian artery downwards, the thickened mediastinal pleura is incised over the descending thoracic aorta. The left superior intercostal vein which crosses it here will probably have been ligated at the time of the original pneumonectomy, but if not it must be divided. The pleural flaps are dissected away from the first part of the descending thoracic aorta, which is then gradually mobilized by blunt dissection just beyond the origin of the left subclavian artery. Care must be taken not to injure the intercostal arteries which arise from the posterolateral surface of the aorta. If their origins are high they will require ligation. A tape is then passed round the upper part of the descending thoracic aorta just beyond the left subclavian artery (**Fig. 38.6**). If one of the intercostal arteries is inadvertently torn, the distal end is secured and ligated. The site of origin from the aorta is occluded with a finger while the dissection to place a tape round the aorta is continued. Then by traction on the tape, the site of leakage is easily identified and is closed with a 4/0 polypropylene stitch.

The anterior flap of pleura is dissected off the distal part of the aortic arch. The vagus and recurrent laryngeal nerves will be seen crossing the

**Figure 38.6**

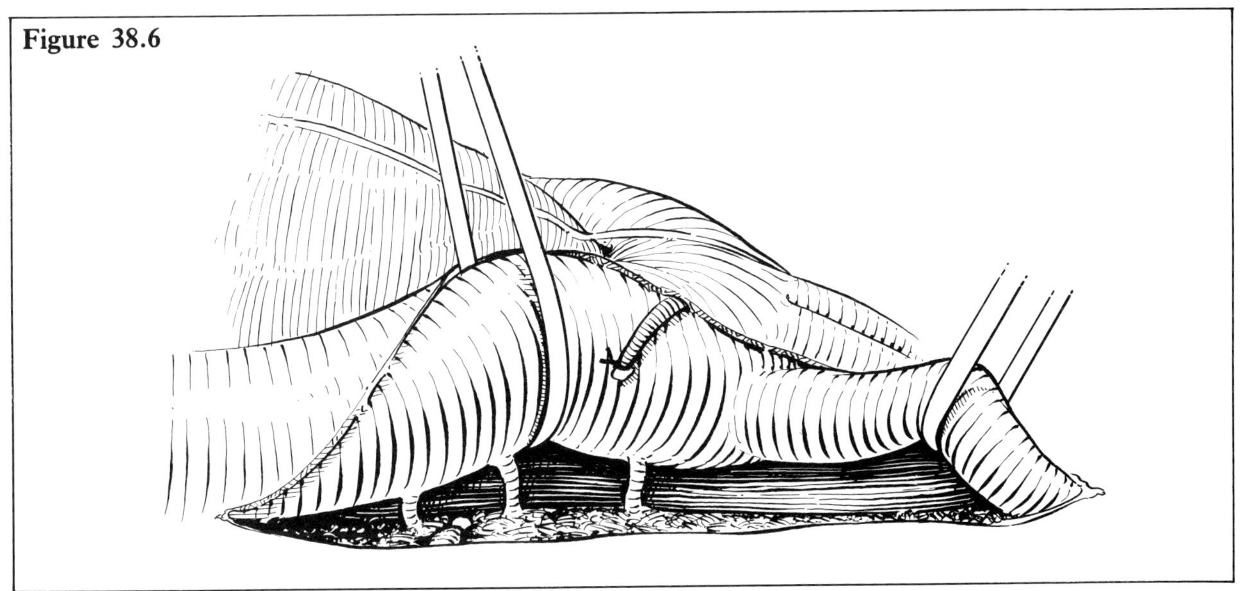

**Figure 38.7**

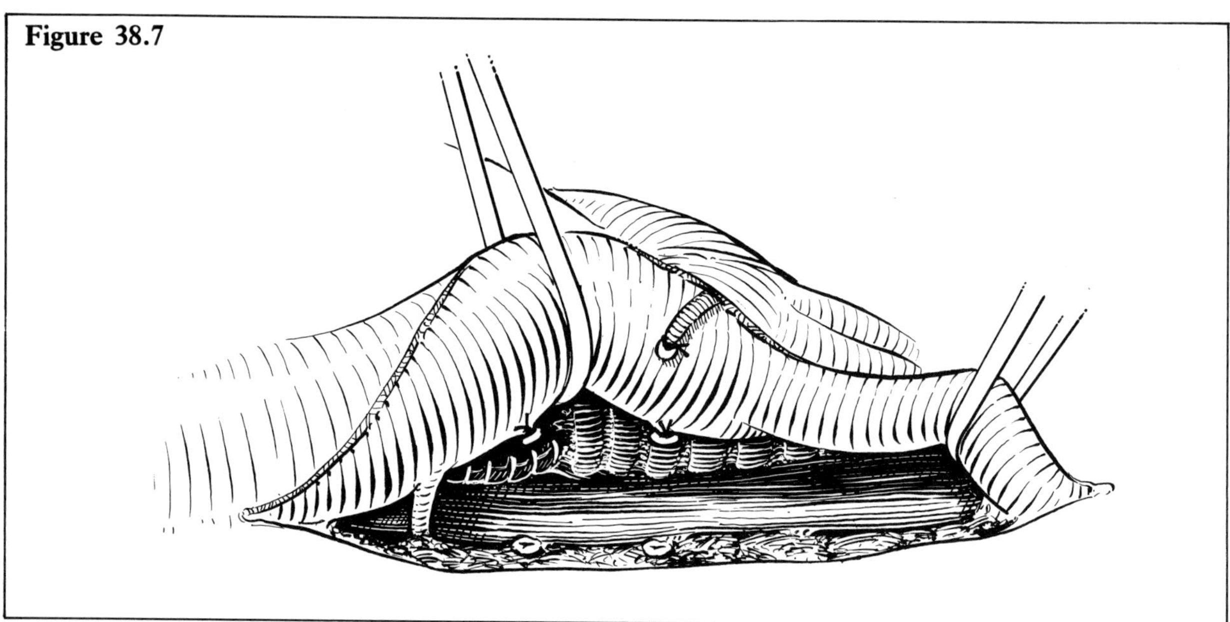

arch immediately anterior to the left subclavian artery and must be preserved. Working partly from below the arch and partly behind it after retracting the subclavian artery forwards, the distal arch is mobilized largely by finger dissection, and a tape passed round it. By forward traction on the aortic tapes the posterior surface of the aorta is now freed from the oesophagus and the lower end of the left side of the trachea (**Fig. 38.7**). The dissection is easier than on the right side because these structures have not previously been dissected. The bronchial stump now comes into view and is treated exactly as described for the right side.

# 39 Late post-pneumonectomy bronchopleural fistula

Because of the extensive pleural sepsis and fibrosis, it is not usually possible to treat these fistulae in the manner described for early fistulae. Long-term drainage of the pleural space will already have been established.

A simple approach which is sometimes effective for a small fistula is endoscopic cauterization. This is carried out by inspection of the fistula with the rigid bronchoscope and the application of 20% caustic soda. The cottonwool bud of a bacterial swab held in the jaws of bronchoscopic biopsy forceps serves as a useful applicator. The cottonwool tip is dipped in 20% caustic soda, lightly wrung out and then applied, and repeatedly replaced by fresh swabs until the whole area turns black. It has been recommended that the caustic soda is neutralized by swabs soaked in acetic acid, but we have found this to be unnecessary as long as any excess fluid in the region is removed by suction.

The procedure should be repeated at two-weekly intervals and is probably worth continuing for up to ten applications. Its success can be determined by removing air from the pleural cavity with a pneumothorax apparatus until a negative pressure is achieved. The pressure is measured a few hours later and if it has not returned to atmospheric levels, it may be assumed that the fistula has closed. If this is the case, the empyema cavity should be treated by irrigation (p. 66), and then the chronic tube track is excised and closed.

If cauterization fails to close the fistula, the problem becomes more difficult to solve and requires major surgical techniques. Since it is likely that the pneumonectomy was carried out for malignant disease, it is undesirable to subject the patient to a major operation when the prognosis may be very limited. It is usual, therefore, to wait at least a year so as to detect early recurrence of the tumour. During this time the patient may be able to live an acceptable—albeit somewhat restricted—life with permanent intercostal tube drainage of the empyema space. The degree of restriction is determined by the size of the bronchopleural fistula, since the air flow through the fistula may seriously impair the patient's ventilation, and by the quantity of purulent drainage, which will determine the frequency of dressing changes during the day.

Excision of the fistula and obliteration of the pleural space by extensive thoracoplasty or the use of vascular pedicle muscle flaps is successful in some cases. Our preferred method for closure of the fistula is re-resection or repair of the bronchial stump via a transpericardial approach. This technique has the advantage that the resutured bronchial stump is excluded from the infected pleural cavity, so that there is a greater chance of healing without the risk of secondary infection of the newly formed suture line.

The approach for either right or left side is through a median sternotomy. The sternum is divided with an oscillating saw which diminishes the risk of opening a pleural cavity. The raw surface of the bone is sealed with bone wax and divided periosteal vessels on both the superficial and deep aspects of the sternum are sealed with diathermy.

The pericardium is opened in the midline and the pericardial fluid is removed with a sucker. The underlying heart is protected with two fingers while the pericardial incision is continued downwards until the diaphragm is reached. Lateral extension of this incision at right angles to the original incision for 3 cm to the right and left opens the pericardium widely, and allows it to be suspended from the wound edge with sutures. The two lobes of the thymus gland are separated as far up as the innominate vein which crosses the upper part of the field. The sternal spreader can now be opened widely to give excellent exposure of the operative field.

To expose the *right* main bronchial stump, the aorta must be retracted to the left and the superior vena cava to the right. First a sling is passed around the ascending aorta. To allow this the pericardium between the ascending aorta and the pulmonary artery is incised and a space opened by blunt dissection between the two. A curved Semb artery forceps is then passed under the ascending aorta and a tape fed into the jaws of the clamp and

Figure 39.1

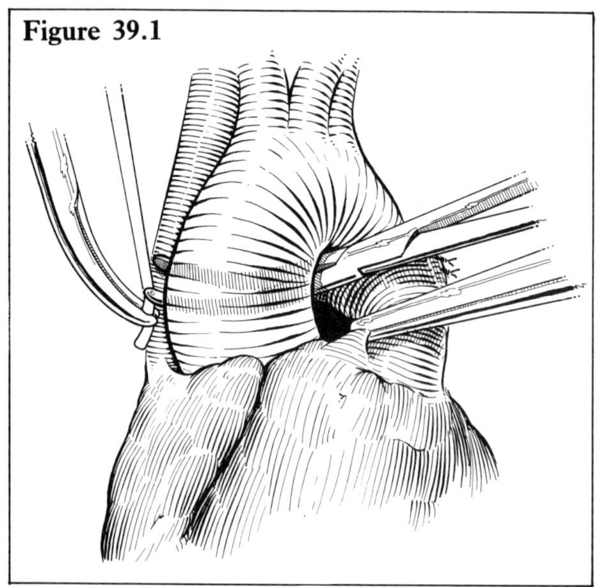

Figure 39.2

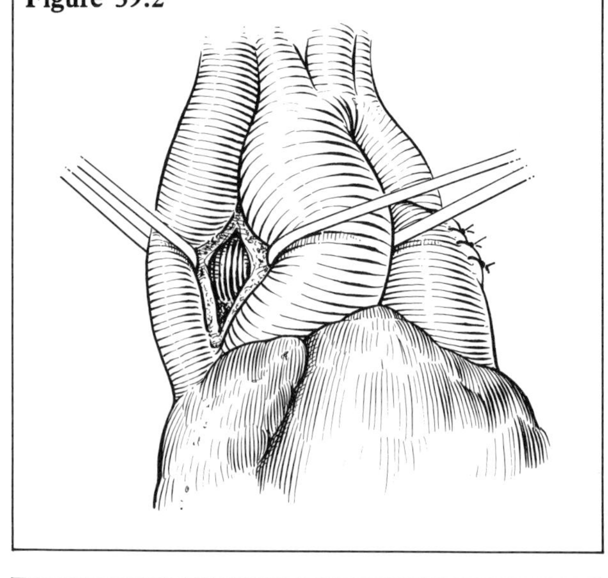

Figure 39.3

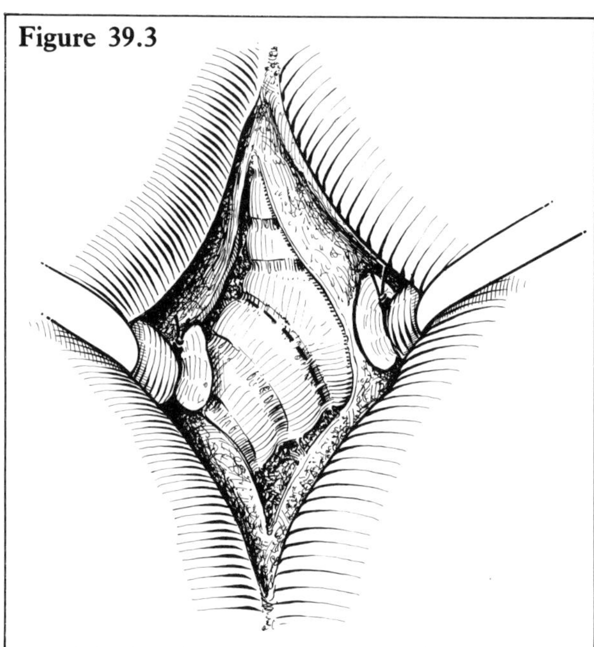

Figure 39.4

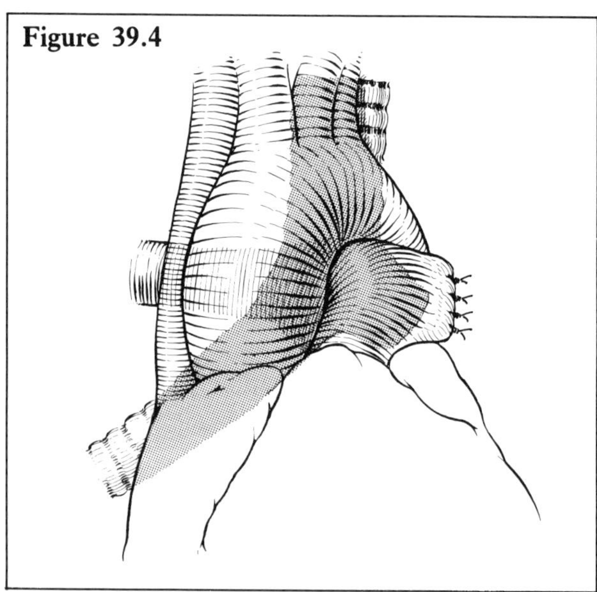

drawn around it (**Fig. 39.1**). Care must be taken to avoid injuring the right pulmonary artery which lies immediately beneath the ascending aorta.

The pericardium is now picked up and incised on the left side of the superior vena cava. Here again the pulmonary artery lies directly beneath it. With a similar technique to that used for the aorta, a tape is passed round the superior vena cava. The ascending aorta is drawn to the left and the superior vena cava to the right. Between the two the right pulmonary artery is seen coursing transversely (**Fig. 39.2**). The pericardium is incised along its upper and lower margins, and a 3-cm length of the artery is dissected free. It is ligated at each end of this portion. Alternatively, it may be divided between arterial clamps and the cut ends closed with a continuous 4/0 polypropylene suture.

Immediately deep to the pulmonary artery the lower end of the trachea and the origin of the right main bronchus will be found. The pericardium is incised upwards along the right border of the trachea and downwards beyond the carina. The fascial sheath of the lower end of the trachea is then opened and the origin of the right main bronchus carefully dissected (**Fig. 39.3**). The bronchus is then divided as high as possible and closed with interrupted figure-of-eight stainless steel wire sutures. The divided bronchial stump is then covered with a flap of pericardium which is attached to both its anterior and posterior surfaces. The distal end of the bronchial stump is also closed with interrupted sutures and displaced towards the pleural cavity by one or more layers of sutures, which will exclude it from the pericardium.

For access to the *left* side, the same incision is used but the retractor must be opened further and the patient rotated about 30 degrees to the right. The anatomical relationships of the major structures are shown in **Fig. 39.4**. The left pulmonary artery is exposed by continuing the pericardial incision between the aorta and main pulmonary artery to the left. A finger can now be passed behind the left pulmonary artery, and thus the pericardium at its lower margin just above the left atrial appendage is identified and incised (**Fig. 39.5**). It is now possible to pass a Semb forceps beneath the left pulmonary artery, which is divided in a manner similar to that on the right.

By intermittent retraction of the left atrium and ventricle to the right the left superior pulmonary vein comes into view (**Fig. 39.6**). It is mobilized and divided between ligatures. Between these two structures the fold of Marshall can be seen running from the posterior aspect of the left atrial appendage to the pulmonary artery. It is divided, after coagulation with diathermy as it usually contains a small vessel.

The aortic arch is retracted upwards with a suitable instrument such as Cummings' retractor. The lower end of the trachea and the origin of the left main bronchus can now be palpated through the posterior parietal peritoneum. Incisions are made along each margin of the origin of the left main bronchus, and its fascial sheath is incised to expose it and the lower end of the trachea (**Fig. 39.7**). The bronchus is closed by direct suture and the stump covered with a flap of posterior parietal pericardium. The distal end of the bronchus is closed off and the pericardium closed over it.

The pericardium can be left open. Two drains should be inserted, one beneath the heart and the

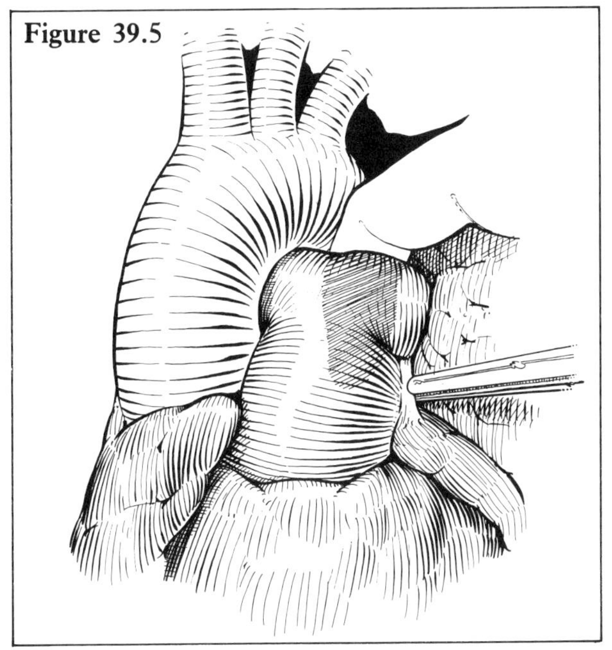
**Figure 39.5**

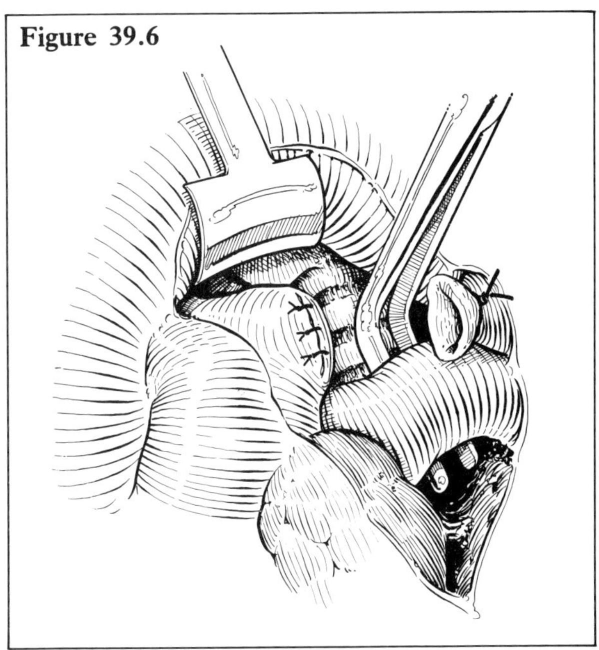
**Figure 39.6**

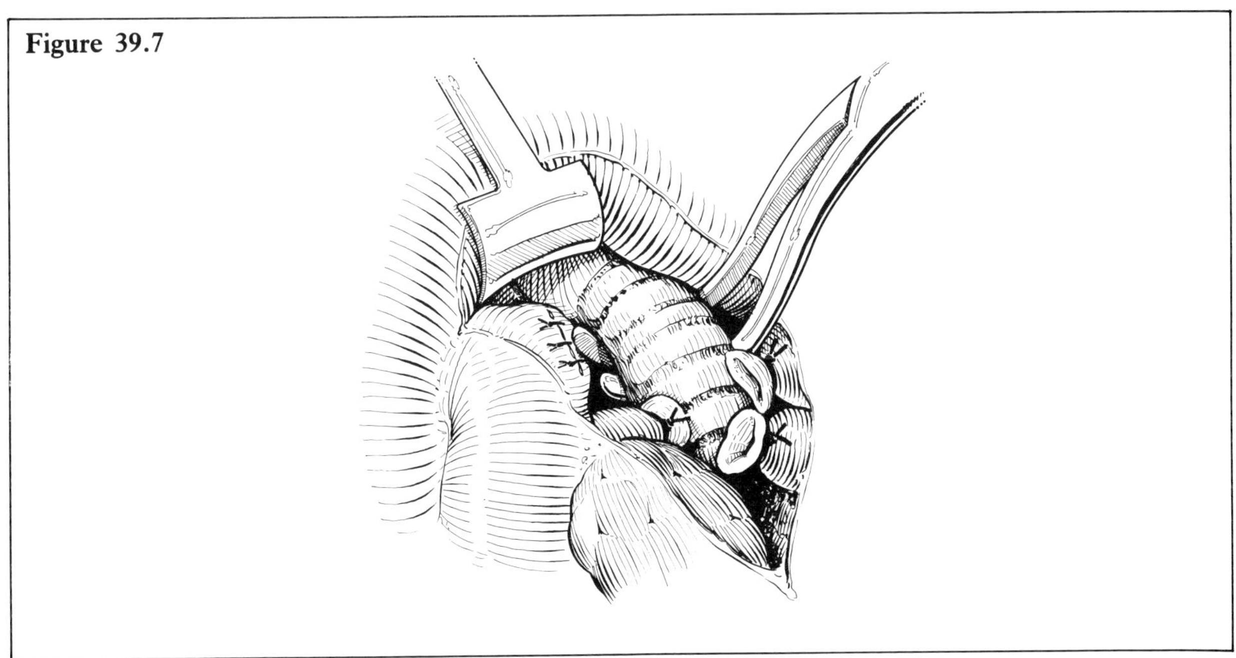
**Figure 39.7**

other anteriorly to it. The two halves of the sternum are approximated with stainless steel wire sutures and the skin and subcutaneous tissue closed.

Successful completion of this operation leaves the patient with an infected pleural cavity. This may be treated by excision and curettage of its walls, and excision and closure of the chronic tube track. Subsequently the space should be treated by irrigation until all infection has been eliminated. The space is then filled with saline containing antibiotics, and in the absence of continued reinfection from an open bronchus, should remain sterile.

If a major thoracic drainage procedure has been carried out previously, an alternative approach is to fill the thoroughly cleaned pneumonectomy space with vascularized chest wall muscle flaps, such as lattisimus dorsi or trapezius. Expert help from a plastic surgeon should be sought in raising these flaps to ensure the best results.

# SECTION 6

# MEDIASTINAL SURGERY

# 40 Anatomy of the mediastinum

The mediastinum is the space between the pleural cavities occupying the centre of the thoracic cavity. It contains the heart and the great vessels, the trachea and its major branches, the oesophagus, the thoracic duct, the thymus gland and the vagus and phrenic nerves (**Figs. 40.1, 40.2**).

**Figure 40.1**

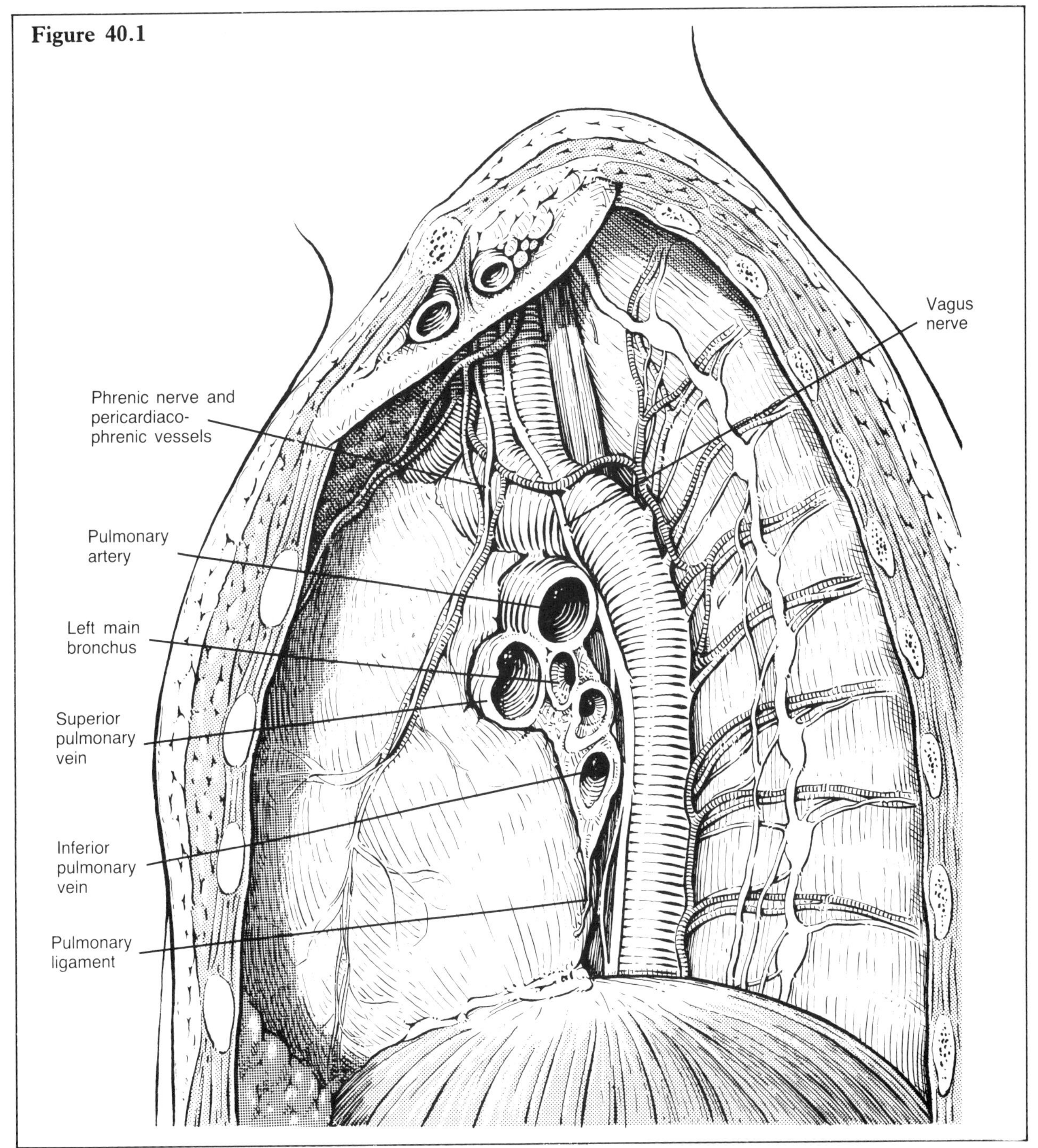

The mediastinum is divided into four compartments: superior, anterior, middle and posterior (**Fig. 40.3**). The important topographical division is an imaginary line between the sternal angle of Louis and the lower border of the fourth thoracic vertebra. Above this line is the superior mediastinum, extending to the thoracic inlet. Below, the mediastinum is divided into three compartments by the fibrous pericardium. In front is the anterior mediastinum and behind it the posterior mediastinum. The contents of the pericardium constitute the middle mediastinum.

There is a minimum of connective tissue between the mediastinal structures to allow free movement. There are two important condensations of connective tissue within the mediastinum: the pretracheal and the prevertebral fascia. The pretracheal fascia extends from the larynx to the arch of the aorta. The prevertebral fascia extends from the base of the skull to the base of the body of the fourth thoracic vertebra. These structures have important clinical implications, as infections within the mediastinum are contained by them. Thus infection in the neck anterior to the pretracheal fascia will be contained within the anterior mediastinum. Infection behind the prevertebral fascia can extend for the full length of the superior mediastinum.

**Figure 40.2**

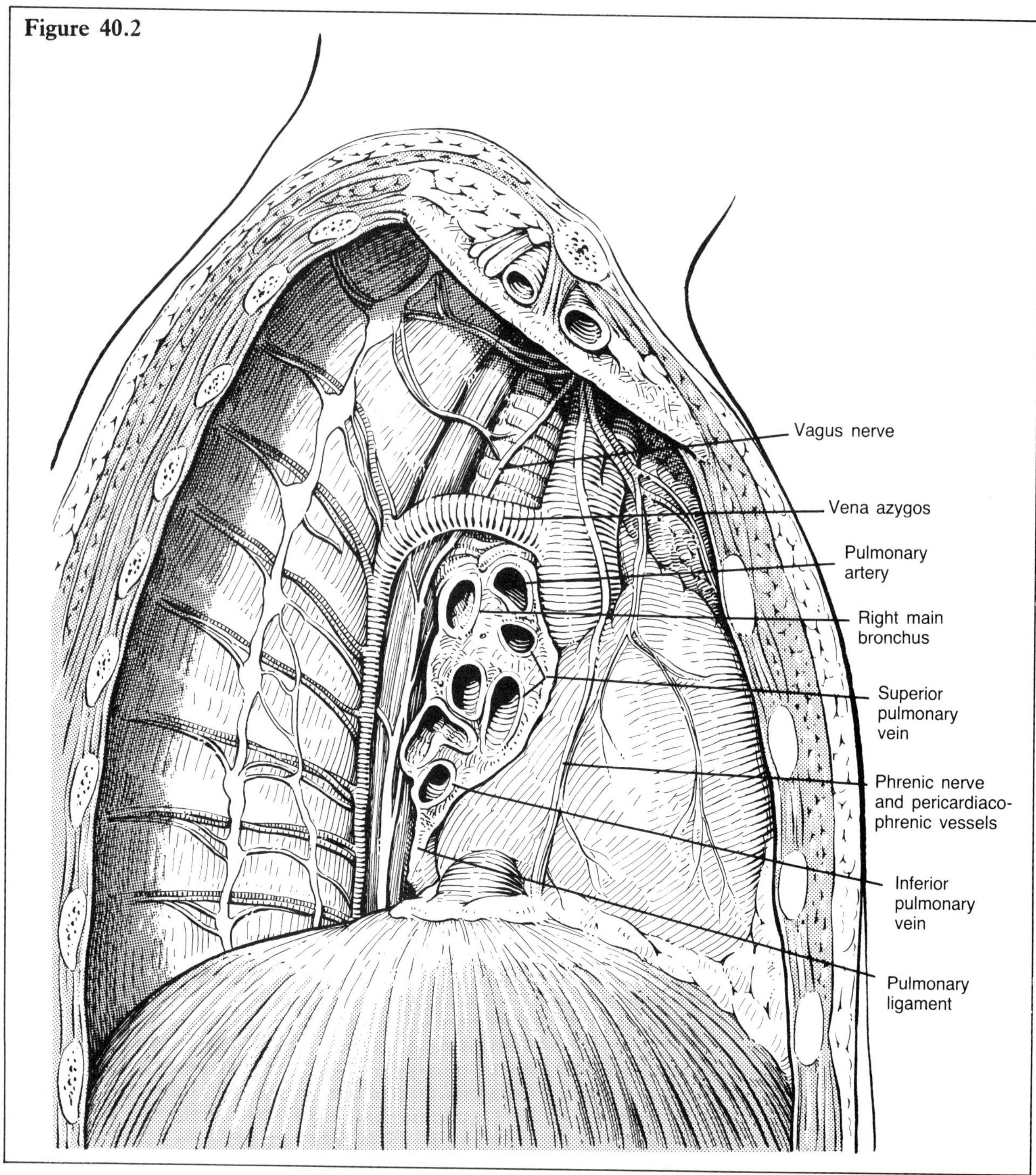

**Figure 40.3**

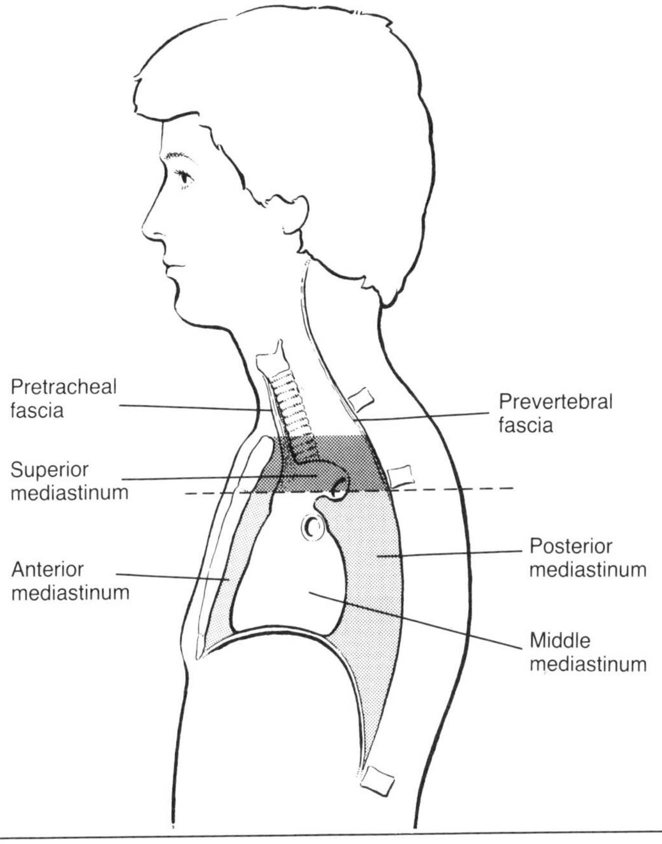

Pretracheal fascia
Superior mediastinum
Anterior mediastinum
Prevertebral fascia
Posterior mediastinum
Middle mediastinum

**Figure 40.4**

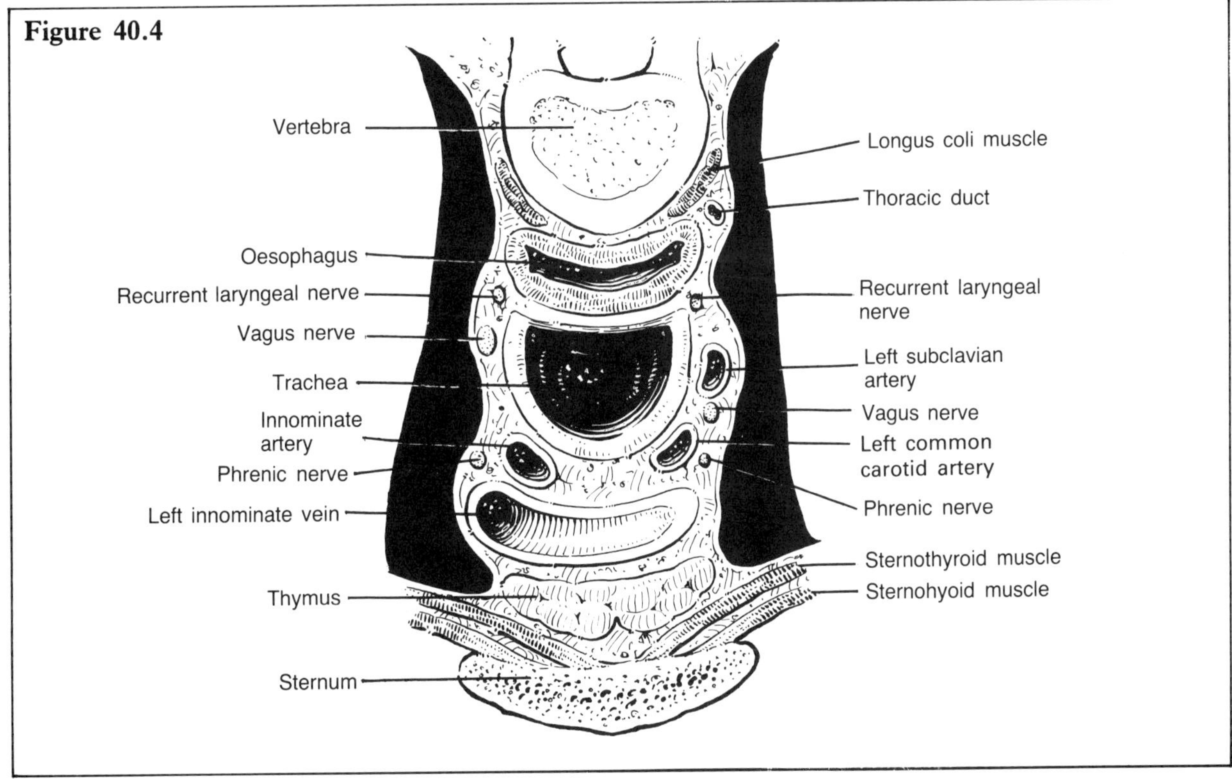


## Superior mediastinum

The superior mediastinum is bounded anteriorly by the manubrium and posteriorly by the anterior surface of the first four thoracic vertebrae. The relationships of the structures contained in this region are illustrated in **Fig. 40.4**. It is important for the surgeon to appreciate the relationships of the major vascular structures surrounding the trachea for the safe conduct of mediastinoscopy.

**Figure 40.5**

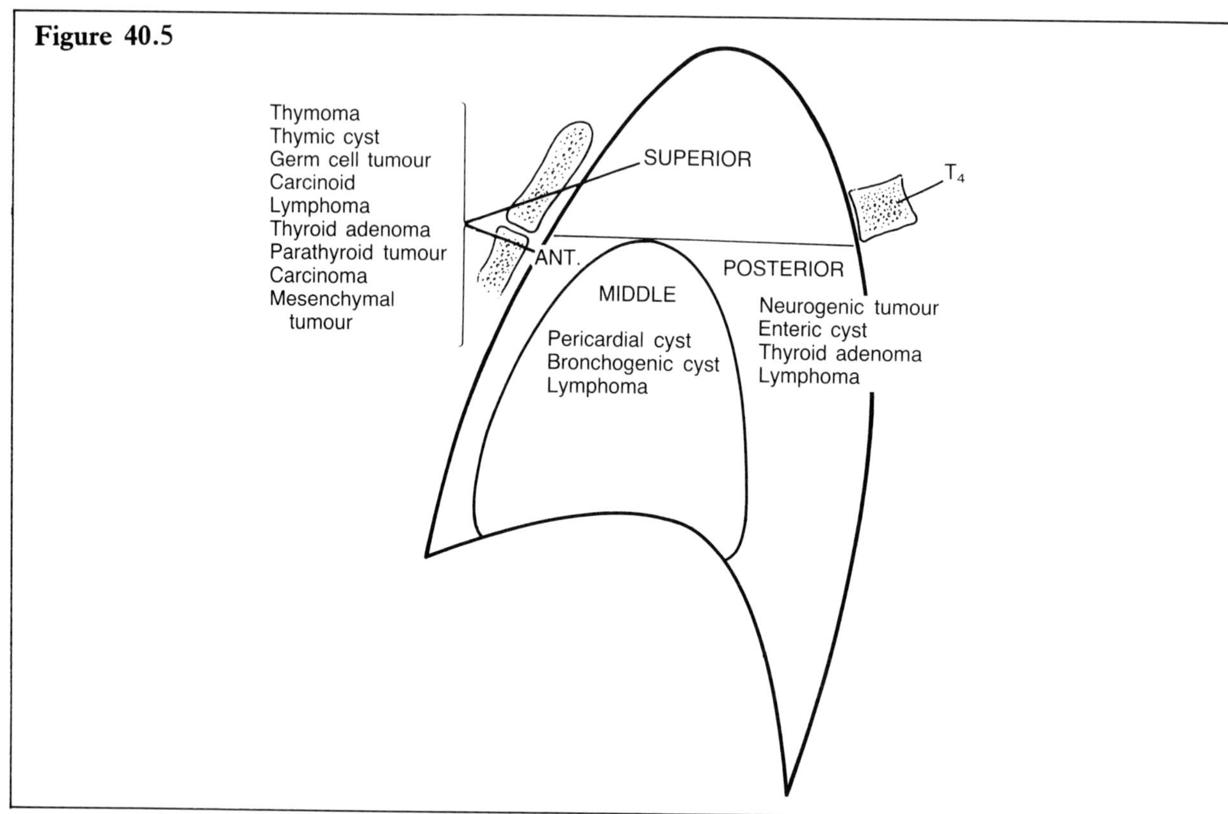


## Posterior mediastinum

The major contents of this region are:

1. Descending aorta.
2. Thoracic duct.
3. Azygos and hemiazygos veins.
4. Oesophagus and vagus nerves.
5. Thoracic duct.

## Anterior mediastinum

This space contains the thymus gland and prepericardial fat. The lower parathyroid glands may lie within this fat.

## Mediastinal neoplasms

The anatomic distribution of the more common primary mediastinal neoplasms and cysts is illustrated in **Fig. 40.5**.

# 41 Mediastinoscopy

Mediastinoscopy is used for the removal of mediastinal lymph nodes for histological examination to detect the spread of bronchial carcinoma, or for biopsy of some mediastinal masses. There has been a resurgence of interest in this procedure since the more widespread and enthusiastic application of the principles of staging of pulmonary tumours prior to attempting resection. The presence of mediastinal lymph-node involvement ($N_2$ disease) has been shown to alter the long-term prognosis for survival to such an extent that many surgeons will not consider proceeding to major pulmonary resection if $N_2$ disease is present. The classically described $N_2$ lymph node stations and their related anatomical structures are shown in **Fig. 41.1**. Group 8 are not shown and lie parallel with the distal oesophagus.

More recent evidence suggests that prior evaluation with CT scanning is very helpful in deciding which patients require mediastinoscopy or a staging procedure. If no nodes are visible with contrast-enhanced mediastinal CT scans, or all nodes are less than 10 mm, mediastinal biopsy is unnecessary.

The presence of superior mediastinal obstruction is not a contraindication to the procedure, as long as caution is exercised. Because of the extent of the disease, only superficial examination is necessary to find the causative tumour which will usually be found lying in the thoracic inlet, where the superior caval vein is being compressed.

Mediastinoscopy is also useful in establishing the cause of mediastinal lymphadenopathy discovered on plain chest radiography or CT scan. Common causes include sarcoidosis and tuberculosis. A specimen should always be sent for culture as well as histological examination to exclude the latter. In general, mediastinoscopy is not a suitable procedure in cases of anterior mediastinal cysts or tumours, partly because a median sternotomy is subsequently necessary to remove the mass, but—perhaps more importantly—because the small amounts of tissue removed by mediastinoscopy are often not of diagnostic value. In such cases an anterior mediastinotomy is more suitable, as a larger tissue sample can easily be obtained.

**Figure 41.1**

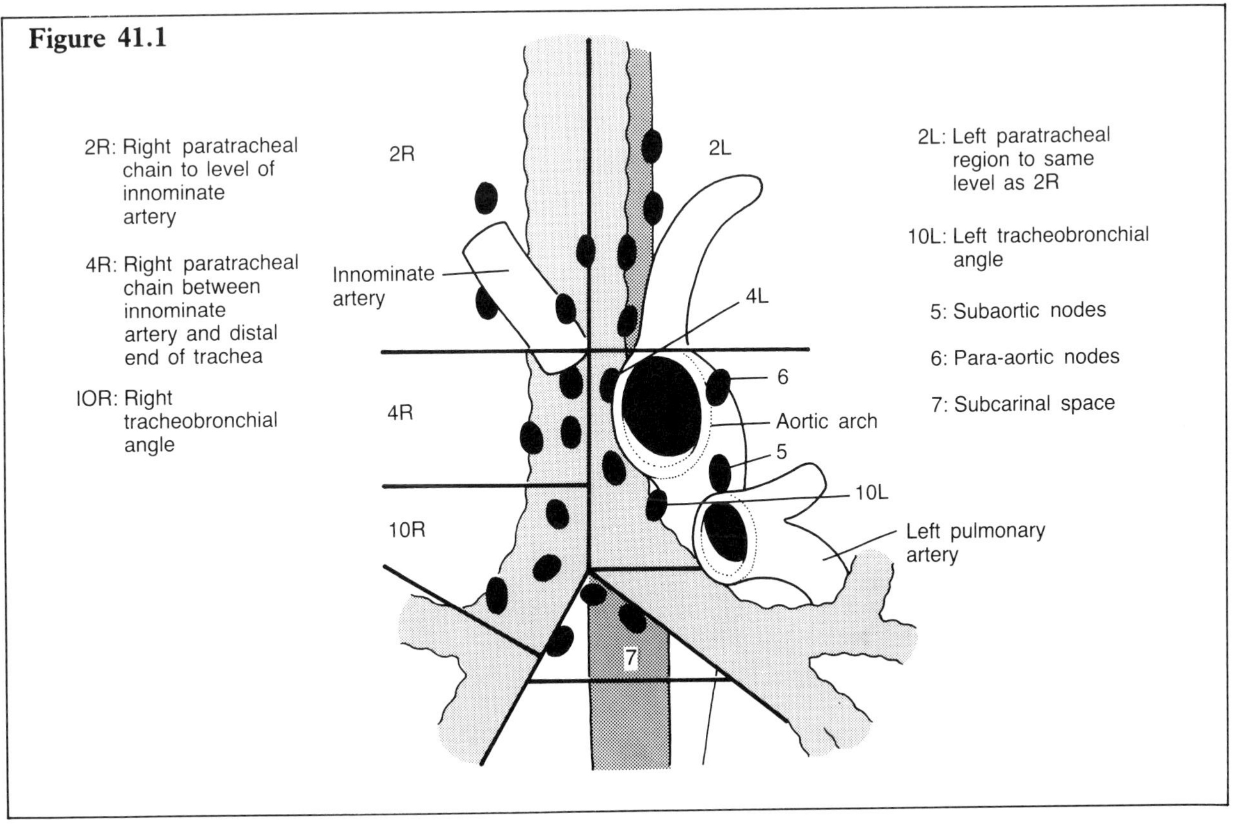

**Figure 41.2**

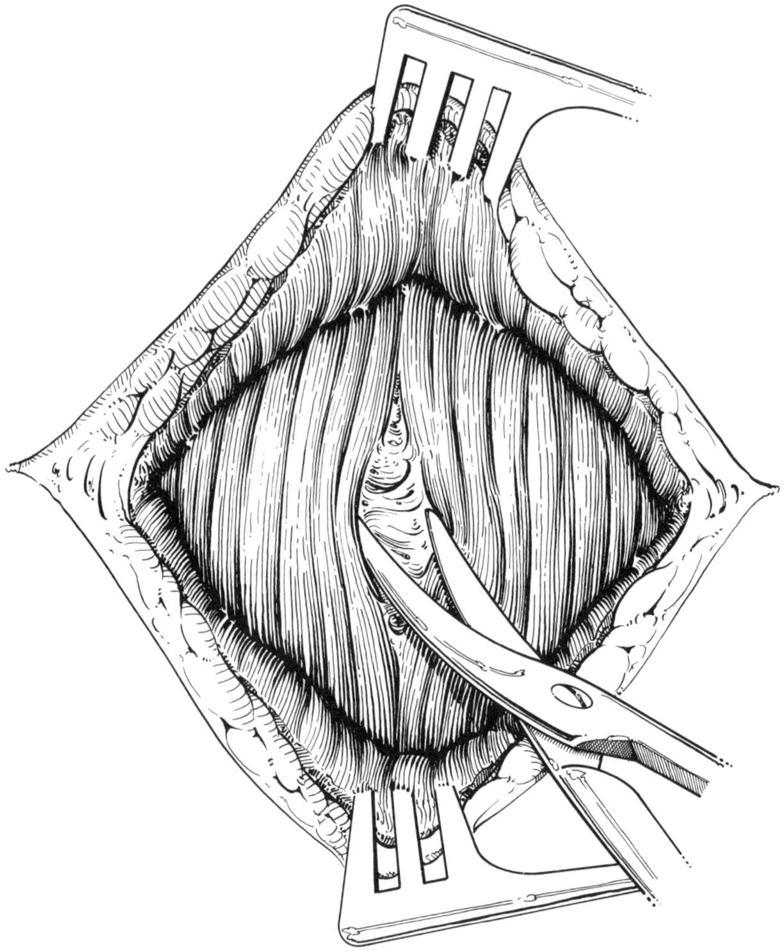

## Procedure

The procedure is carried out under general anaesthesia. A cushion is placed between the scapulae, and the head lowered to drop the shoulders and project the trachea forwards. A 25-mm transverse incision is then made 1 cm above the upper border of the manubrium. The platysma muscle is divided with diathermy. A small mechanical retractor is inserted and the midline between the sternothyroid muscles defined (**Fig. 41.2**). This layer is incised with diathermy, and with a little blunt dissection beneath it, the anterior wall of the trachea is identified. If a common inferior thyroid vein is present it will be necessary to divide it (**Fig. 41.3**).

Next the pretracheal fascia is elevated and incised (**Fig. 41.4**). Blunt dissection now extends downwards along the trachea, and behind the innominate artery (**Fig. 41.5**). The dissection is gradually extended along both sides of the trachea, particularly on the right. In this way a bloodless paratracheal tunnel is developed, into which the mediastinoscope can then be inserted. Dissection is continued with the tip of a metal sucker that has a diathermy end to it, or with a blunt dissector.

**Figure 41.3**

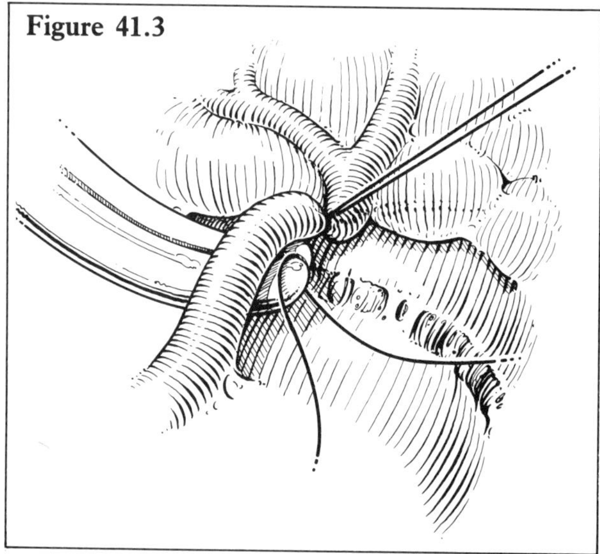

Individual lymph nodes that have been identified by CT can be dissected out in this way as far down as the right tracheobronchial angle and the carina. The lymph nodes in the right paratracheal group are contained within a firm, fibrous envelope, and this must be disrupted before the individual nodes can be identified. If individual lymph nodes have

**Figure 41.4**

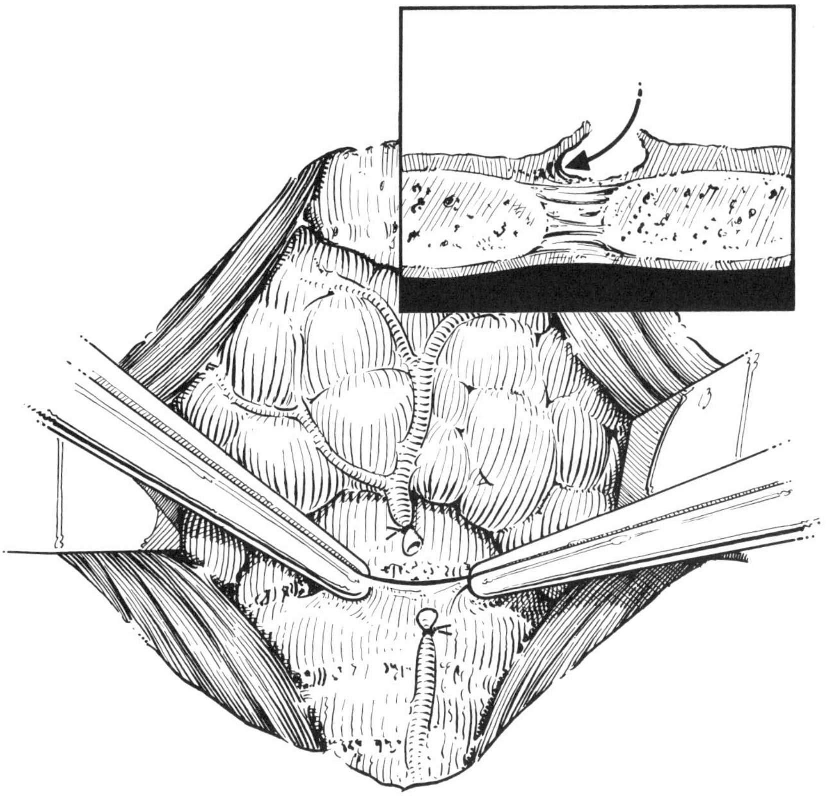

**Figure 41.5(a)**

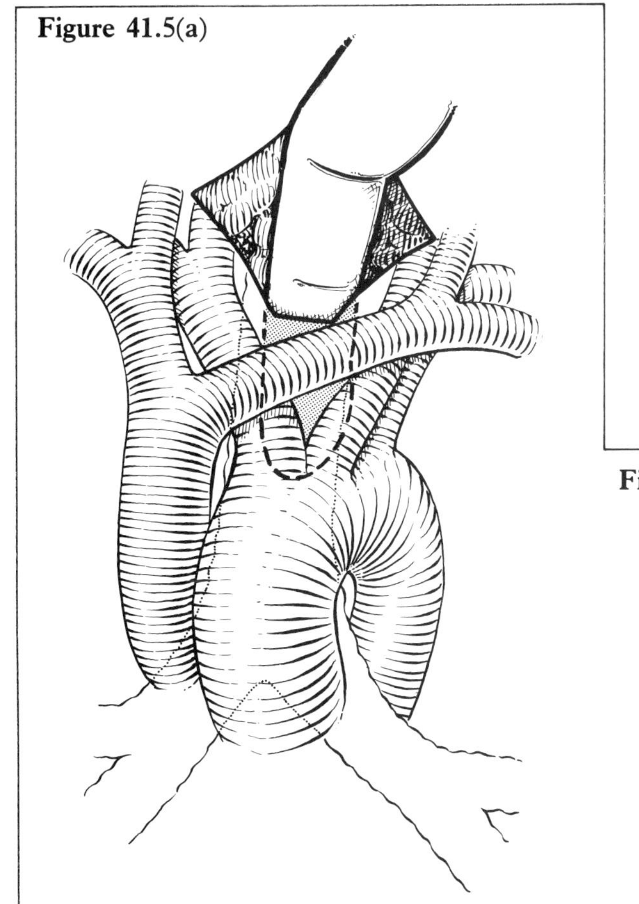

not been found but a large mass is present, a biopsy may be obtained from it. This, however, should be preceded by aspiration with a large needle to exclude a vascular structure, particularly the superior vena cava to the right of the trachea, which may be adherent to the tumour. Indeed if there is any doubt about the nature of a structure to be biopsied it is wise to exclude a vascular structure by prior aspiration as described. The superior vena cava can often be identified by the venous pulse within it.

As many as possible of the abnormal lymph nodes should be biopsied or removed. These nodes

**Figure 41.5(b)**

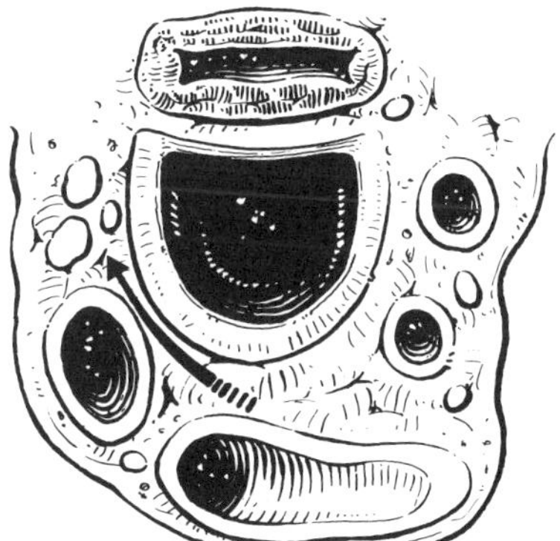

may be discrete, 1 cm or more in diameter, and firm, or they may be matted together and firm or hard. It is frequently possible to enucleate a complete lymph node with a finger.

In addition to carrying out biopsies of tissue as described, it is possible to section the vagus nerve through the mediastinoscope as it crosses the trachea obliquely, from anterior to posterior, in its midportion. This may be indicated in patients with hypertrophic pulmonary osteoarthropathy to relieve the severe pain that they usually experience in their wrists or knees.

On completion of the procedure, haemostasis is secured by diathermy of any discrete bleeding points, or by temporary packing if bleeding is more troublesome. The pretracheal muscles and the platysma are then approximated with absorbable sutures, and the skin incision closed with a subcuticular stitch of the same material or skin clips. Drainage of the wound is seldom necessary.

## Complications

Injudicious use of the biopsy forceps may result in haemorrhage from the superior vena cava, azygos vein, brachiocephalic artery, arch of the aorta or even the right pulmonary artery. Pneumothorax may also result and therefore a routine chest radiograph should be taken after the procedure. Damage to the recurrent laryngeal nerves may occur, possibly from excessive dissection around the sides of the trachea.

If major haemorrhage occurs the wound should be packed. If the bleeding is well controlled by packing and judicious control of the blood pressure then little else may be necessary. However, if bleeding cannot be controlled by this method a posterolateral thoracotomy should be carried out on the side from which the biopsy causing the haemorrhage was taken, and the bleeding site controlled directly.

# 42 Anterior mediastinotomy

Anterior mediastinotomy gives access to abnormalities of the mediastinum lying in front of the great vessels and also to those that lie below and lateral to the carina. In particular the subaortic fossa, the site of lymphatic spread from left upper lobe tumours, can be examined. These are all areas that cannot be approached (or can only be approached with great difficulty) via a cervical mediastinoscopy. This procedure has an additional advantage in that the pleura can easily be opened and biopsies can be obtained from the hilar region of the lung. Because this is a unilateral procedure, the area of interest must be identified and localized to one or other side by means of tomography or CT scanning beforehand.

**Figure 42.1**

## Procedure

The patient lies supine and a transverse incision is made 15 mm from the midline for 4-5 cm overlying the third intercostal space (**Fig. 42.1**). It is deepened through the pectoral muscles (**Fig. 42.2**) and a self-retaining retractor inserted so as to expose the third intercostal space (**Fig. 42.3**). Alternatively, 3 cm of the second costal cartilage may be excised subperichondrially. If the costal cartilage is excised great care is required on the deep surface, since the perichondrium is closely adherent to the costal cartilage, and if the rugine is allowed to stray from the correct plane the pleura may be entered inadvertently. It should be noted that excision of

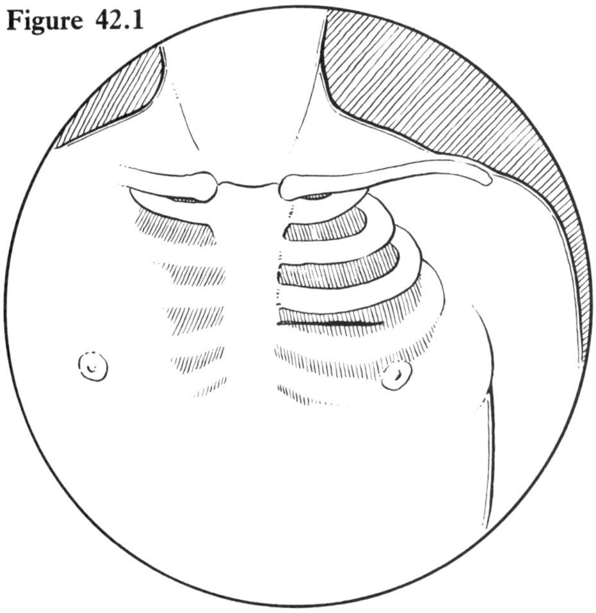

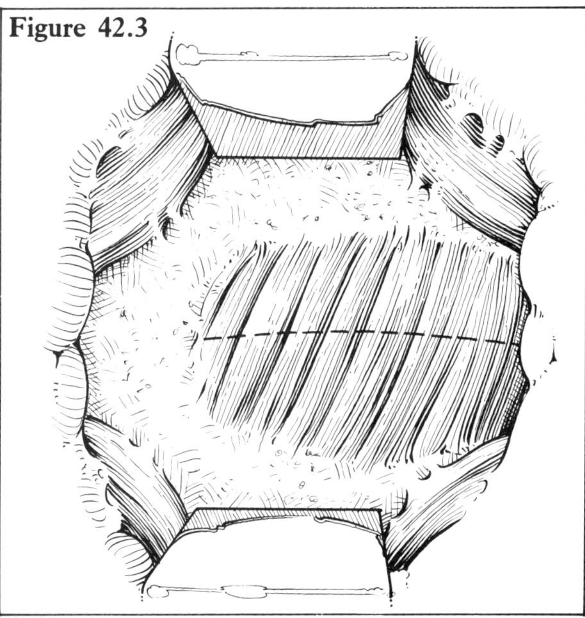
**Figure 42.3**

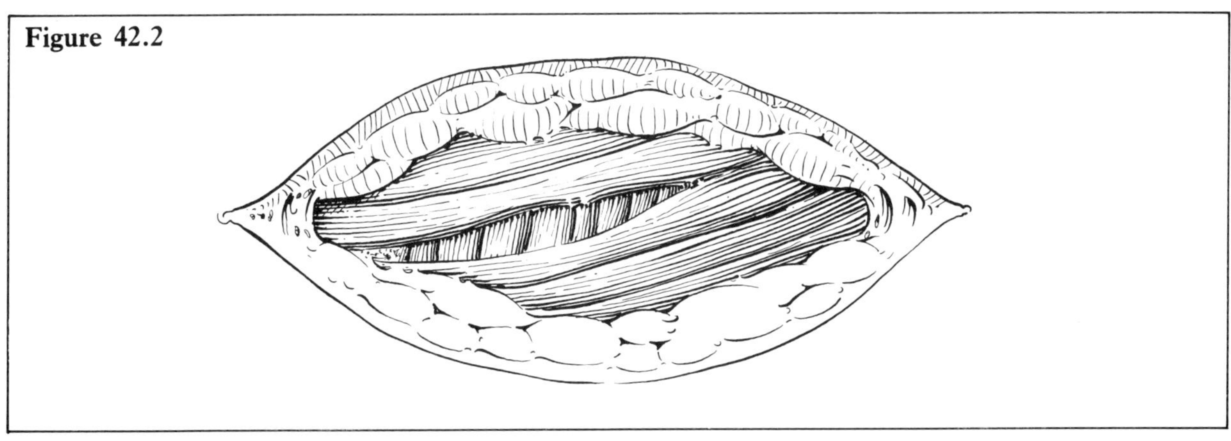
**Figure 42.2**

Figure 42.4

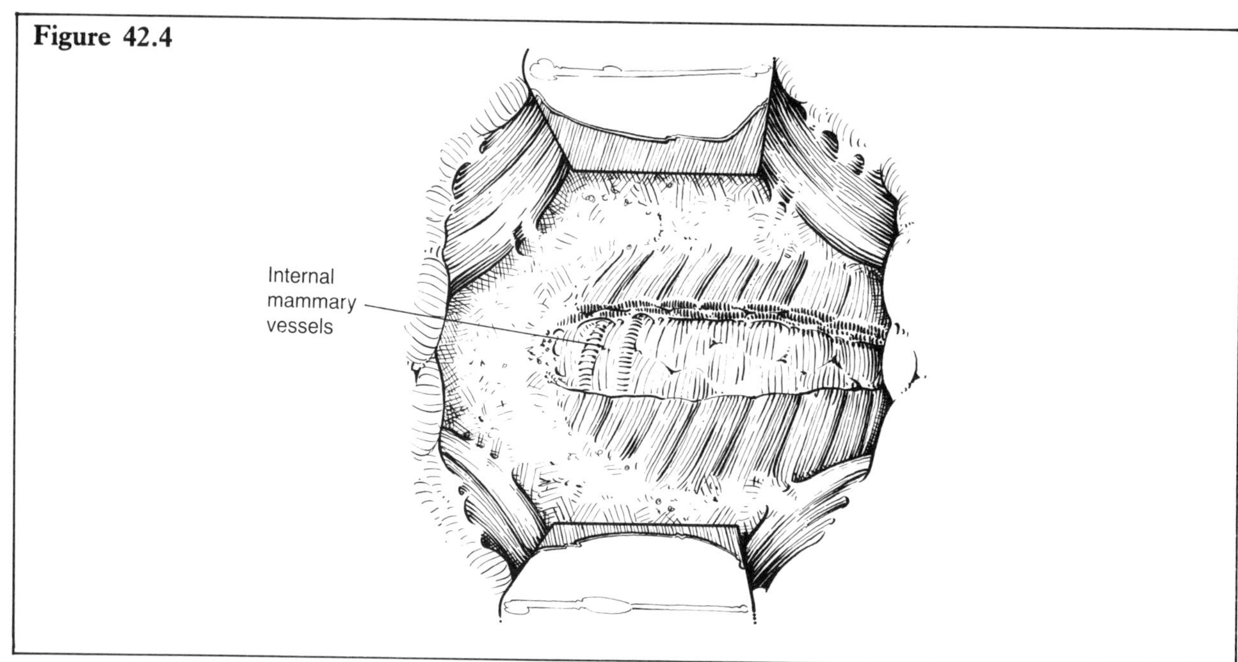


the costal cartilage may result in a lung hernia postoperatively. This is unlikely if the intercostal muscles are incised and the costal cartilages left intact.

At the medial end of the operative field the internal mammary vessels will now be seen (**Fig. 42.4**). They are best divided between sutures at this stage (**Fig. 42.5**), since otherwise they are liable to be torn. The space beneath the sternum is now developed by blunt dissection in both a cephalad and a caudad direction. This allows the pleura to be displaced laterally.

A retrosternal mass in the anterior mediastinum is now easily accessible. A large biopsy, at least 2 cm × 1 cm × 1 cm, should be obtained. With many tumours in this position, enough tissue is needed to enable the histopathologist to assess the architecture of the tumour as well as the cell type. This is particularly important in the case of lymphomas, mediastinal seminomas and some thymomas.

Further posteriorly on the right side, the right paratracheal lymph nodes are accessible between the superior vena cava and the ascending aorta (**Fig. 42.6**). Care must be exercised when taking a biopsy from this region, since if a mass is present, it can be difficult to determine whether the superior vena cava has been displaced. Aspiration should be carried out if there is any doubt, although this procedure is not infallible; sometimes the superior vena cava is stretched into a ribbon-like structure over the mass, and a needle will pass through it without yielding any blood.

On the left side this approach gives access to the lymph nodes of the subaortic fossa (**Fig. 42.7**).

If further information is sought, the pleura can be opened and the corresponding pulmonary hilum

Figure 42.5

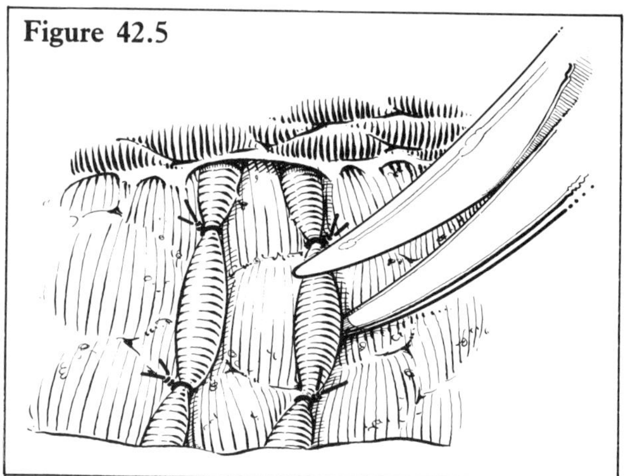

Figure 42.6

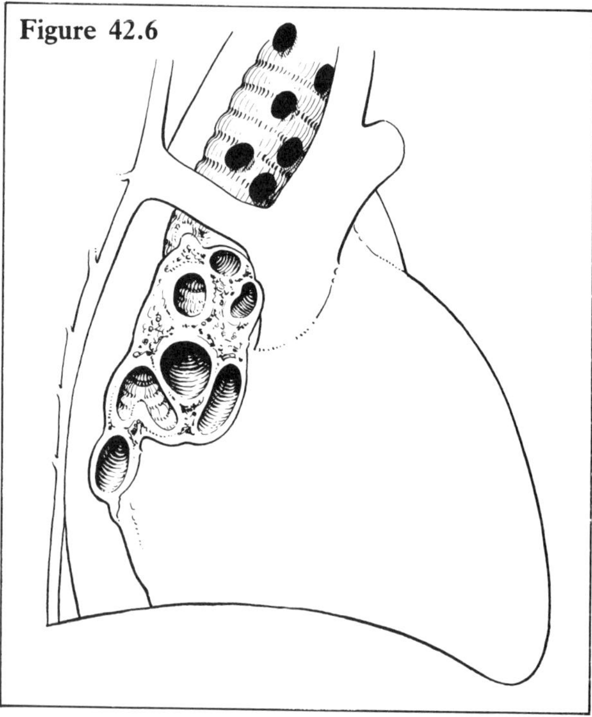

Figure 42.7

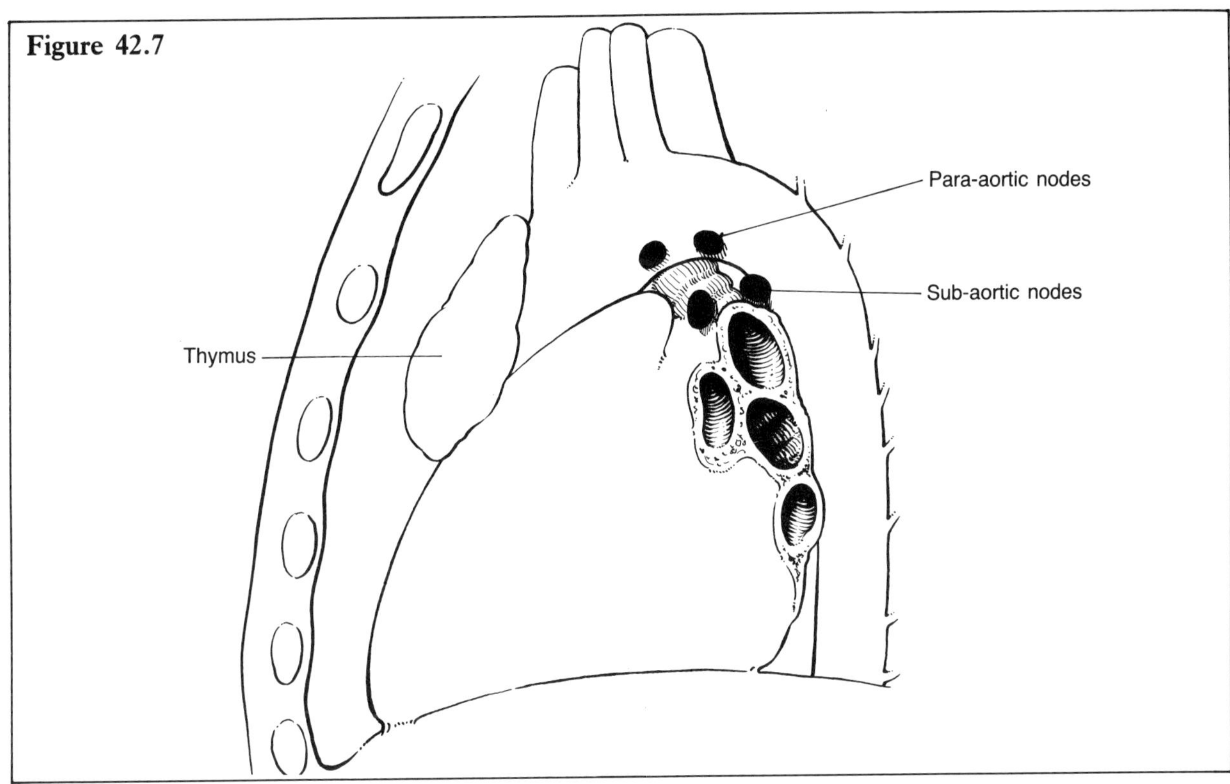


and lung itself can be palpated. If there is a local pulmonary lesion, it too may be biopsied.

When the examination has been completed, any intrapleural air can be aspirated through a small tube while the wound is closed around it. The tube may then be withdrawn while the anaesthetist hyperinflates the lungs. This obviates the need for an intrapleural drain.

If the operator thinks that it is advisable to drain the anterior mediastinal area, a vacuum drain is brought out through a small incision below the wound. If the pleura has been opened, a size 16 Argyle catheter should be passed into the pleural cavity and connected to an underwater seal. In any case a postoperative chest radiograph must be taken to exclude pneumothorax.

# 43 Thymectomy

Thymectomy is indicated in the treatment of myasthenia gravis and for thymic tumours which may or may not be associated with myasthenia. Patients with myasthenia gravis may have impaired ventilatory capacity and only a poor ability to cough. Therefore every effort must be made to avoid pulmonary complications. Minimal tracheal trauma and sparing administration of intravenous fluids are important ways to maintain good respiratory function. The endotracheal tube should be inserted carefully and removed as soon as possible after the end of the operation when the patient's ventilation is adequate.

Specific points in the management of anaesthesia for the myasthenic patient are worthy of mention in the light of some recent advances. Such patients have a reduced margin of safety when muscle relaxants are used. Techniques of anaesthetic management have varied from those using no specific relaxants, normally combined with a reduced preoperative dose of anticholinesterase drugs immediately preoperatively, to relaxant techniques with the possibility of impaired neuromuscular function necessitating a postoperative period of artificial ventilation.

The advent of the muscle relaxant atracurium, which is dependent upon rapid degradation 'Hoffman' elimination, together with the availability of enflurane, allows an anaesthetic technique that produces minimal disturbance to the patient. It is possible to continue the anticholinesterase therapy up to the time of operation. Induction is with a minimal dose of thiopentone, following which neuromuscular transmission is monitored by displaying the output from a train-of-four stimulator (Datex relaxograph). Muscle relaxation is then secured with incremental aliquots of atracurium while observing the degree of neuromuscular blockade. The patient is intubated and anaesthesia maintained with nitrous oxide and oxygen and added enflurane. Minimal enflurane is given, but if the neuromuscular blockade needs reinforcing an increase in the concentration of enflurane will achieve this without any additional atracurium. With this technique residual neuromuscular blockade is not a problem and the patient should be able to resume oral anticholinesterase within three hours of completion of the operation. It is advisable to nurse the patient for the first 48 hours postoperatively in the intensive care unit, where the facility to ventilate is readily to hand.

**Figure 43.1**

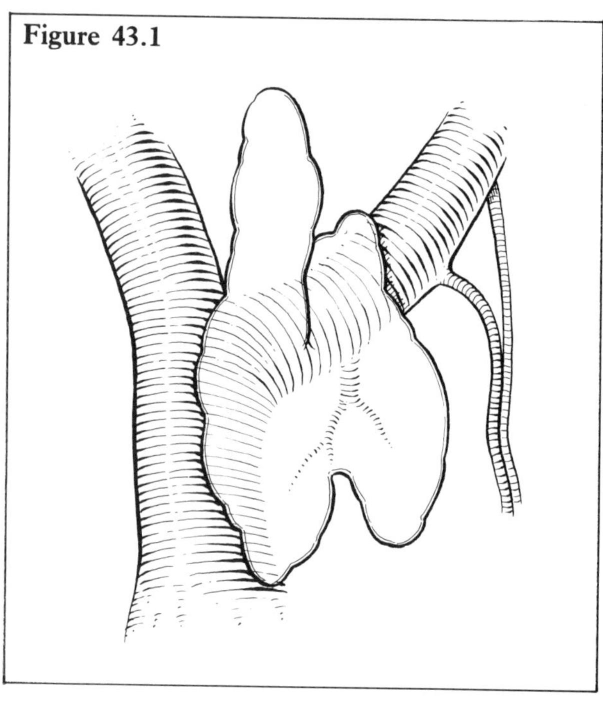

## Procedure

The thymus gland is H-shaped, the two lower poles extending downwards on to the pericardium, the upper poles reaching to the thyroid gland (**Fig. 43.1**). The incision extends from 25 mm below the suprasternal notch to the lower margin of the xiphisternum (**Fig. 43.2**); it is carried down to the bone, using diathermy to incise the periosteum. The origins of the pectoral muscles sometimes cross the midline, and some muscle fibres may be divided. The sternum is frequently curved, and so the operator must ensure that the incision remains in the middle of the sternum by palpating the intercostal spaces on either side. The bone is divided with a mechanical saw, preferably an oscillating type which is less likely to damage the soft tissues. Bleeding from the bone marrow is controlled with bone wax. A sternal spreader is inserted to give an opening of 7-8 cm. The thin layer of fascia overlying the gland is incised vertically, and the lower poles are freed by blunt dissection (**Fig. 43.3**). All the fibrofatty tissue anterior to the pericardium, between the two pleural margins laterally and as far as the diaphragm inferiorly should be removed with the gland, as it may contain thymic tissue. The small arteries supplying the gland which arise from the internal mammary arteries are coagulated with diathermy.

Figure 43.2

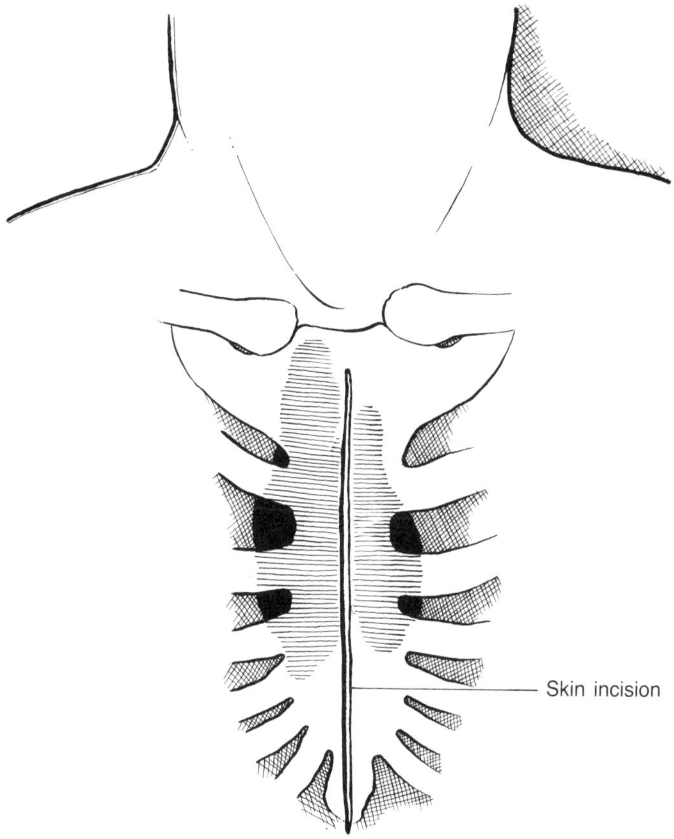

Figure 43.3

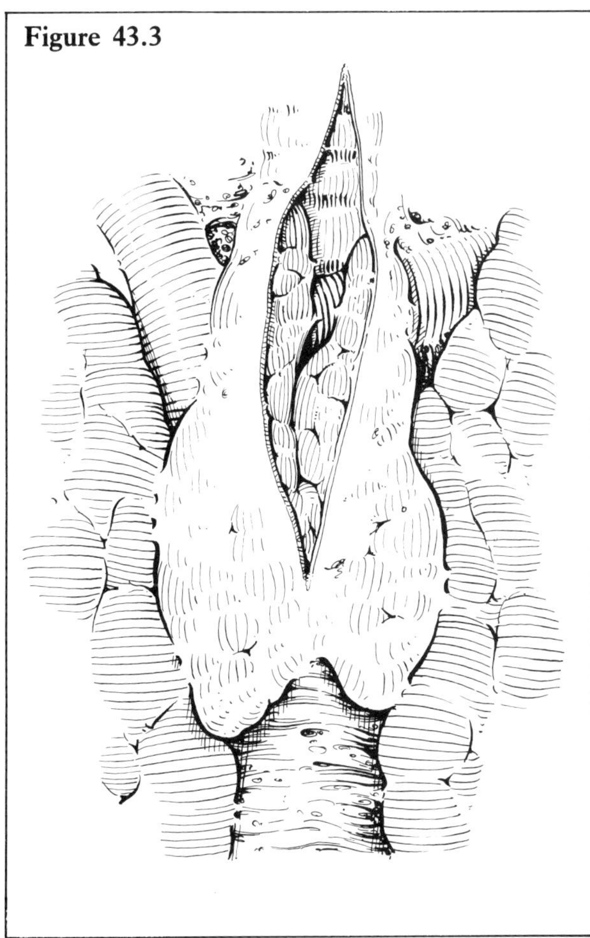

Figure 43.4

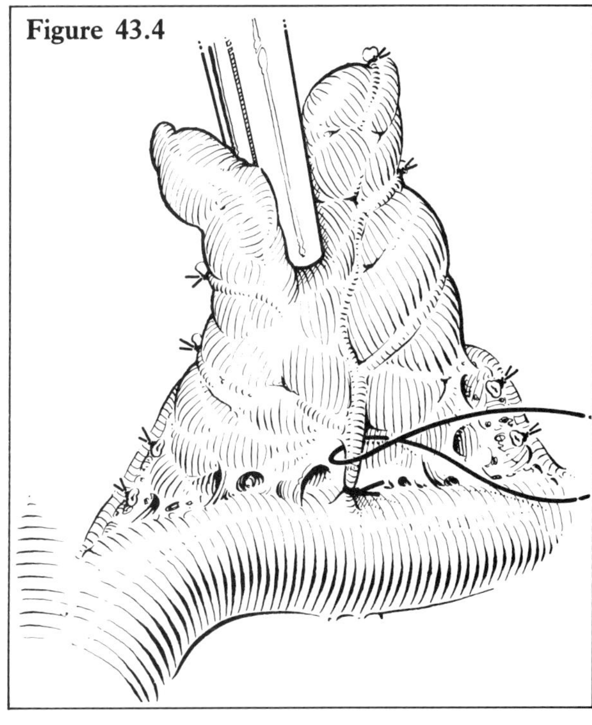

The large vein that drains from the central portion of the gland into the left brachiocephalic vein is divided between ligatures (**Fig. 43.4**). Dissection then continues upwards to free the upper poles of the gland, which are removed intact by blunt dissection. The left upper pole quite commonly splits into two portions, one running anterior to the left brachiocephalic vein and the other behind it. Fibrofatty tissue in this upper portion of the incision must also be removed. Great care should be taken not to open either pleural cavity. The gland is now free and is removed.

Before closure a further careful inspection of the anterior mediastinal space is made as far down as the diaphragm and as far laterally as the pleural margins for any other thymic tissue. Bleeding points are coagulated with diathermy. If the pleural cavities have not been opened, a single silicone anterior mediastinal drain is all that is necessary.

## Closure

The two halves of the sternum are approximated by six stainless steel wire sutures which penetrate the body of the sternum on each side (see p. 37). Alternatively, the wire may be passed around the body of the sternum, very close to its lateral margin so as to avoid the internal mammary artery. In either case the points of penetration on the deep surface of the sternum must be carefully inspected for bleeding before the sutures are tied. Such bleeding is best controlled by thread sutures passed through the periosteum on the undersurface of the sternum adjacent to the penetrating wire.

The sternum is closed by twisting the wires through four turns. The redundant wire is cut, leaving a 1-cm length which is then bent over, flattened against the sternum and tucked under the cut edge of the periosteum so that the end will not project through the skin. The pectoral muscles are

**Figure 43.5**

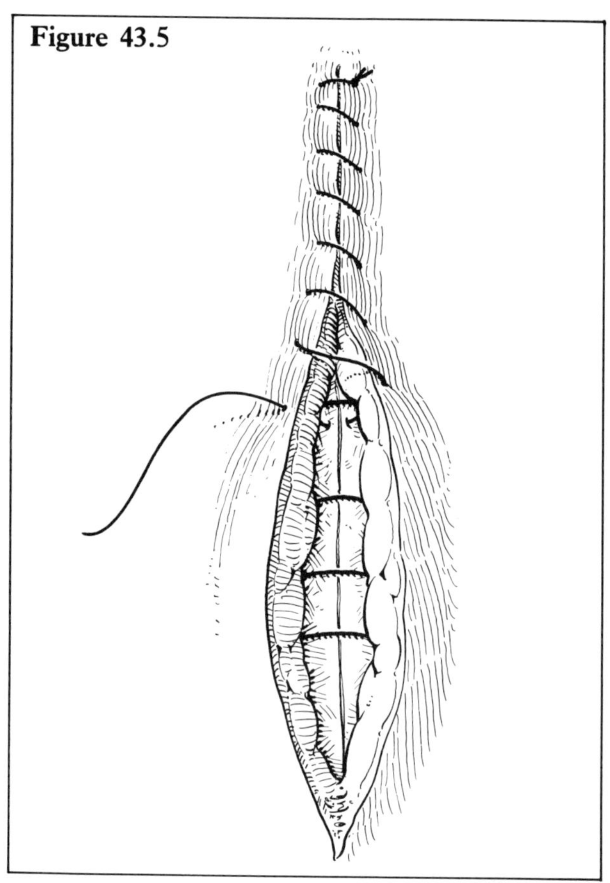

approximated with a continuous nylon suture which must pick up the outer periosteal layer of the sternum (**Fig. 43.5**). This prevents a dead space in which fluid might collect and which might cause delayed healing, discharge or infection. The skin is closed by any standard technique.

# 44 Excision of mediastinal neurogenic tumour

Mediastinal neurogenic tumours lie mainly in the paravertebral region at any level in the chest, and are usually incidental radiological findings. They should be removed because they may extend through an intervertebral foramen and compress the spinal cord (**Fig. 44.1**). Rarely, they may develop sarcomatous degeneration. CT scanning is valuable in determining whether the tumour has extended into the spinal canal. If so, the operation should be preceded by a laminectomy to remove the intraspinal extension. If CT scanning or myelography are not available, an intraspinal extension may be missed and only discovered at operation. In this case an emergency laminectomy is necessary, because oedema and vascular thrombosis affecting the residual portion of tumour may rapidly cause spinal cord ischaemia.

## Procedure

With the patient in the lateral position, a posterio-lateral thoracotomy is performed. Usually the rib space overlying the middle of the tumour is opened, but for lesions at the apex an incision in the fourth intercostal space is more suitable. The lung is deflated by the anaesthetist and retracted gently to the side.

Next, the parietal pleura is incised around the margins of the tumour. These tumours are frequently quite vascular and therefore as much dissection as possible should be carried out with diathermy. Even when there is no intraspinal extension, the tumour is firmly fixed and its mobilization may be difficult. Traction is best achieved by passing three or four heavy thread sutures on a large needle through the tumour and collecting all the ends in a single haemostat (**Figs. 44.2, 44.3**).

The ideal plane of dissection is deeper than may at first be apparent. The layers of compressed tissue surrounding the tumour should be picked up and incised serially until the yellow surface and whorled fibres of the tumour can be clearly seen. As the tumour is freed, additional thread sutures are passed through it to increased traction. The numerous vessels that enter the tumour should be identified without damaging them, coagulated and divided (**Fig. 44.4**).

**Figure 44.1**

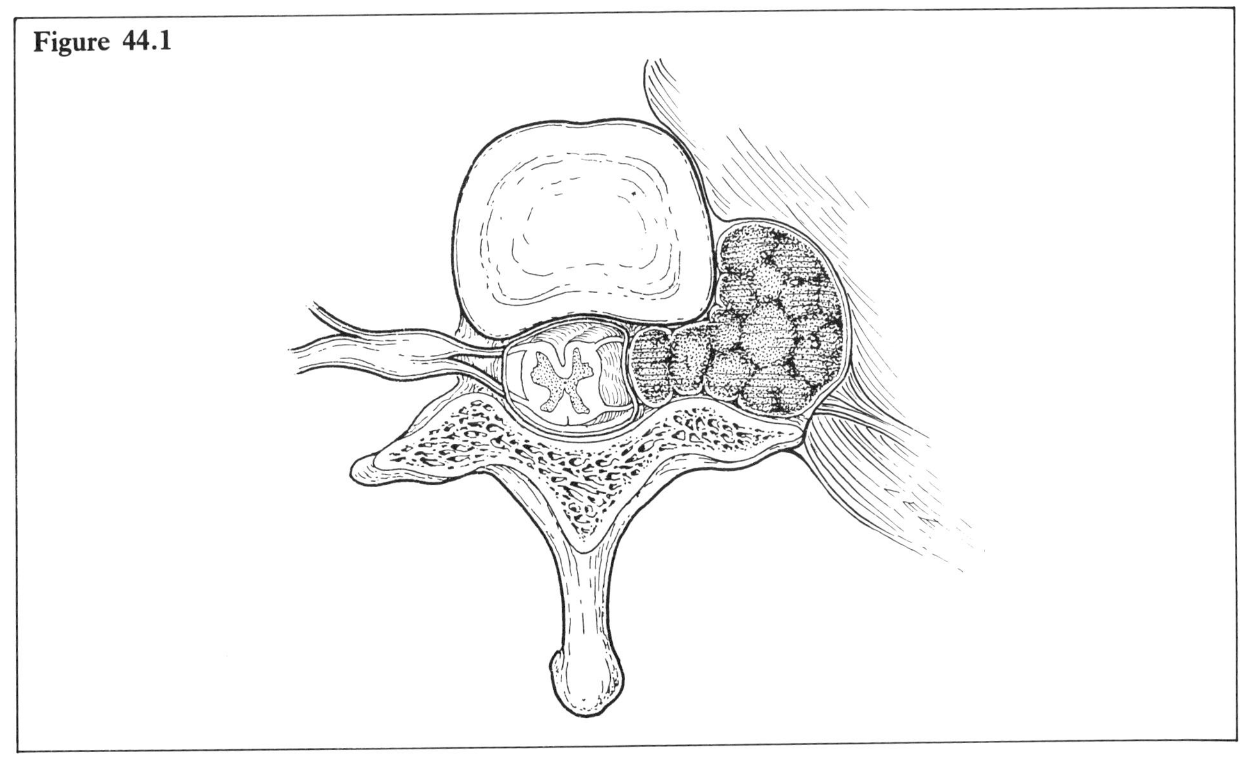

Figure 44.2

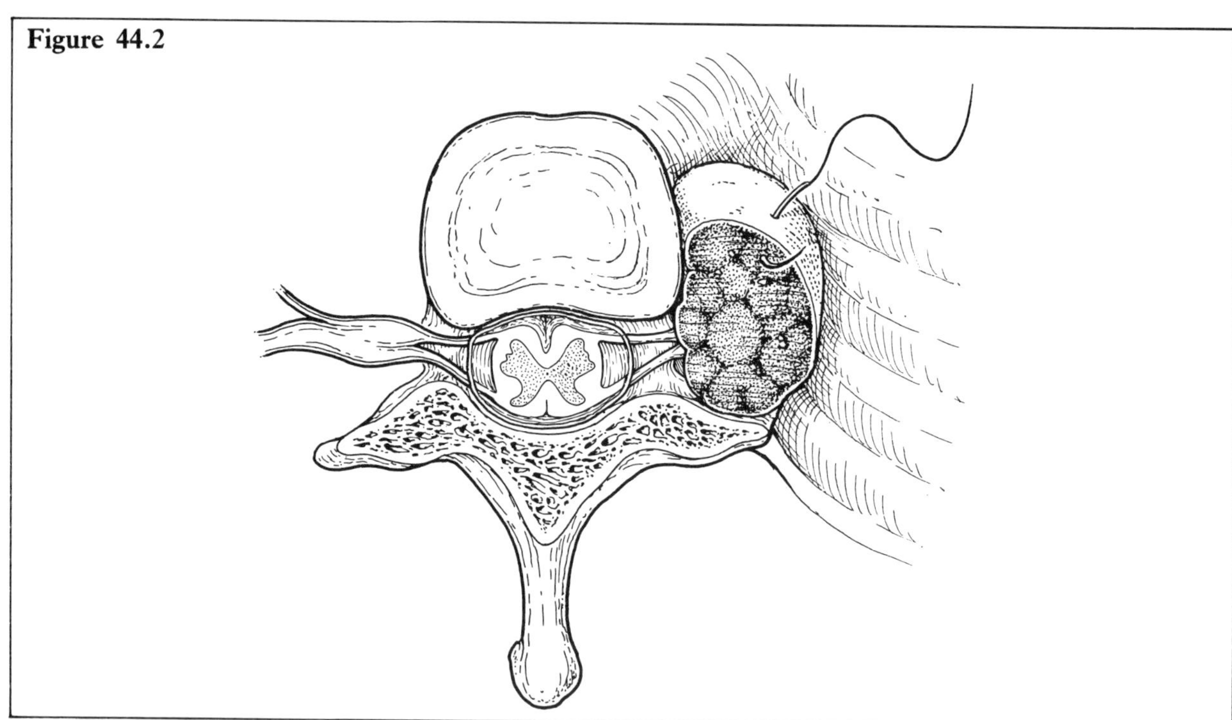

Figure 44.3

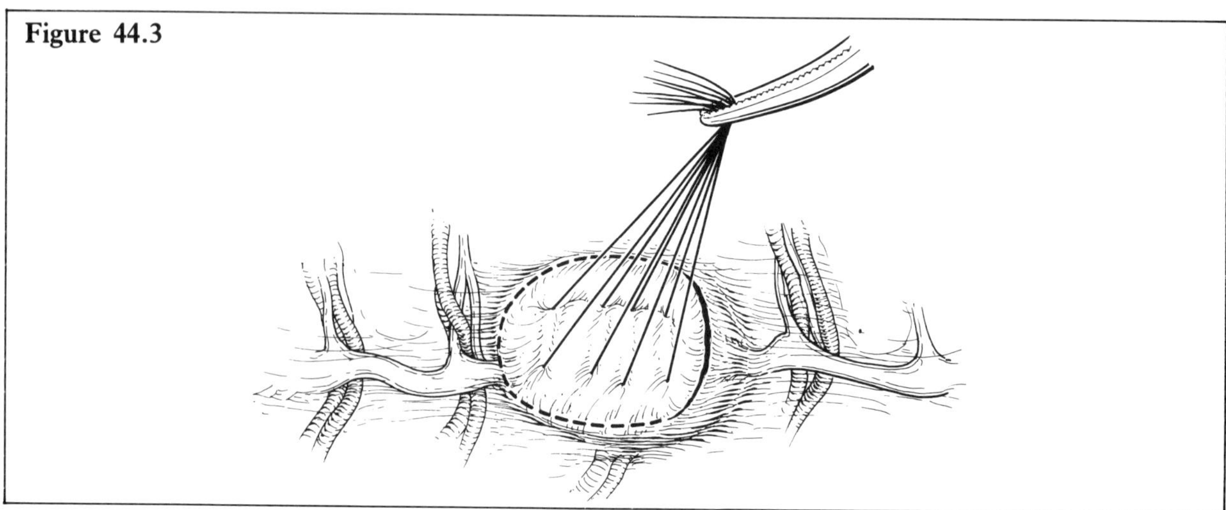

Figure 44.4

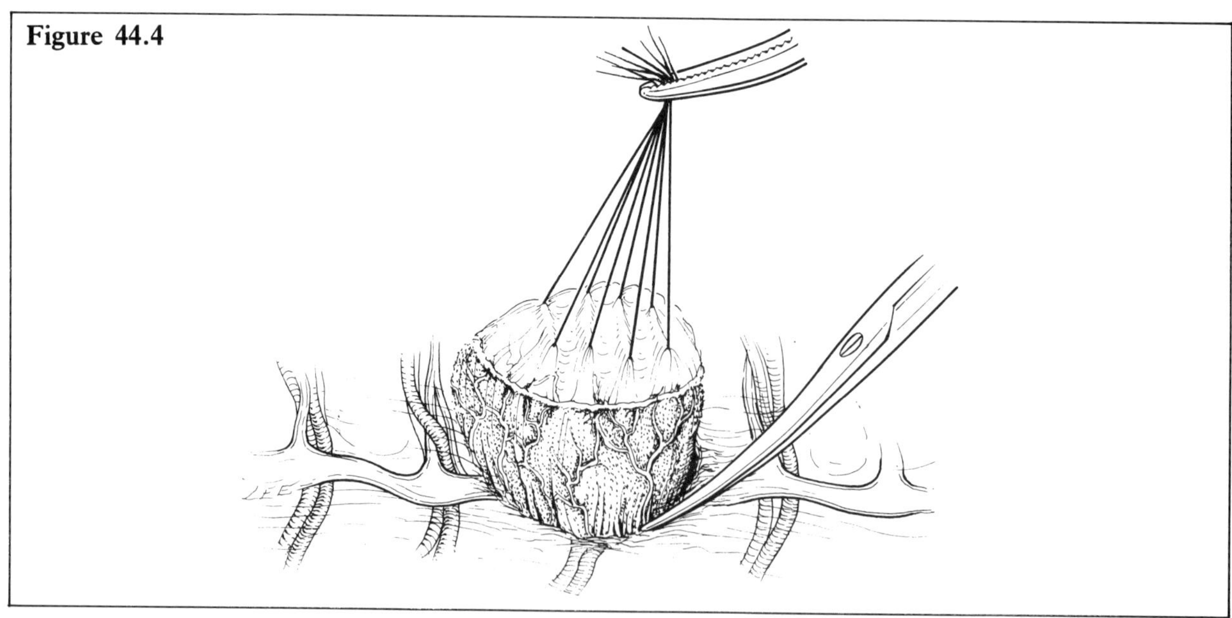

Because many of these tumours arise from the sympathetic chain, which spreads out over the surface of the tumour, it is often helpful to divide this structure below the tumour and exert traction on its upper end.

The azygos vein must be kept in view and protected on the right side, as must the aorta on the left. The dissection proceeds centripetally all around the tumour until finally only its attachment in the region of the intervertebral foramina remains. The tumour may have extended into several foramina, which hold it firmly, and must be dislodged partly by instrumental dissection and partly by blunt dissection using pressure with the index finger. The assistant is warned to exert gentle traction to avoid tearing the tumour or the veins passing through the intervertebral foramen. With care these veins can be identified and secured with a clip as they leave the tumour. Each intervertebral foramen is treated in the same way in turn, and the tumour finally lifted out.

Bleeding from an intervertebral foramen must not be treated by blind diathermy or by packing, as these procedures may damage the spinal cord or its blood supply. Bleeding may cease after a piece of oxidized cellulose has been laid in the foramen for 10 minutes.

Intrapleural haemostasis is now achieved and the incision closed after the insertion of a single pleural drain and re-expansion of the lung.

If there is any possibility of continued bleeding into the extradural space a neurosurgeon should be alerted. Neurological examination of the lower limbs must be carried out every 15 minutes for 3 hours and then hourly for 12 hours.

# 45 Excision of other mediastinal cysts and tumours

## Indications for operation

1. An undiagnosed mass in the anterior mediastinum.
2. A dermoid cyst.
3. A teratoma or other germ cell tumour.
4. A thymic tumour.

Thymic lymphomas and seminomas are best treated with radiotherapy or chemotherapy, and when the diagnosis is suspected a mediastinoscopy, or anterior mediastinotomy and biopsy, is the appropriate procedure. Calcified thymic cysts are harmless and it is unnecessary to remove them.

### Bronchogenic cysts

Bronchogenic cysts derive from cell rests isolated during the main pulmonary branching that occurs during separation of the lung bud from the primitive foregut; they are therefore found closely associated with the trachea, main bronchi or oesophagus, or within the lung itself. The cysts are usually round or ovoid, and are not usually multiloculate. Bronchial epithelial elements including ciliated areas can usually be found within them, and indeed are the key to the diagnosis. Cysts with a communication to the airway may become infected, and haemorrhage may occur into them. In any case removal is recommended. This can be accomplished by simple enucleation; any connection with an airway should be secured with a ligature.

### Enteric cysts

Enteric cysts are also referred to as *reduplication cysts* or *enterogenous cysts*; they originate from the dorsal division of the foregut. These cysts may be found at any level of the posterior mediastinum, lying next to the oesophagus. They are smooth-walled, and contain in their walls some or all of the components of the upper gastrointestinal tract, although often bearing cilia. They may contain gastric mucosa, and may secrete hydrochloric acid with consequent ulceration, haemorrhage or perforation. Connection with the oesophagus (albeit of pinhole size) is not uncommon, and suture ligation of the base should be carried out. Occasionally enteric cysts may communicate with the spinal cord; these cases are usually associated with spinal abnormalities.

## Procedure

A median sternotomy is performed (see p. 36). If the tumour is small, it is dissected out together with the anterior mediastinal fat and if necessary with part of the thymus gland (see Chapter 43). The drainage of the tumour is likely to be via the thymic vein, and this must be identified and ligated (see **Fig. 43.4**, p. 165).

Large tumours present a difficult problem as they may fill the anterior mediastinal space and abut firmly against the posterior surface of the sternum. The two halves of the sternum cannot then be easily separated. Moreover, there is likely to be obstruction of the veins around the tumour causing considerable haemorrhage.

After the sternum has been split with an oscillating saw, each half is elevated in turn with a small Langenbeck retractor. It is often possible to free the tumour from the back of the sternum by blunt dissection with the finger, pushing in the angle between the tumour and the posterior surface of the sternum (**Fig. 45.1**). If this cannot be done, each half of the sternum should be retracted further

**Figure 45.1**

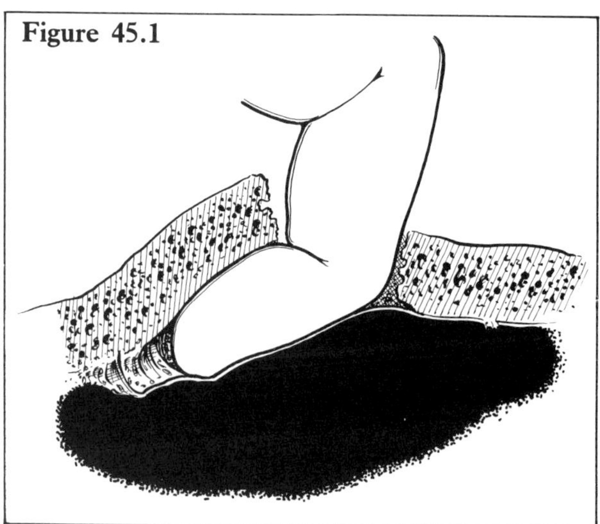

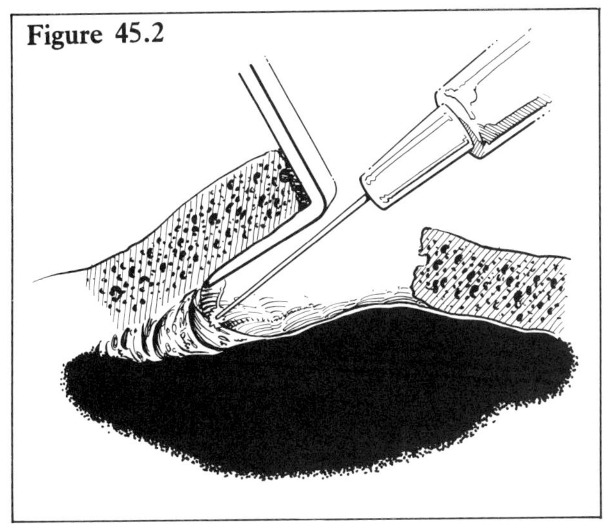

**Figure 45.2**

and diathermy used to incise along the posterior surface of the sternum and costal cartilages, keeping to a plane superficial or deep to the posterior periosteum (**Fig. 45.2**). Bleeding is controlled by packing. The procedure is repeated beneath the other half of the sternum. It will then be possible to insert a sternal spreader.

The mass is inspected and its limits defined. A malignant tumour may involve the anterior pericardium and may spread into the pleural cavities (as far back as the phrenic nerves on each side) and the upper lobes of the lung. Above, the brachiocephalic vein may be involved, and to the right of this, the superior vena cava. The inflammatory reaction around an infected dermoid cyst may involve the same structures and produce a similar appearance. A biopsy and frozen section may be helpful at this stage, but the interpretation of frozen sections of thymic tumours and lymphomas is extremely difficult, and the result should be regarded with caution. If a tumour is extensive, both pleural cavities should be opened to assess operability. If the lung or either phrenic nerve is involved, resection is probably not justified.

Dissection of resectable tumours should begin between the mass and the anterior surface of the pericardium. If a separation cannot be achieved the pericardium is opened with a transverse incision at the lower level of the tumour. Excision is contraindicated if the tumour has ulcerated through the pericardium, or if there are multiple intrapericardial metastases.

If there are no metastases, the incision in the pericardium should be extended at each end vertically upwards anterior to the phrenic nerves. In this way the superior vena cava, pulmonary artery and aortic arch are exposed without risk of their being damaged (**Fig. 45.3**). Excessive traction must not be exerted on the tumour at this stage, because if the vena cava or brachiocephalic veins are invaded, a tear may result which could be difficult to repair. Tumour invasion of the great veins is an indication to abandon the procedure. If,

**Figure 45.3**

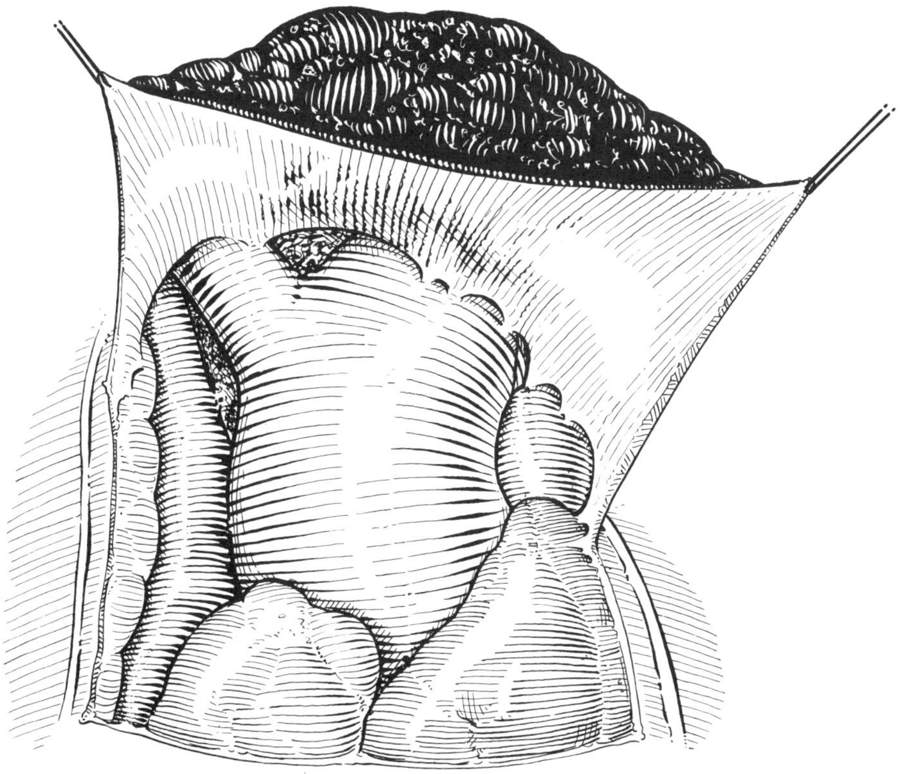

however, the left brachiocephalic vein is minimally involved it can be dissected out on each side of the tumour immediately behind the sternoclavicular joint and ligated. The central portion can then be removed with the tumour. It is not necessary to reconstruct the vein.

Haemostasis must now be secured. The excessive venous bleeding that characterizes tumours obstructing the great veins will now have ceased, but the whole operation field should be rendered as dry as possible. A size 28 or 32 Argyle drain is placed in the anterior mediastinum and brought out immediately to one side of the lower end of the incision. If a pleural cavity has been opened during the course of the operation it should be drained in the usual way. The two halves of the sternum are then approximated and the incision closed as described on p. 166.

Occasionally the tumour is very large and tense, filling the anterior mediastinum completely, and after dissection has confirmed that it cannot be removed, attempts to close the sternum may result in profound hypotension. If this problem is encountered the wire sutures should be tied starting from below, and it will usually be found possible to close the lower half of the sternum. The upper half may then be left open and the muscles and skin closed over it. Healing is usually quite satisfactory and the sternum rapidly becomes stable.

# 46 Intrathoracic goitre

The thyroid gland arises from the dorsal surface of the oropharynx and during embryonic development may be carried downward into the superior mediastinum. More commonly the gland develops in the neck, but a pathological enlargement of the lower pole extends into the thorax and, expanding, becomes trapped there. Although aberrant thyroid tissue may arise within the mediastinum, as witnessed by a blood supply originating at that site, this is an unusual occurrence.

The upper part of the goitre may be visible and palpable in the neck. The mediastinal extension is commonly found anteriorly and to the right of the trachea, but the bulk of it often lies behind the trachea.

Some patients may present with gradually worsening stridor, accompanied occasionally by dysphagia. If there is haemorrhage into a cyst within the goitre enlargement may be rapid, producing critical airway and oesophageal obstruction. Occult, advanced malignant change may also occur, particularly in the elderly.

The treatment of choice is excision. Access is almost always satisfactory through a cervical incision; it is rarely necessary to split the manubrium and upper sternum.

## Procedure

The patient is fully anaesthetized and intubated with an endotracheal tube. A small sandbag is placed under the centre of the shoulders and the patient's head rested on a rubber ring. The neck is extended as far as possible (**Fig. 46.1**). After the skin has been prepared from mandible to mid-chest with a topical antiseptic, the head is draped in a separate 'head' towel over the endotracheal tube.

Some surgeons find the initial dissection facilitated by infiltration of the subcutaneous tissue with 1:10 000 adrenaline solution (10 ml diluted to approximately 50 ml in normal saline). We do not practise this technique, although we have no criticism of it.

A curved incision is made with a broad-bladed scalpel in a skin crease from the posterior margin of one sternomastoid muscle to the posterior margin of the other. The centre of the incision is two fingers' breadth above the sternal notch (**Fig. 46.2**). The incision must follow the skin crease. There is a tendency to curve it upwards at the ends which results in ugly scarring. The incision is deepened through the platysma muscle using the diathermy

**Figure 46.1**

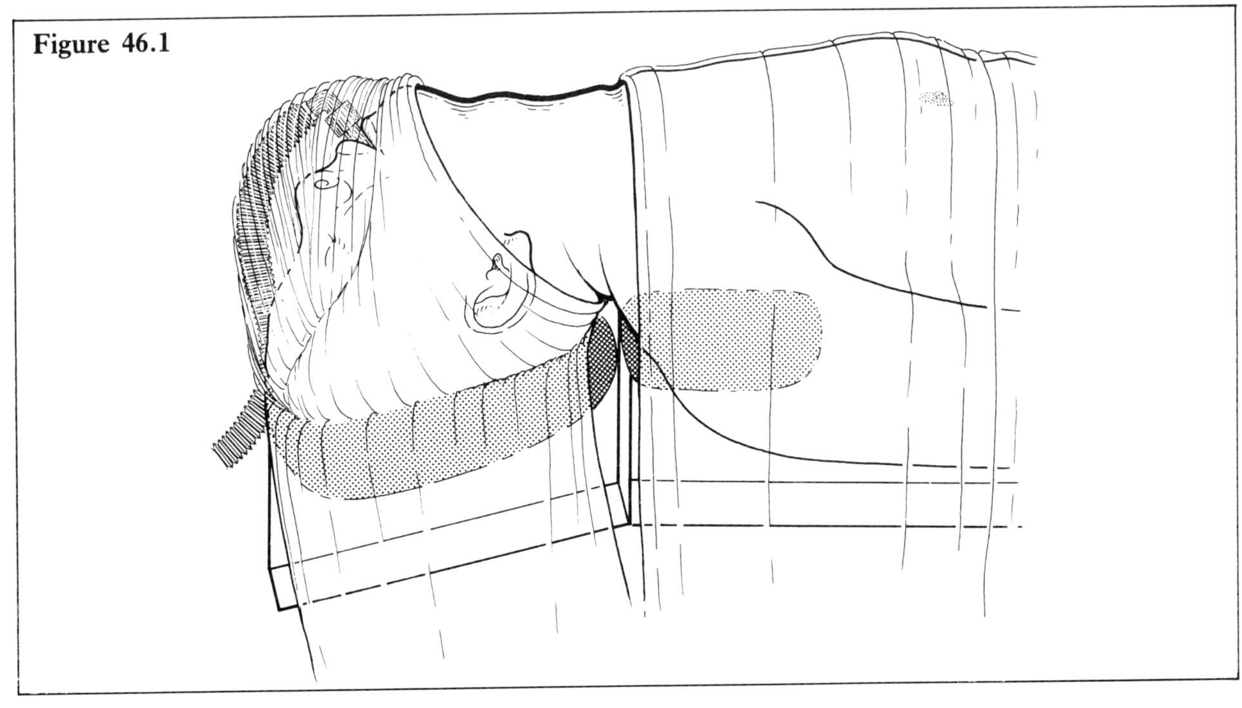

**Figure 46.2**

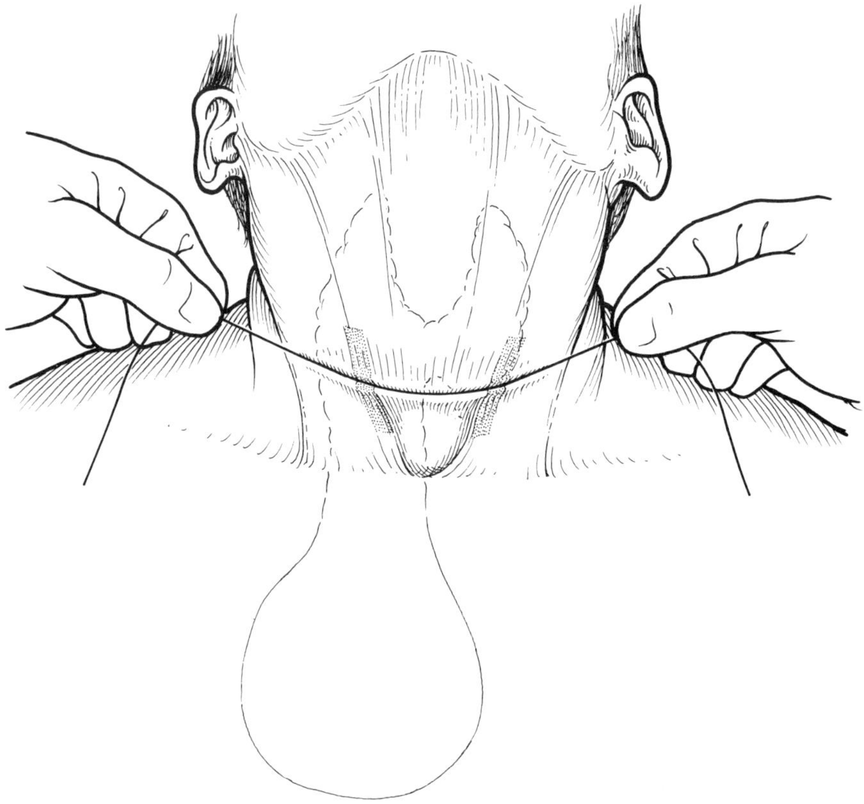

point to expose the underlying sternohyoid and sternothyroid muscles. A pair of tissue-holding forceps is placed on the superficial fascia at the upper edge of the wound and elevated by the assistant. The direction of elevation must be truly vertical to the deeper structures, to prevent 'button-holing' of the skin. The full-thickness flap including the platysma muscle is developed evenly by sharp dissection to the upper margin of the thyroid cartilage. All small vessels are cauterized with the diathermy, larger ones are tied with a fine absorbable ligature. Much of the separation of this flap may be accomplished by stroking the subcutaneous fat from the underlying muscle with the handle of the scalpel or a swab-covered finger (**Fig. 46.3**). The most adherent areas are usually

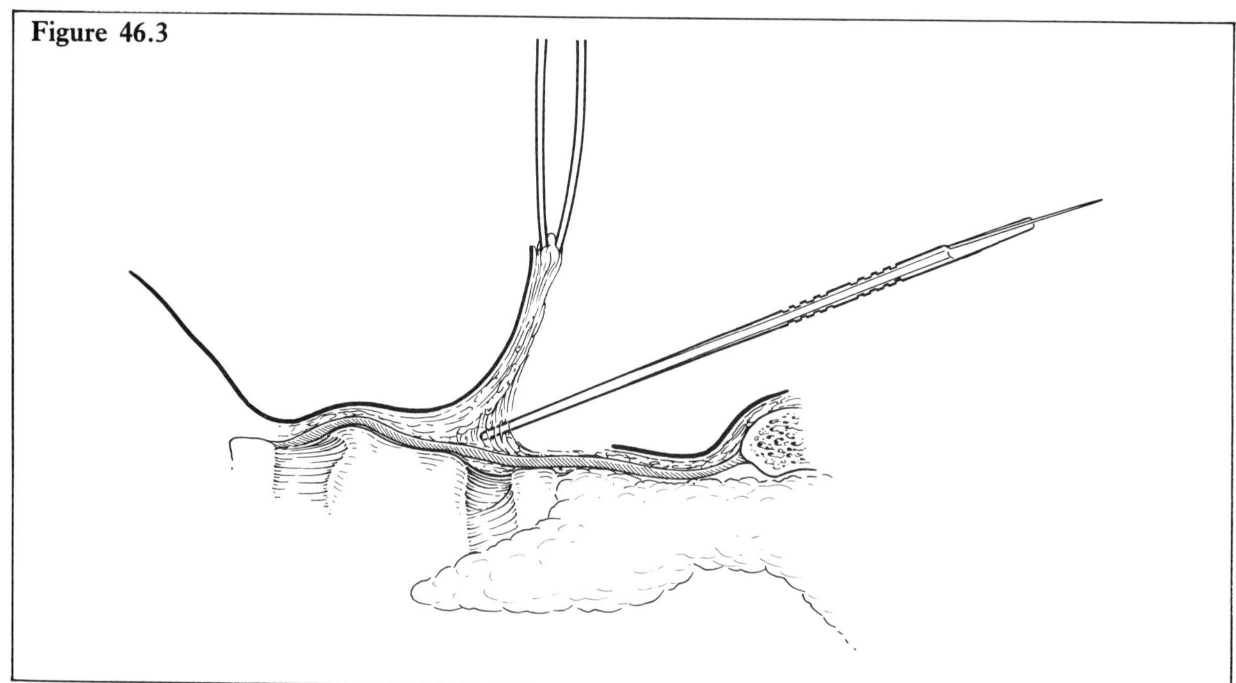

**Figure 46.3**

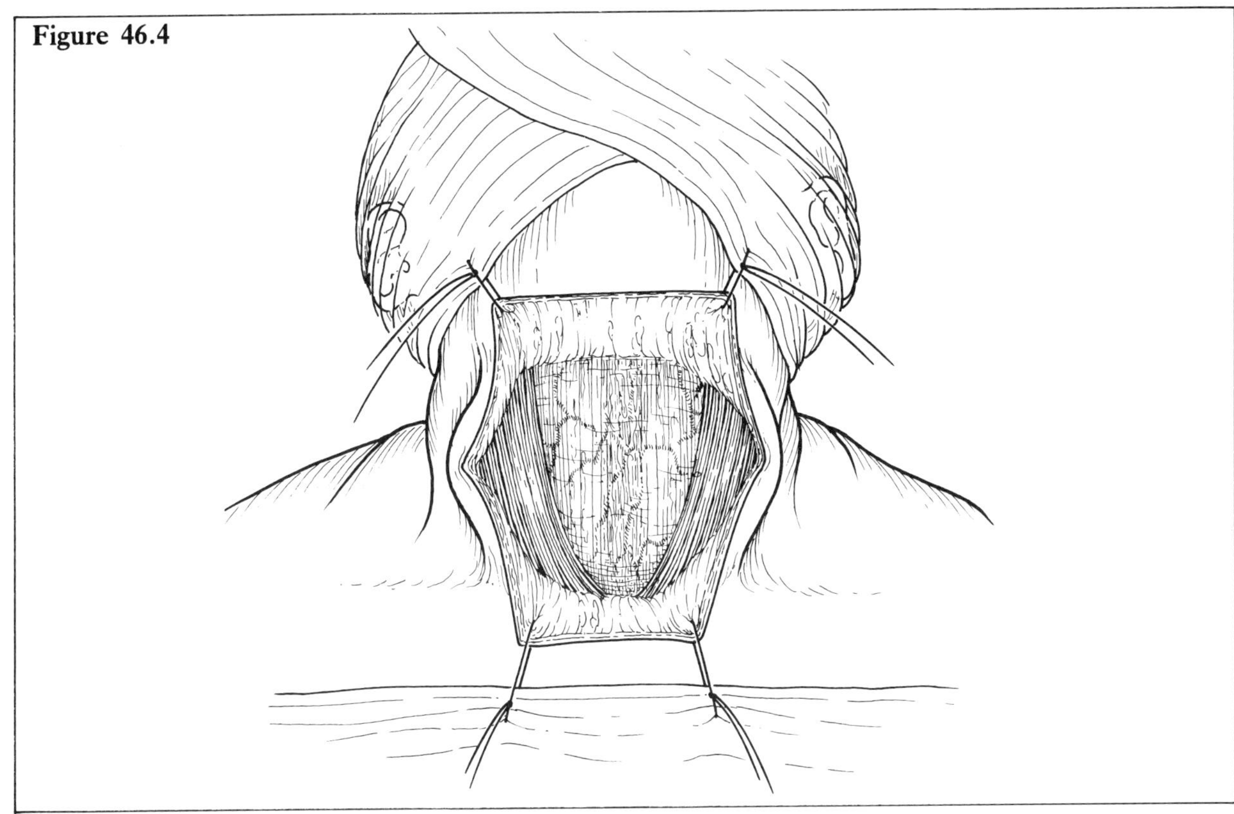

Figure 46.4

over the sternomastoid muscles if the epimysium is inadvertently opened. The lower skin flap is developed to the sternal notch in the same way.

The wound edges are then held apart, either with a thyroidectomy retractor or with stay sutures placed through the subcutaneous tissues and sutured to the skin towels. The latter may be preferred as it leaves the operative field less cluttered (**Fig. 46.4**).

The strap muscles are then separated in the midline (**Fig. 46.5**). If a significantly large part of the goitre is in the neck, it may be necessary to divide the muscles transversely between arterial clips and oversew with an absorbable suture. The sutures should be left uncut and may be used for retraction (**Fig. 46.6**).

The thyroid gland will then be encountered with the isthmus lying across the trachea. Often the cervical part of the thyroid gland is of normal size. With finger dissection the space around the intrathoracic portion of the gland is opened (**Fig. 46.7**). The bulk of it frequently lies to the right-

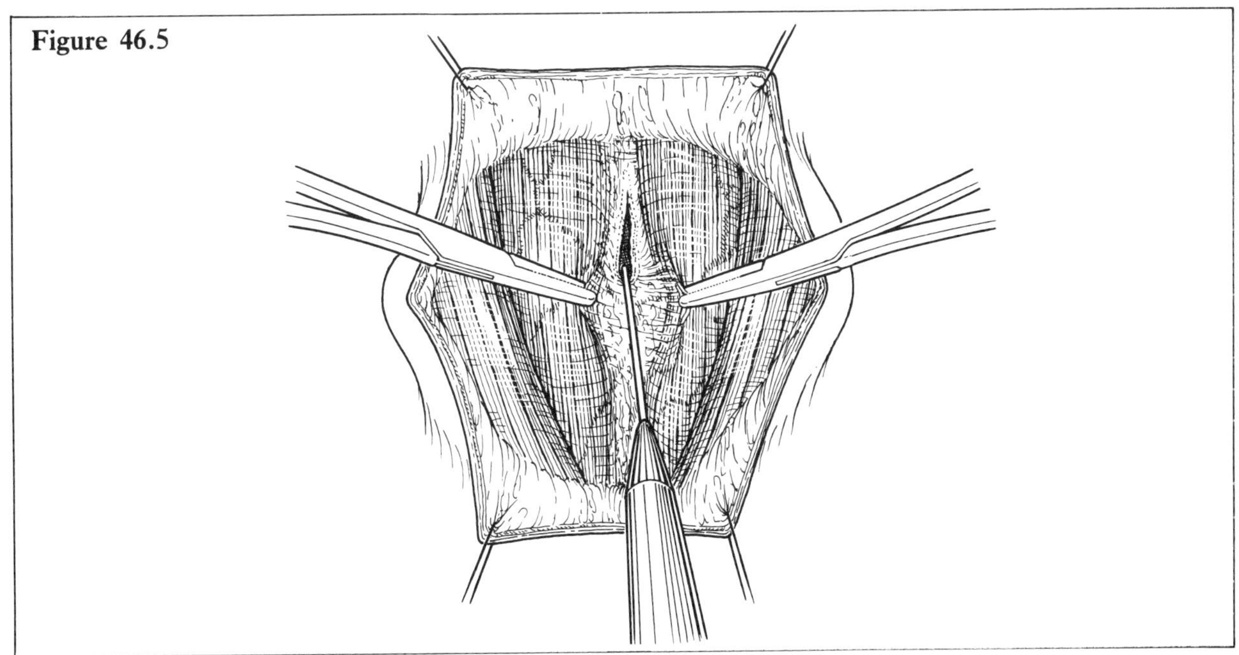

Figure 46.5

hand side of the trachea and often extends posterior to it. At first sight it will often appear to be too large to deliver into the neck, but with care and persistent dissection this can usually be accomplished. There are no vascular attachments to the thyroid gland within the mediastinum and therefore dissection can be carried out in a blind fashion. A dessertspoon may help to lever the gland into the neck without rupturing it. If the goitre is solid enough, it may be possible to pull it into the

**Figure 46.6**

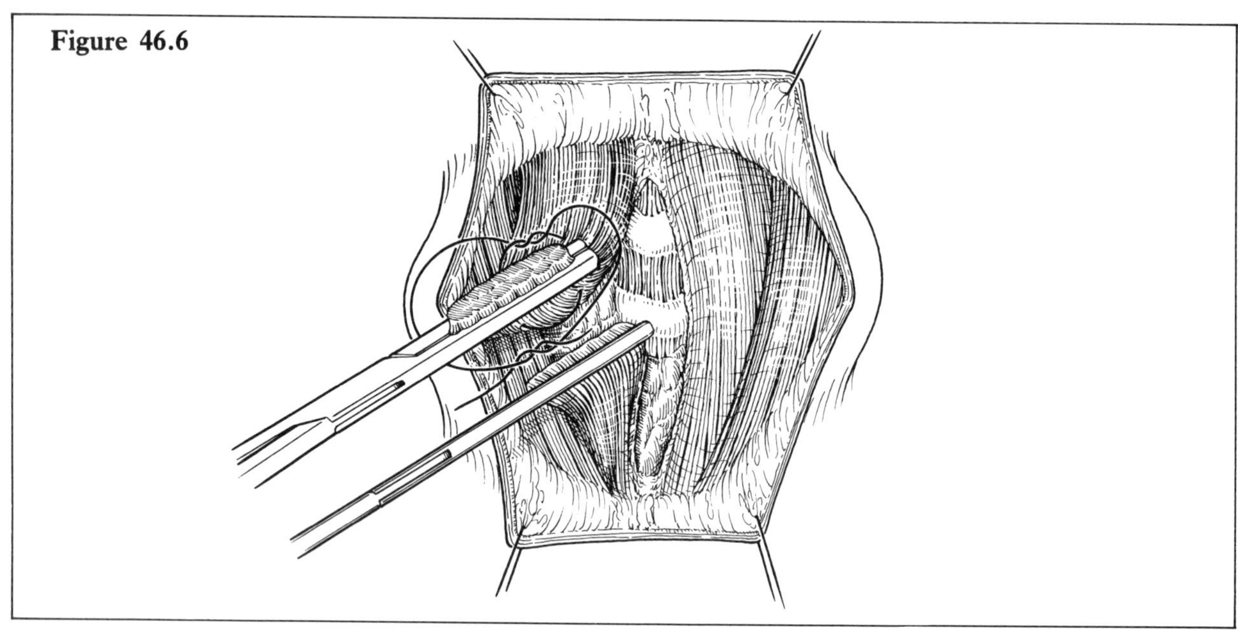

**Figure 46.7**

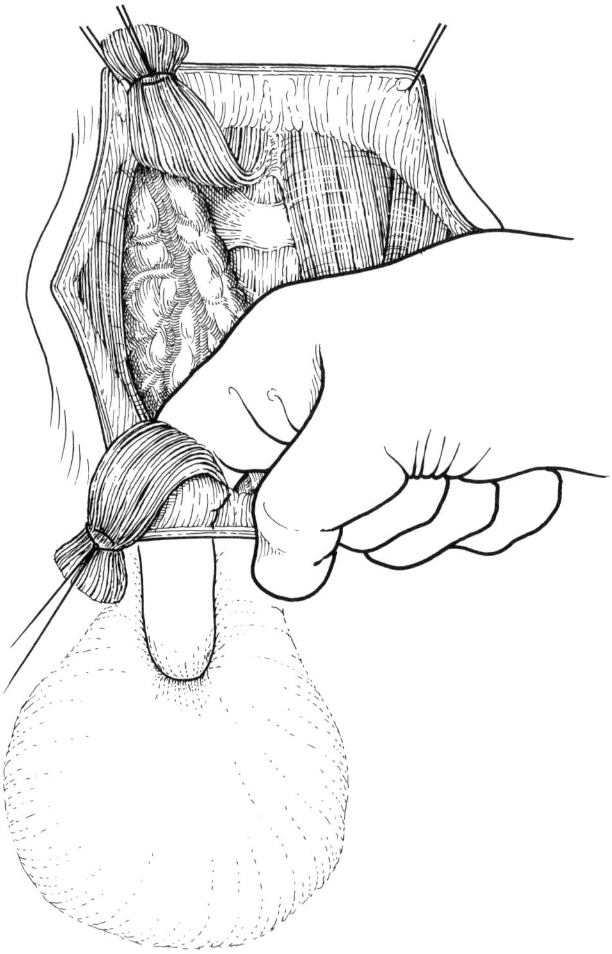

**Figure 46.8**

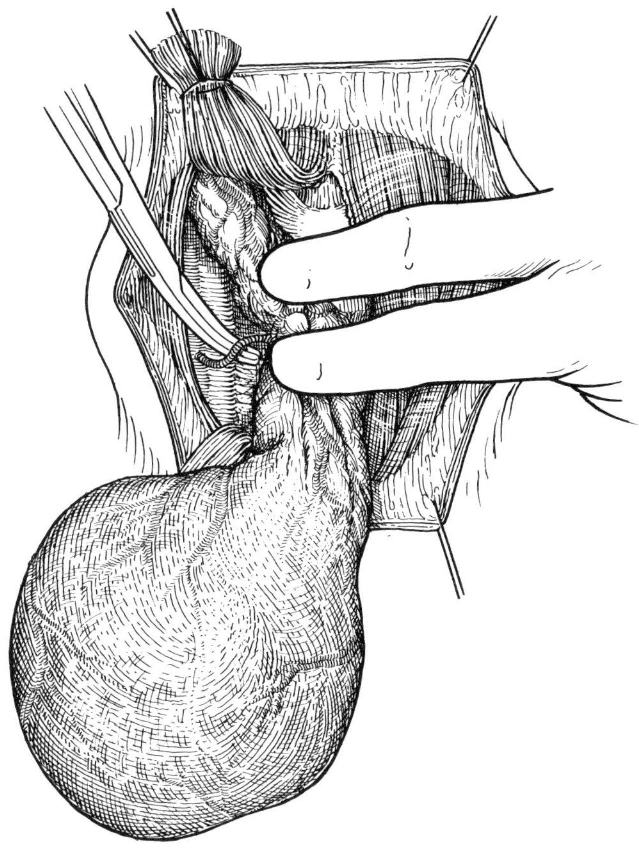

neck after impaling it with a myomectomy screw. Neither of these techniques is usually necessary. Occasionally the gland may rupture, but this is of little consequence provided care is taken to extract all of it when the bulk of the tissue has been removed. If the thyroid enlargement is malignant, it must not be allowed to rupture, and it will be necessary to split the manubrium to allow further access. It is very rarely necessary to split the whole sternum. The thyroid gland extends into the posterior mediastinal compartment, where further access is not enhanced by opening the anterior mediastinal space. Once the goitre has been delivered into the neck a standard, subtotal thyroidectomy is performed. If one lobe is of normal size and consistency, there is no need to remove it.

First the middle thyroid vein is divided between ligatures close to the thyroid gland (**Fig. 46.8**). If the vein is not divided early in the procedure it may be avulsed from the internal jugular vein. The upper pole is mobilized and divided between ligatures, the proximal end being doubly ligated. One of these must be a suture ligature to prevent loss of control of the superior thyroid artery (**Fig. 46.9**). There may be a cluster of inferior thyroid veins entering the posteroinferior margin of the gland; these are ligated, together with the inferior thyroid artery. During this part of the procedure great care must be taken not to damage the

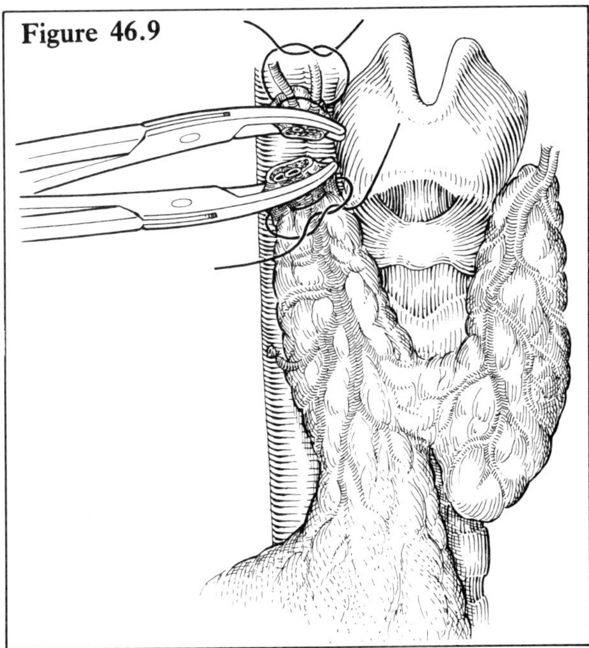
**Figure 46.9**

recurrent laryngeal nerve which lies in the tracheo-oesophageal groove. To avoid damage, the loose fascial tissue between the carotid sheath and the thyroid gland should be swept away with a small gauze sponge mounted on a Kocher or Roberts clamp (**Fig. 46.10**). When dissection is complete the isthmus of the thyroid gland is separated from the pretracheal fascia and a clamp passed behind

Figure 46.10

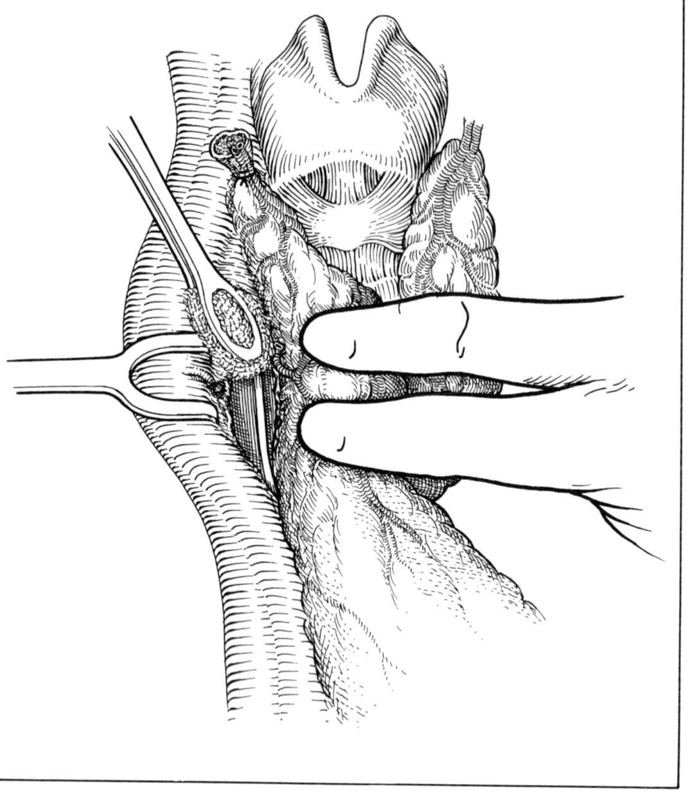

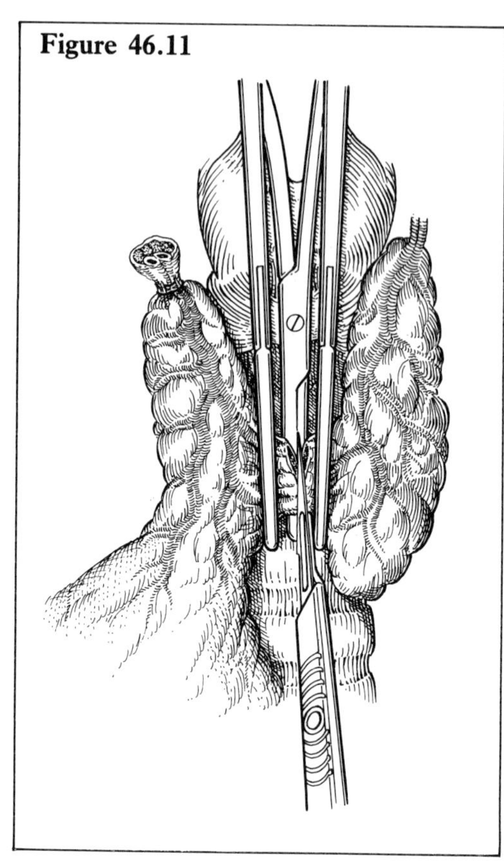

Figure 46.11

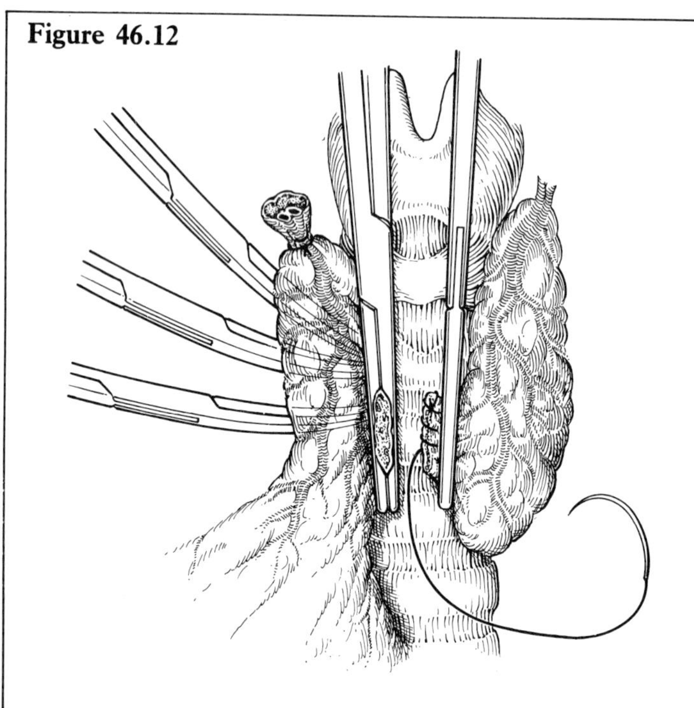

Figure 46.12

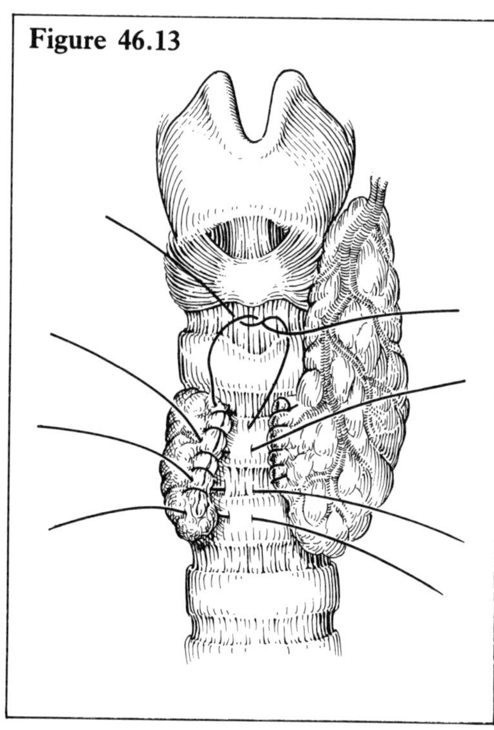

Figure 46.13

it. It is clamped on each side and divided with a scalpel (**Fig. 46.11**). Each end is then oversewn with an absorbable suture. The proposed line of excision of the gland from its lateral tracheal attachments is marked with a series of short artery clamps (**Fig. 46.12**); the gland is excised above the clamps and removed. The thyroid remnant is firmly oversewn with a 3/0 absorbable suture, to prevent haemorrhage. These stitches pick up the adventitia overlying the trachea (**Fig. 46.13**).

### Procedure for the malignant thyroid gland

If the thyroid enlargement is malignant, a total thyroidectomy should be performed, provided the tumour is not anaplastic or with extensive local invasion. In the latter two cases only palliation can be achieved, and the object is to debulk the tissue to relieve airway or oesophageal compression.

When a curative resection is thought possible every care should be taken to excise the entire gland. In these circumstances, the recurrent laryngeal nerves should be sought and preserved, as they are more at risk from trauma in this radical procedure.

## Closure

Extreme care should be taken to achieve absolute haemostasis prior to closure. A vacuum drain is passed into the residual mediastinal cavity. If the strap muscles have been divided, they are reapproximated by tying together the sutures that were used to oversew the ends. A second vacuum drain is left beneath this layer and brought out through a separate stab wound in the neck (**Fig. 46.14**). The strap muscles are then loosely approximated in the midline.

The platysma muscle is repaired with an absorbable suture. The skin is closed, either with a continuous, subcuticular monofilament nylon suture or with skin clips. If clips are used a clip remover must be attached to the patient's pillow at all times for speedy removal should bleeding occur — airway compression by a rapidly expanding haematoma may be fatal. Similarly, if a subcutaneous nylon suture has been used the ends must be left protruding from the skin for easier removal.

At the end of the procedure the vocal cords should be inspected by the anaesthetist to confirm that they are undamaged. A postoperative chest radiograph is essential to exclude a pneumothorax which may result from the intrathoracic dissection.

If skin clips have been used, alternate ones may be removed on the third postoperative day and the remainder on the fourth postoperative day. The drains are removed on the second postoperative day or when all drainage has ceased.

**Figure 46.14**

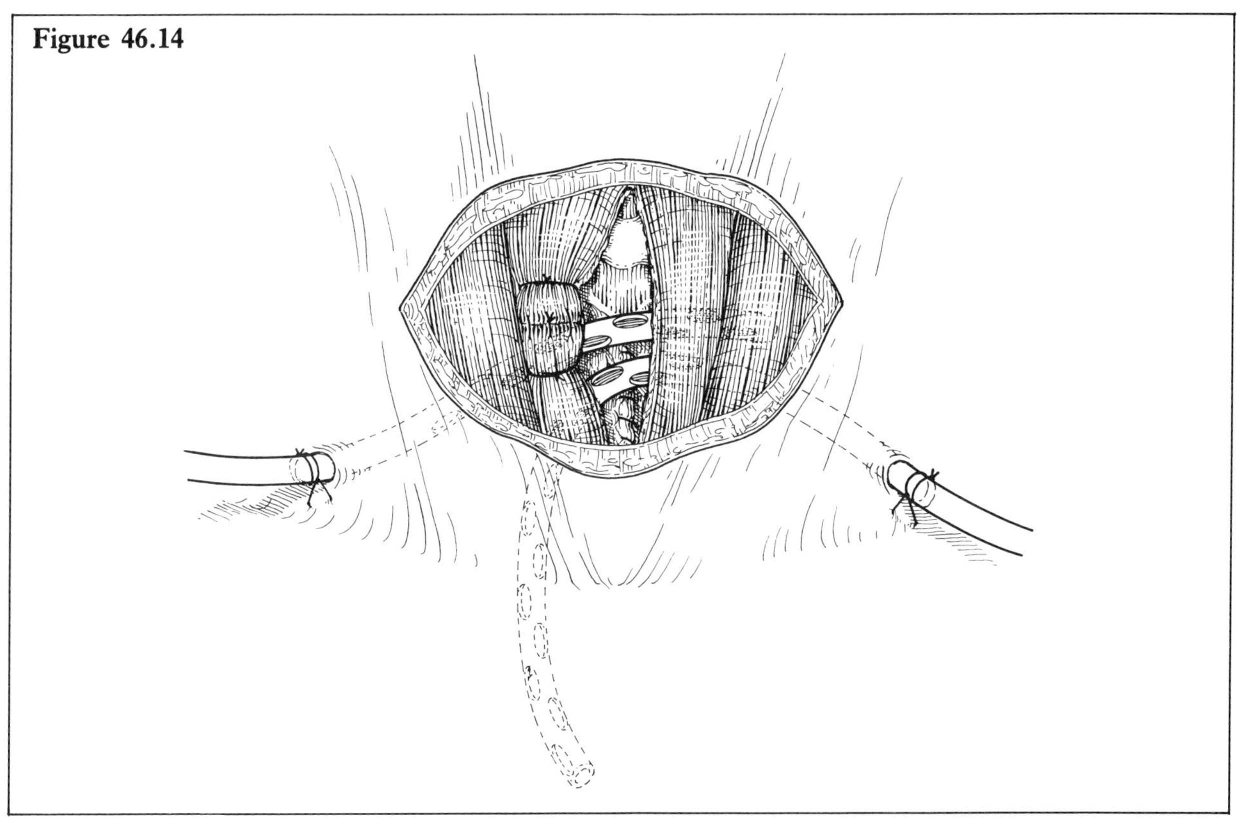

# 47 Pericardial drainage

A pericardial effusion may occur in association with many different disease processes. Many effusions will resolve spontaneously as the causative disease abates. Others may be drained by simple needle aspiration via a subxiphisternal approach (**Fig. 47.1**). To avoid penetration of the right ventricle an ECG electrode should be attached to the needle and the ECG monitored, to indicate contact with the heart.

Needle aspiration is inadequate treatment for acute purulent pericarditis, as the pus is usually loculated. Subxiphisternal exploration and insertion of a pericardial drainage tube is preferable, and can be performed under local anaesthesia. A vertical incision approximately 3 cm long is made just to the left of the xiphisternum (**Fig. 47.2**). The wound is deepened through the linea alba and blunt dissection is carried up between the xiphisternal and anterior costal origins of the diaphragm. The pericardium lies directly behind this and can then be incised after elevating it with a hook (**Fig. 47.3**).

It is desirable to avoid entering the pleural spaces, as an empyema may result. All accessible intrapericardial loculations are broken down and pus aspirated. Specimens are kept for culture. A large drainage tube is then passed into the pericar-

Figure 47.1

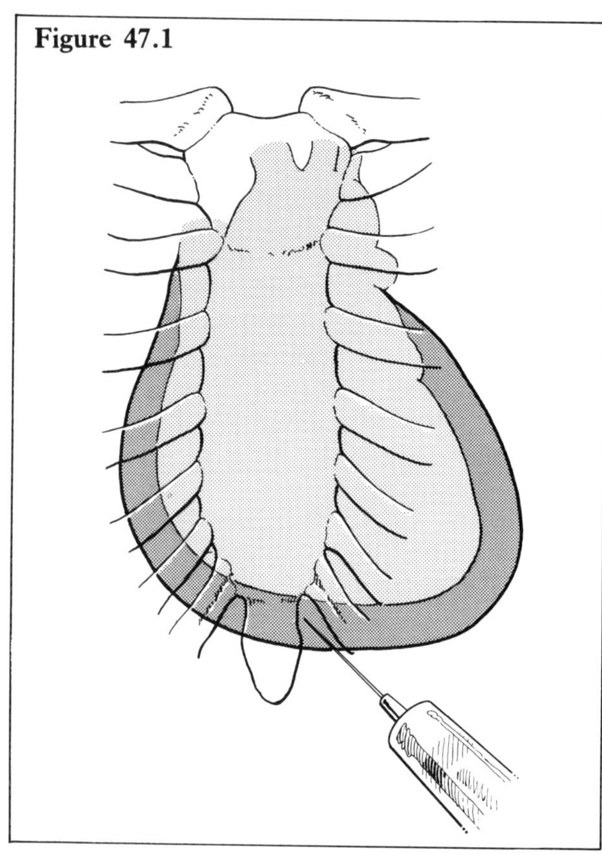

Figure 47.2

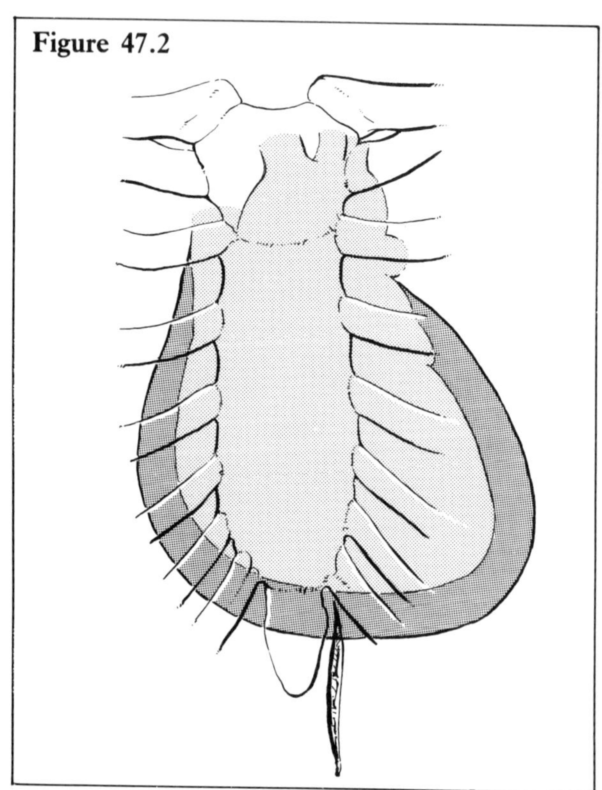

Figure 47.3

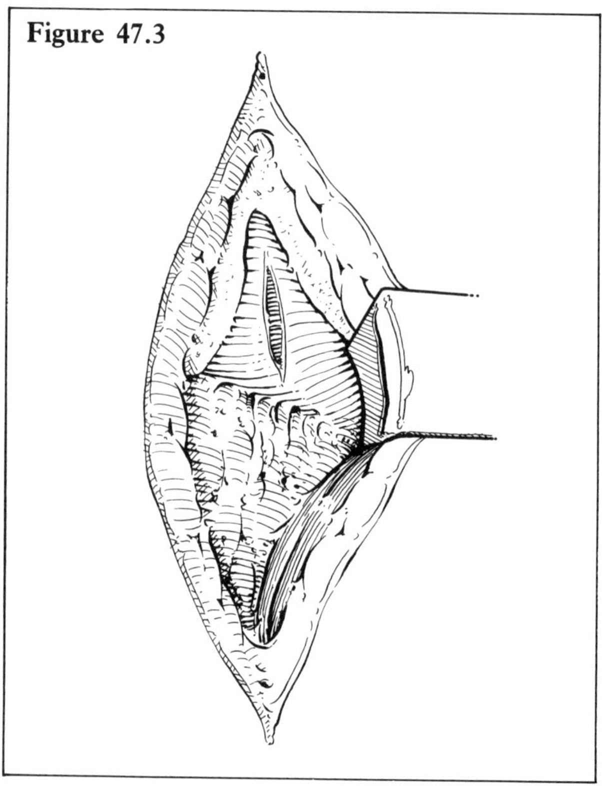

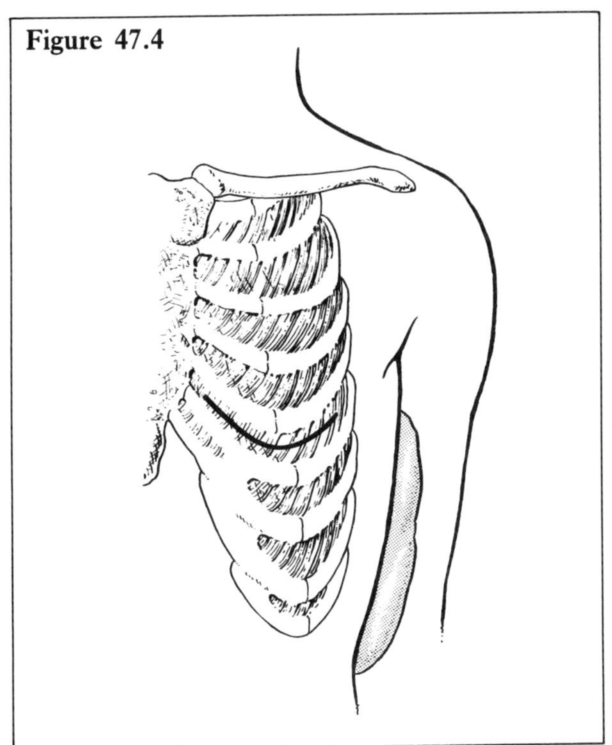
Figure 47.4

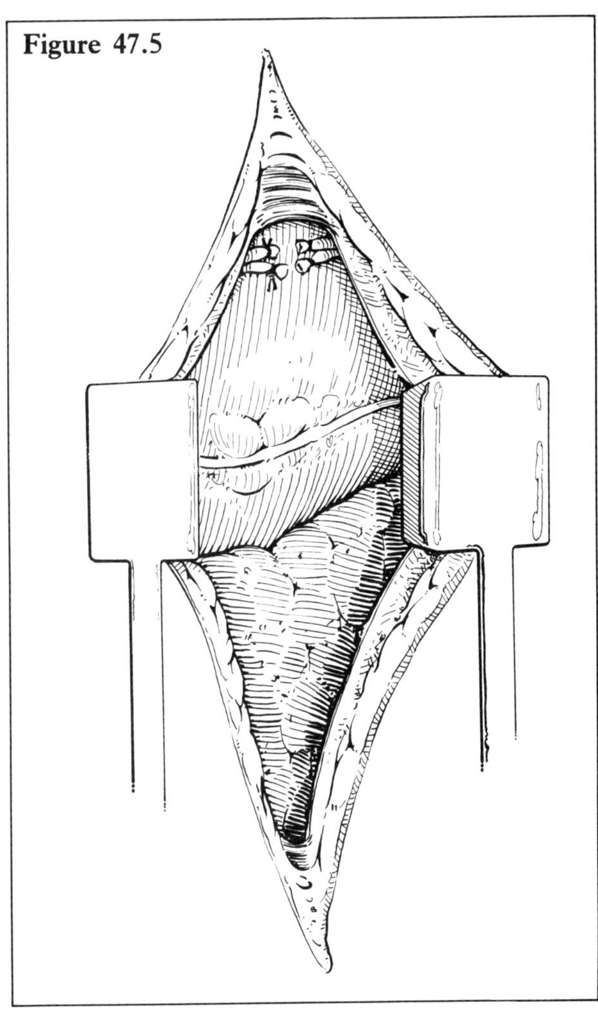
Figure 47.5

dial cavity and brought out through the wound. The drain is kept on 50 mmHg (7 kPa) suction until all drainage has ceased.

A few cases need formal exploration and drainage. The main indications are as follows:

1. Cardiac tamponade that cannot be relieved by needle aspiration or tube drainage.
2. To obtain pericardium for biopsy.

## Procedure

The patient is anaesthetized and placed supine on the operating table. The left side of the chest is elevated by a sandbag (**Fig. 47.4**). A short anterior thoracotomy incision is made over the sixth intercostal space. This is deepened through the muscle layer until the chest wall is reached. The pleural cavity is entered by incising the intercostal muscle

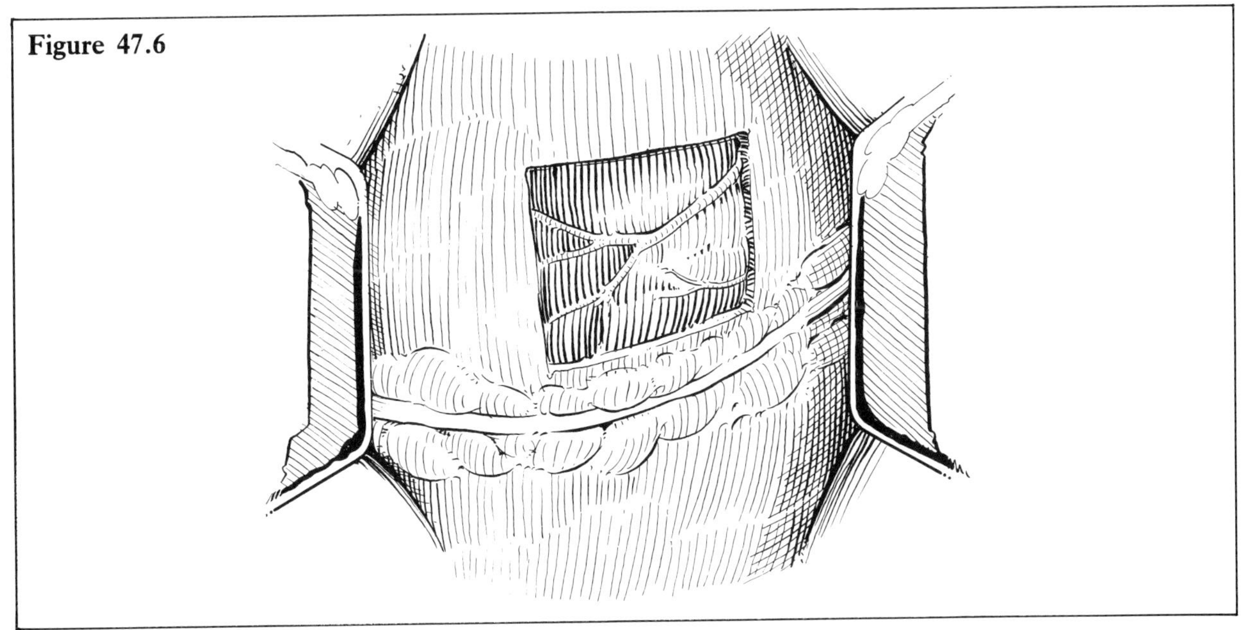
Figure 47.6

between the fifth and sixth ribs (**Fig. 47.5**). Care must be taken when the retractor is opened, to prevent damage to the internal mammary artery and vein; sometimes it is necessary to ligate these vessels.

The pericardium is incised anterior to the phrenic nerve, and a piece of pericardium approximately 3 cm × 3 cm is excised and sent for pathological examination (**Fig. 47.6**). The effusion is allowed to drain and samples sent for culture and cytology. Any loculations are broken down.

### Closure

The pericardial fenestration is left open and a drain is fixed in the pleural space with a basal hole to encourage free drainage. The ribs are approximated with pericostal sutures, and the remainder of the wound is closed as described on p. 35.

SECTION 7

# OESOPHAGEAL SURGERY

# 48 Surgical anatomy of the oesophagus and related structures

The oesophagus is a muscular tube, approximately 25 cm long, extending from the pharynx to the stomach. It is closely applied to the front of the vertebral column throughout most of its length. It leaves this position to pass through the diaphragm at the level of the tenth thoracic vertebra (**Fig. 48.1**). This forward angulation may be very pronounced in some patients; this must be remembered during endoscopy using the rigid instrument and during dilatation of a distal stricture, or a perforation may result. In the posterior mediastinum the oesophagus passes from the right side of the thoracic vertebrae to the left (**Fig. 48.2**).

There are three areas of constriction at which foreign bodies may be held up: these are at the cricopharyngeus muscle (12–13 cm from the incisor teeth); where the oesophagus is crossed by the aortic arch (22–25 cm from the incisor teeth); and where it traverses the diaphragm (37–39 cm from the incisor teeth).

Immediately anterior to the oesophagus in the cervical region and the superior mediastinum is the membranous portion of the trachea. Lying in the groove between the two structures are the recurrent laryngeal nerves (**Fig. 48.3**).

In the posterior mediastinum the oesophagus passes behind the left main bronchus and the left atrium. Patients with left atrial enlargement may complain of mild dysphagia because of compression at this point. In the lower part of the posterior mediastinum the thoracic duct lies behind and to the right of the oesophagus. Higher up, the duct passes behind the oesophagus and crosses to the left at about the level of the fifth thoracic vertebra, then continues upwards on the left side. During dissection of the oesophagus its presence should be

**Figure 48.1**

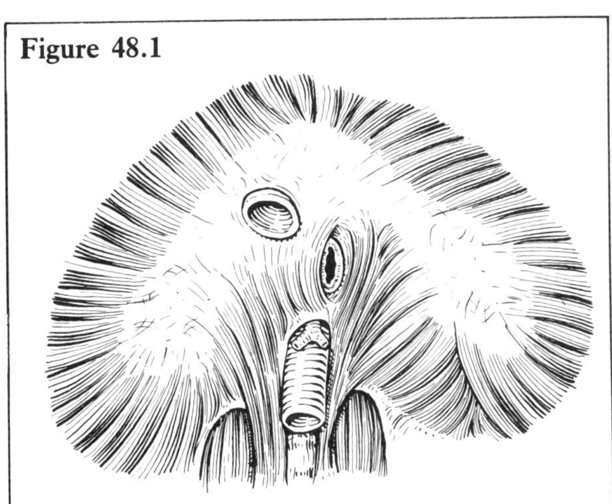

**Figure 48.2**

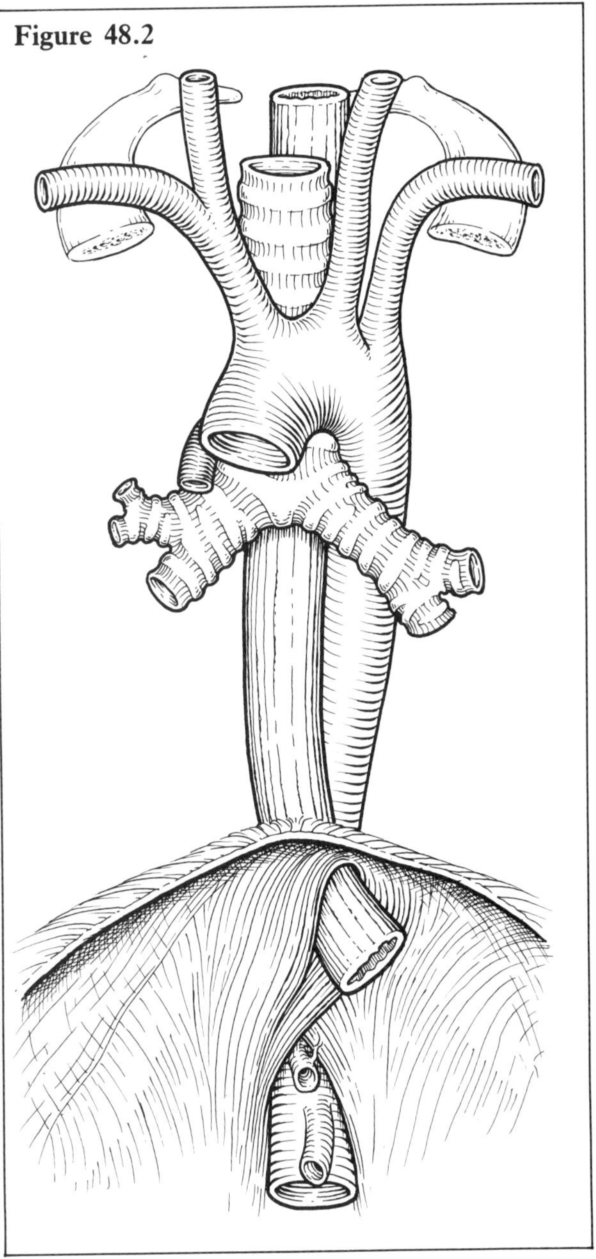

**Figure 48.3**

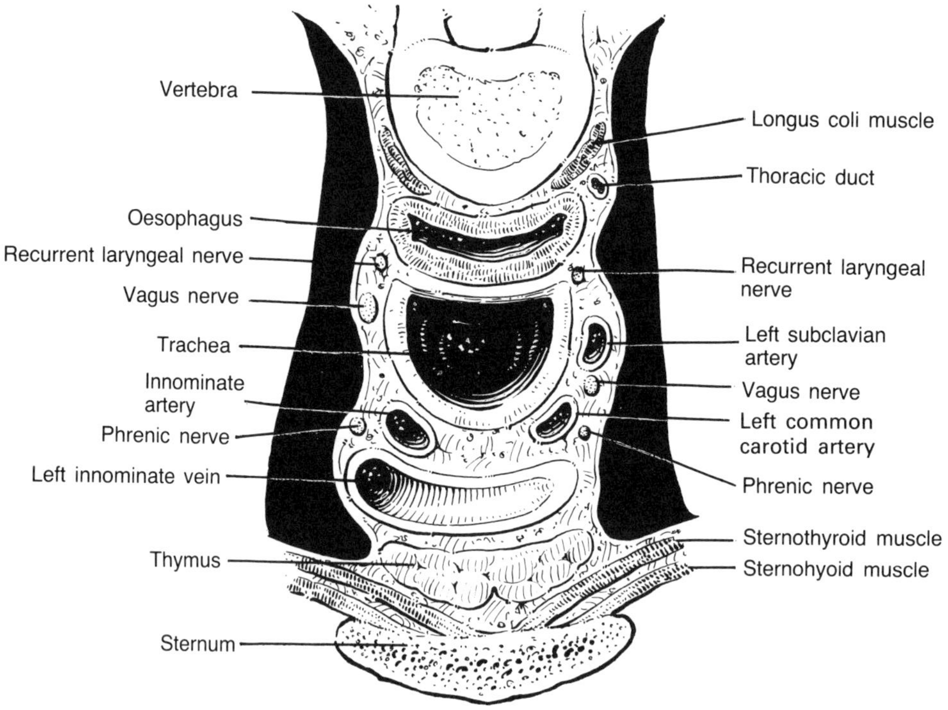

Vertebra
Longus coli muscle
Thoracic duct
Oesophagus
Recurrent laryngeal nerve
Vagus nerve
Recurrent laryngeal nerve
Trachea
Left subclavian artery
Innominate artery
Vagus nerve
Phrenic nerve
Left common carotid artery
Left innominate vein
Phrenic nerve
Sternothyroid muscle
Thymus
Sternohyoid muscle
Sternum

remembered, as a chylothorax can be an exceedingly troublesome postoperative complication.

The parietal pleural and peritoneal reflections on to the oesophagus give rise to the phreno-oesophageal ligaments (**Fig. 48.4**). Between the two layers lies areolar tissue with fine blood vessels. These important structures are often difficult to dissect accurately. Great care is required so that the vagus nerves are not injured.

The wall of the oesophagus consists of an external longitudinal muscle coat, an internal circular muscle coat and the oesophageal mucosa. A thickened band of circular muscle, the cricopharyngeus, guards the upper end. At the distal end there is an area of high pressure which can be demonstrated by manometry; unlike the cricopharyngeus, however, this high-pressure zone (HPZ) is not anatomically distinct.

The normal antireflux mechanism is complex and has the following distinct components. First, and most important, is the intra-abdominal portion of the oesophagus. The resting intra-abdominal pressure is higher than that within the thorax, and as the lumen of the oesophagus reflects the intrathoracic pressure, this section is kept closed except when a bolus of food passes through it. Secondly, the right crus of the diaphragm which loops round the oesophagus (**Fig. 48.2**) can be shown to exert pressure on it. This high-pressure area is often indistinct from that at the distal end of the oesophagus. Thirdly, the angle of insertion of the gastro-oesophageal junction encourages it to close as the stomach fills. Finally the high-pressure zone within the oesophagus, already alluded to, plays its part. Any surgical method to restore gastro-oesophageal competence must take into account all of these mechanisms.

**Figure 48.4**

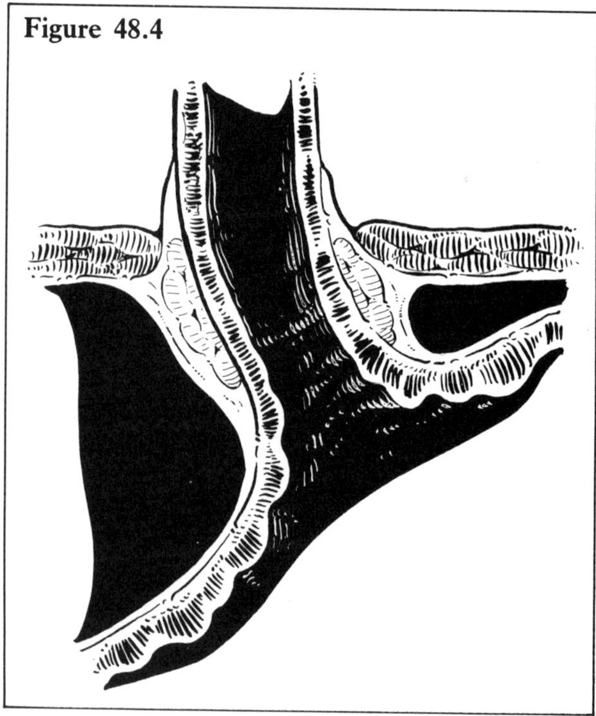

# 49 Oesophagoscopy and dilatation

For oesophagoscopy both flexible and rigid instruments are available and are complementary. As in bronchoscopy, each instrument has its merits, and the surgeon in training should endeavour to become familiar with both.

The rigid instrument (**Fig. 49.1**) is preferred for the removal of foreign bodies, obtaining large biopsy specimens and the dilatation of difficult strictures.

The flexible endoscope (**Fig. 49.2**) allows examination of the stomach and duodenum and in particular the gastro-oesophageal junction from below. It can be used with topical anaesthesia and mild sedation whereas the rigid endoscope can only be safely used with a general anaesthetic.

## Rigid Oesophagoscopy

The patient should have a barium swallow prior to the examination and should be starved for at least six hours. A general anaesthetic with the use of an endotracheal tube is recommended. The patient is positioned supine on the operating table with the head on a flexible extension (**Fig. 49.3**). The neck is flexed on the trunk and the head

**Figure 49.1**

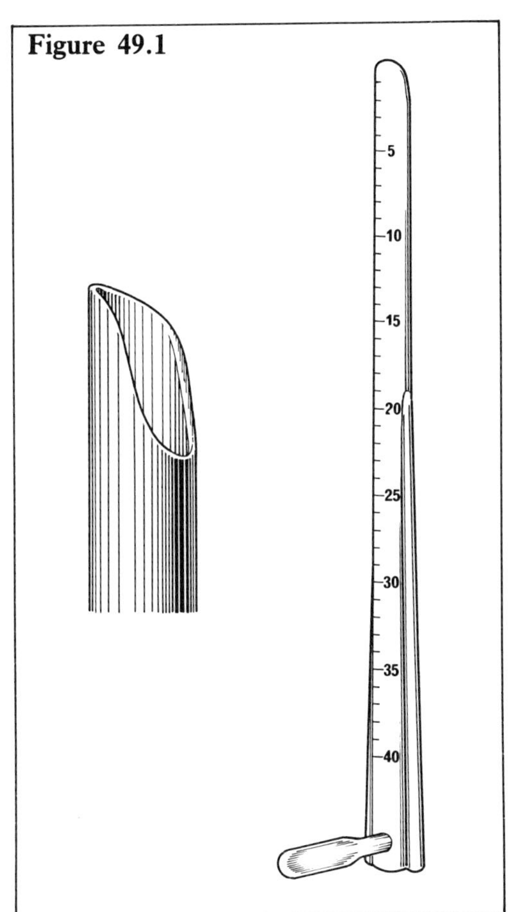


**Figure 49.2**

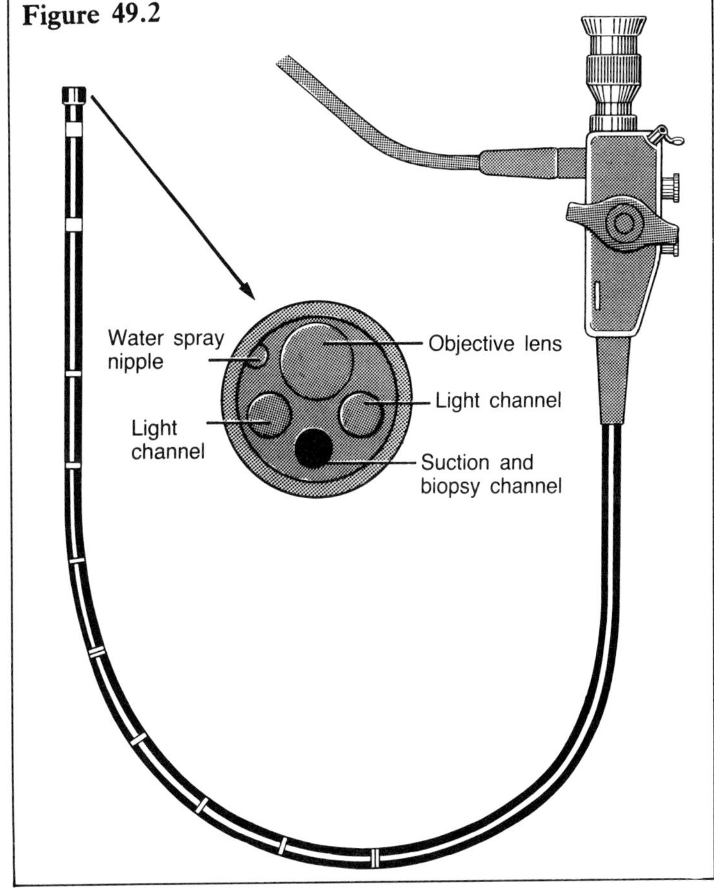


**Figure 49.3**

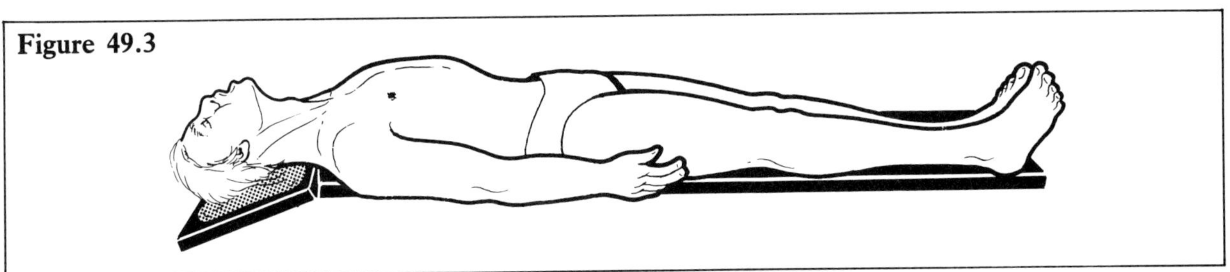

extended on the neck to give a position that is often likened to that of 'sniffing the morning air'!

The operator's thumb is used as a fulcrum to protect the upper lip, maxilla and upper teeth. The tongue is levered forward with the tip of the endoscope which is then passed to the back of the oropharynx behind the endotracheal tube, until the cricopharyngeus muscle is seen (**Fig. 49.4**). It is most important from this point onwards not to push the endoscope too hard, and to keep the lumen of the oesophagus in sight at all times. Failure to do so is likely to result in a tear of the oesophageal mucosa and perforation.

To pass the endoscope beyond the cricopharyngeus muscle it should be gently rotated from side to side. This will allow the beak of the instrument to open the sphincter without pushing. Once the endoscope has entered the body of the oesophagus the neck is extended and the endoscope will pass easily onward towards the gastro-oesophageal junction.

Commonly the dilatation of a stricture and biopsy of the area are performed together. If this is so we recommend that the dilatation is done first; otherwise perforation is more likely because the wall of the oesophagus may be weakened by the biopsy.

**Figure 49.4**

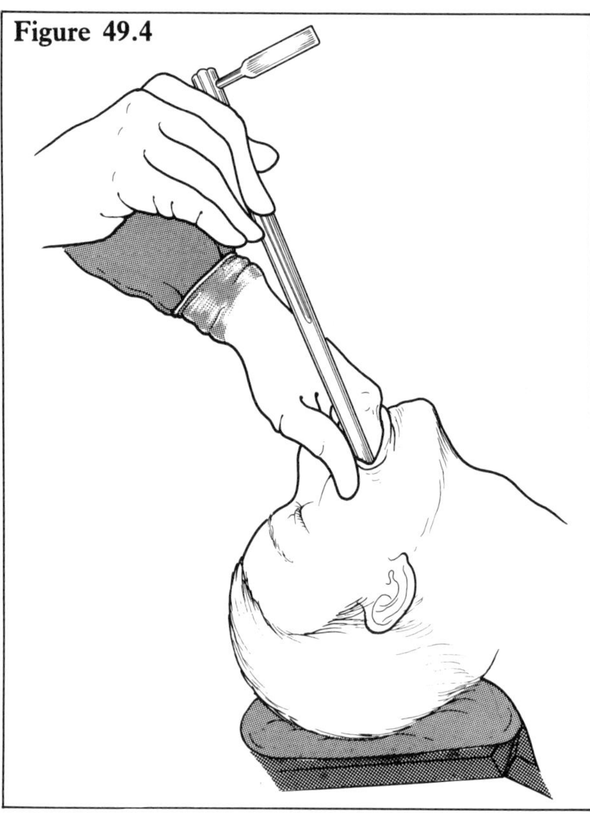

## Dilatation of an oesophageal stricture

Several types of dilators are available for use with the rigid endoscope. The most commonly used ones are the Hurst–Maloney mercury-loaded bougies, the Chevalier–Jackson gum-elastic bougies mounted on a metal guide wire, and the Earlam bougies made of a stiff but deformable silastic also mounted on a metal guide wire (**Fig. 49.5**). The Earlam bougies have a more rounded distal end and are perhaps less likely to result in a perforation than the Chevalier–Jackson type.

Whichever type is used it is important to keep the lumen in sight and never to push blindly. A

**Figure 49.5**

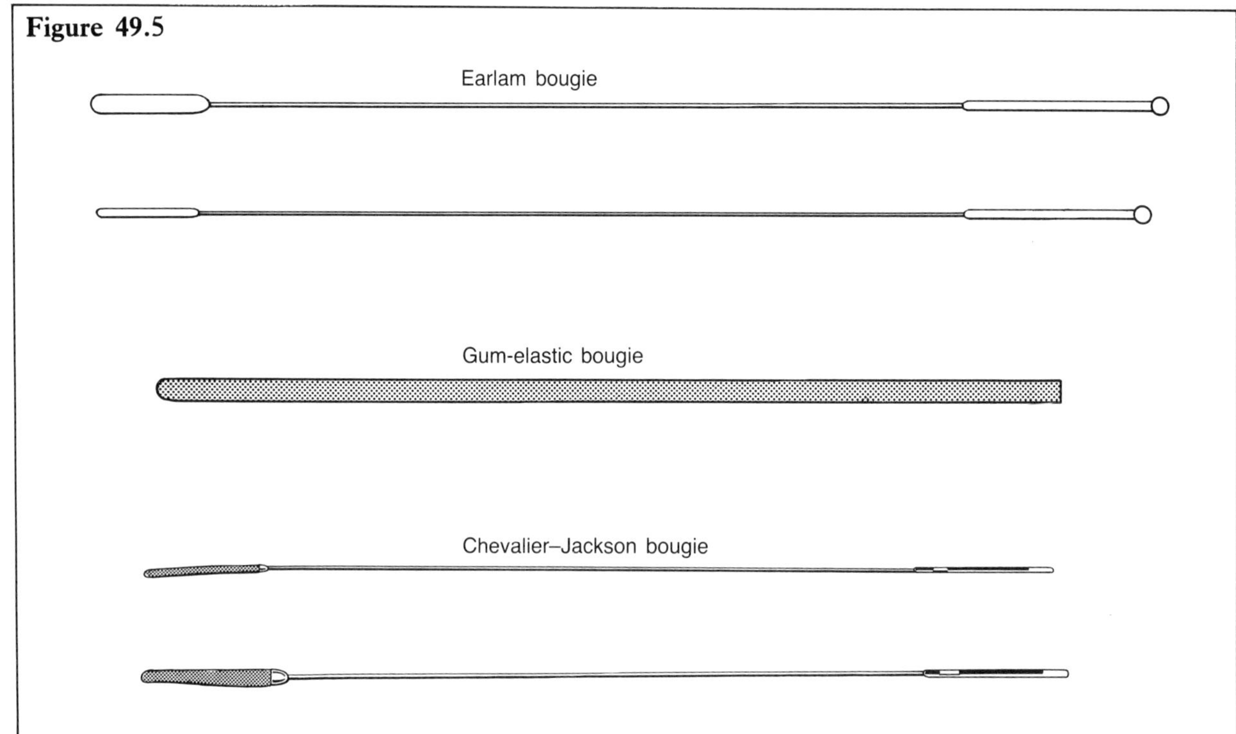

narrow stricture can often be negotiated by varying the angle of flexion of the tip of a dilator and rotating it from side to side while exerting gentle pressure. Perforation should then rarely (if ever) occur.

## Flexible oesophagoscopy

Before beginning the procedure it is essential to give the patient a full explanation of what is about to happen in order to obtain increased cooperation.

The oropharynx is anaesthetized with a local anaesthetic spray. With the patient lightly sedated and lying on the left side with the head slightly flexed, the endoscope is introduced through a mouth guard to prevent damage to the instrument. The patient is asked to swallow the instrument as it is introduced. The process is therefore in part a passive and in part an active one on behalf of both the patient and the endoscopist. Once the endoscope has passed beyond the cricopharyngeus muscle it can usually be passed with ease onward to the stomach.

### Dilatation using the flexible endoscope

Two methods of dilatation are available. For peptic or malignant strictures dilatation may be carried out over a guide wire using the Eder–Puestow system (**Fig. 49.6**).

For cases of achalasia a system of balloon dilatation is available (**Fig. 49.7**). The balloon dilators are passed across the stricture over a guide wire, then inflated with air to a pressure of 250 mmHg (33 kPa) for three minutes.

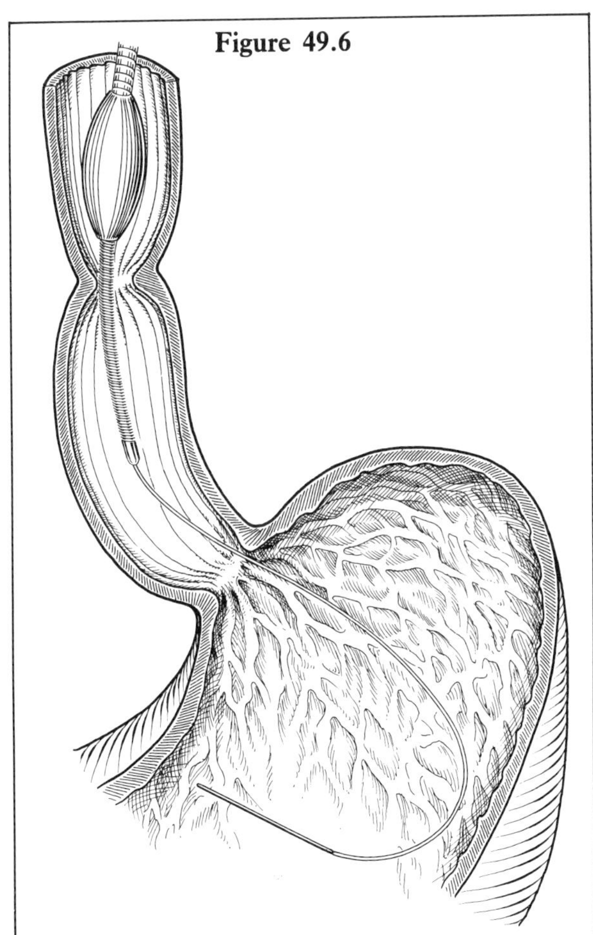

**Figure 49.6**

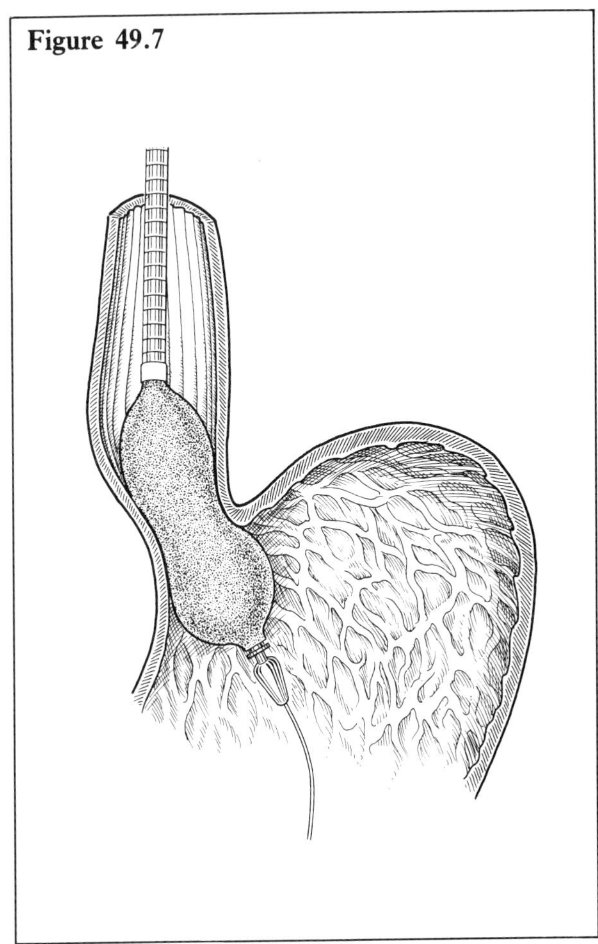

**Figure 49.7**

# Operations for benign oesophageal disease

# 50 Heller's operation for achalasia of the cardia

Heller's operation should be performed whenever achalasia is diagnosed, irrespective of the presence of symptoms, to prevent the complications associated with aspiration of the oesophageal contents into the lungs. If the operation is carried out early enough it may reduce the incidence of late development of carcinoma of the oesophagus.

When the condition is found to be associated with a hiatal hernia, repair of the hernia should be carried out at the same time. Some authorities consider that an antireflux procedure should always be performed after a cardiomyotomy. However, the inferior oesophageal sphincter does not play an important part in the control of reflux, and after the limited operation described here the cardia usually remains competent.

## Procedure

A double-lumen endotracheal tube is inserted to permit deflation of the lungs. The incision is a left anterolateral thoracotomy entering the pleural cavity through the bed of the sixth or seventh rib. As the line of the incision does not cross the scapula, it follows the anterior two-thirds of the course of the rib.

The lung is deflated and retracted upwards, thus exposing the inferior pulmonary ligament which is divided with scissors or with diathermy close to the lung (**Fig. 50.1**). The small arteries in it are coagulated with diathermy. The incision stops at the lower margin of the inferior pulmonary vein which can be identified by a lymph node situated

**Figure 50.1**

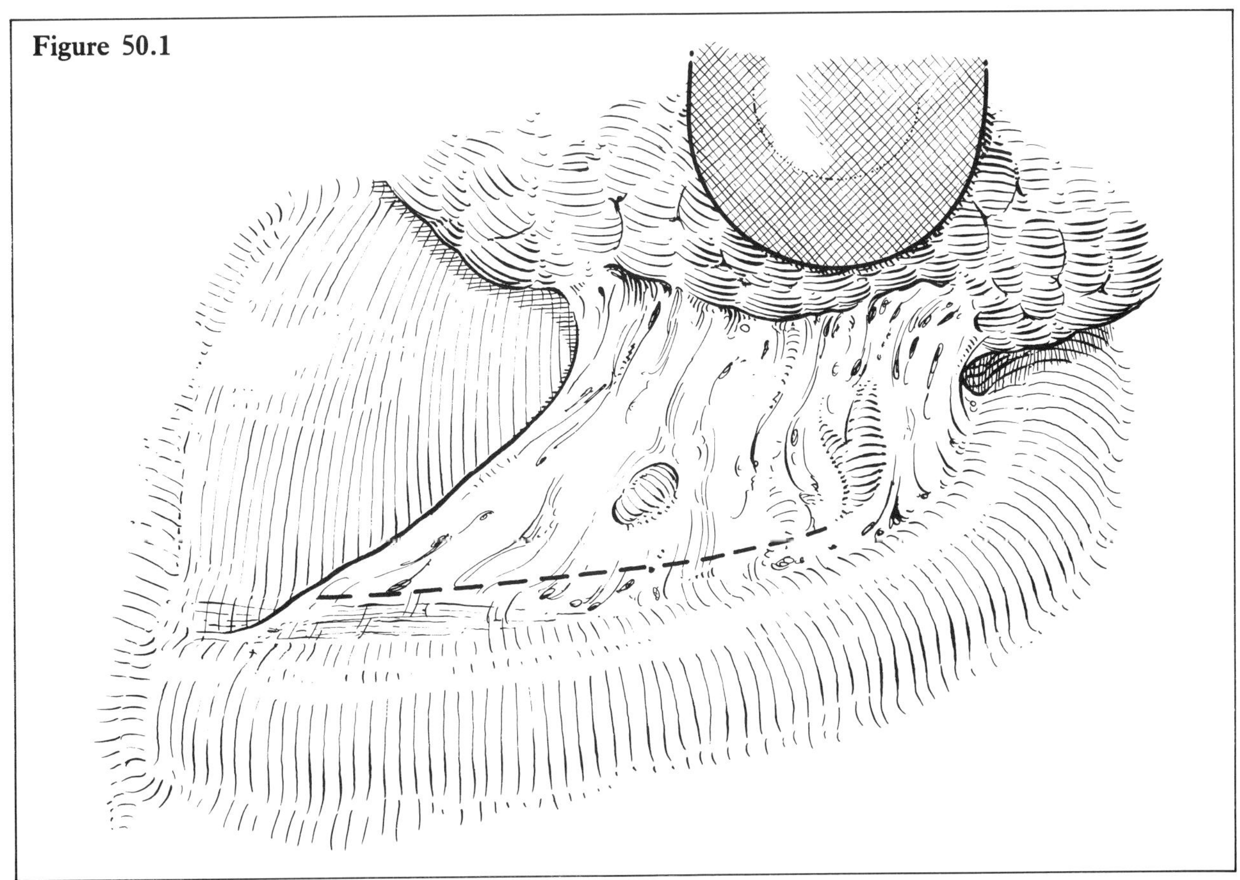

immediately below it. The enlarged, thick-walled oesophagus is mobilized with a finger from the inferior pulmonary rein to the level of the diaphragm (**Fig. 50.2**). This dissection should be kept close to the muscle wall of the oesophagus. A 12-mm moistened linen tape is then passed around it; this is less traumatic than the narrow nylon tape that is commonly used. By exerting traction on the tape, the oesophagogastric junction is drawn up into the thorax, and the narrowed segment of oesophageal wall is clearly seen.

The fingers of the left hand are now placed behind the oesophagus so that their pulps, invaginating the posterior wall, put the anterior wall on the stretch. Using a scalpel with a large blade, a 5-cm incision is made in the long axis of the oesophagus extending on to the stomach (**Fig. 50.3**). As this incision is deepened through the longitudinal muscle fibres, the deeper circular muscle comes into view. Bleeding is largely controlled by increasing the pressure of the fingers of the left hand. One or two of the larger vessels may require ligation. Diathermy is to be avoided because of the risk of causing necrosis of the mucosa and subsequent perforation. As the circular muscle fibres are divided the blade of the knife is rotated so that it cuts almost parallel to the surface. With increasing pressure from behind, the deepest muscle fibres tear and the mucosa bulges through. Any remaining constricting bands show up clearly and are divided. The incision through the circular muscle must extend to the whole length of the incision in the

**Figure 50.2**

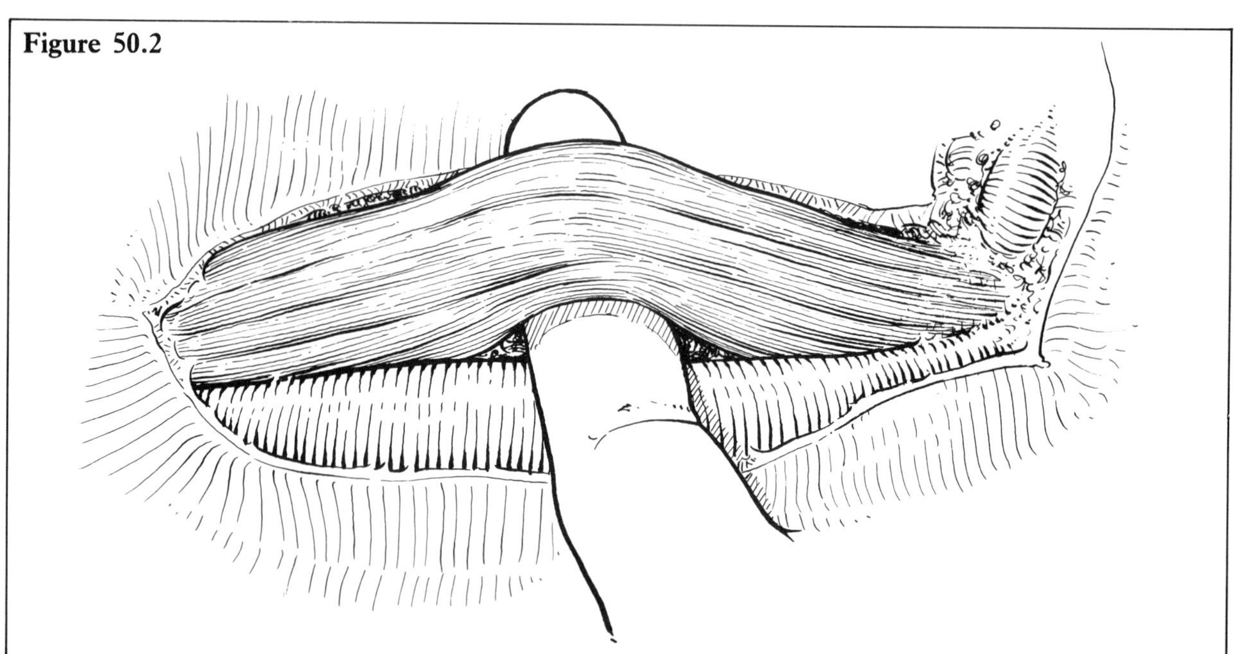

**Figure 50.3**

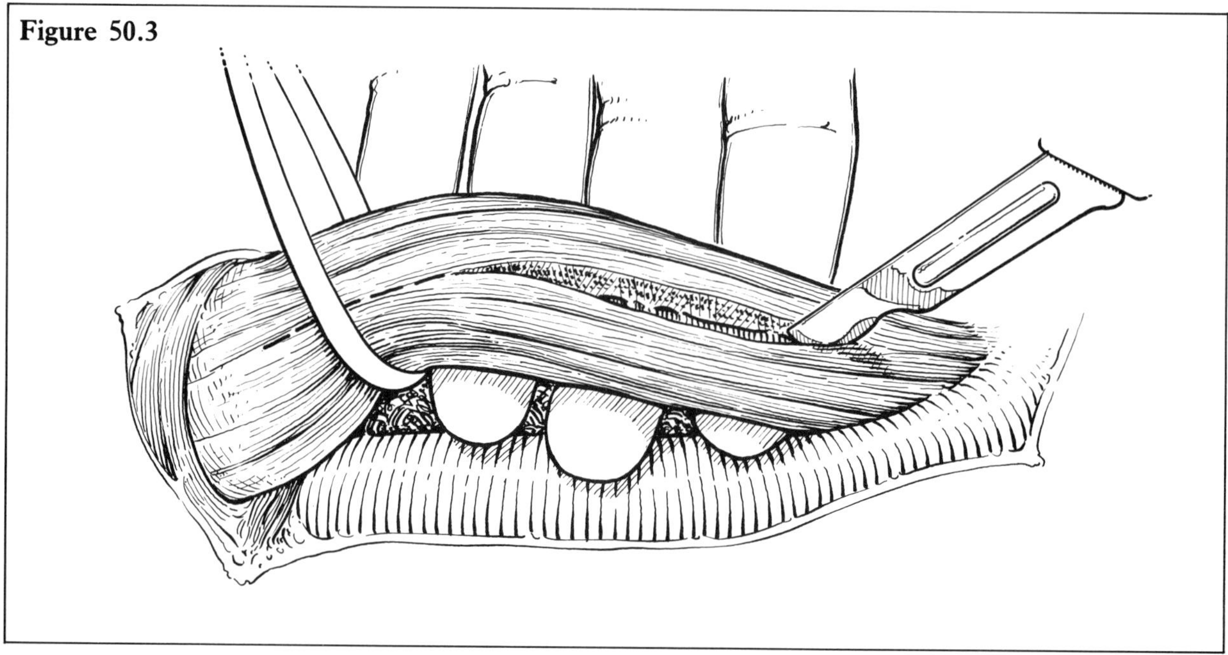

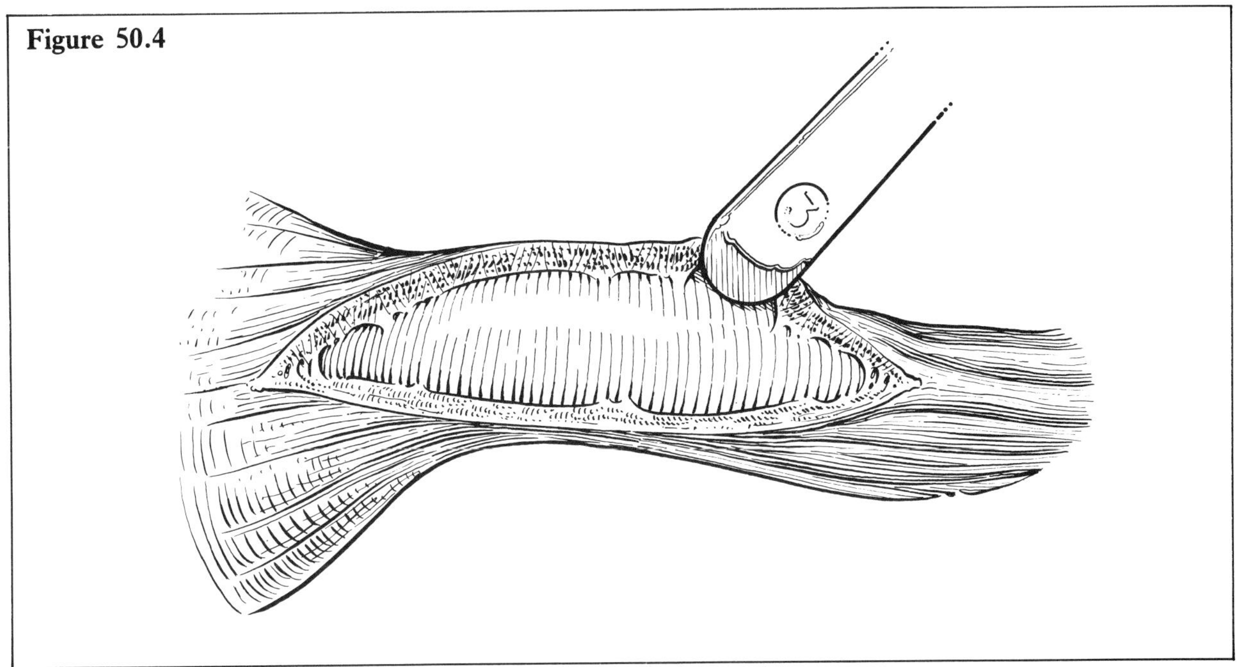

Figure 50.4

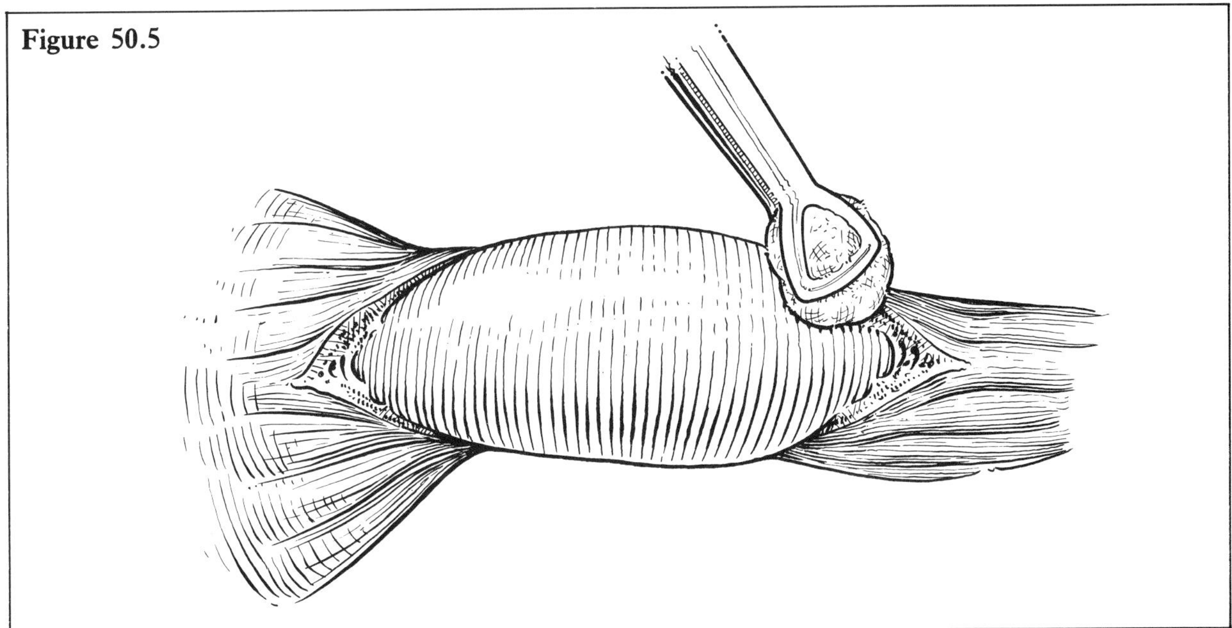

Figure 50.5

longitudinal muscle (**Fig. 50.4**). The muscle is then swept back on either side with a small pledget to free the mucosa for 50% of its circumference (**Figs. 50.5, 50.6**). Any remaining bleeding is controlled by pressure for five minutes with a swab.

A nasogastric tube is not required, and indeed could ulcerate the thin mucosa.

Some surgeons advise inflation of the oesophagus by the anaesthetist at the end of the procedure, to detect residual constricting bands or perforations. Using the technique described above this procedure is unnecessary; it is also dangerous, since it might rupture the oesophagus.

The oesophagus is returned to its bed, the lung re-expanded and the chest closed, with a single drain left in the pleural cavity.

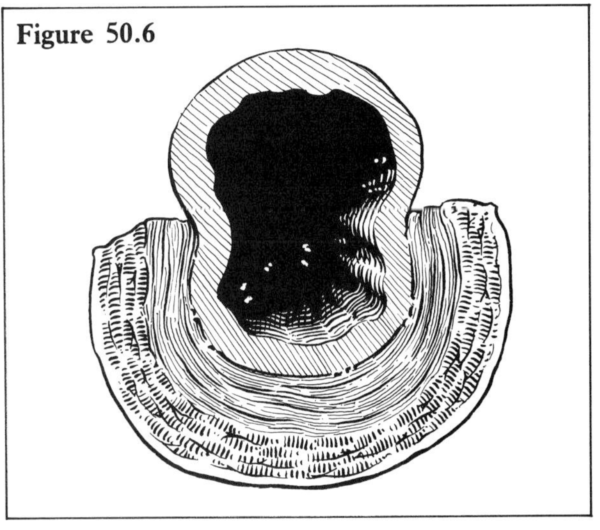

Figure 50.6

**Figure 50.7**

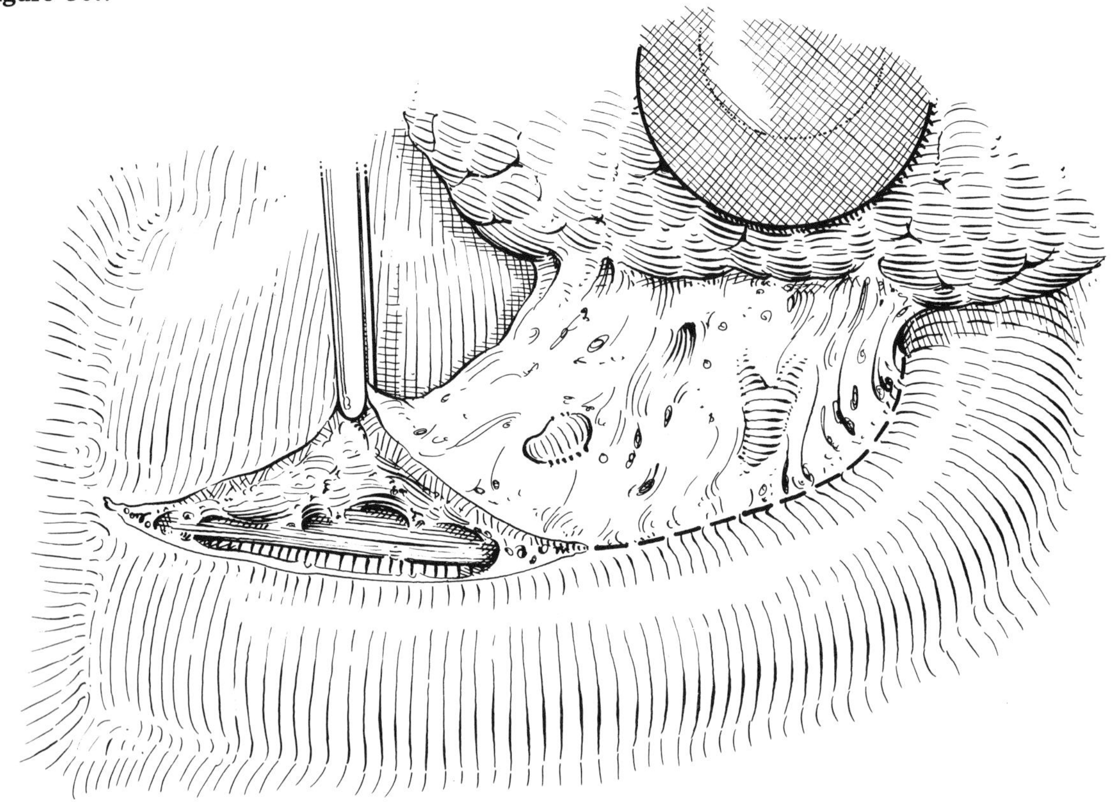

**Figure 50.8**

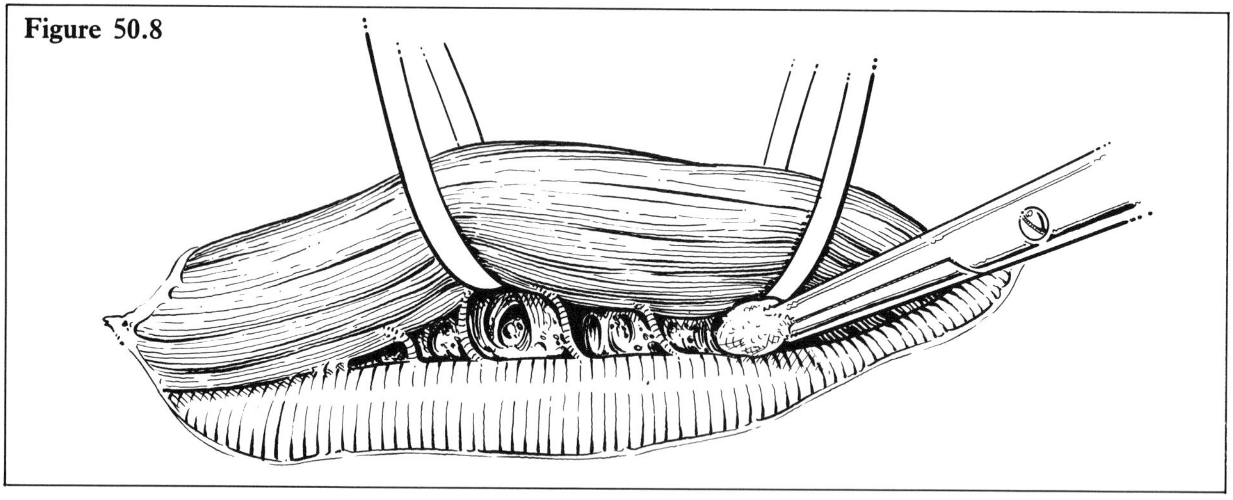

**Figure 50.9**

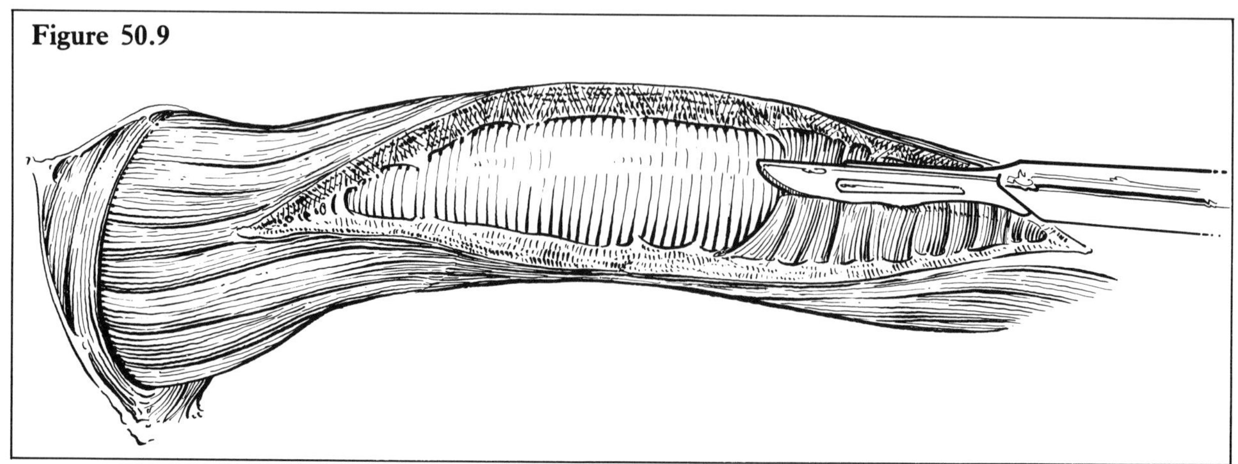

## Extended myotomy

The indication for this operation is dysphagia caused by diffuse oesophageal spasm. Manometric studies are necessary to confirm the diagnosis and to determine the extent of the spasm.

The first steps in the operation are the same as for Heller's operation (described above). However, at the upper limit of the division of the pulmonary ligament, the pleural incision is continued behind the inferior pulmonary vein and the hilum of the lung, and in front of the descending thoracic aorta as far up as the aortic arch (**Fig. 50.7**). The oesophagus is dissected from its bed a short distance above the level of the inferior pulmonary vein and a second tape passed around it here (**Fig. 50.8**). The dissection is at right angles to the oesophageal wall so that the entering vessels are preserved. Complete mobilization of the oesophagus is unnecessary.

Using the belly of the scalpel, the incision in the longitudinal muscle is extended up to the aortic arch. The circular muscle comes into view. The handle of a scalpel is passed deep to the circular muscle, freeing a centimetre at a time from the mucosa; these fibres are then divided. The procedure is repeated until the aortic arch is reached (**Fig. 50.9**).

The operation is completed as described for Heller's operation.

# 51 Excision of pharyngeal pouch

The pharyngeal pouch emerges in the midline, posteriorly between the transverse and oblique fibres of the cricopharyngeus muscle (**Fig. 51.1**). As it enlarges it descends behind the oesophagus and usually deviates to one or other side. It may extend a variable distance into the mediastinum.

## Indications

Indications for this operation are dysphagia, noisy eructation with meals, nocturnal cough or recurrent pneumonia from inhalation of the pouch contents into the lungs. The patients are often elderly, but as the operation is not a stressful procedure, advanced age should not be considered a contraindication.

The operation is performed on the side to which the pouch is seen to deviate in the anteroposterior view of the barium swallow. If the pouch remains central, either side is satisfactory.

A preliminary oesophagoscopy may be performed to empty the sac of food contents and to exclude the presence of a carcinoma in its wall. The opportunity is taken to pass a large bougie into the oesophagus. The pouch frequently lies in a direct line with the pharynx, and unless this is realized there is a danger of perforating it with the instrument or the bougie. To find the oesophageal lumen the patient's neck must be extended as far as possible and the head lowered so that the oesophagoscope is pointing anteriorly. Sometimes the oesophageal lumen cannot be detected at this stage and then oesophagoscopy should be abandoned.

Figure 51.1

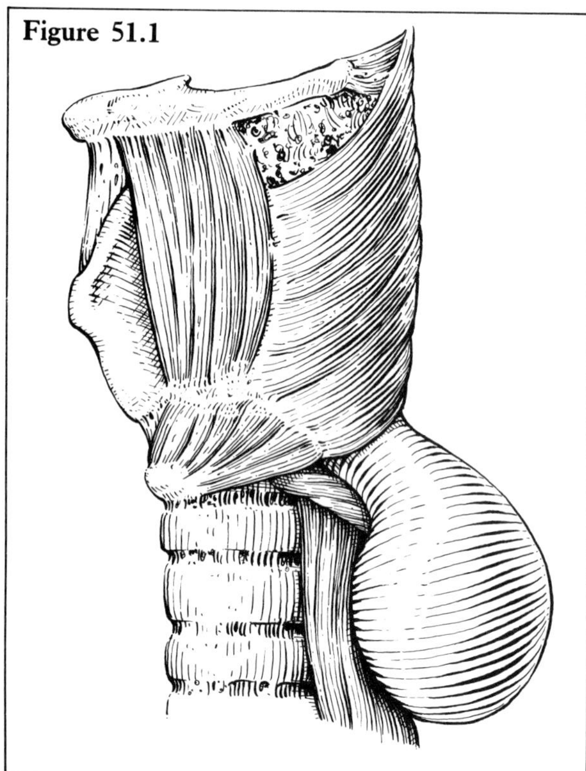

## Procedure

The patient lies supine with the head turned to the opposite side. The skin is incised along the anterior border of the sternocleidomastoid muscle for a distance of 5 cm. The incision should extend from a point two fingers' breadth above the clavicle to the level of the hyoid bone (**Fig. 51.2**). The

Figure 51.2

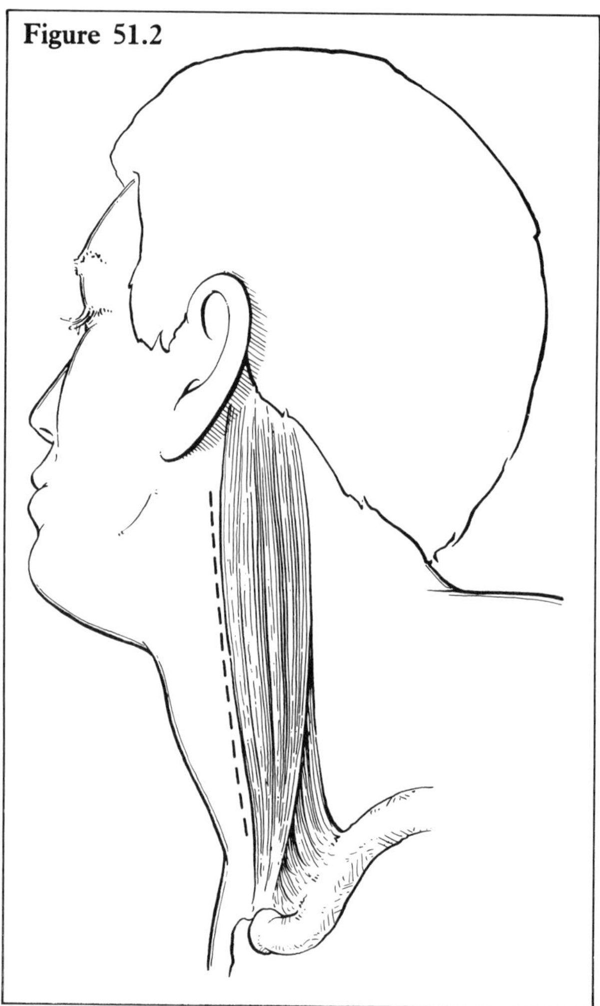

platysma muscle is divided in the same line. The external jugular vein is seen and can usually be preserved. A self-retaining retractor is inserted and the deep cervical fascia along the anterior border of the sternomastoid muscle is incised throughout its length (**Fig. 51.3**). The omohyoid muscle in the lower part of the incision is divided.

The sternomastoid muscle is retracted laterally, exposing the carotid sheath and internal jugular vein (**Fig. 51.4**). One or two small vessels require ligation. The lateral lobe of the thyroid gland is observed medially, and the middle thyroid vein running into the internal jugular vein is divided between ligatures. The carotid sheath is retracted

**Figure 51.3**

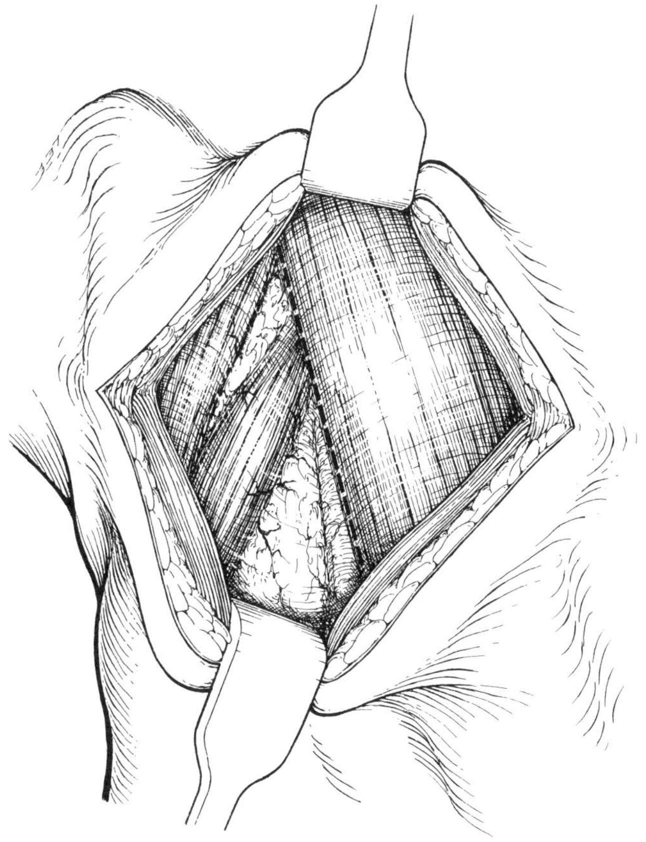

**Figure 51.4**

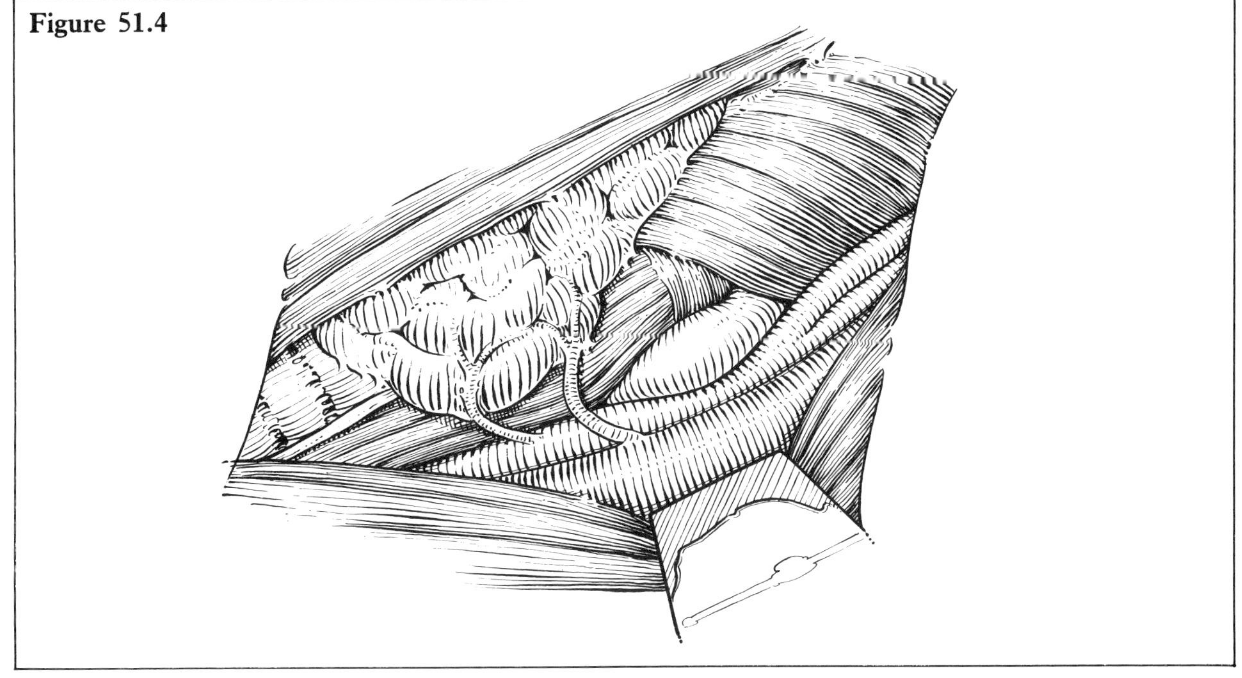

laterally together with the sternomastoid muscle, and the thyroid gland and trachea retracted medially. Blunt dissection behind the trachea brings the oesophagus into view, and the dissection continues behind it both upwards and downwards and across the midline to the opposite side.

If it was not possible to place a bougie in the oesophagus at an earlier stage the anaesthetist is asked to do so now. The surgeon should assist by placing a finger behind the upper end of the oesophagus, which will prevent the bougie from entering the pouch. An alternative procedure is to allow one bougie to rest in the pouch and for the anaesthetist to pass another alongside it, which will usually enter the oesophagus. Another procedure said to be helpful in identifying the pouch is to pack it with ribbon gauze at the time of oesophagoscopy.

The trachea is now retracted a little more forward and to the opposite side. This brings the back of the oesophagus into view. The muscle fibres are divided by sharp or blunt dissection and the outline of the mucosal pouch soon becomes visible. It is then grasped with a small Duval forceps and mobilized completely with blunt dissection until its neck can be seen all around (**Fig. 51.5**). This identification is greatly helped by the oesophageal bougie. It is not possible to rotate the oesophagus sufficiently to the opposite side to allow the whole of the pouch to be directed towards the operator.

**Figure 51.5**

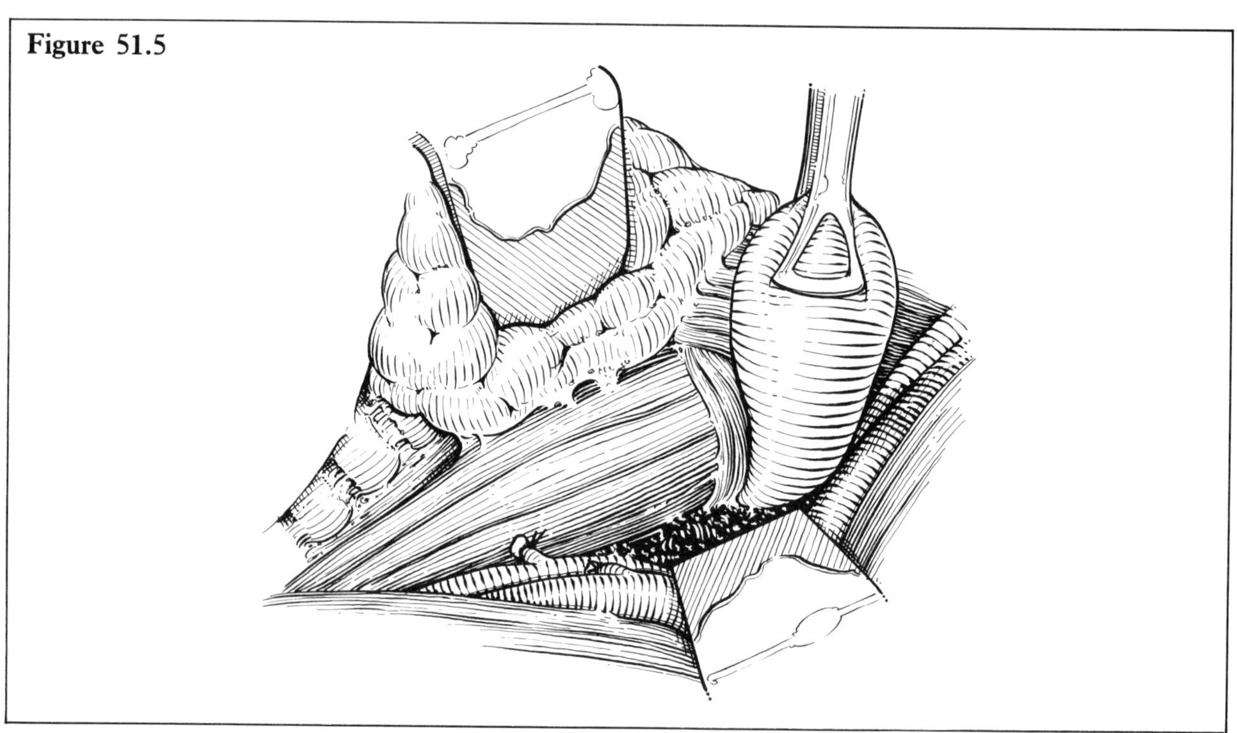

**Figure 51.6**

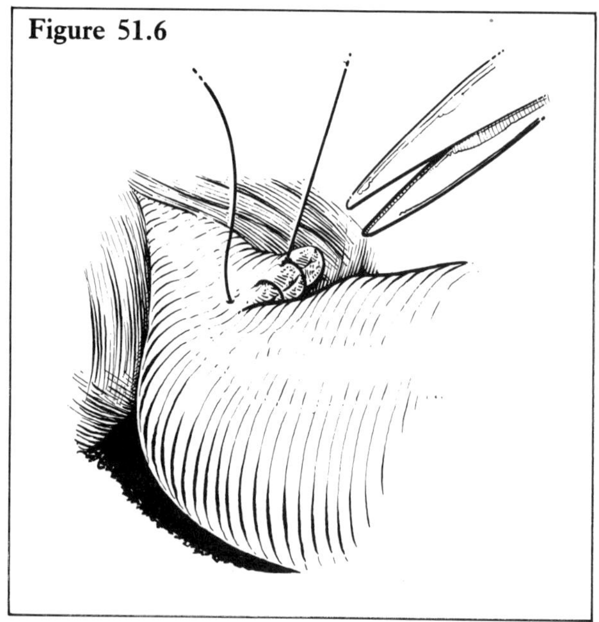

If a stapler is available (TA30 with 3.5-mm staples), it is slipped over the sac, pressed firmly against the oesophageal bougie and fired. The redundant mucosa is excised.

In the absence of a stapler the best way to excise the sac is to incise the neck with scissors a short distance at a time, suturing the edges after each cut with non-absorbable monofilament sutures (**Fig. 51.6**). These sutures can then be used to exert traction to bring the far side of the neck into view. The oesophageal bougie ensures that the oesophageal lumen is not narrowed and also that none of the sac is left behind. When the suture line is completed the sutures are all cut short (**Fig. 51.7**).

Haemostasis is now secured; if this is perfect no drain is necessary. Otherwise, or if the operator is doubtful about the integrity of the suture line, a short vacuum drain is passed through the skin and sternomastoid muscle from just above the clavicle into the retro-oesophageal space. The operative site is dusted with antibiotic powder.

**Figure 51.7**

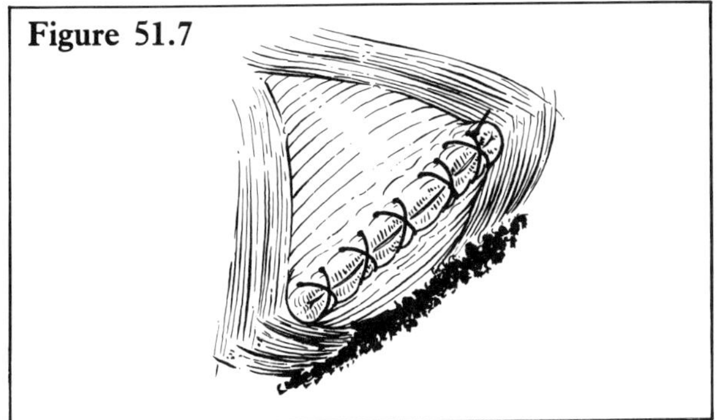

### Closure

The sternomastoid muscle is reattached to the deep cervical fascia, and the platysma repaired with absorbable sutures. Any technique may be used for the skin. Our own preference is for an absorbable subcuticular suture.

The drain is removed on the day after operation, when the patient may start taking liquids. If, however, the surgeon fears the development of a fistula (manifested by saliva emanating from the drain track), the drain should be cut short and left *in situ* for five days. A subsequent leak from the suture line will follow the drain track and the fistula will gradually heal spontaneously.

# 52 Operations for hiatal hernia

There are two varieties of hiatal hernia, which are symptomatically and anatomically distinct. The common form is the sliding hiatal hernia (**Fig. 52.1**), in which there is failure of the sphincteric action for the prevention of gastro-oesophageal reflux at the cardia, resulting in oesophagitis which may progress to stricture formation in the lower oesophagus. The reflux of gastric contents may also spill over into the lungs, causing recurrent episodes of pneumonia or pulmonary fibrosis.

The para-oesophageal hernia (**Fig. 52.2**) is much less common. Venous congestion in its wall may be responsible for persistent bleeding, causing severe anaemia. An ulcer may develop in the herniated stomach wall, or at the neck of the sac, and this may perforate or be responsible for episodes of acute haemorrhage. The portion of the stomach within the chest may become obstructed and distend, giving rise to recurrent attacks of pain and vomiting. In rare cases it may rupture into the chest, usually a rapidly lethal complication.

Recent physiological studies have shown that the reflux-preventing mechanism at the cardia is a complex one, involving not only the position, length and strength of the lower oesophageal sphincter but also the crura of the diaphragm and the size of the hiatal orifice. Simple reduction of the hernia and repair of the hiatus is followed by a high incidence of recurrence of the hernia.

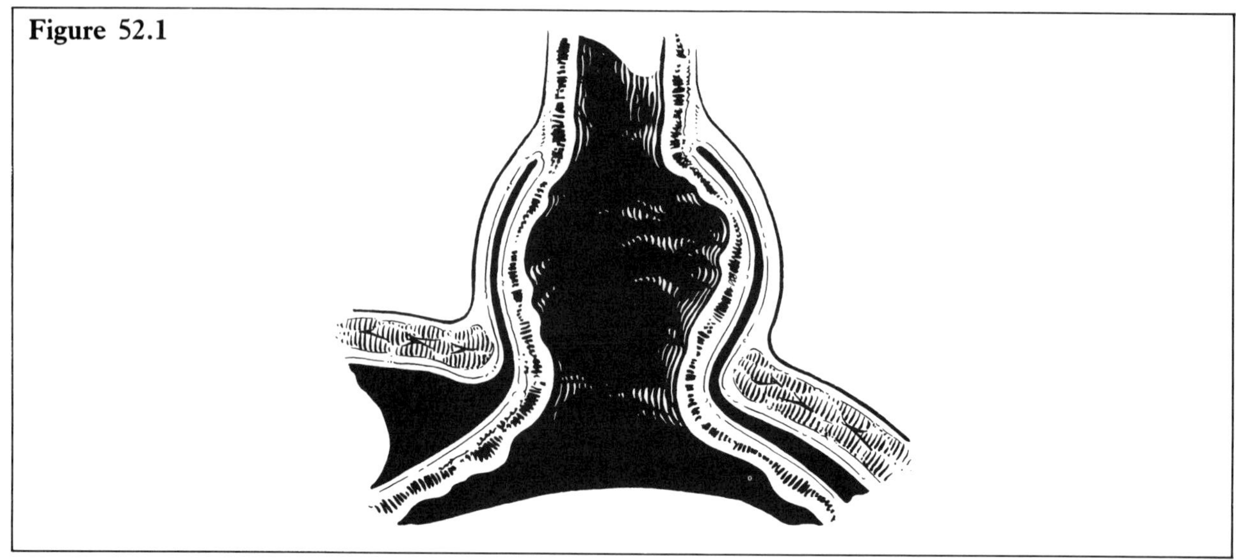
**Figure** 52.1

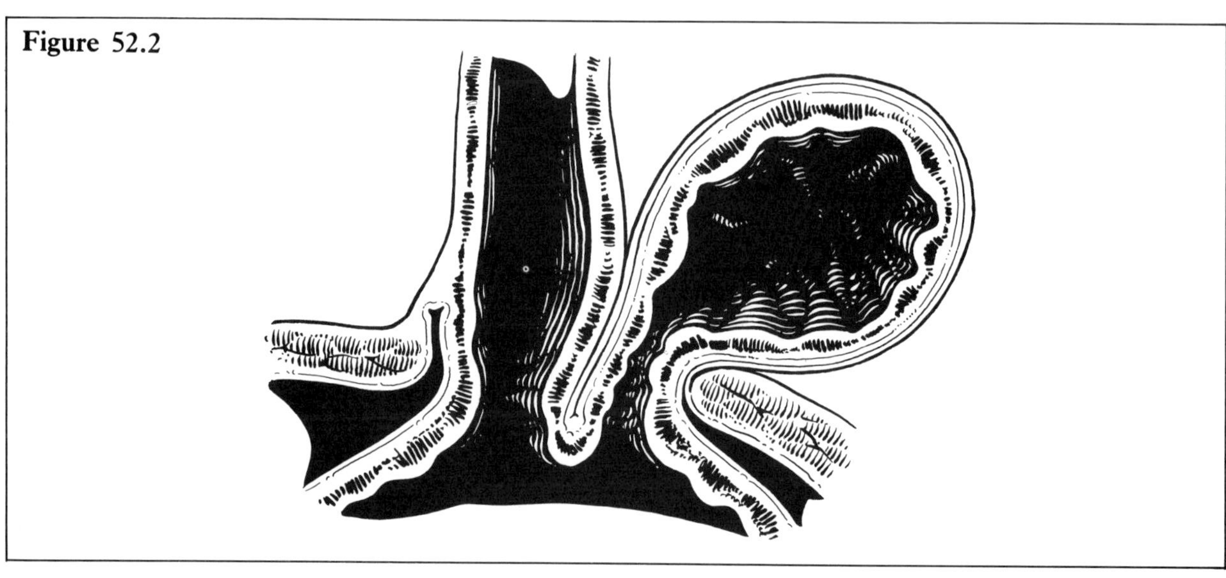
**Figure** 52.2

Current operations such as the Nissen and Belsey procedures are therefore directed towards creating an artificial 'flutter valve' which will prevent gastro-oesophageal reflux and which closes more tightly the higher the gastric pressure rises. A much improved method of fixation of the stomach below the diaphragm is the basis of the Hill operation, which also has a very low recurrence rate.

### Preoperative assessment

A careful history must be taken to exclude disease of the stomach, duodenum and gallbladder as sources of the symptoms. A barium swallow demonstrates the hernia, oesophageal strictures and any other oesophageal disease, as well as permitting study of the stomach and duodenum. Where the symptoms are suggestive, a cholecystogram is also carried out. Oesophagoscopy with either a rigid or flexible instrument is essential for determining the level of the hernia, while the degree of the oesophagitis is confirmed by biopsy. Oesophageal manometry is also strongly advised as it permits an assessment of oesophageal motor function, which is diminished in some conditions such as scleroderma and increased in others such as diffuse muscular spasm. Oesophageal manometry also permits an assessment of the tone and length of the lower oesophageal sphincter and of its position in relation to the diaphragm. An overnight oesophageal pH study is invaluable, because it enables detection of patients with gastro-oesophageal reflux whose symptoms occur solely in the upright position. These patients suffer from aerophagia, and they are not benefited by an antireflux procedure which simply replaces their reflux by gastric distension.

### Indications for operation

1. Severe symptoms not responding to medical treatment. Here it must be emphasized that weight reduction will abolish the symptoms in the majority of patients.
2. Stricture formation.

The reasons for operative repair of para-oesophageal hernia have been referred to above.

## Nissen fundoplication

The incisions for these oesophageal operations can give rise to more severe and more persistent pain than those for most operations in the thorax. The reasons for this are not fully understood but it is generally agreed that lower intercostal incisions are more likely to be followed by persistent pain. The sixth or seventh intercostal space rather than a lower one should be chosen whenever possible, and indeed all operations for benign conditions of the oesophagus (and most of those for malignant disease) can be performed satisfactorily through these approaches.

The patient is placed in the right lateral position, and a left anterolateral thoracotomy is performed, stripping the lower border of the seventh rib. The incision should continue forward almost to the costal margin. The pulmonary ligament is divided up to the level of the inferior pulmonary vein and the mediastinal pleura incised over the oesophagus up to the level of the aortic arch.

The oesophagus is mobilized from its bed together with its investing fascia which is carefully preserved, and a linen tape passed around it (**Fig. 52.3**). Care should be taken in the lower part of

**Figure 52.3**

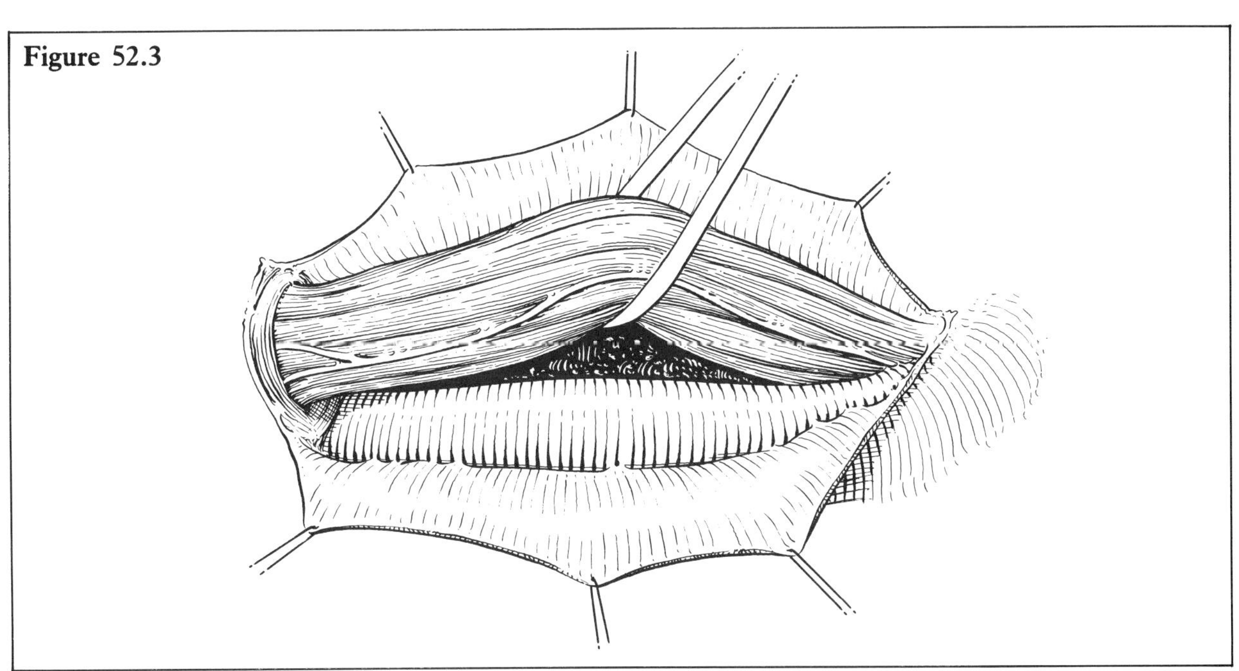

the incision to avoid opening the right pleural cavity. This mobilization is by blunt dissection at right angles to the length of the oesophagus. The aortic and mediastinal vessels that enter it can thus be clearly seen and divided between ligatures. The vagus nerves overlying the oesophagus are carefully preserved. Mobilization is continued up to the level of the aortic arch.

Attention is now directed to the diaphragm, and the margins of the hiatus are exposed by sharp dissection which continues on to the superior surface of the diaphragm (**Fig. 52.4**). On the right side of the oesophagus the diaphragmatic fibres become tendinous, and by picking them up and incising them the peritoneal cavity is entered. The peritoneal incision is continued backwards around both sides of the oesophagus, taking care to preserve the vagus nerves. With traction on the lower end of the oesophagus the stomach and lesser sac come into view. The fundus of the stomach is lifted up, which exposes the highest of the vasa brevia. These vessels are serially divided until the fundus is quite free (**Fig. 52.5**). Care must be taken not to injure the spleen. If there are peritoneal adhesions around the upper end of the spleen these should be divided, because traction on them may tear the splenic capsule.

A size 50 or 60 Hurst–Maloney bougie (or any similar-sized bougie) is now passed by the anaesthetist down the oesophagus and into the stomach (**Fig. 52.5**). The fundus of the stomach is lifted and a trial made of wrapping it around the lower oesophagus (**Fig. 52.6**). The anterior and posterior walls should meet over the lesser curvature without tension. If this cannot be achieved the

**Figure 52.4**

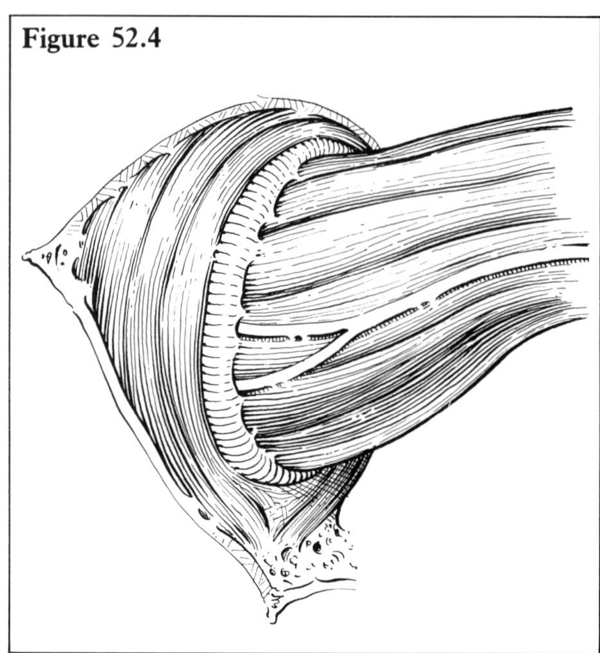

mobilization must be increased, if necessary by dividing some branches of the left gastroepiploic artery. If there is a large pad of fat at the cardia preventing the gastric approximation it should be carefully removed, taking great care not to damage the vagus nerves.

A single 3/0 polypropylene suture is now used to attach the lateral border of the fundus to the left posterolateral wall of the oesophagus about 3 cm above the oesophagogastric junction. The advantage of retaining the oesophageal fascia now becomes apparent, since the sutures do not hold well in the longitudinal muscle of the oesophagus. The anterior and posterior walls of the stomach

**Figure 52.5**

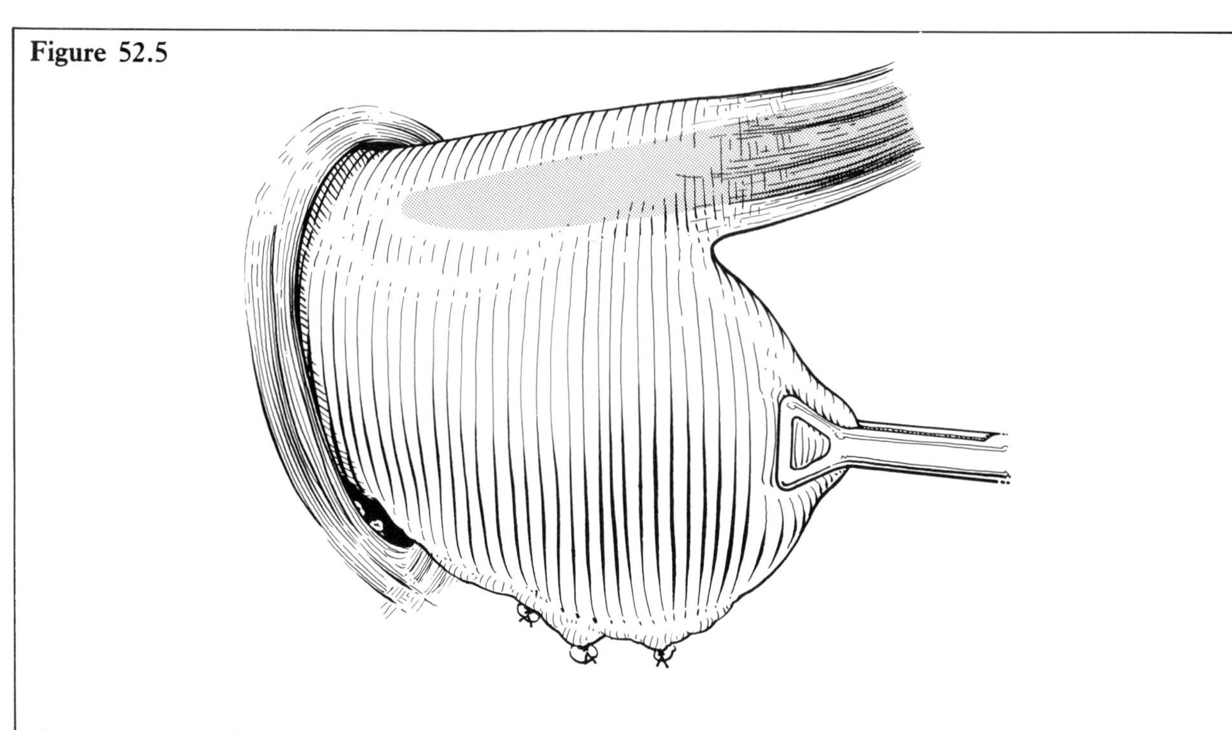

Figure 52.6

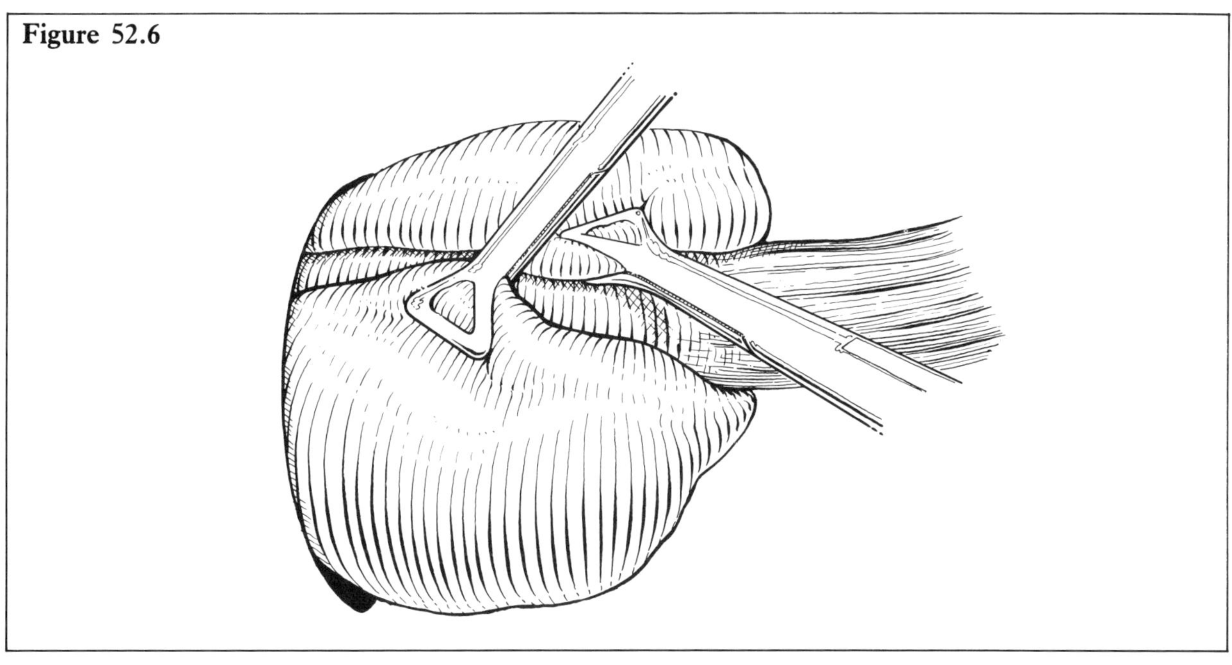

Figure 52.7

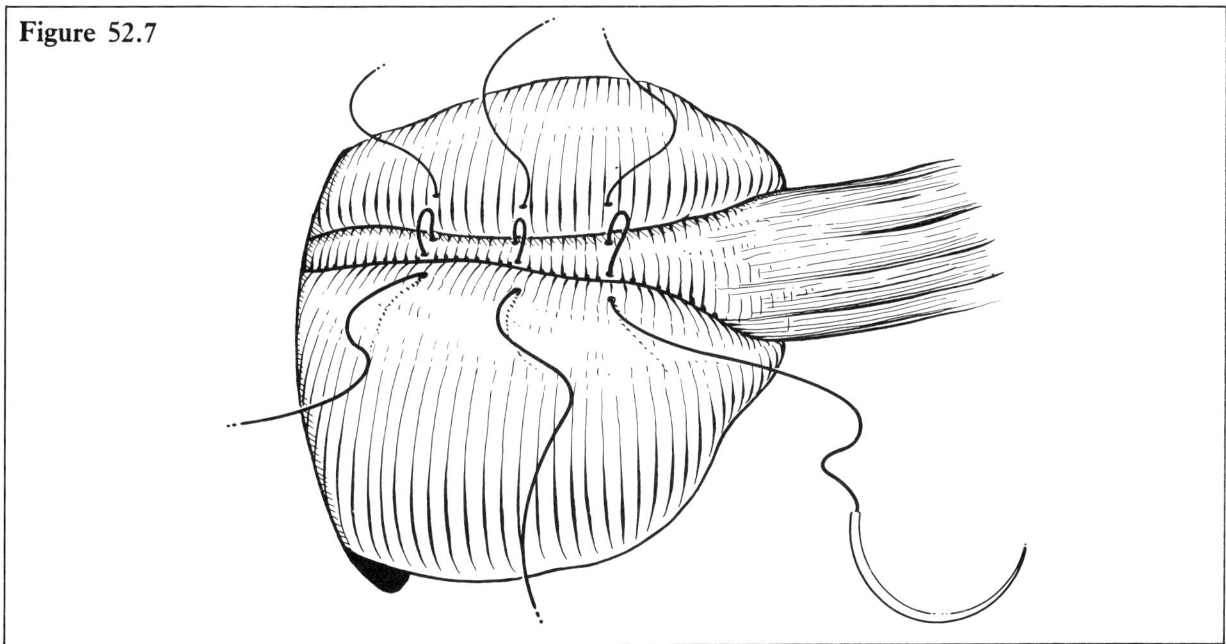

Figure 52.8

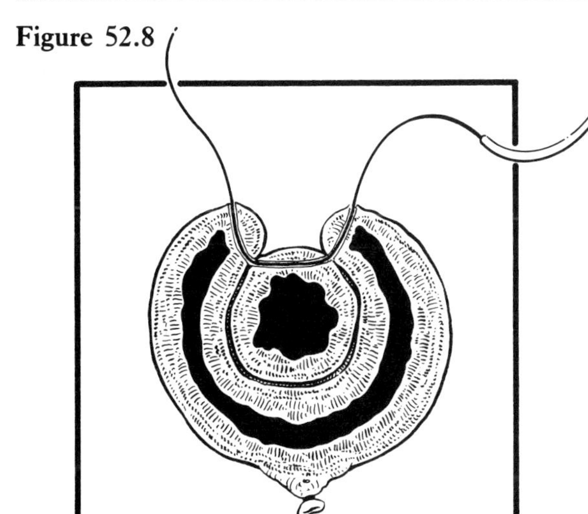

are brought around the lower end of the oesophagus and sutured together using three interrupted 3/0 polypropylene sutures (**Figs. 52.7, 52.8**). These are tied by an assistant while the surgeon keeps the gastric walls in approximation.

A series of interrupted sutures is now used to unite the upper edge of the stomach to the wall of the oesophagus, so preventing the tube of stomach from sliding down again (**Fig. 52.9**). Three sutures are placed through the divergent limbs of the right crus horizontally to narrow the hiatus (**Fig. 52.9**). The large bougie is removed. Interrupted sutures are now placed to approximate the margins of the hiatus to the oesophageal wall above the fundoplication. If this cannot be achieved, the sutures may unite the crus to the upper end of the

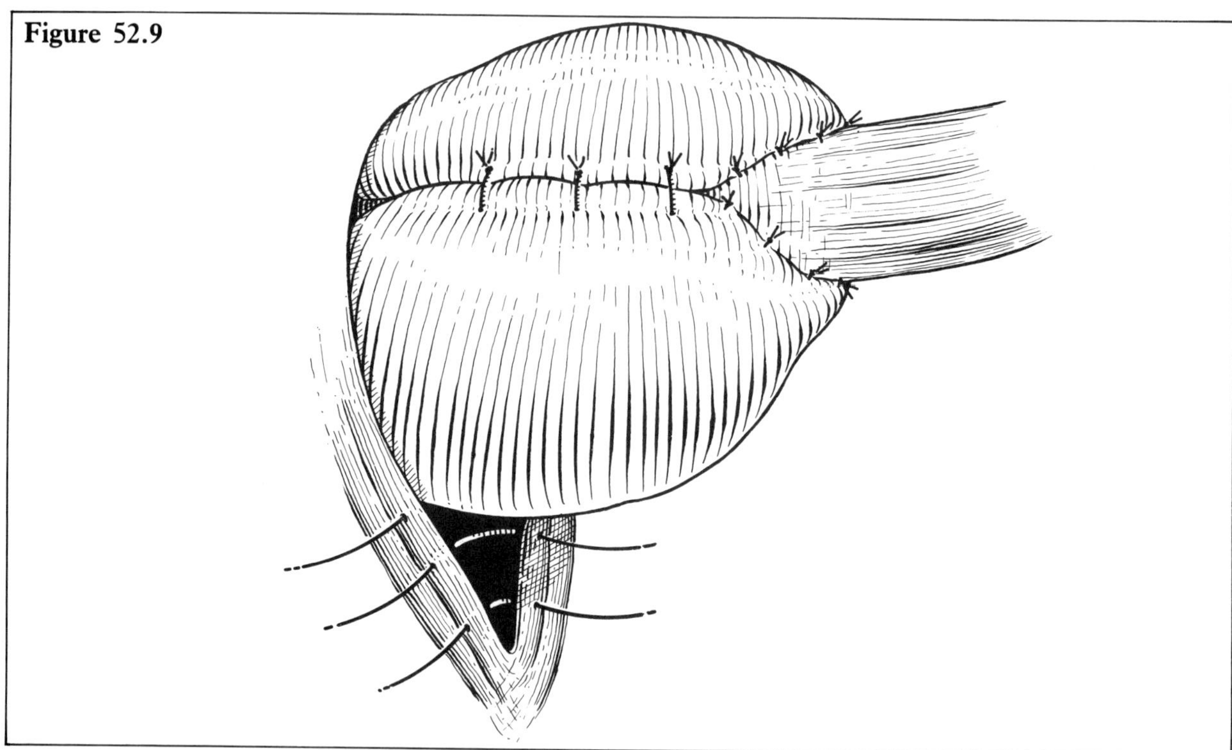

**Figure 52.9**

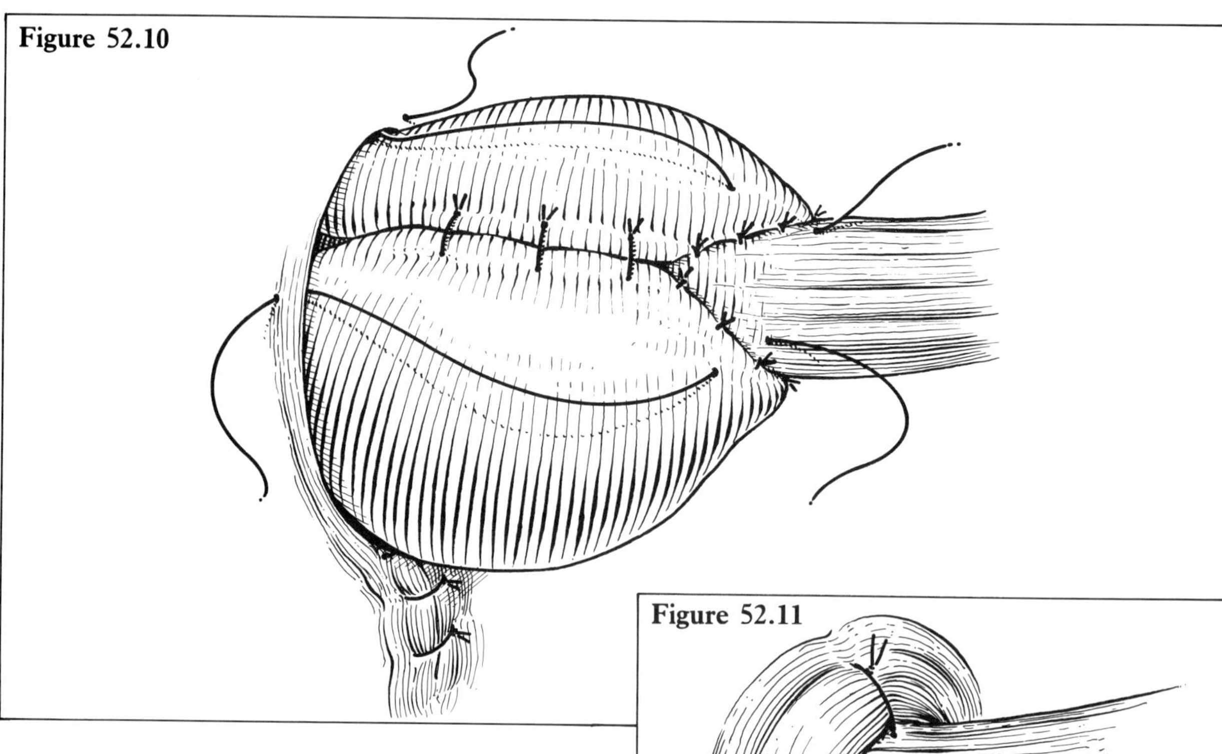

**Figure 52.10**

**Figure 52.11**

sutured collar of the stomach (**Fig. 52.10**). Finally the crural sutures are tied. The posterior stitch is tied first, followed by the adjacent anterior one. Each time the width of the hiatus is checked, so that it still admits the tips of the index and middle fingers. It is often not necessary to tie the third and most anterior suture (**Fig. 52.11**).

The chest is closed, leaving one tube in the left pleural cavity. If the right pleura has been opened a second tube may be passed across the mediastinum into that space.

### Postoperative management

A nasogastric tube is unnecessary. The intercostal drainage tube is removed on the first postoperative day, after which the patient is mobilized and given vigorous physiotherapy, as basal atelectasis is liable to occur. Oral fluid may be given after the first 24 hours and a light diet after 48 hours.

### Re-operations

The fibrosis resulting from previous operations on the hiatus may make it necessary to carry out this operation both from above and below the diaphragm. Although a radial incision in the diaphragm extending from the hiatus to the sixth costal cartilage results in division of phrenic nerve fibres and paralysis of half the diaphragm, we have not found it to have a significant effect on respiratory function, and it is the ideal approach in these cases. Where the scarring is less severe a circumferential incision along the anterior half of the diaphragm gives an adequate exposure of the upper abdominal contents.

## Belsey Mark IV repair

The Belsey procedure also creates a new flutter valve. However, whereas the Nissen operation is of almost universal application, the Belsey procedure is unsuitable for cases of advanced oesophageal fibrosis or severe oesophagitis without a gastroplasty, because in these cases the degree of shortening of the oesophagus may prevent adequate reduction with consequent failure of the operation.

### Procedure

The lower oesophagus and cardia are fully mobilized as described above, and the lesser sac opened. The cardiac pad of fat is carefully removed.

The repair consists of three steps:

1. Narrowing the hiatus posteriorly.
2. A series of sutures to approximate the fundus of thc stomach to the oesophagus.
3. Sutures to return the lower end of the oesophagus to the abdomen.

#### Narrowing the hiatus

The oesophagus is held forward by the sling to expose the crura. Two or three sutures are placed deeply in the muscle to narrow the posterior part of the opening, but are left untied at this stage (**Fig. 52.12**).

#### Invagination of the oesophagus into the stomach

Four mattress sutures of 3/0 polypropylene are passed transversely through the oesophagus just above the cardia and vertically through the wall of the stomach about 25 mm below the cardia. These four sutures encompass about three-quarters of the circumference of the oesophagus and stomach (**Fig. 52.13**). The bites through the oesophageal wall should be mainly through the overlying fascia and

**Figure 52.12**

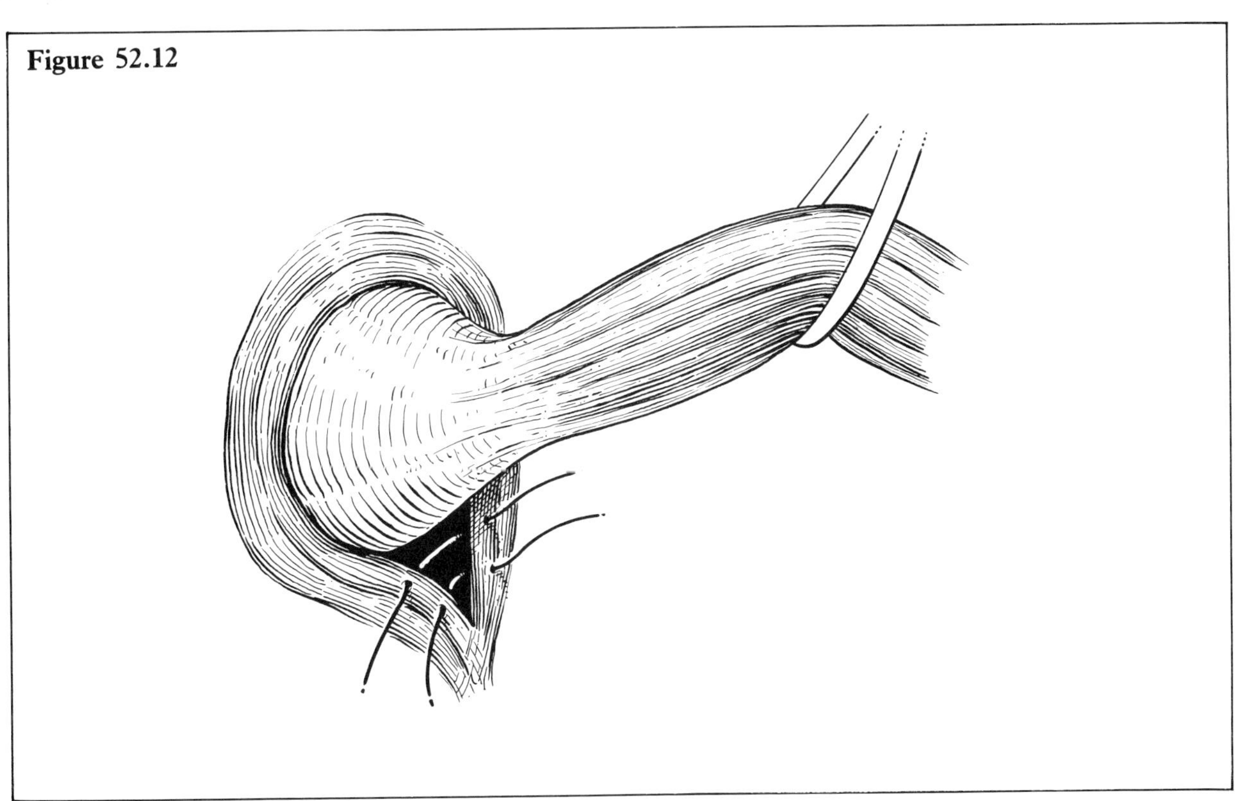

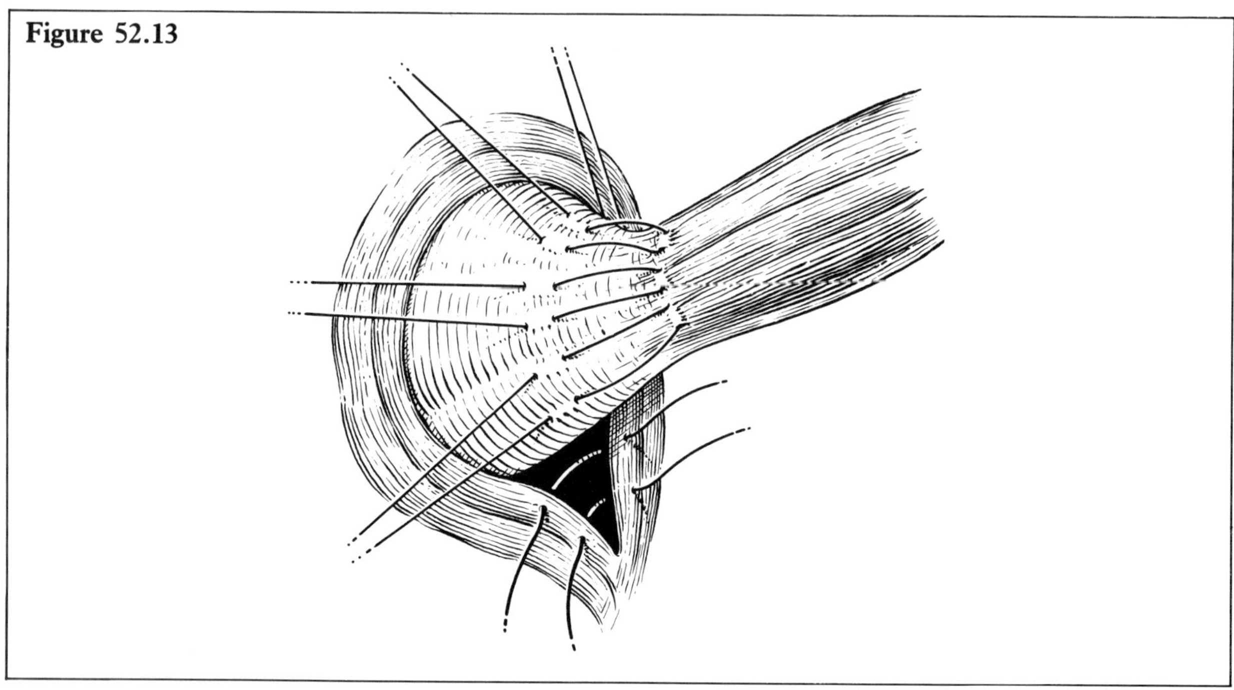
Figure 52.13

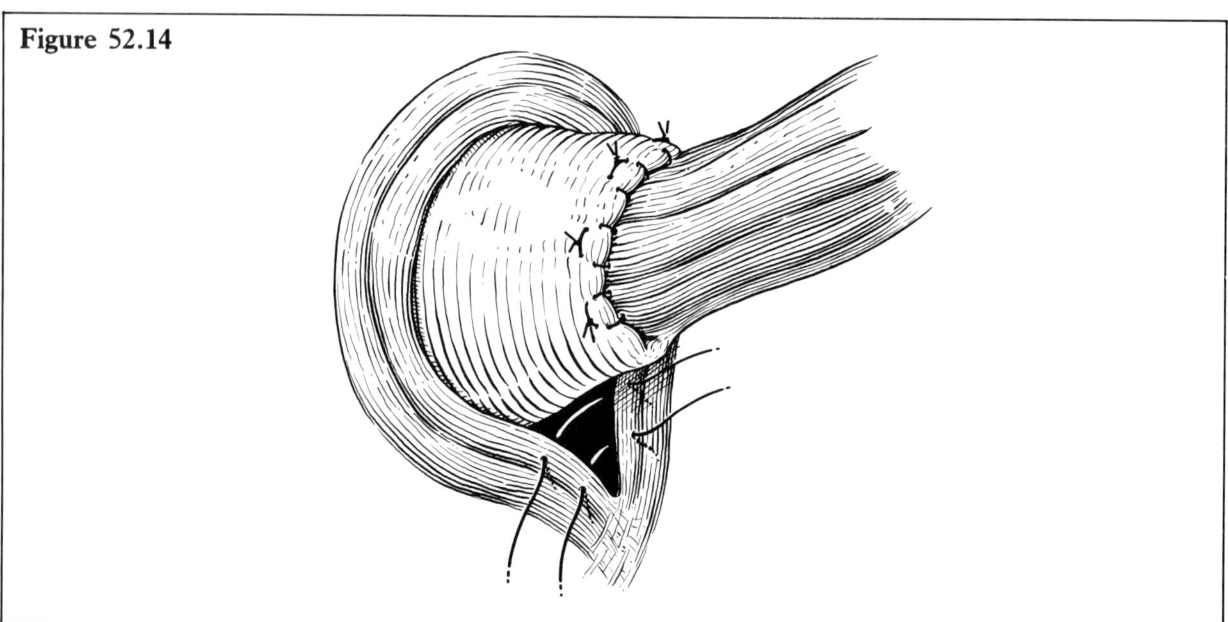
Figure 52.14

only superficially through the muscle. Care must be taken to ensure that the vagus nerves are left between the sutures or underneath them and not incorporated. The sutures are now tied (**Fig. 52.14**).

### Reduction of the hernia

Four similar mattress sutures are now inserted; they are passed through the oesophagus immediately above the previous suture line and through the stomach about 1 cm below it. They are then passed through the diaphragm from below upwards, about 1 cm away from the hiatal margin (**Figs. 52.15, 52.16**). These sutures are tightened while downward traction is applied to the oesophagus, thus returning the stomach to the abdomen (**Fig. 52.17**).

A size 50 bougie is passed into the stomach by the anaesthetist, to ensure that the hiatus is not narrowed excessively. The previously placed crural sutures are now tied (**Figs. 52.18, 52.19**).

### Closure

The chest closure and postoperative management are as previously described for the Nissen repair.

## Hill repair

The Hill repair (or median arcuate posterior gastropexy) was designed, like the previously described operations, to restore the lower oesophageal sphincter mechanism.

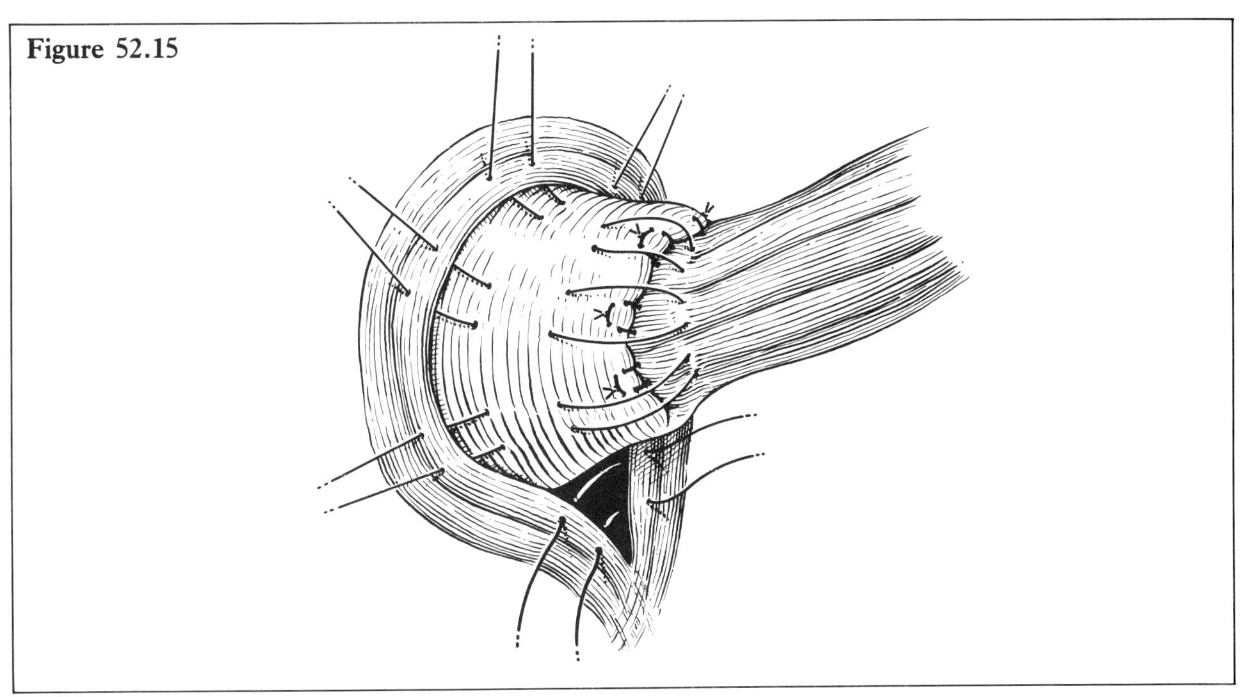
Figure 52.15

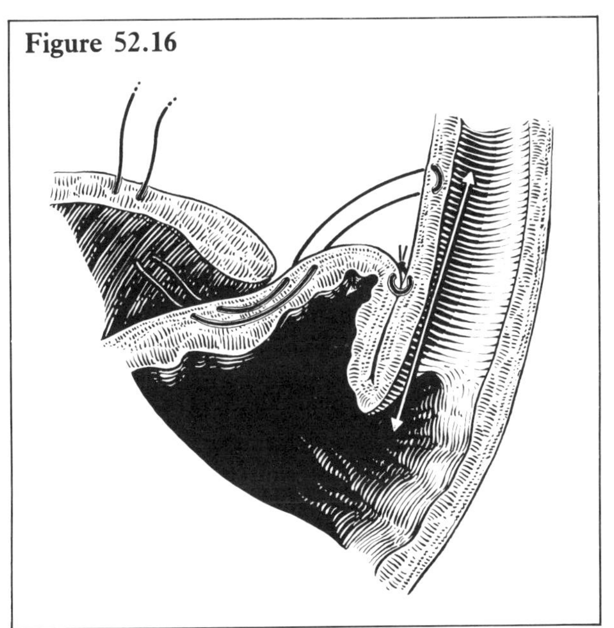
Figure 52.16

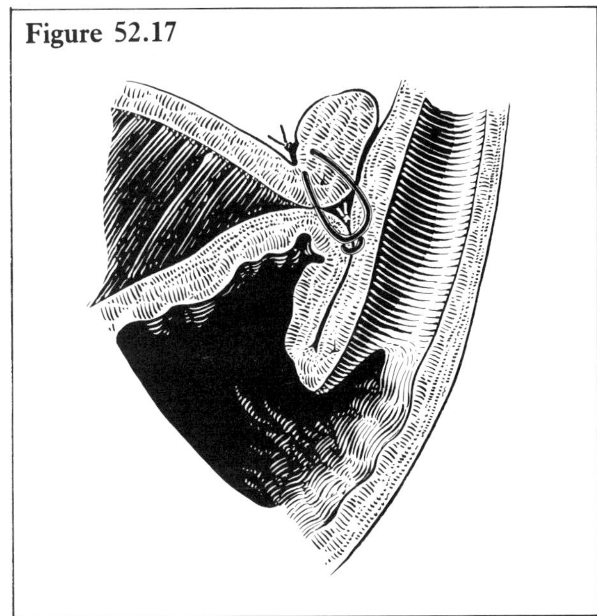
Figure 52.17

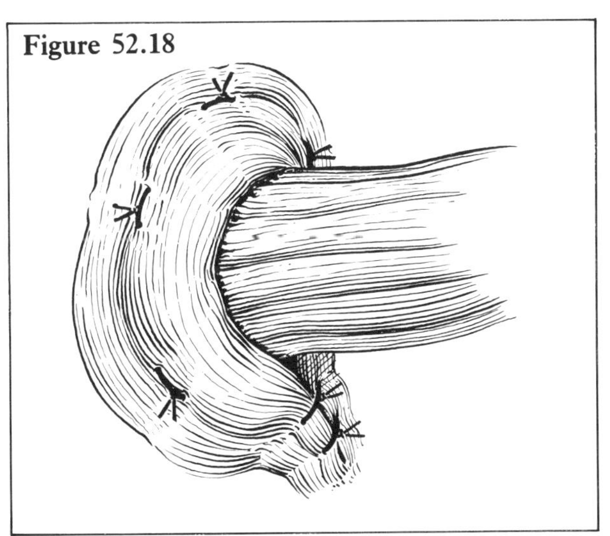
Figure 52.18

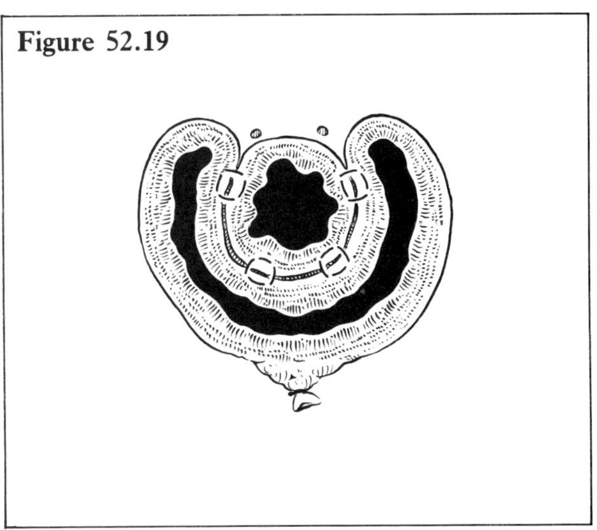
Figure 52.19

## Procedure

A left paramedian incision is made, beginning high up in the notch between the xiphoid and left costal margin.

The left triangular ligament is divided, allowing retraction of the left lobe of the liver out of the operative field. This reveals the phreno-oesophageal ligament and lesser omentum, which are then divided (**Fig. 52.20**). The phreno-oesophageal membrane attaching the fundus and greater curvature of the stomach to the diaphragm is next divided (**Fig. 52.21**). It may be necessary to divide one or two short gastric vessels to achieve adequate mobility of the fundus (**Fig. 52.22**). The posterior phreno-oesophageal ligament is finally divided by

**Figure 52.20**

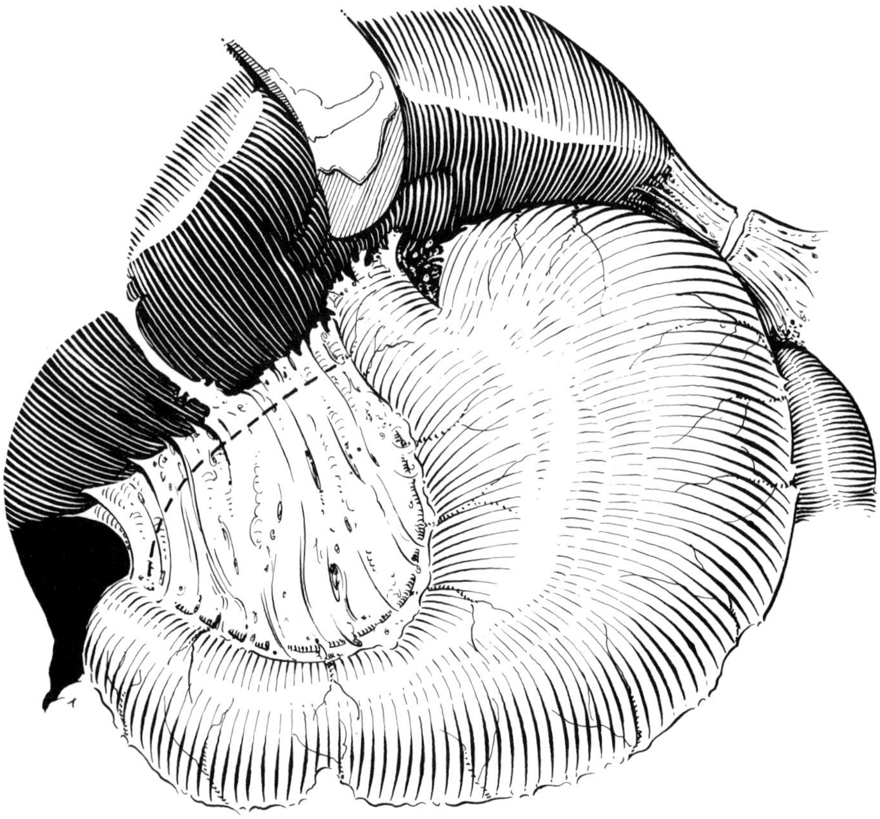

**Figure 52.21**

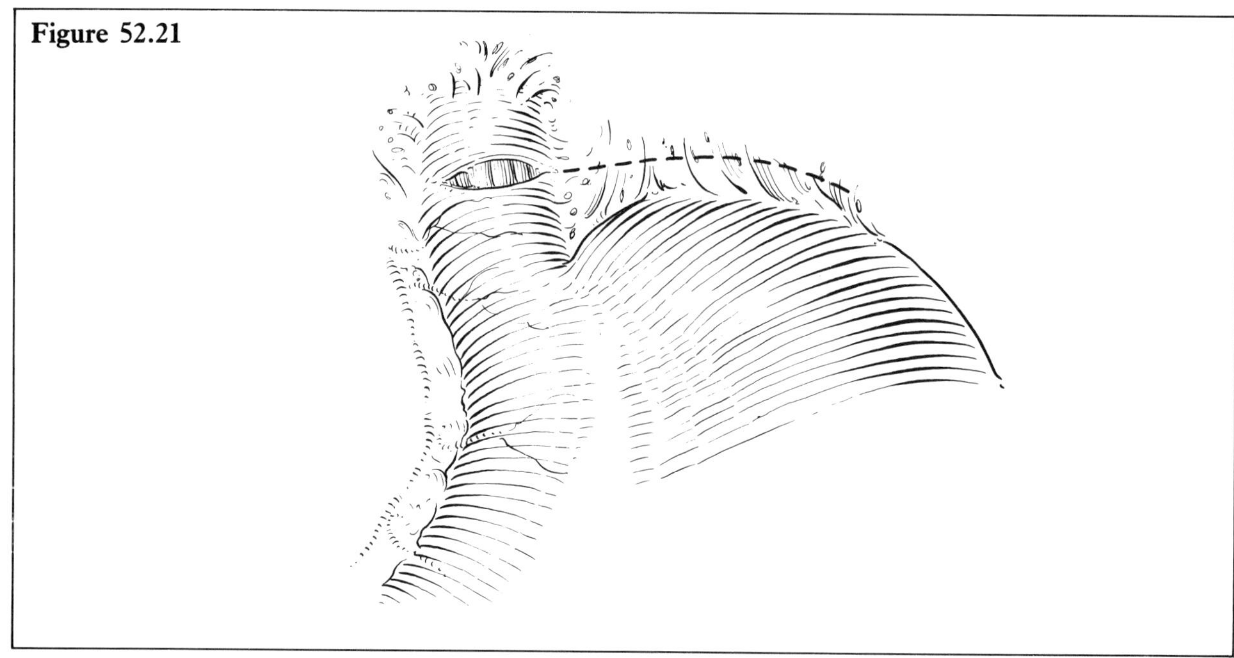

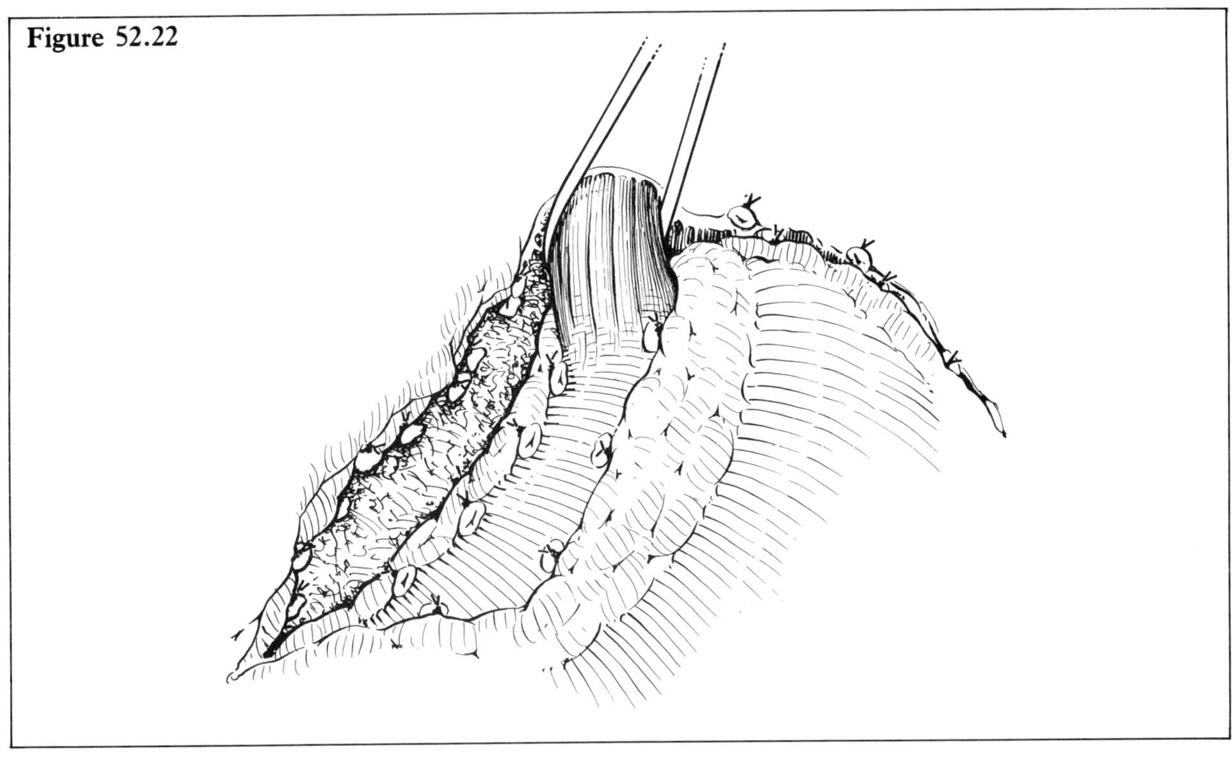
**Figure** 52.22

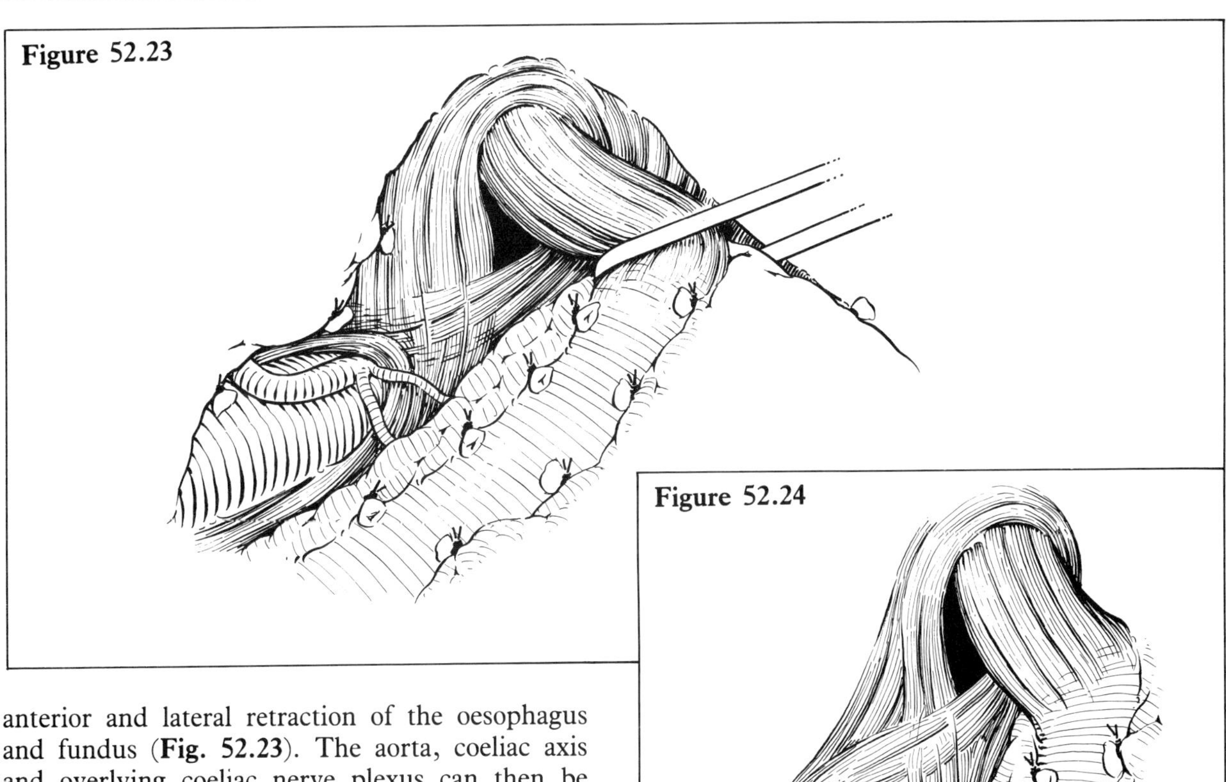
**Figure** 52.23

**Figure** 52.24

anterior and lateral retraction of the oesophagus and fundus (**Fig. 52.23**). The aorta, coeliac axis and overlying coeliac nerve plexus can then be identified by palpation. Underneath these structures the median arcuate ligament can be palpated over the psoas muscle. The inferior margin of the ligament is then dissected clear of the underlying psoas muscle and a Goodsell cervical dilator placed beneath it and passed cephalad. There should be no resistance in this plane (**Fig. 52.24**).

The crura of the hiatus are then approximated with mattress sutures, taking broad bites to include the fascia propria and peritoneum (**Fig. 52.25**).

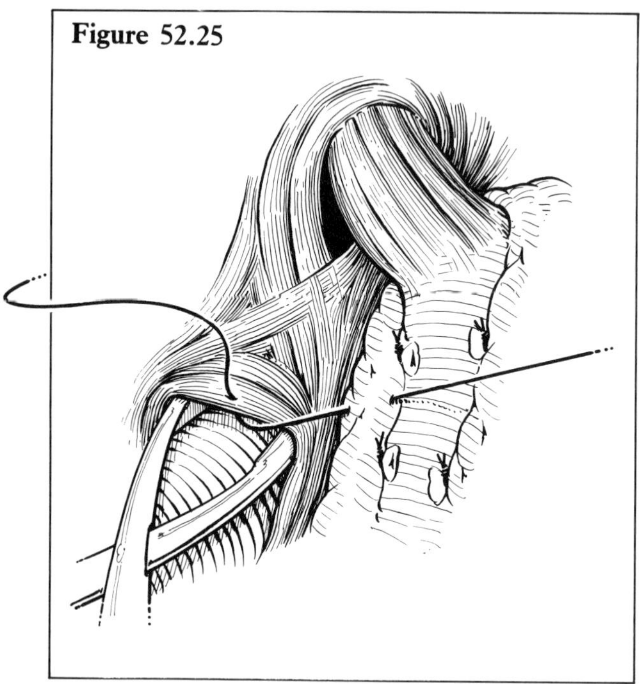
Figure 52.25

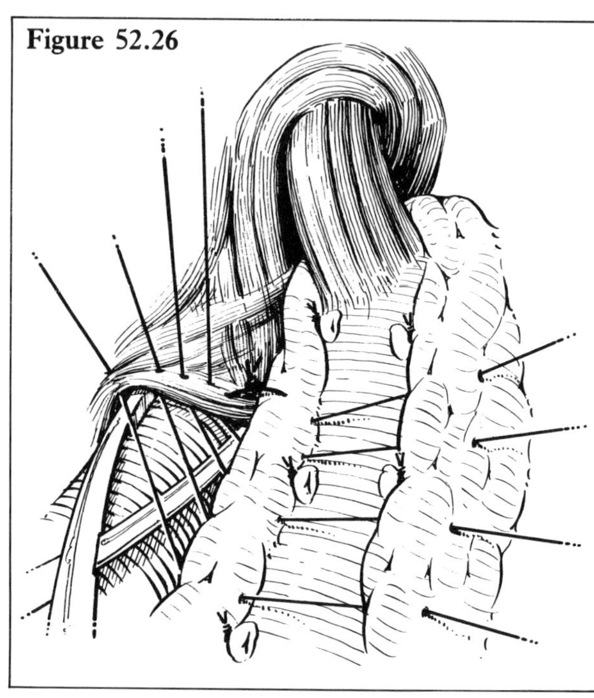
Figure 52.26

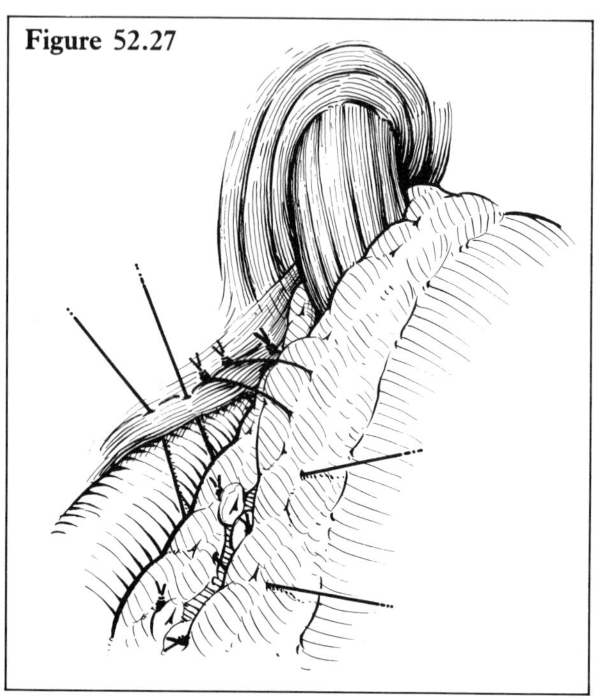
Figure 52.27

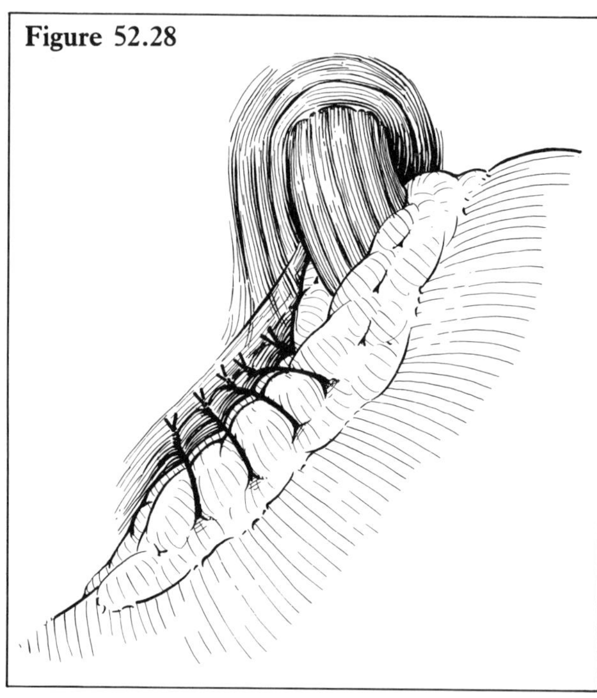
Figure 52.28

These sutures are tied gently, so that a finger can still be inserted alongside the oesophagus at the hiatus. Three or four more sutures are then placed deeply through the anterior and posterior phreno-oesophageal bundles, taking care not to injure the vagal nerves. The sutures are then passed through the median arcuate ligament and preaortic fascia (**Figs. 52.26, 52.27**).

The tension applied to the most cephalad of these sutures determines the calibration of the lower oesophageal sphincter pressure. A further suture, referred to as the imbricating suture, is passed through the anterior and posterior phreno-oesophageal bundles at the level of the gastro-oesophageal junction.

In a further refinement of the method, an oesophageal manometry tube is passed into the stomach. The first two sutures are loosely tied and pulled up until a pressure of 50–55 mmHg (7 kPa) is achieved. The remaining sutures are then tied (**Fig. 52.28**).

### Closure

The abdomen is closed in layers with no intra-peritoneal drain.

# 53 Surgical procedures for oesophageal stricture

Untreated chronic gastro-oesophageal reflux will result in oesophagitis with ulceration and healing by fibrosis. This ultimately results in a stricture, which may be accompanied by acquired shortening of the oesophagus. The prudent use of antacid therapy, and an early antireflux operation if the medical treatment fails, will prevent this. Sadly, many patients do not present until stricture formation has occurred.

## Preoperative assessment

A barium swallow will indicate the presence of an irreducible hernia in acquired shortening; this is apparent when the patient is upright. Preoperative endoscopy, preferably with the flexible endoscope, will reveal the presence of a columnar-lined oesophagus, the level of the oesophagogastric junction and the diaphragmatic hiatus. A stricture can be identified, and dilated with either the balloon dilatation system in combination with the flexible endoscope, or using the gum-elastic bougies and mercury-filled bougies up to 60 French gauge via the rigid instrument (see pp. 188, 189).

For some patients the long-term use of endoscopic dilatation is an acceptable form of therapy, but for others it is less than ideal. Several surgical techniques are available for the management of this problem; the two most frequently used techniques are described below.

## Collis gastroplasty

The chest is entered via a left posterolateral thoracotomy through the sixth or seventh intercostal space. The wound is opened well forwards to the attachment of the diaphragm to allow optimal access. The oesophagus is then mobilized as described on pp. 203–4 after the lung has been allowed to collapse.

The hiatal attachments are divided and the greater and lesser sacs entered. The hepatogastric omentum is divided and the upper part of the greater curve is mobilized. The stomach is then drawn up into the chest and held. The fat pad at the gastro-oesophageal junction is dissected away and removed. Great care is taken to preserve the vagal nerves, particularly the left one which lies anteriorly.

A size 50 Hurst–Maloney bougie is then passed well into the stomach. A GIA stapling device is then placed parallel with the edge of the bougie and the oesophagus, on to the body of the stomach (**Fig. 53.1**). The division of the stomach along this

**Figure 53.1**

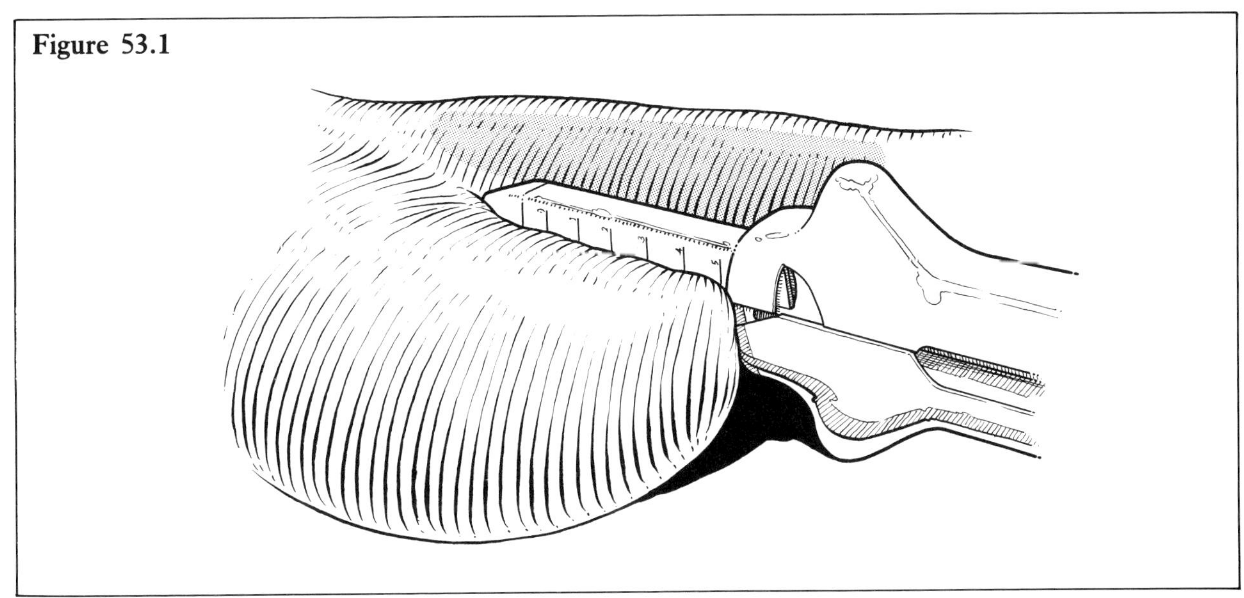

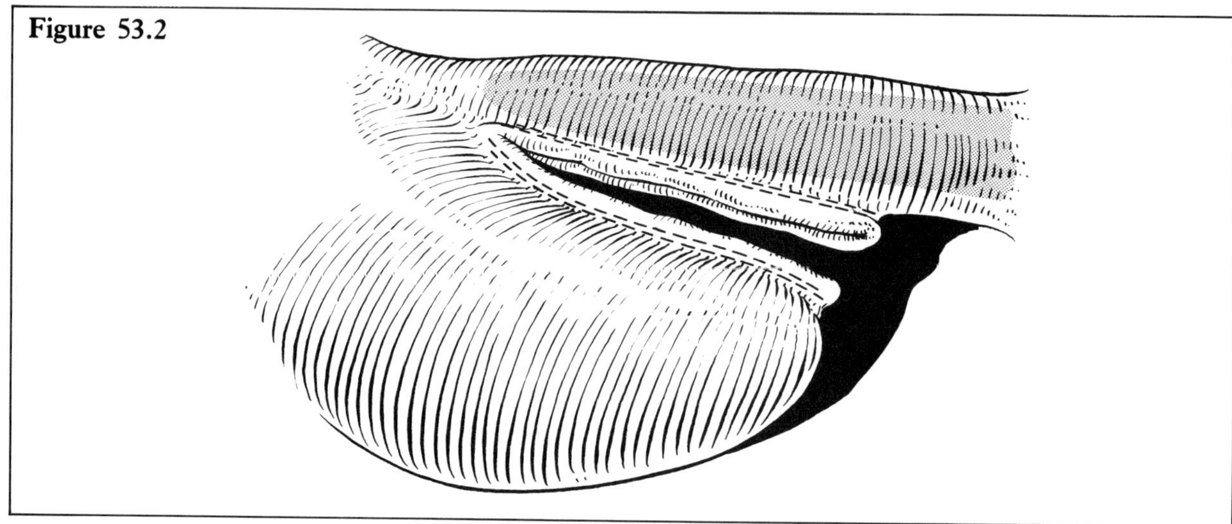

Figure 53.2

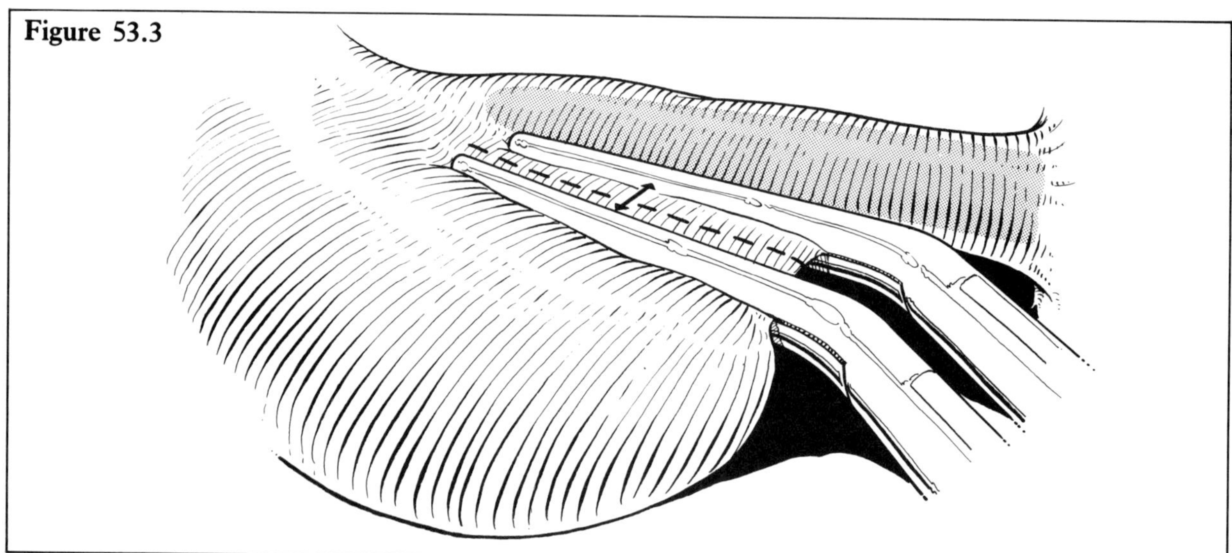

Figure 53.3

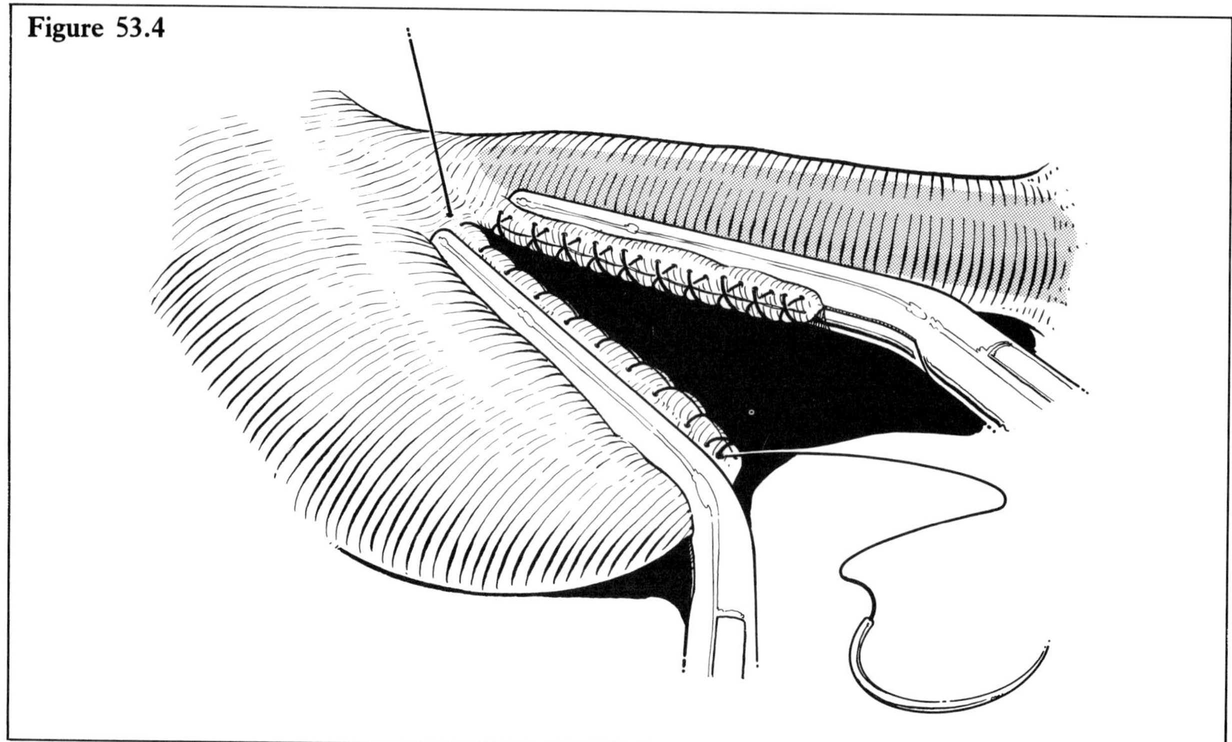

Figure 53.4

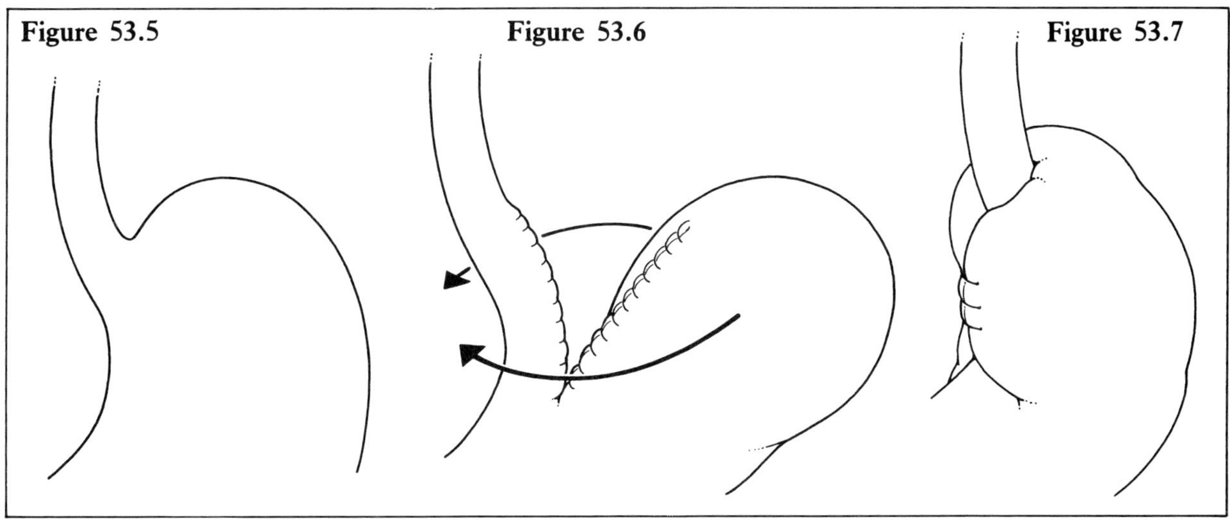
**Figure 53.5** **Figure 53.6** **Figure 53.7**

line will give rise to a 5-cm long gastric tube (**Fig. 53.2**). This can also be achieved by using two soft bowel clamps placed 2–3 cm apart (**Fig. 53.3**), cutting between them and oversewing the cut edges with an 'all coats' non-absorbable suture (**Fig. 53.4**). Whichever method is used the suture line should then be oversewn using a serosal inverting suture. The final result is to produce an extra length of oesophagus about which an antireflux procedure may be constructed (**Figs. 53.5–7**). Either a Nissen or a Belsey repair may be used.

### Postoperative care

Prophylactic antibiotics should be given to cover the operation, but can be stopped after 24 hours. Nasogastric drainage is not necessary as ileus is rare. Clear fluids should be allowed after 24 to 48 hours, and the patient may rapidly advance to a solid diet.

Postoperative dilatation may be necessary because the stricture is still present, and is usually accomplished by the passage of a size 50 Hurst–Maloney bougie.

## Oesophagogastroplasty

In this procedure the narrowed segment is enlarged directly. Around the repair an antireflux procedure must be performed which also supports the repaired tissue.

The oesophagus and stomach are mobilized as described on pp. 203–4 and a tape is passed around the oesophagus. A vertical incision is then made across the narrowed segment (**Fig. 53.8**). Stay

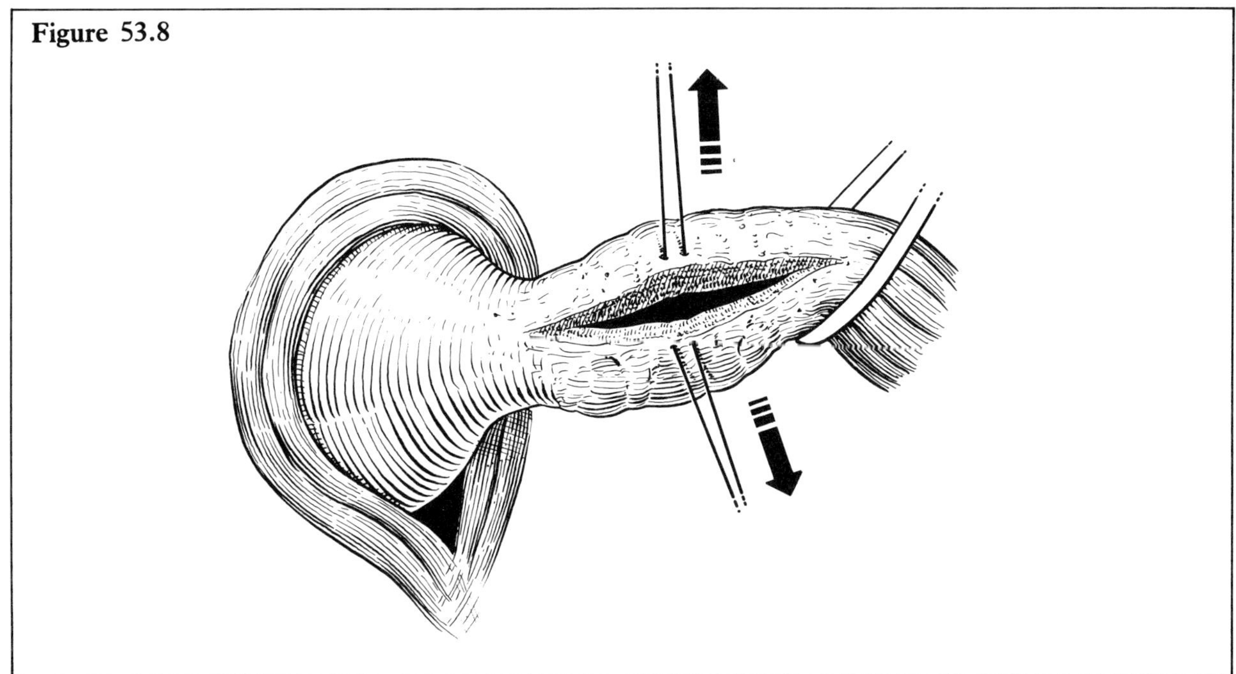
**Figure 53.8**

sutures are placed at the midpoint on each side of the incision and used as traction sutures. These serve to distract the lateral margins, converting the longitudinal incision into a transverse one (**Fig. 53.9**). Further interrupted sutures are then passed from the superior margin to the inferior margin (**Fig. 53.9**); these are tied to complete the repair (**Fig. 53.10**). A Nissen fundoplication is then carried out around the widened oesophagus (**Fig. 53.11**).

This operation is not satisfactory in the shortened oesophagus, where it may be impossible to reduce such a repair below the diaphragm.

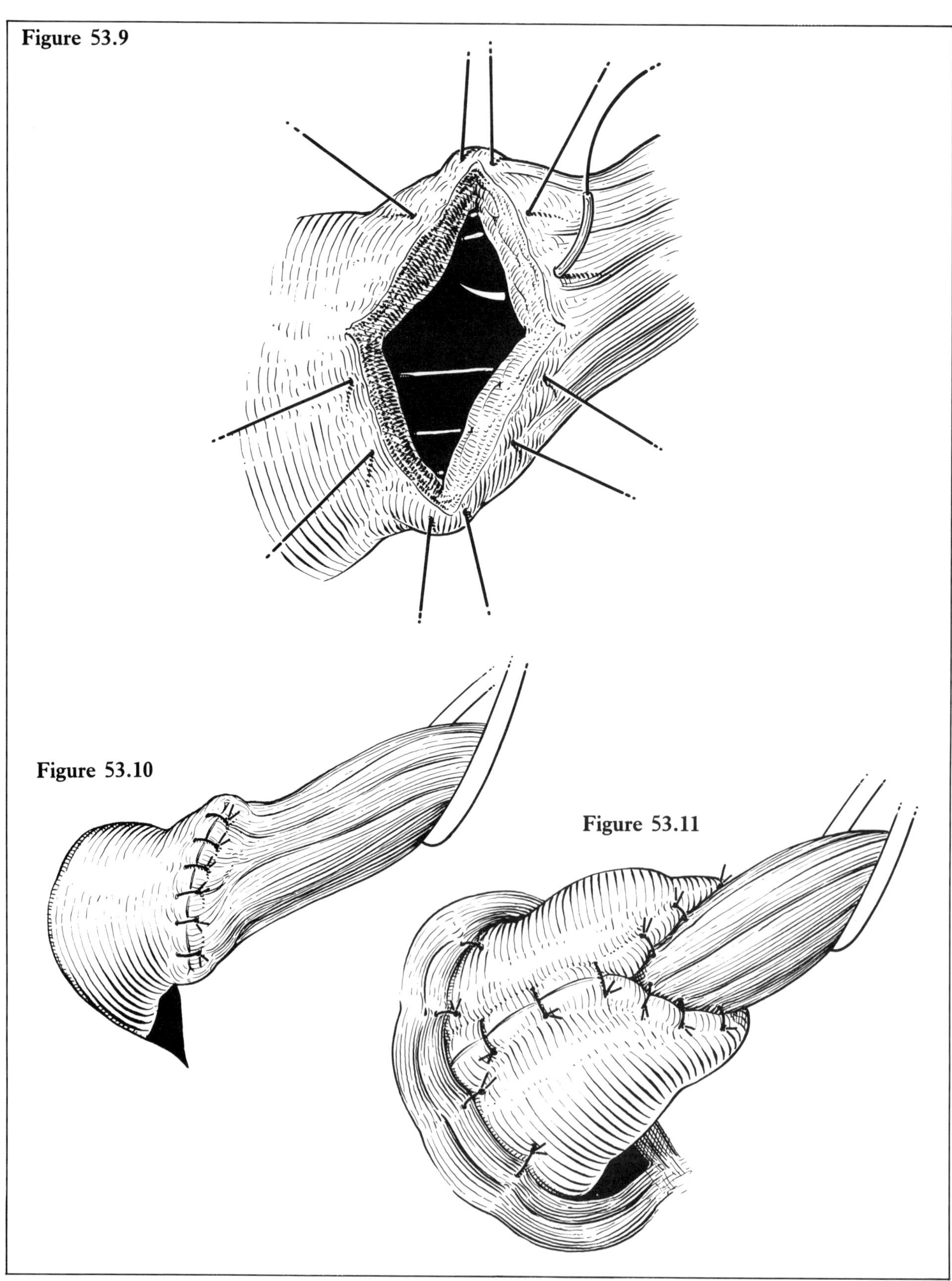

**Figure 53.9**

**Figure 53.10**

**Figure 53.11**

# 54 Surgical treatment of perforation and spontaneous rupture of the oesophagus

Perforation of the oesophagus occurs most commonly after instrumentation. Other causes are less common, and include impaction of swallowed foreign bodies, penetrating wounds of the neck (and rarely the chest), malignant ulceration and spontaneous rupture.

The key to successful management of this potentially fatal condition is early recognition. Treatment delayed beyond 12 hours results in a rapid increase in the resultant mortality, which is reported as 80–100% in several series. With prompt treatment it should be possible to achieve a mortality of 30% or less in specialist units.

## Spontaneous rupture of thoracic oesophagus

Spontaneous rupture occurs more frequently in men than women, and usually in late middle age. There is often a history of retching, which may or may not be productive, but is almost always associated with the sudden onset of severe chest pain. Rupture most commonly occurs in the lower third of the oesophagus. The pleural and mediastinal soiling rapidly produce a shocked patient.

A plain chest radiograph will usually reveal a pleural effusion. Air can be seen within the mediastinum and may track up into the neck. It may also permeate into the abdomen.

The most important investigation for management is the barium swallow. During the study the patient should lie on the side on which the chest pain occurs, to allow the radio-opaque material to drain through the perforation, as a small leak may otherwise be missed.

## Management

Only intramural dissections and small cervical instrumental perforations should be managed conservatively. The treatment consists of broad-spectrum intravenous antibiotics (which must include metronidazole), no oral intake, and adequate analgesia. When pain has subsided, the systemic signs have abated, and the barium swallow shows no leakage, oral food may be cautiously introduced.

A large cervical perforation, or one in which a large pool of barium collects in the neck, should be treated by inserting a vacuum drain into the space after approaching it by the technique described on pp. 198–200 and illustrated in **Figs. 51.2–51.5**. A residual abscess after conservative treatment is managed similarly. The drain can be removed after a week, and the resulting fistula will close spontaneously.

All other perforations should be operated on as soon as possible.

Resuscitation of shocked patients and antibiotic treatment are begun immediately. If the patient is profoundly hypotensive through septic cardiovascular collapse and loss of fluid into the chest, rehydration should be carried out expeditiously using colloid solutions but operation must not be delayed. Crystalloid solutions should be avoided, as increased pulmonary permeability often accompanies such severe sepsis, resulting in the likelihood of adult respiratory distress syndrome.

## Procedure

Several procedures are available but the essential features of all are to drain the pleural space, to expand the lung, and to prevent further contamination of the pleural space. The side to be operated on is determined by the radiographic site of the pleural exudate, or of the leak or the side of pain, or a combination of these features. The pleural space is approached by a posterolateral thoracotomy through the bed of the sixth or seventh rib (pp. 24–26).

The mediastinal pleura is incised widely, from the arch of aorta on the left or the azygos vein on the right to the diaphragm (**Fig. 54.1**). The torn edges of the oesophagus are identified and any obviously dead tissue removed. The mucosa is identified (**Fig. 54.2**), a step facilitated by the passage of an oesophageal bougie which can then

Figure 54.1

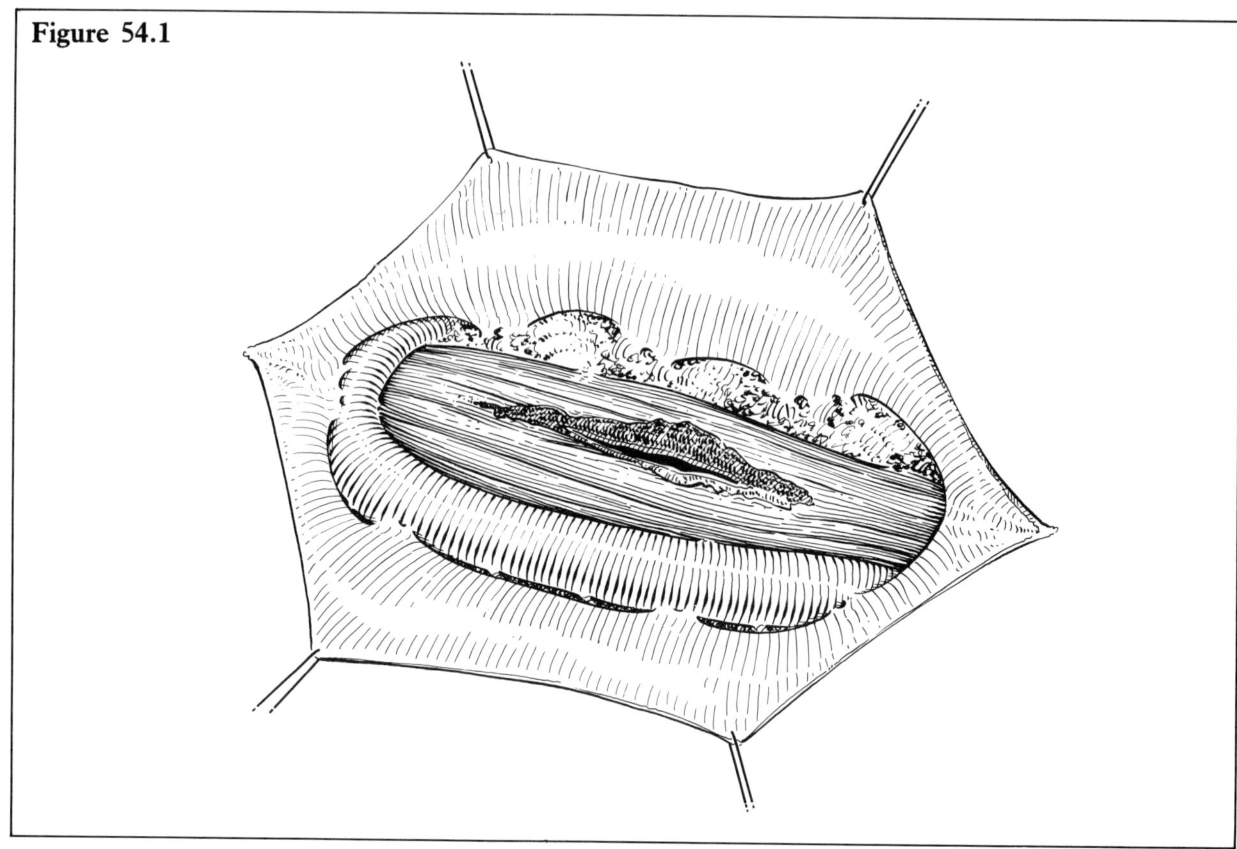

Figure 54.2

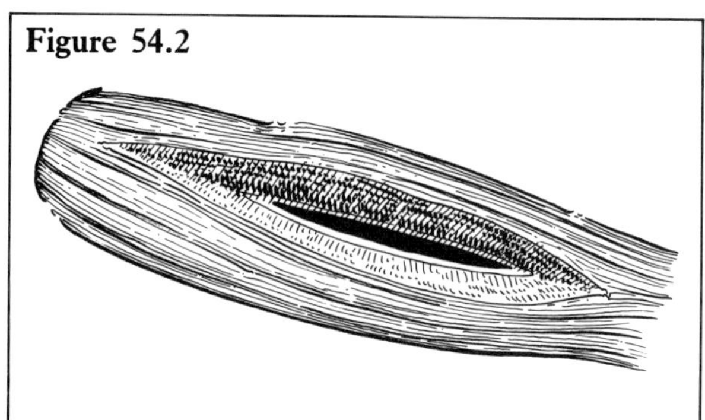

Figure 54.3

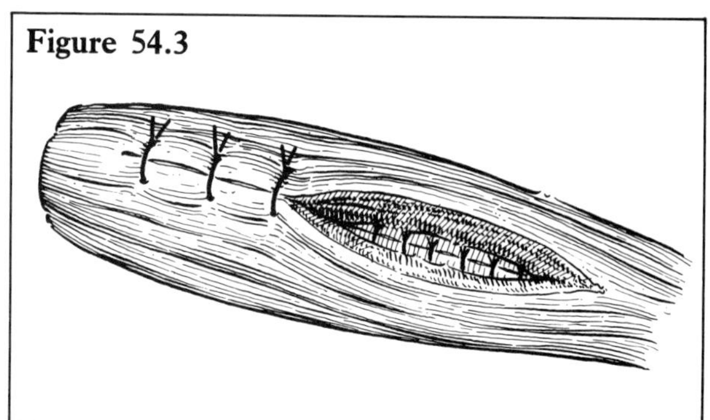

Figure 54.4

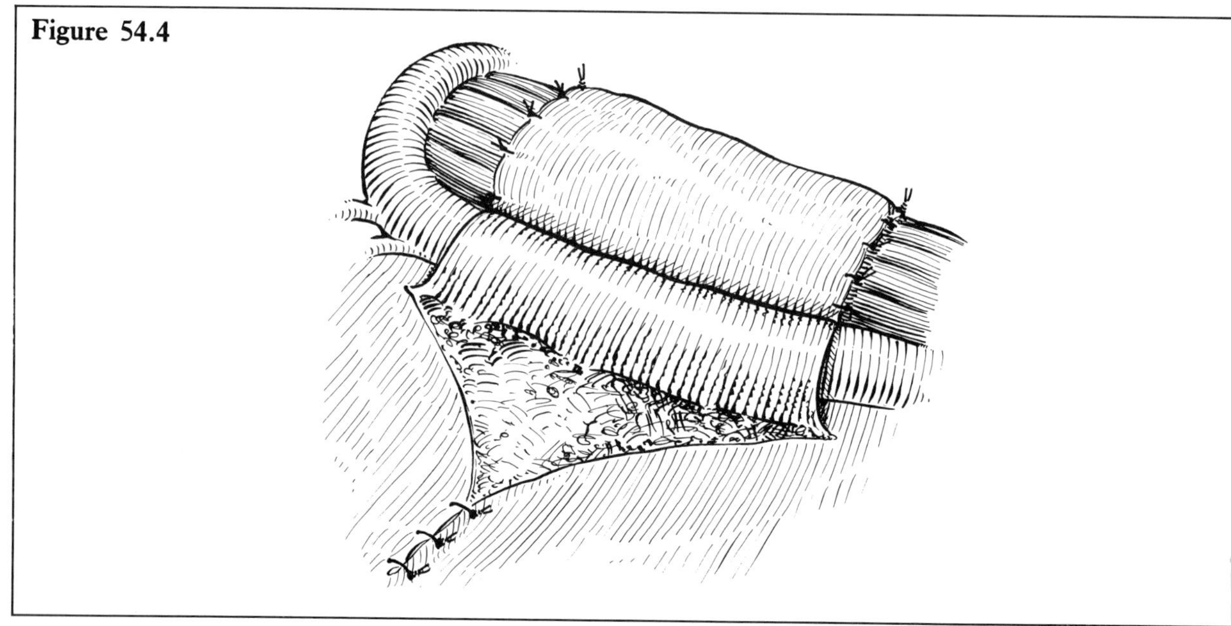

Figure 54.5

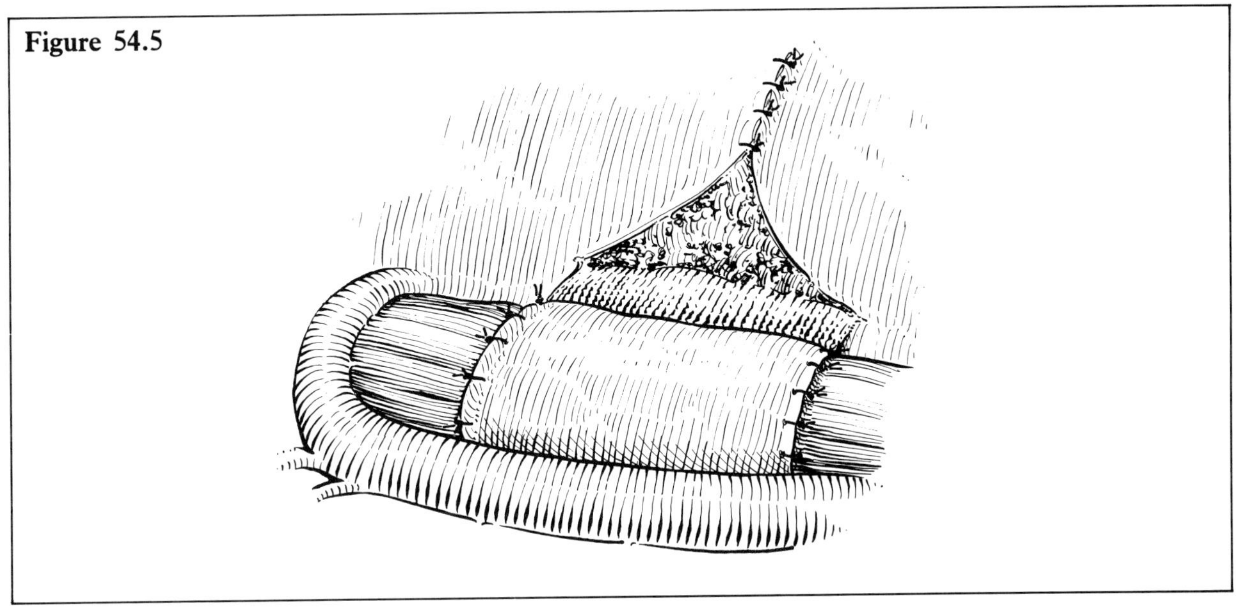

Figure 54.6

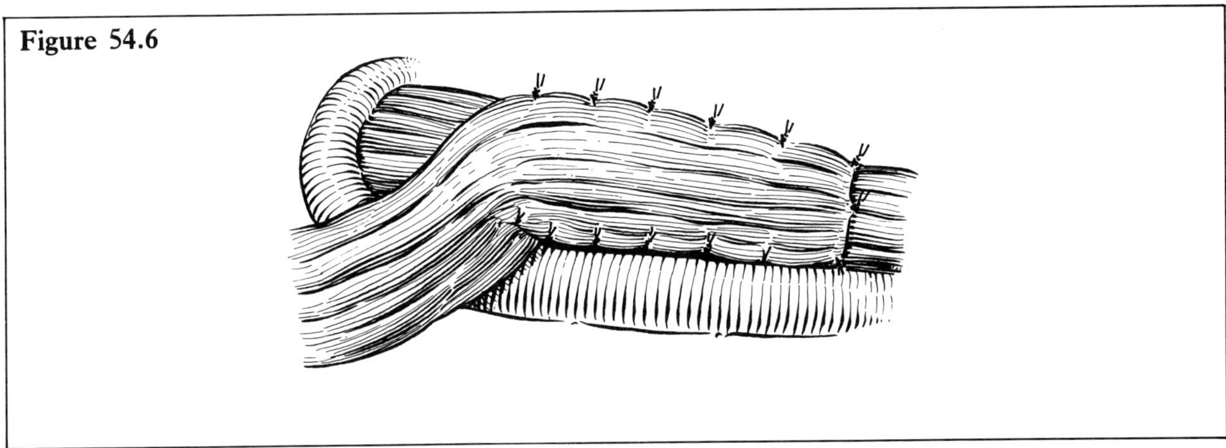

be identified in the mediastinum. In recent or short perforations direct suture of both mucosa and muscular layers may be possible (**Fig. 54.3**), but in late perforations any suturing is limited to a single full-thickness layer of interrupted polypropylene or wire sutures. The repair is reinforced with a strip of pleura (**Fig. 54.4**), pericardium (**Fig. 54.5**), diaphragm, or intercostal muscle bundle (**Fig. 54.6**).

### Repair of long perforations

We have adopted the following technique for excessively long perforations where much of the thoracic oesophagus may be destroyed. Careful and complete debridement of the thorax is carried out. The lung is freed as completely as possible. Only the lateral surface of the oesophagus is exposed, and the deeper aspect is left undisturbed. A nasogastric tube is passed into the stomach via the mouth by the anaesthetist with the direct guidance of the surgeon. A full-length intercostal muscle bundle is then taken down, with its vascular pedicle carefully preserved. It is then tacked on to the surface of the cut edges of the oesophagus longitudinally with interrupted sutures (**Fig. 54.6**).

### Postoperative care

The chest is closed over three tube drains. Two should be placed at the apex of the chest and the third at the base. Oral fluid is avoided and antibiotics are continued for seven days. By this time the systemic signs of infection have usually settled. The chest drains are left in place until there is no movement in the fluid levels in the tubing in the underwater seal bottle and all drainage has ceased, suggesting that the lung is firmly adherent to the chest wall.

Two weeks postoperatively a barium swallow is performed, and if contamination of the pleural space does not occur a diet consisting largely of solids can be given. If there is a leak but it is confined to the tube drain tract, then it is still safe to feed the patient. The leak will invariably cease with time provided that there is no distal obstruction. A distal obstruction would normally have been excluded during the preoperative investigations, but if this had been rendered impossible by the urgency of the case, it should be excluded early in the postoperative course.

# 55 Surgical management of leiomyoma of the oesophagus

These benign neoplasms are the most common tumour found in the wall of the oesophagus. They occur usually in the lower part of the oesophagus where the wall consists of smooth muscle; frequently they are incidental findings at the time of surgery for other conditions.

Occasionally leiomyomas may cause dysphagia. Contrast radiographic studies will reveal a smooth filling defect. At endoscopy no mucosal lesion is visible, and no biopsy should be taken as a breach of the mucosal wall may lead to an oesophageal leak after surgical removal. Occasionally they may present as massive tumours in the posterior mediastinum, and at this advanced stage diagnosis may not be easy, although a combination of CT with contrast enhancement will confirm the diagnosis.

The indication for operation is usually the lack of absolute certainty about the diagnosis in the absence of histological confirmation. Multiple tumours may be present. Rarely, sarcomatous change may occur.

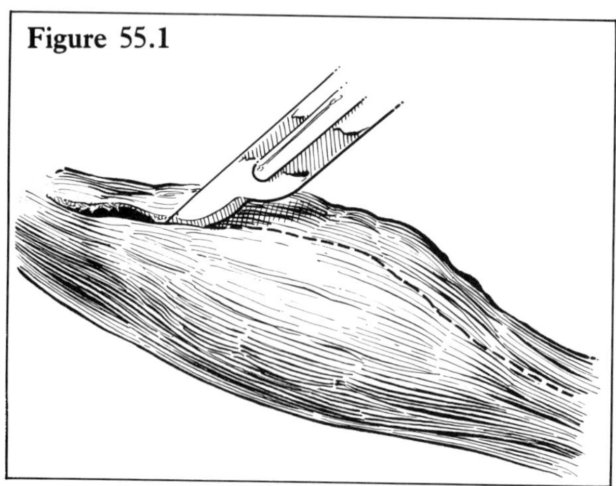

**Figure 55.1**

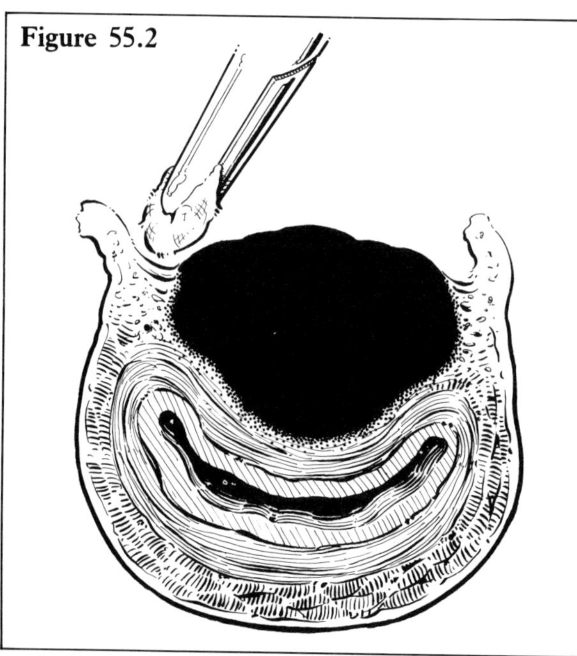

**Figure 55.2**

## Procedure

Since these tumours lie in the lower part of the oesophagus where the smooth muscle is to be found, the chest should be opened through a lateral thoracotomy through the sixth or seventh intercostal space.

The oesophagus is mobilized at the level of the tumour. The outer, thin adventitial layer and muscular layer are incised (**Fig. 55.1**). The leiomyoma can almost always be enucleated with blunt dissection, leaving the mucosa intact (**Fig. 55.2**). If the mucosa has been breached it should be repaired with an absorbable suture. If the muscle walls are not too ragged they may be approximated with interrupted sutures (**Fig. 55.3**). Very rarely, with extremely large tumours, it may be necessary to carry out a local resection and reconstruction.

The chest is closed over a single drain. A normal diet can be taken on the day following surgery if there is no fear of a leak. If a leak is suspected a barium study should be carried out before oral intake is permitted.

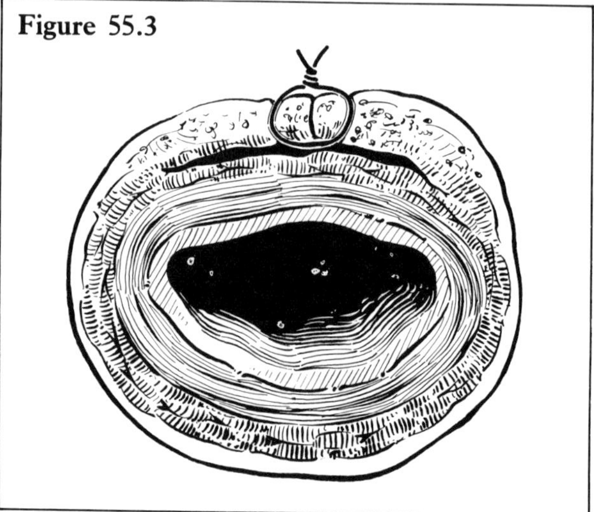

**Figure 55.3**

# Operations for malignant oesophageal disease

# 56 Investigations and preoperative preparation

Carcinomas may occur at any level of the oesophagus; those at the cardia frequently extend into or arise from the stomach. Patients present with increasing dysphagia, and may have suffered considerable weight loss and even dehydration at the time they are first seen. The majority of these tumours are not curable because of extension outside the oesophagus, metastases to regional lymph nodes or to the liver or peritoneum. The object of the operation is therefore to restore swallowing, although a small percentage of patients do survive five years.

The patients are often elderly, but assessment of their suitability for a resection is based more on the state of the cardiovascular and respiratory systems and the patient's general condition, than on age *per se*. In patients unsuitable for resection (which includes all those with distant metastases) a bypass procedure leaving the primary tumour *in situ* or permanent intubation are preferable.

## Investigations

A chest radiograph and routine blood screen is obtained. A barium swallow, with examination of the stomach if adequate barium will pass beyond the stricture, should be carried out. This is followed by oesophagoscopy, which will also establish the level and fixity of the tumour. A biopsy is obtained at the same time to establish the diagnosis. In cases with severe obstruction it may be possible to dilate the stricture to enable the patient to swallow in the days before operation. A bronchoscopy is necessary to determine whether the tumour has invaded the trachea or a main bronchus, and also to exclude the diagnosis of a carcinoma of the bronchus invading the oesophagus.

Liver metastases may be excluded by ultrasound or CT scan of the upper abdomen, although both false-positive and false-negative results are common. Recent studies have also demonstrated that neither CT nor magnetic resonance scans can give reliable information on the extent of local intrathoracic spread. In the light of this, we do not routinely employ preoperative CT scanning.

## Preoperative preparation

There is no clear evidence that delaying the operation to restore the patient's nutrition is beneficial. Dehydration should be corrected by intravenous fluid administration, and anaemia by blood transfusion. If there is pulmonary infection from spillage into the lungs, a period of physiotherapy and antibiotic administration is necessary.

The site and extent of the tumour will determine not only the surgical approach, but also the most appropriate part of the gastrointestinal tract to be used for reconstruction. It has long been recognized that submucosal spread is common and often extensive; a proximal clearance of 10 cm is therefore recommended.

We prefer a left thoracoabdominal approach for lesions of the gastro-oesophageal junction and distal oesophagus. If the stomach involvement is not too extensive, particularly along the lesser curve, then we would choose to use stomach as the oesophageal substitute. If the stomach is extensively involved then colon or jejunum is preferable as the stomach remnant is unlikely to be long enough.

For middle third tumours a two-stage procedure is necessary to allow adequate proximal clearance of the tumour. The stomach is again our first choice for reconstruction, as the tumour usually does not reach the gastro-oesophageal junction.

If a good clearance cannot be obtained, or the proximal extent of the tumour is greater, then a three-stage operation with anastomosis in the neck is more suitable. The stomach may not be long enough to reach this far; if this is the case, the colon should be used.

Recently blind oesophagectomy with cervical anastomosis has regained popularity. Concern was expressed that such a blind technique would lead to extensive haemorrhage; however, this has proved to be unfounded.

# 57 Left thoracoabdominal approach for malignant disease

The patient is positioned in the right lateral position with hips rotated backwards about 45 degrees (**Fig. 57.1**). An exploratory laparotomy is first performed through an oblique excision extending from the tip of the seventh intercostal cartilage to the midline about halfway between the xiphisternum and the umbilicus.

A careful search for peritoneal, hepatic and coeliac nodal metastases is made. If they are present, the prognosis is poor and the surgeon should abandon a major resection and either place an oesophageal tube to allow swallowing or perform a conservative palliative resection.

The region of the cardia is now palpated and the mobility of the tumour assessed. Minor degrees of involvement of the crus or tail of the pancreas may still allow resection, but if the tumour is firmly fixed a radical operation should be abandoned.

### Thoracic extension

If no metastases are found, the incision is extended and the chest opened by a left posterolateral incision through the seventh or eighth rib bed and the operability of the primary tumour assessed. If it appears to be removable the costal margin is divided. It is advisable to remove a 1–2 cm segment of costal margin to facilitate the repair at the end of the operation. The diaphragm is incised radially (**A** in **Fig. 57.2**) and the anterior edge of the hiatus divided. Branches of the pericardiophrenic artery are suture-ligated and the sutures left long to be used as diaphragmatic retractors (**Fig. 57.2**). Alternatively, a

**Figure 57.1**

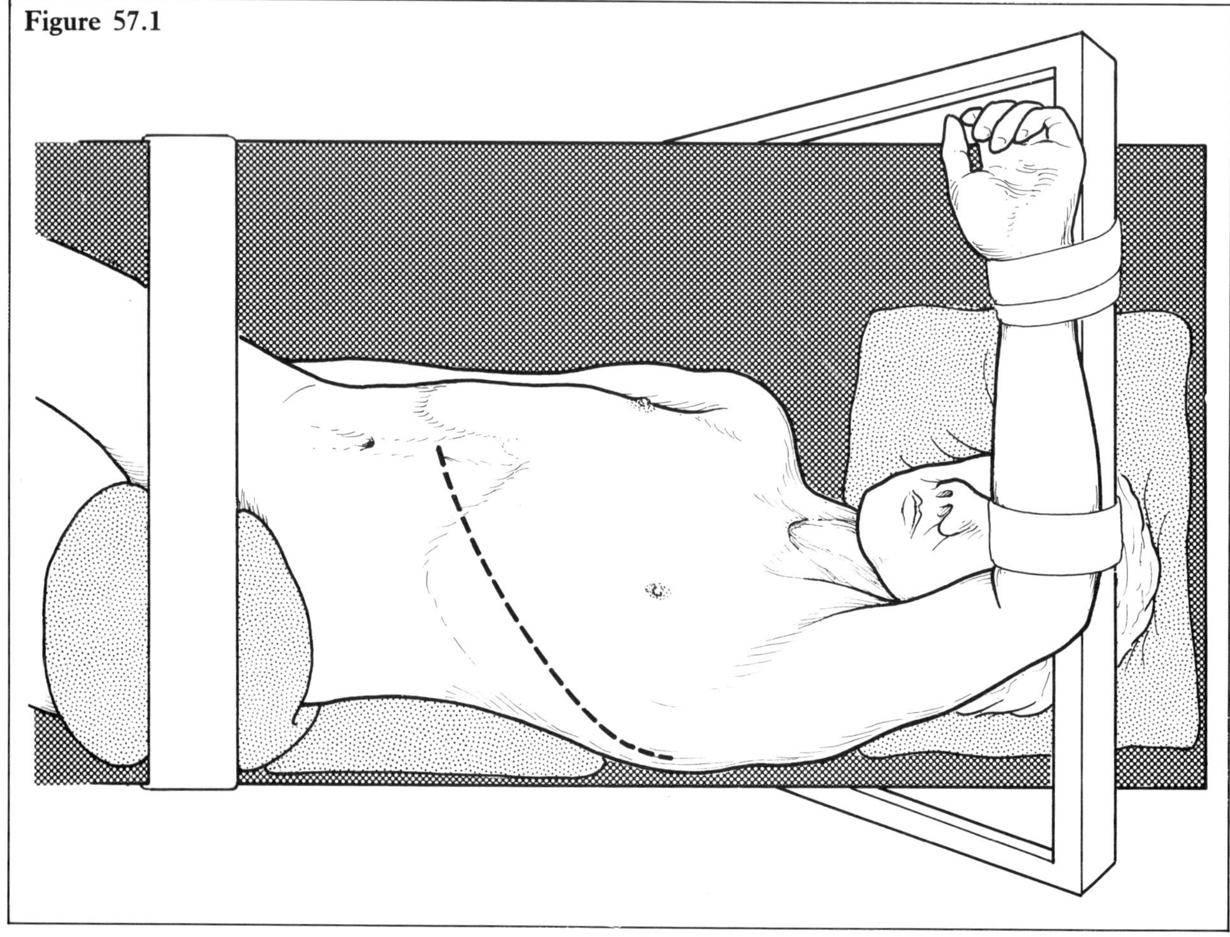

**Figure** 57.2

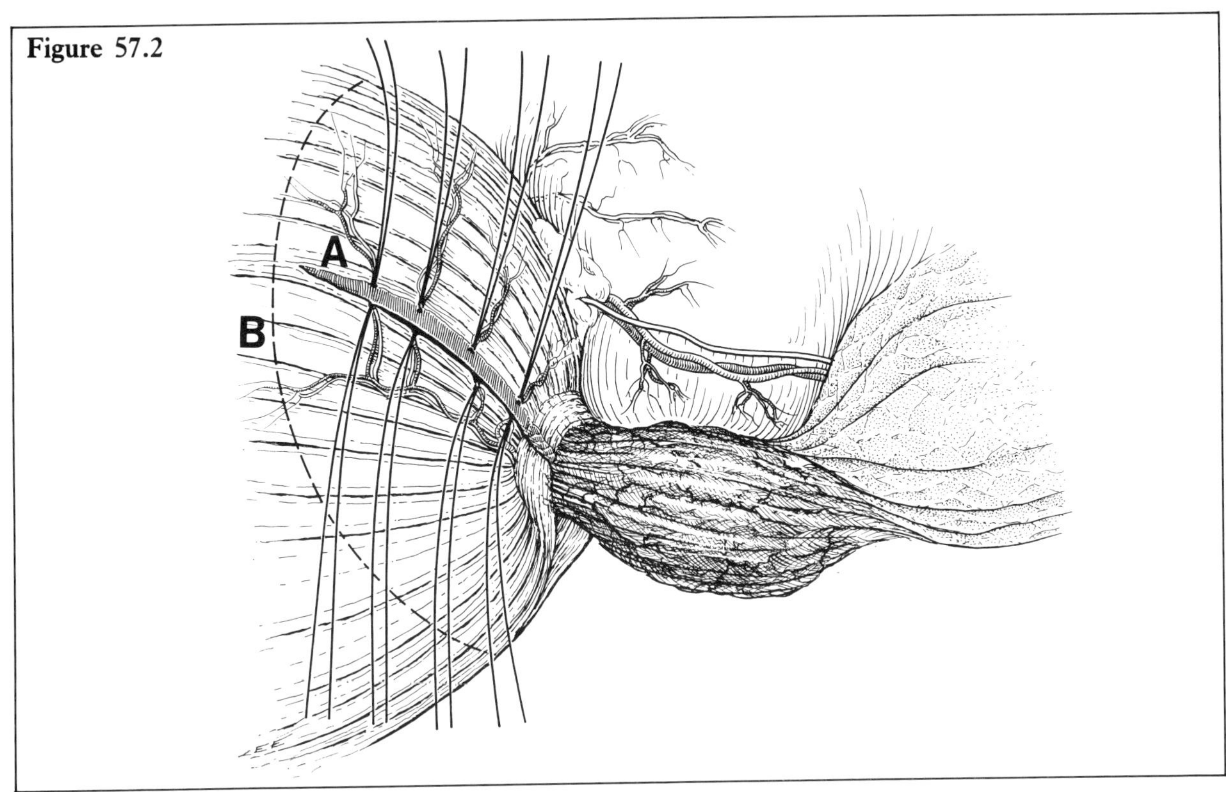


**Figure** 57.3

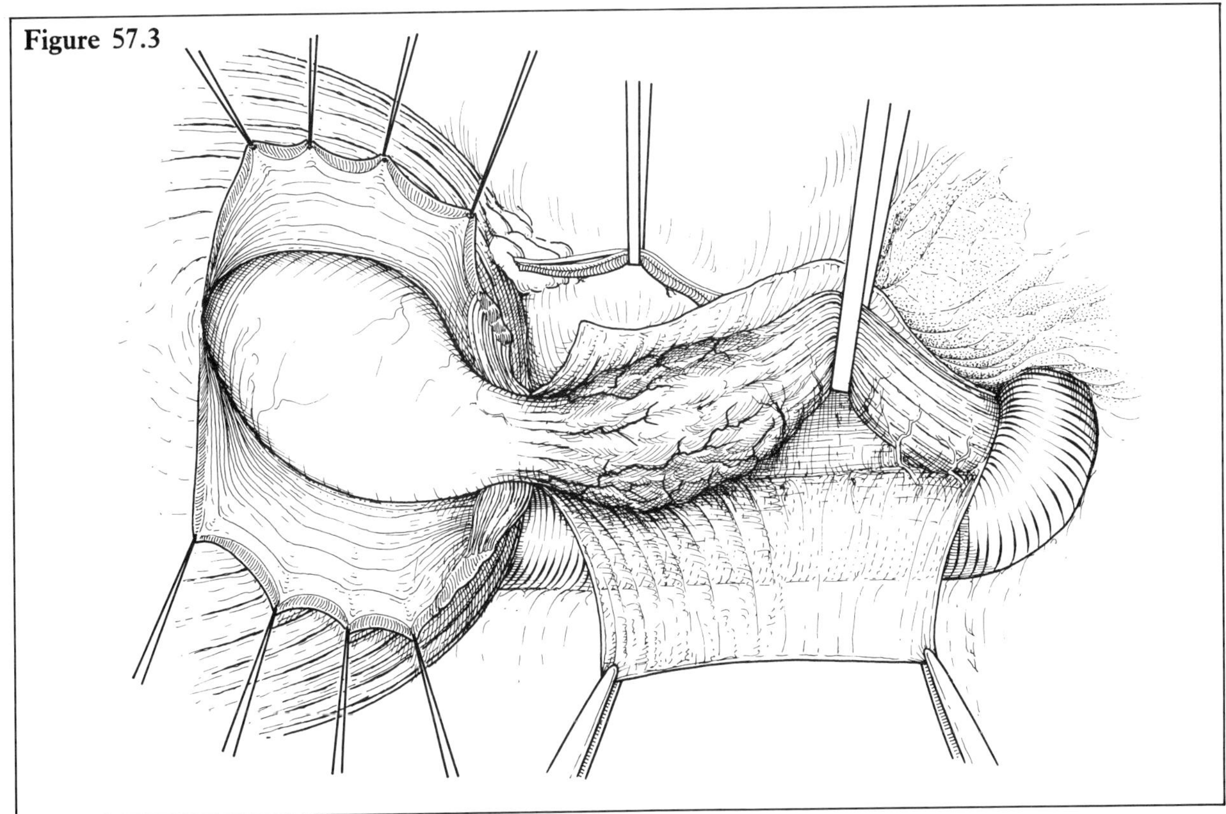

circumferential incision approximately 2 cm from the costal attachment may be used (B in **Fig. 57.2**). We usually prefer the former incision.

### Mobilization of the oesophagus

The pulmonary ligament is divided and the mediastinal pleura incised over the oesophagus as far as the aortic arch. The oesophagus is mobilized above the tumour and a sling placed around it (**Fig. 57.3**). The oesophageal vessels are carefully dissected and ligated The tumour is mobilized, keeping the plane of the dissection close to the aorta on the left and if necessary opening the pleural cavity on the right.

The lesser sac is opened through the greater

omentum and the attachments between the omentum and the lower pole of the spleen are divided between clamps and ligated (**Fig. 57.4**). The tail of the pancreas is mobilized, and if it is involved by tumour the pancreas is divided with diathermy central to the involved area between soft clamps. The cut surface is closed with a series of mattress sutures which must be tied gently, otherwise they will cut through the substance of the pancreas (**Fig. 57.5**). The sutured end of the pancreas is then buried beneath the posterior peritoneum with a few interrupted sutures. The lesser omentum is detached from the right side of the oesophagus and the hilum of the liver, and then divided parallel to the bile duct as far down as the pylorus. There is often a hepatic branch of the left gastric artery within the lesser omentum which should be divided between ligatures. The greater omentum is detached from the greater curvature of the stomach, taking extreme care to leave the gastroepiploic arch intact (**Fig. 57.4**). The branches of this artery to the omentum are divided between arterial clamps and ligated, or are divided by a stapling device. The dissection continues as far as the pylorus.

Next the cardia is freed from the hiatus (**Fig. 57.6**). If the tumour has transgressed the serosa in this region a portion of the hiatus is removed with it. The stomach is turned upwards and the left

**Figure 57.4**

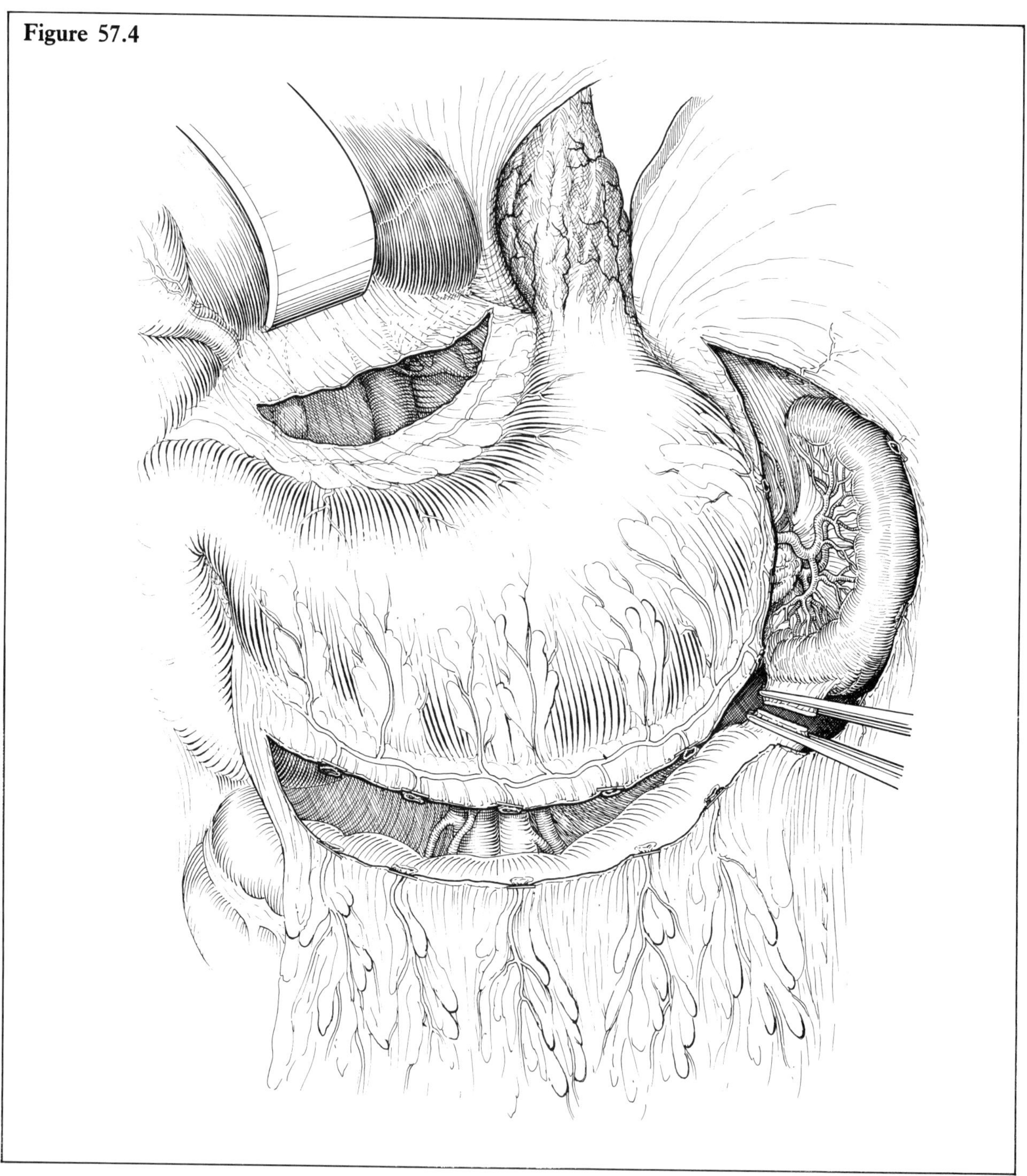

**Figure** 57.5

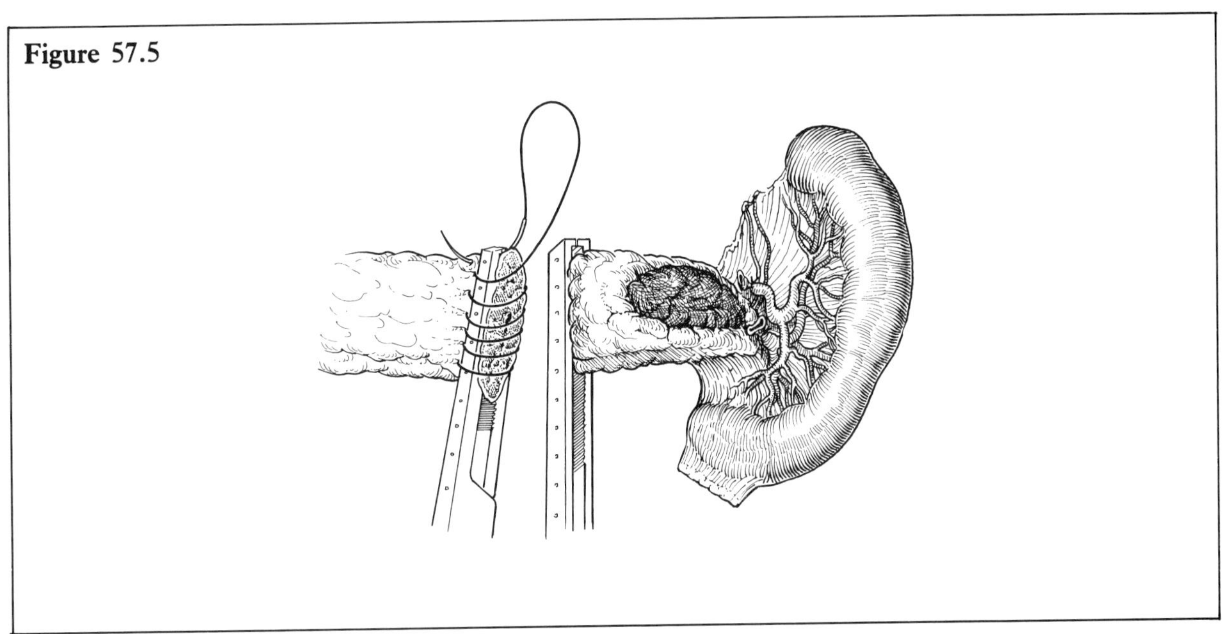

**Figure** 57.6

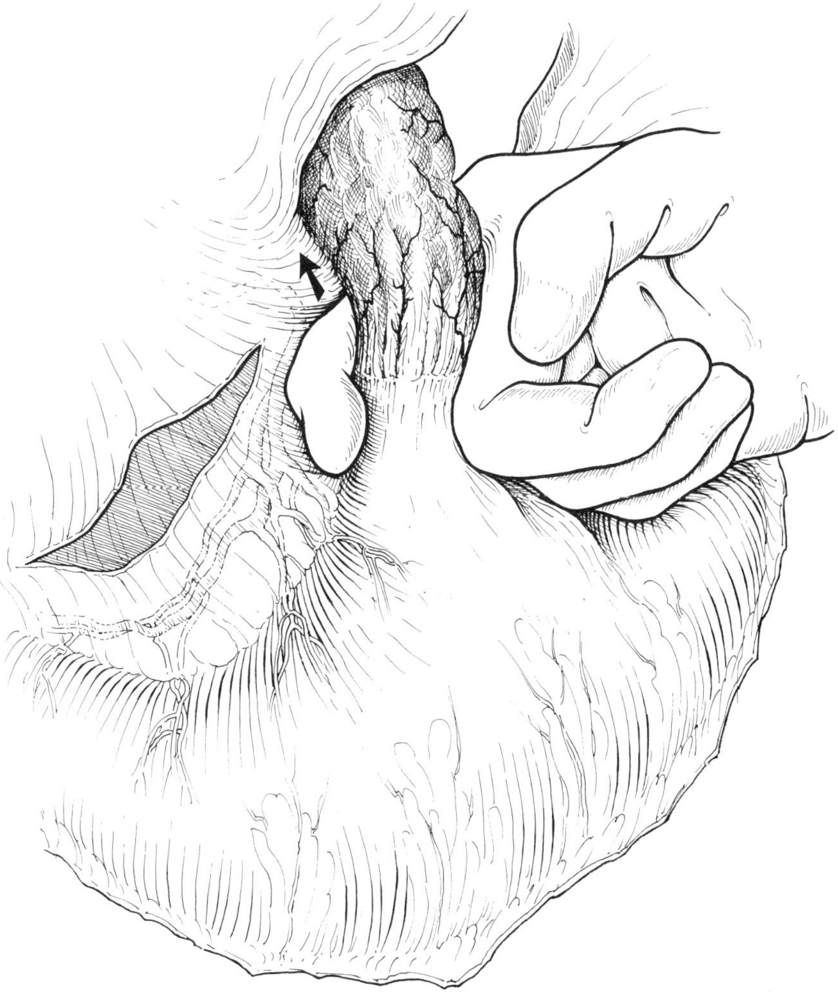

**Figure 57.7**

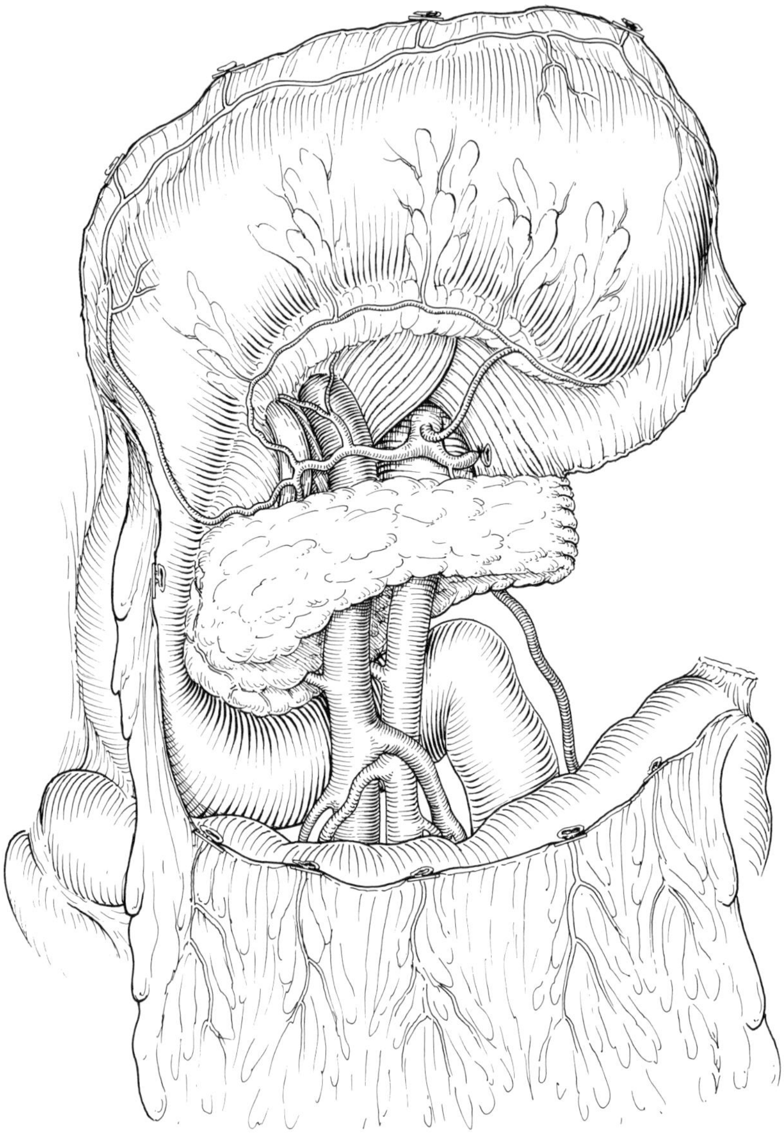

**Figure 57.8**

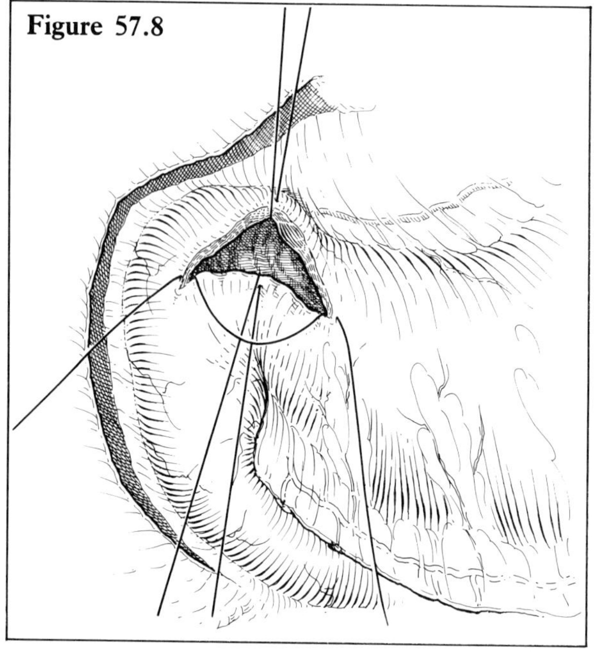

**Figure 57.9**

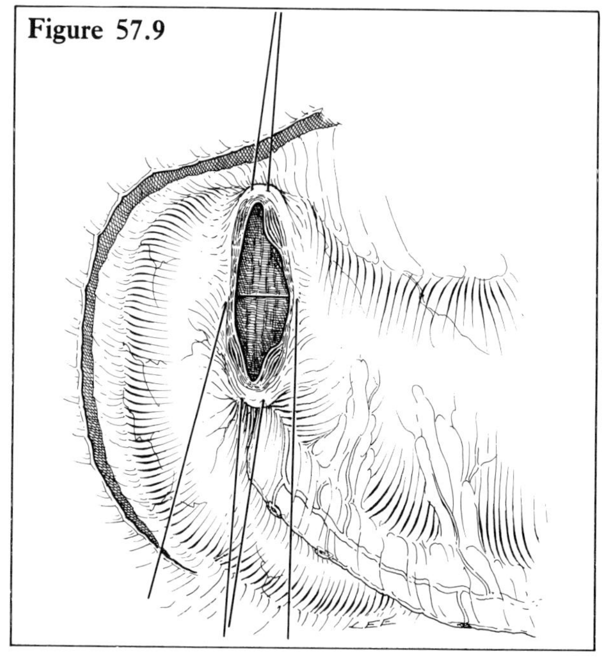

gastric artery sought at its emergence from the coeliac axis at the upper border of the pancreas (**Fig. 57.7**). The origins of the three branches of the coeliac axis should be separately identified so that the left gastric artery alone is divided. The lymph nodes around the coeliac axis are removed.

During the dissection the vagus nerves are divided, and gastric stasis may result. Different authors give differing advice on how to manage this problem. The possibilities include pyloroplasty, pyloromyotomy, digital dilatation or no treatment. The technique of pyloroplasty is illustrated in **Figs. 57.8–10**; however, we believe that the procedure is unnecessary and may result in severe and troublesome biliary reflux. We are of the opinion that as a rule no procedure is necessary, but if the surgeon is concerned, then a pyloromyotomy is adequate (**Fig. 57.11**).

### Formation of gastric tube

The next step is the formation of a gastric tube. With the thumb and index finger of the left hand, the junction of the right and left gastric arteries is grasped at the middle of the lesser curvature. With a little blunt dissection the margin of the stomach is freed from the vascular arcade, which is divided between ligatures. Two long clamps are placed across the stomach from the termination of the left gastroepiploic artery to the prepared point on the lesser curvature, and the stomach divided between them (**Fig. 57.12**). The proximal end is covered with a swab and turned upwards over the costal

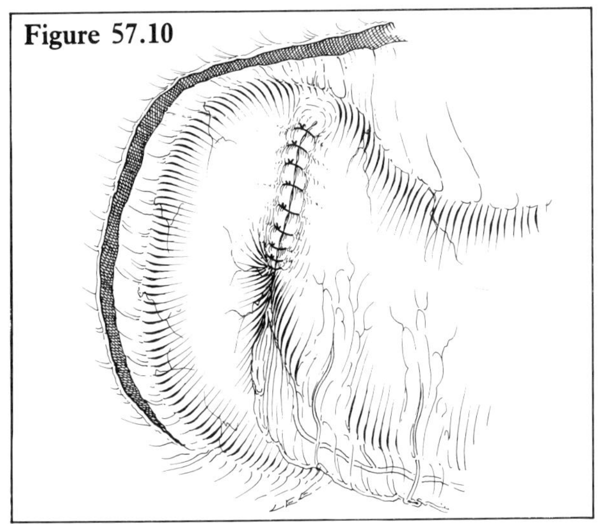

**Figure 57.10**

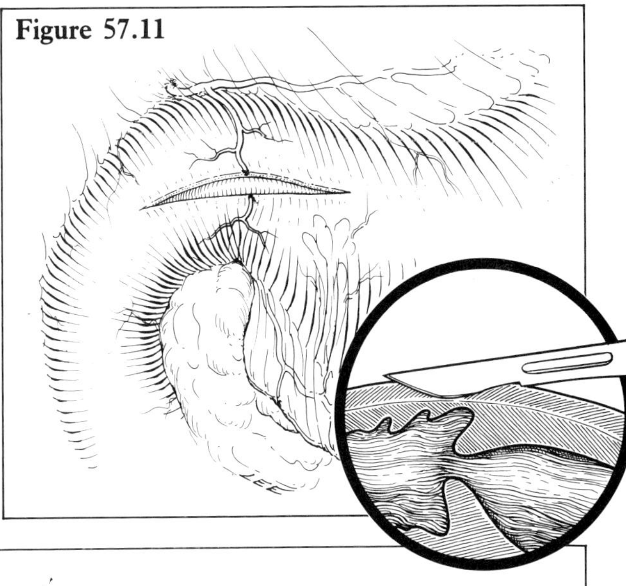

**Figure 57.11**

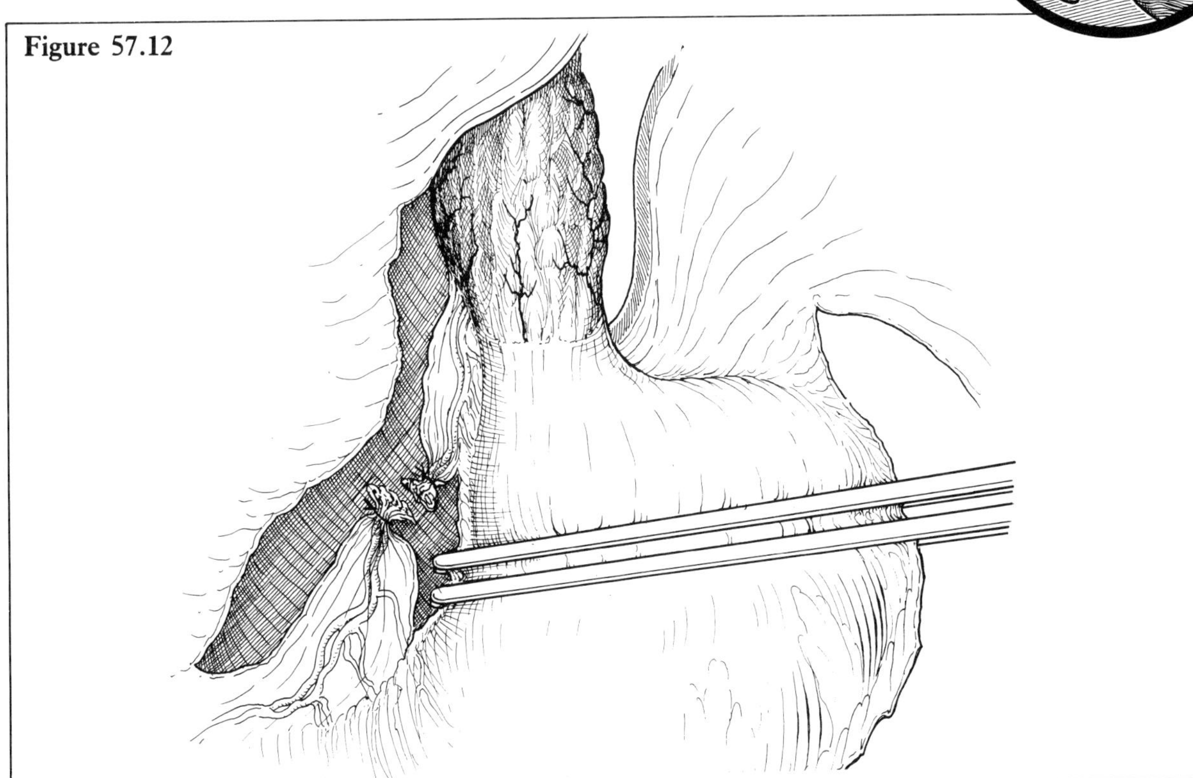

**Figure 57.12**

Figure 57.13

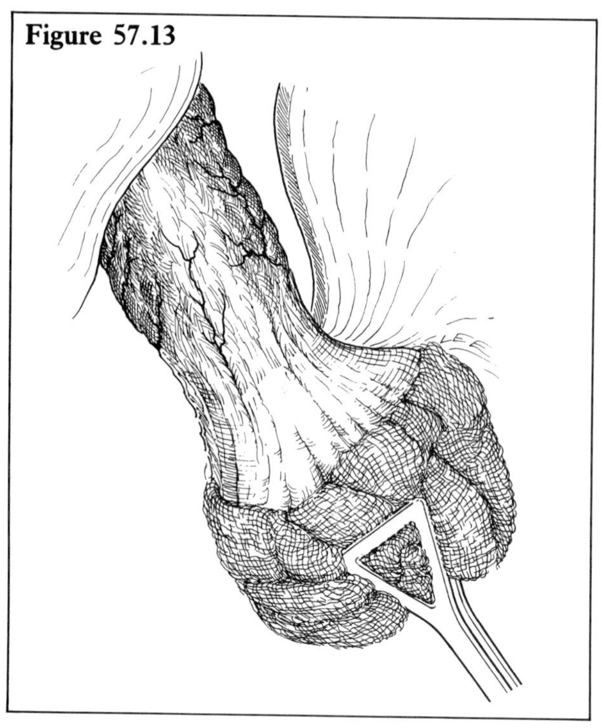

margin (**Fig. 57.13**). The distal end is closed with a continuous suture of 2/0 catgut (**Fig. 57.14**). The clamp is removed and the cut edge buried with fine interrupted sutures (**Fig. 57.15**).

The tube of stomach is now tested for length by passing it upwards into the thorax along the bed of the oesophagus. It should reach 10 cm above the upper margin of the tumour, and indeed will usually reach to the apex of the chest (**Fig. 57.16**).

### Oesophagogastric anastomosis

A suitable point is chosen about 2 cm from the tip of the tube of stomach for the anastomosis. It should lie as far away as possible from the previous gastric suture line.

Three or four mattress sutures are inserted to unite the serosa of the stomach with the posterior wall of the oesophagus, and tied (**Fig. 57.17**).

A 30 mm incision is made transversely in the stomach about 1 cm below the line of junction with the oesophagus, and the stomach contents sucked out. Bleeding is controlled by suction.

Figure 57.14

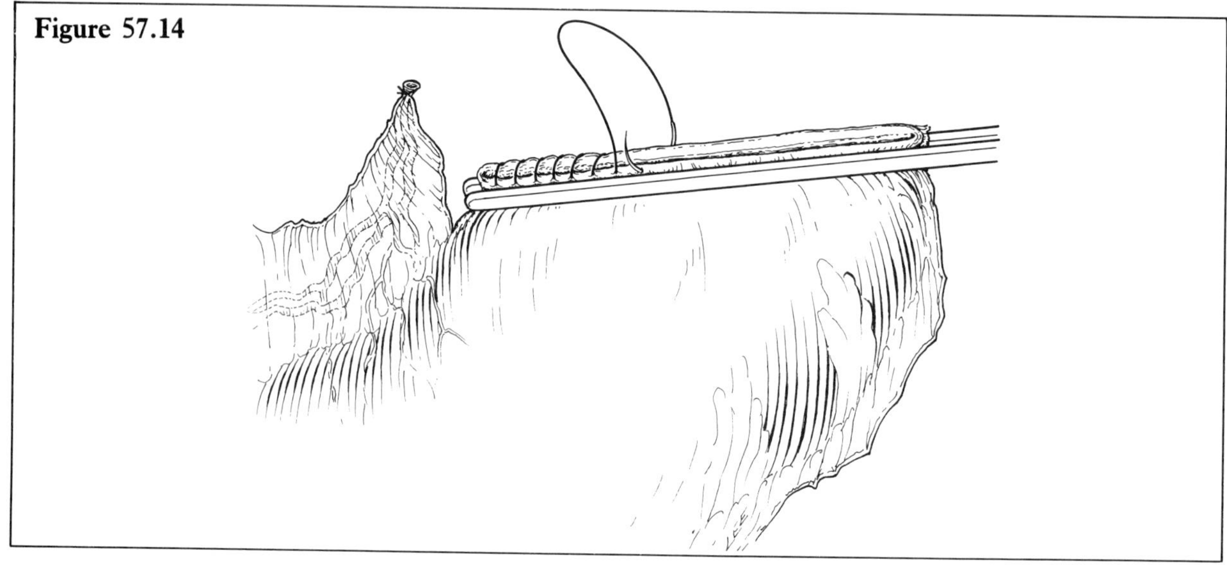

Figure 57.15

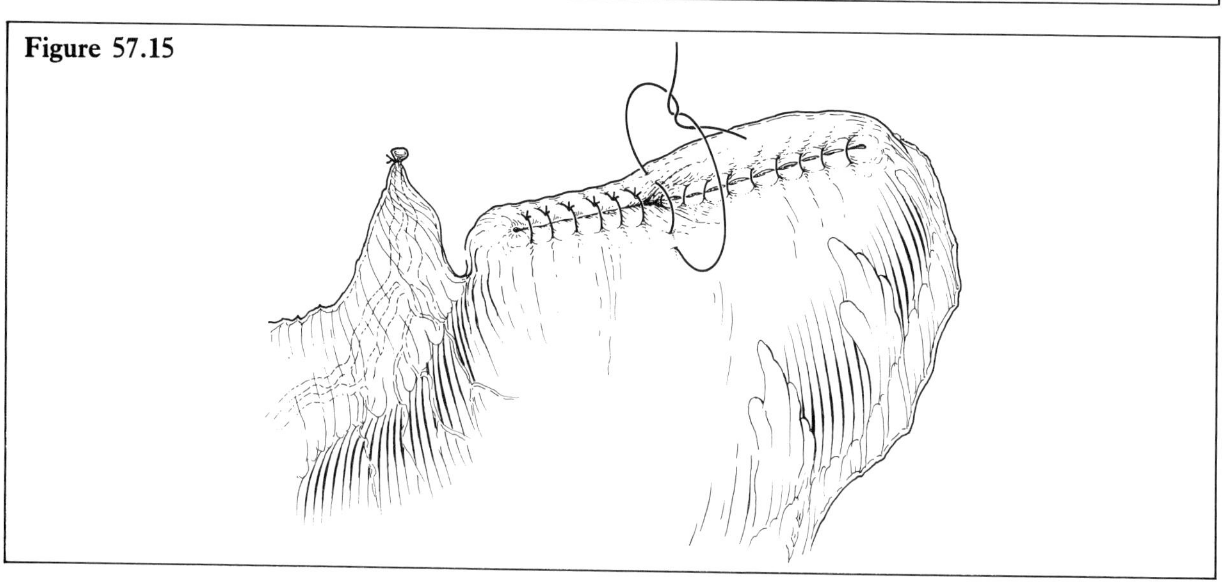

**Figure 57.16**

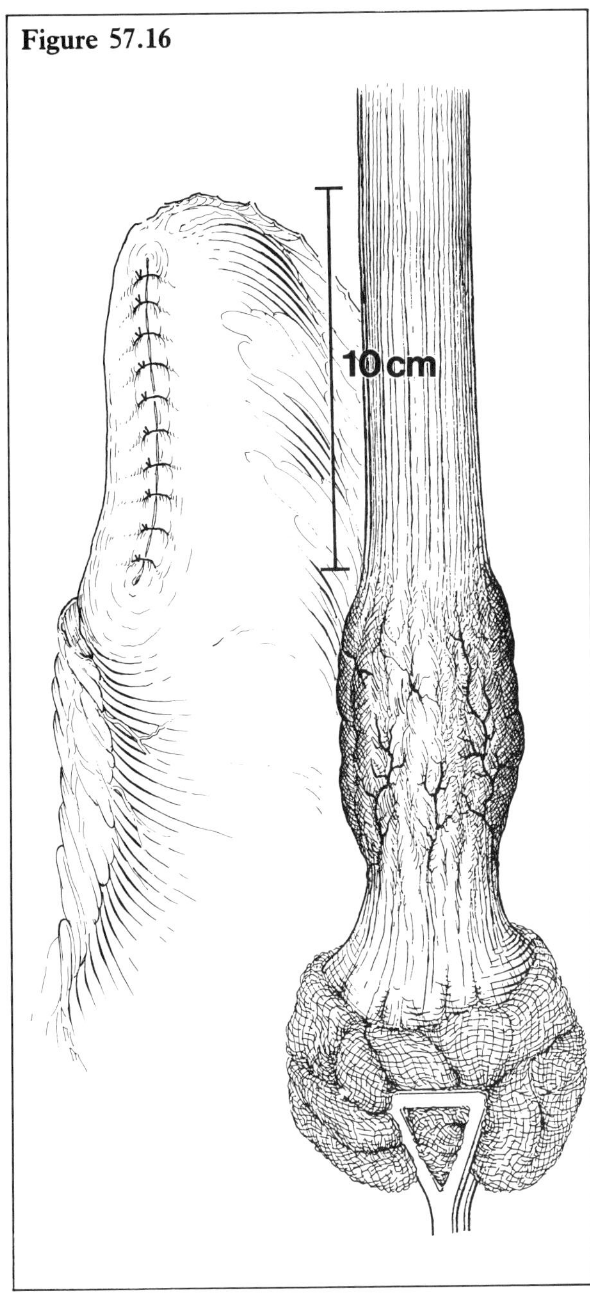


**Figure 57.17**

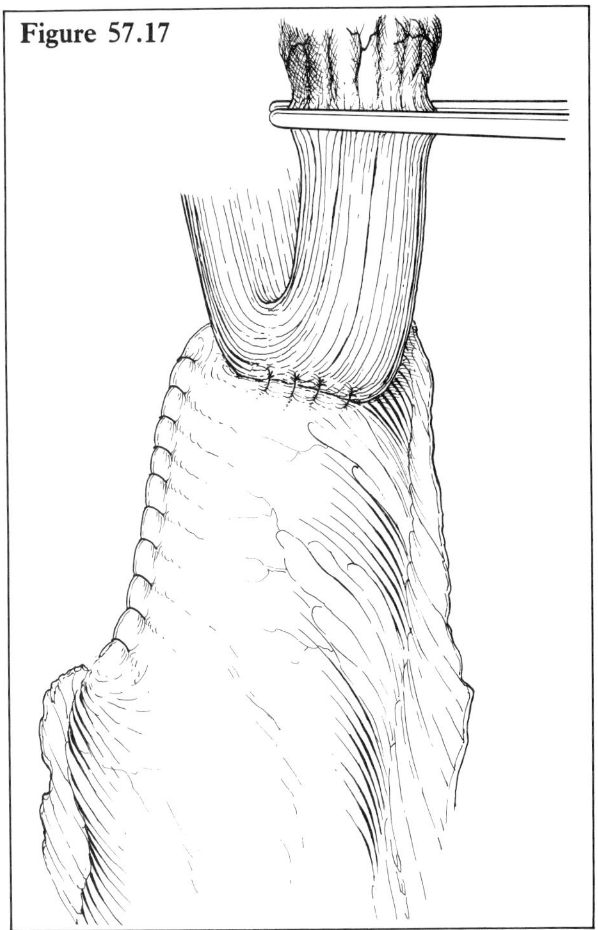

**Figure 57.18**

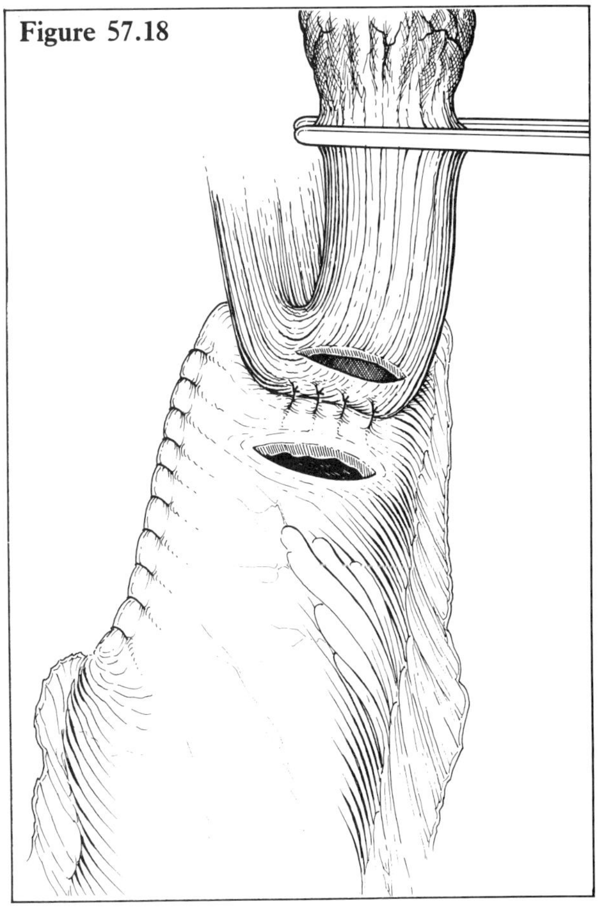

The oesophagus is cross-clamped a short distance below the site of the proposed anastomosis to avoid soiling from its contents. The posterior wall is then incised transversely 1 cm from the posterior suture line (**Fig. 57.18**); this incision should be the same length as that in the stomach. If the diameter of the oesophagus is small it is possible to enlarge it somewhat by dividing it obliquely. This must not be exaggerated as it will jeopardize the blood supply.

The ends of the incisions are united with a traction suture (**Fig. 57.19**); this travels from outside the oesophagus into its lumen, picking up the mucosa, and then from the mucosa of the stomach to its serosa. It must be stressed that it is essential to include the mucosa with each bite of the needle. A third suture is placed across the

**Figure 57.19**

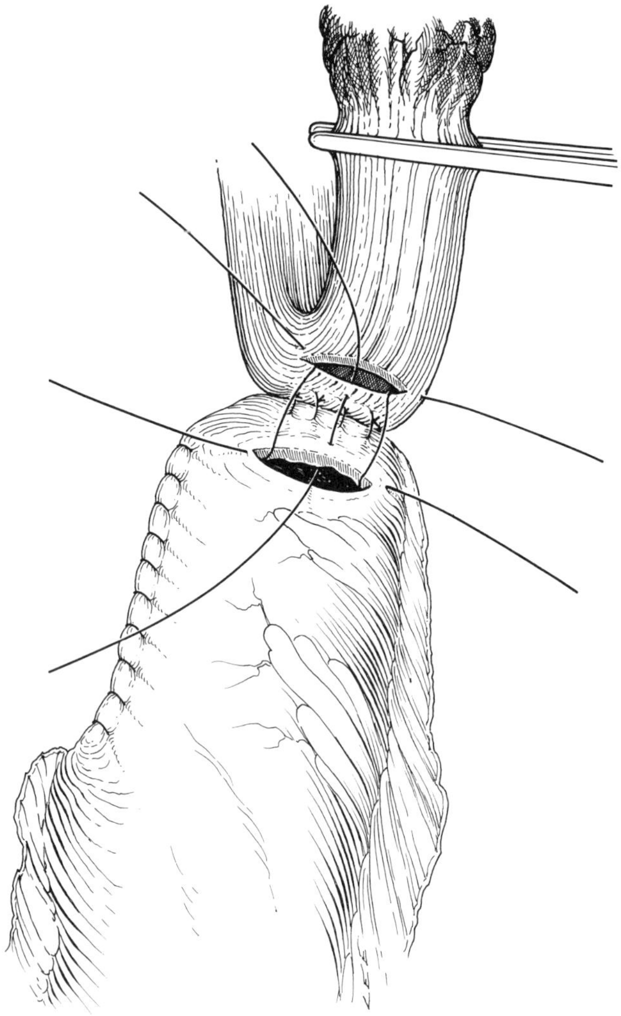

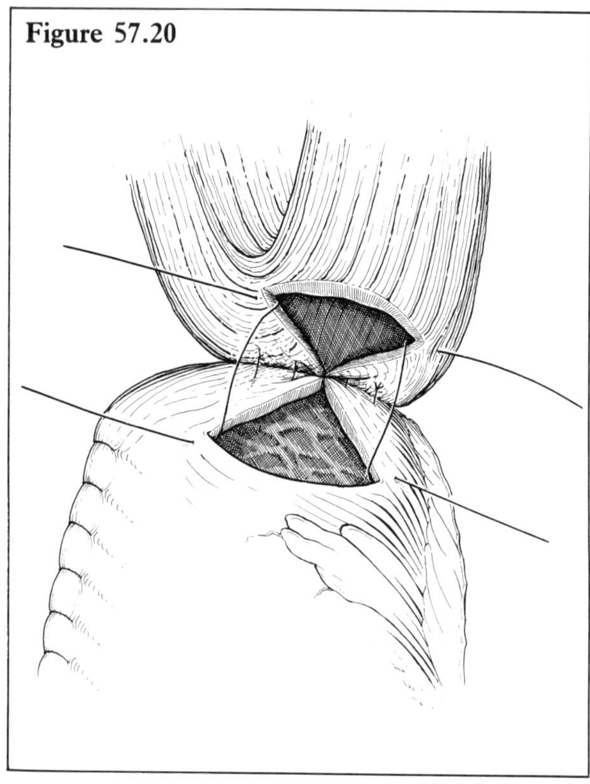

**Figure 57.20**

middle of the incision, picking up the full thickness of the walls of both viscera, and tied (**Fig. 57.20**). The posterior walls of the stomach and oesophagus are then united by a row of similar sutures, the knots of which remain in the lumen (**Fig. 57.21**); 3/0 polypropylene is a suitable suture material for this purpose.

The anterior wall of the oesophagus is transected with scissors and a nasogastric tube is passed across the posterior half of the anastomosis into the stomach. A similar row of sutures is now placed to unite the anterior walls of the stomach and the oesophagus, and the two corner sutures are tied (**Fig. 57.22**). When possible, a second row of interrupted mattress sutures is used to bury the first layer (**Figs. 57.23, 57.24**).

### Closure

The first step in closure is to repair the diaphragm with thread sutures. The first of these is placed behind the stomach to approximate the two crural pillars. A series of 3/0 polypropylene sutures then unite the serosa of the stomach to the margins of an opening which is left in the diaphragm for

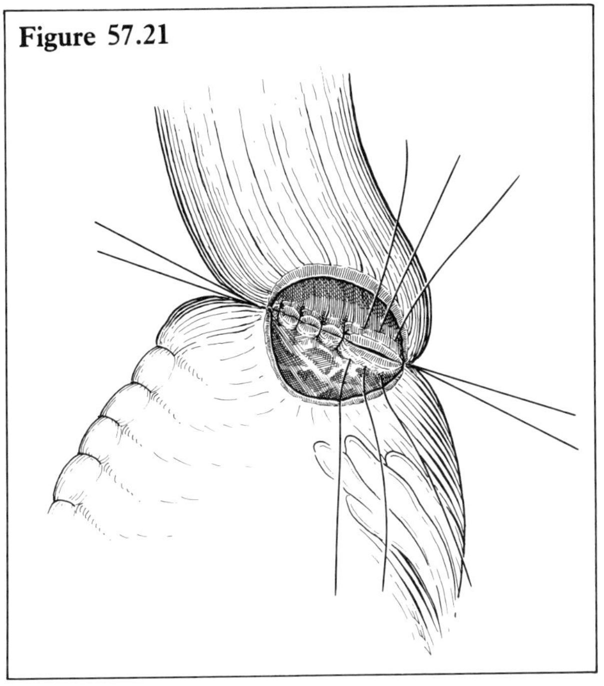
Figure 57.21

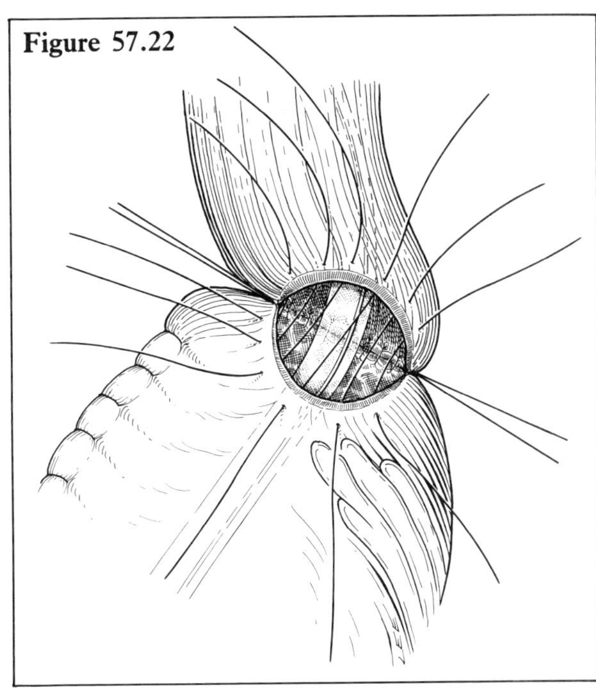
Figure 57.22

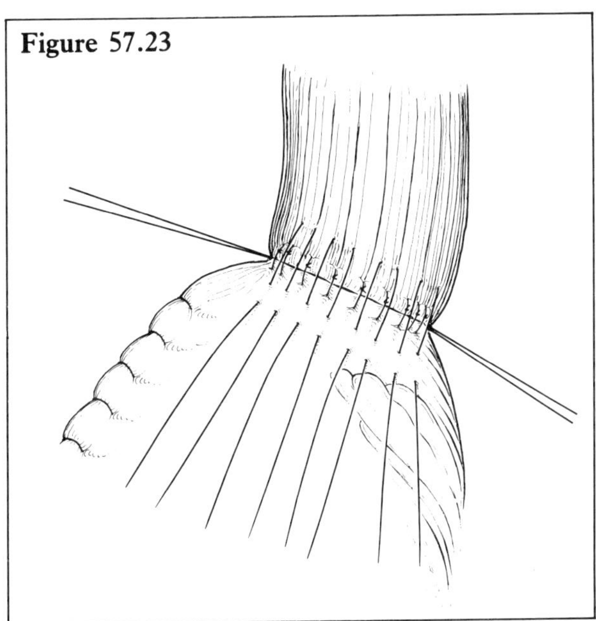
Figure 57.23

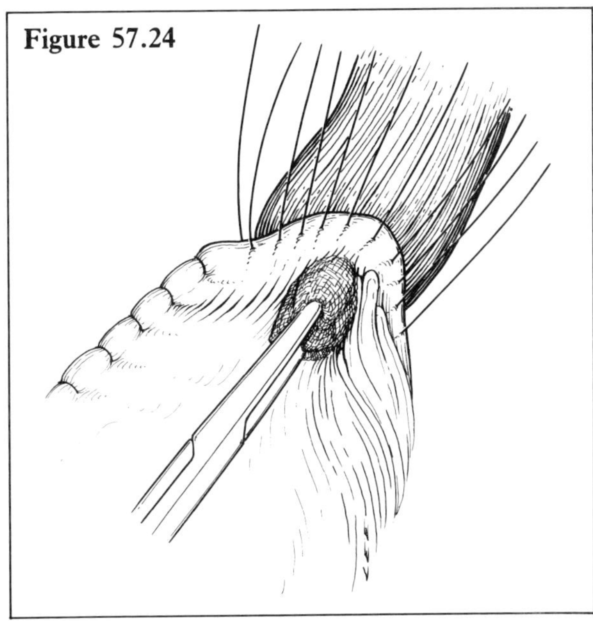
Figure 57.24

the passage of that organ. The remainder of the diaphragm is closed with interrupted thread sutures. Before the peripheral part can be sutured it is necessary to relax or remove the rib spreader.

The divided costal cartilage is united with a series of heavy, non-absorbable mattress sutures.

Two drains are passed into the pleural space. The left lung is re-expanded. The thoracic and abdominal incisions are closed in layers with continuous nylon sutures.

## Postoperative management

Patients undergoing this procedure often lose a considerable amount of fluid during the course of the operation, and usually require 4 to 5 litres in the 24-hour period of the operation and immediate recovery period. The central venous pressure is used to monitor fluid loss. It should be maintained at between 5 and 10 cm$H_2O$, and the urine flow at 50 ml per hour. Blood loss is combated by transfusion. The chest tubes are removed as soon as drainage has fallen below 150 ml per day and the chest radiograph shows that the lung is fully expanded. This is usually attained on the first postoperative day.

The nasogastric tube is allowed to drain freely into a bag and is removed as soon as bowel sounds are heard. Small amounts of fluid can then be given orally while the remainder is supplied by intravenous infusion. Free fluids may be given a day later and a light diet started after three to four days. Early mobilization is essential. Vigorous physiotherapy is given from the first postoperative day, and the patient is kept well propped up in bed to diminish the risk of aspiration of gastric contents.

If the patient develops fever and a pleural effusion, especially a haemopneumothorax, a breakdown of the anastomosis is likely. A barium swallow should then be carried out to determine the extent of the leak. Small leaks will often heal after satisfactory pleural drainage has been established; but larger ones may require refashioning of the anastomosis, or even cervical oesophagostomy and gastrostomy followed by a later reconstruction of the pathway with colon.

# 58 Two-stage oesophagogastrectomy

## Abdominal stage

The purpose of this stage is to mobilize the stomach, after a thorough search for intra-abdominal metastases.

The patient is placed supine on the operating table. An upper midline incision is made, extending around and below the umbilicus for 2–3 cm. Alternatively, if the subcostal angle is wide, a transverse abdominal incision transecting the rectus muscles is used (**Fig. 58.1**). The diaphragm and subcostal margins are retracted with a broad-bladed 'third hand' retractor. The colon and greater omentum are then drawn out of the wound to reveal the stomach. The lesser sac is opened through the gastrocolic omentum. The lienocolic ligament is divided between clamps, and the stomach mobilized with division of the branches of the gastroepiploic vessels as previously described (**Fig. 58.2**). The left triangular ligament is divided

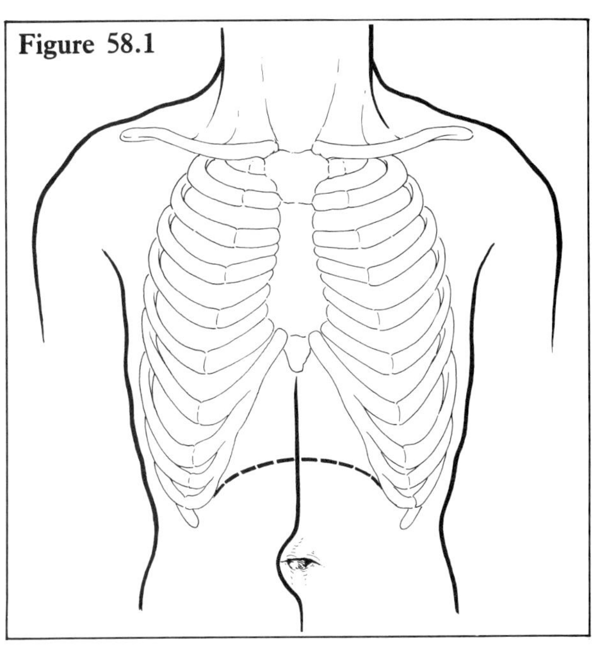

**Figure 58.1**

**Figure 58.2**

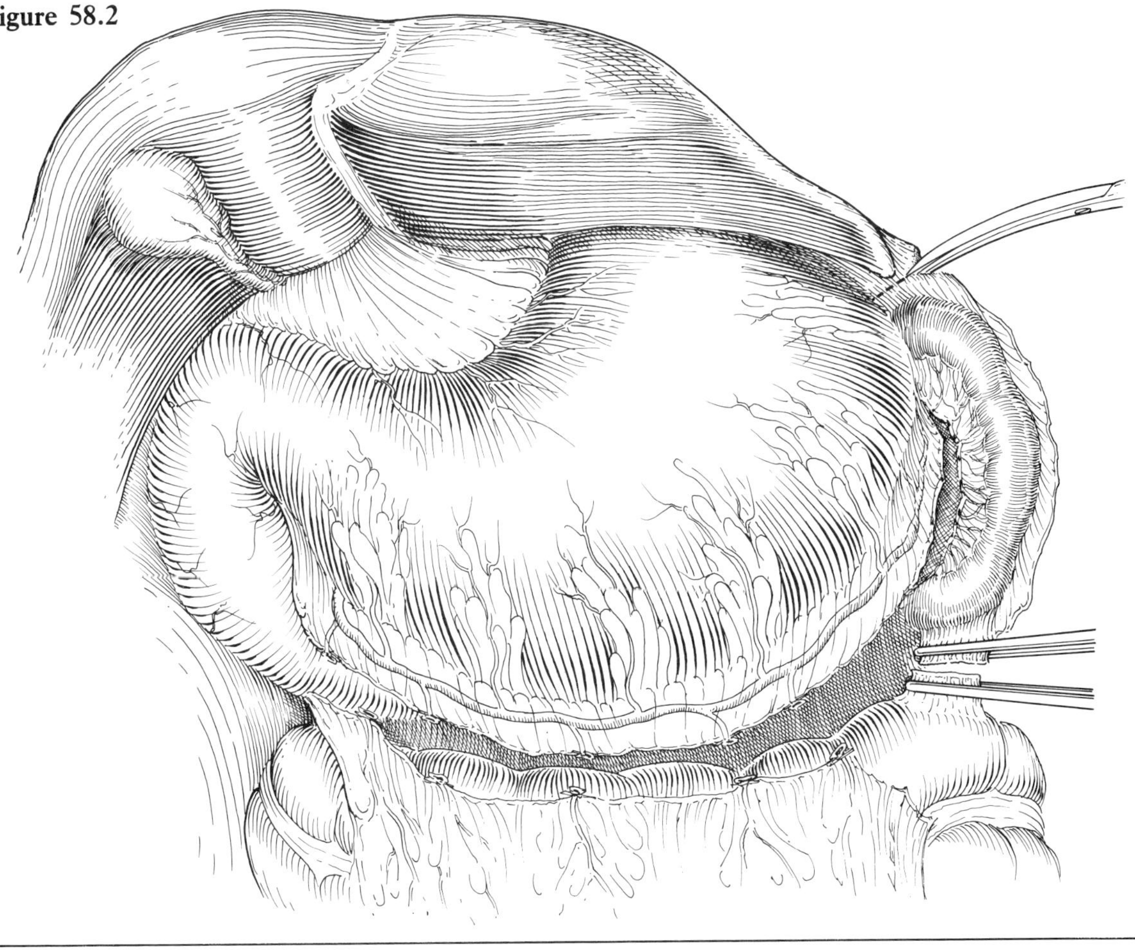

and the lesser omentum is divided close to the liver (**Fig. 58.3**). A large broad retractor is used to retract the left costal margin. The stomach is drawn downwards and to the right and the vasa brevia are divided, taking great care not to injure the spleen. The higher vasa brevia are now at some considerable distance from the operator and it is convenient to divide them between Ligaclips (stainless steel clips mounted on long forceps). The stomach is mobilized as far as the pylorus, but the right gastric vessels are preserved. The stomach is now turned upwards and the left gastric artery

**Figure 58.3**

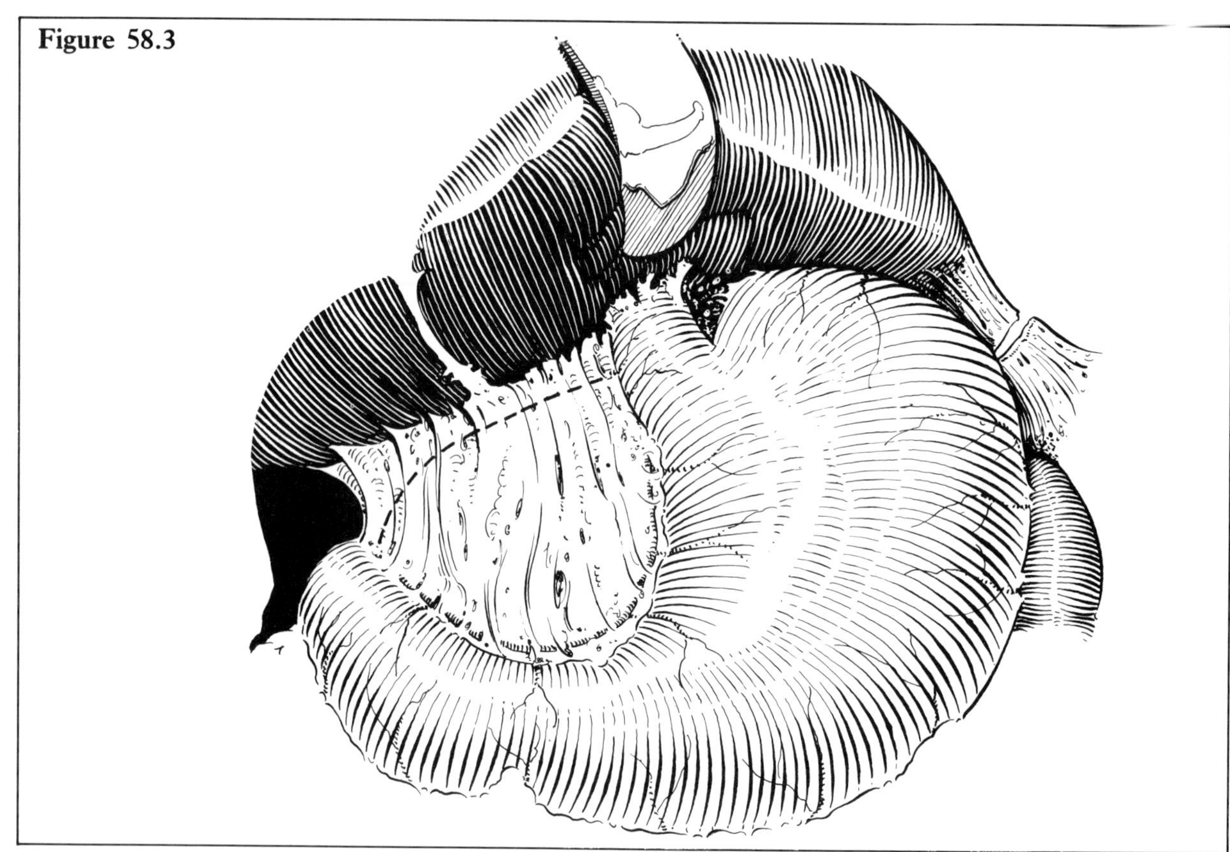

**Figure 58.4**

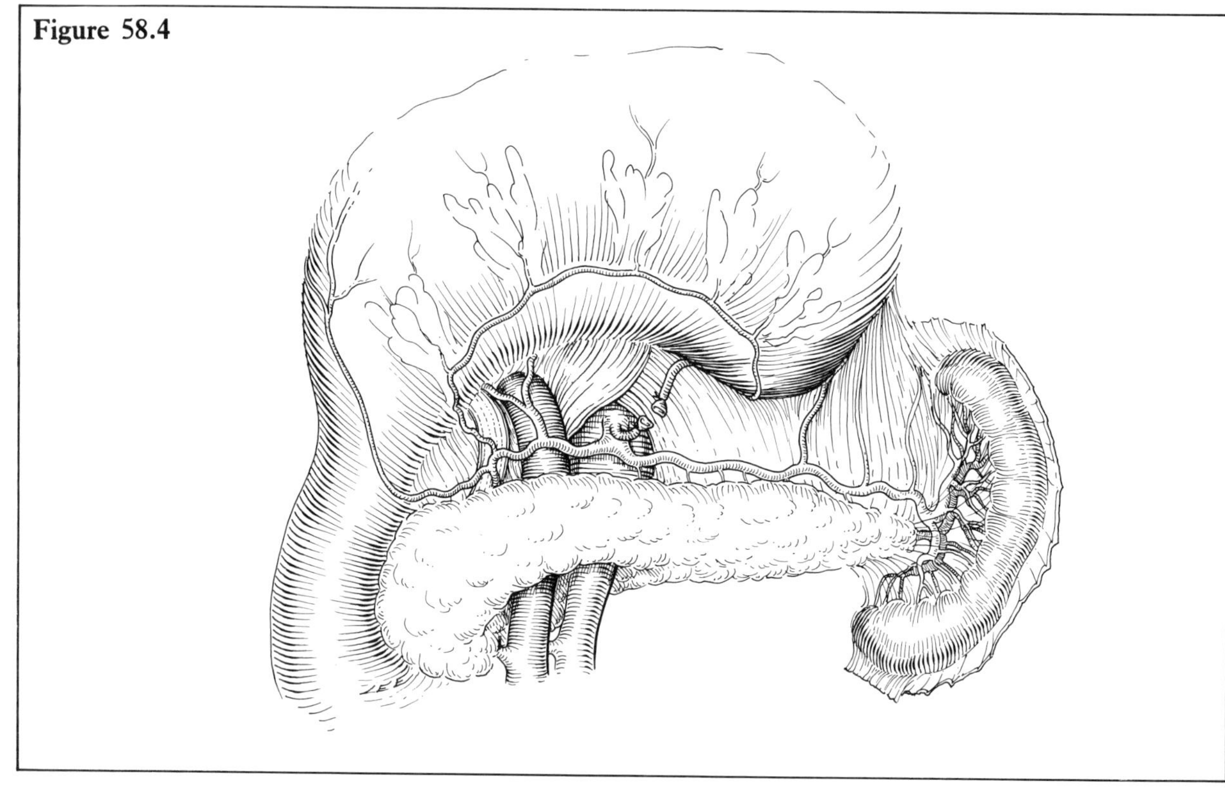

divided at its origin (**Fig. 58.4**).

Next, the oesophagus is freed from the oesophageal hiatus by division of the overlying peritoneum, and the vagus nerves are divided above the cardia (**Fig. 58.5**). By blunt dissection the oesophagus can now be mobilized for some distance up into the mediastinum, where the tumour may be felt. To increase gastric mobility the peritoneum on the right side of the duodenum is mobilized (Kocher's manoeuvre, **Fig. 58.6**). If necessary, the first three parts of the duodenum are mobilized with the head of the pancreas. Haemostasis is

**Figure 58.5**

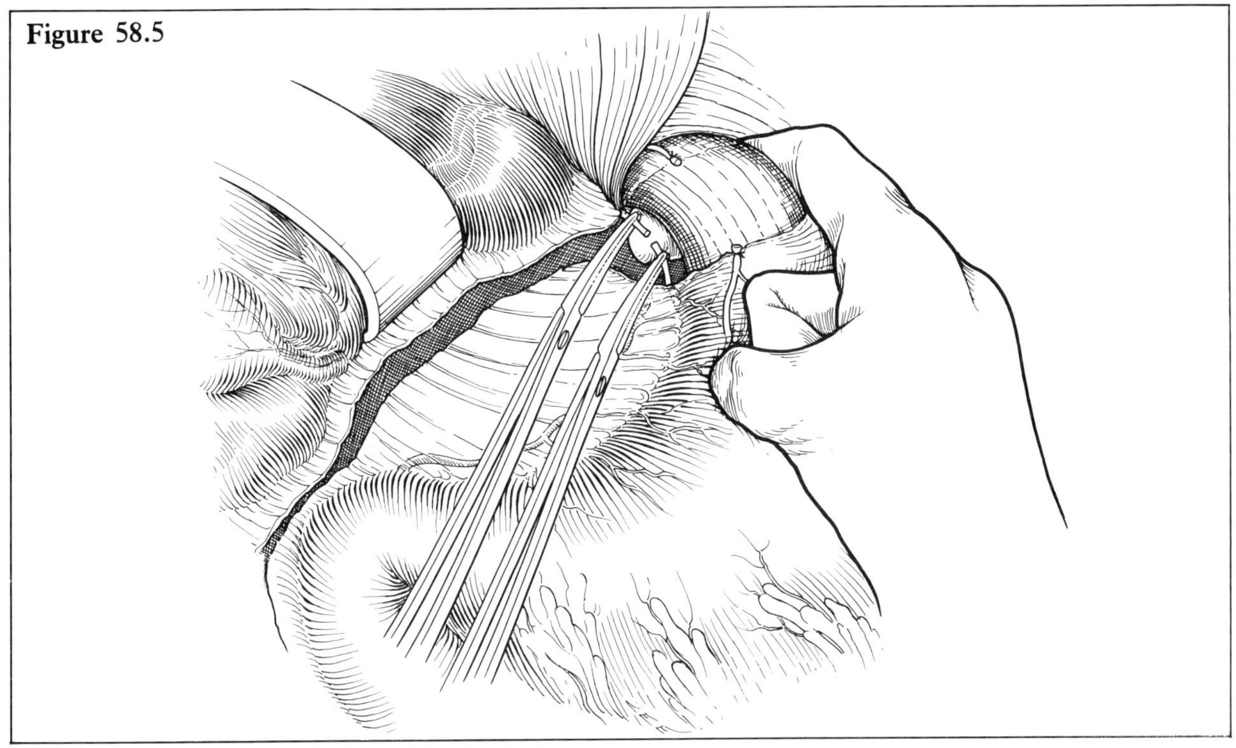

**Figure 58.6**

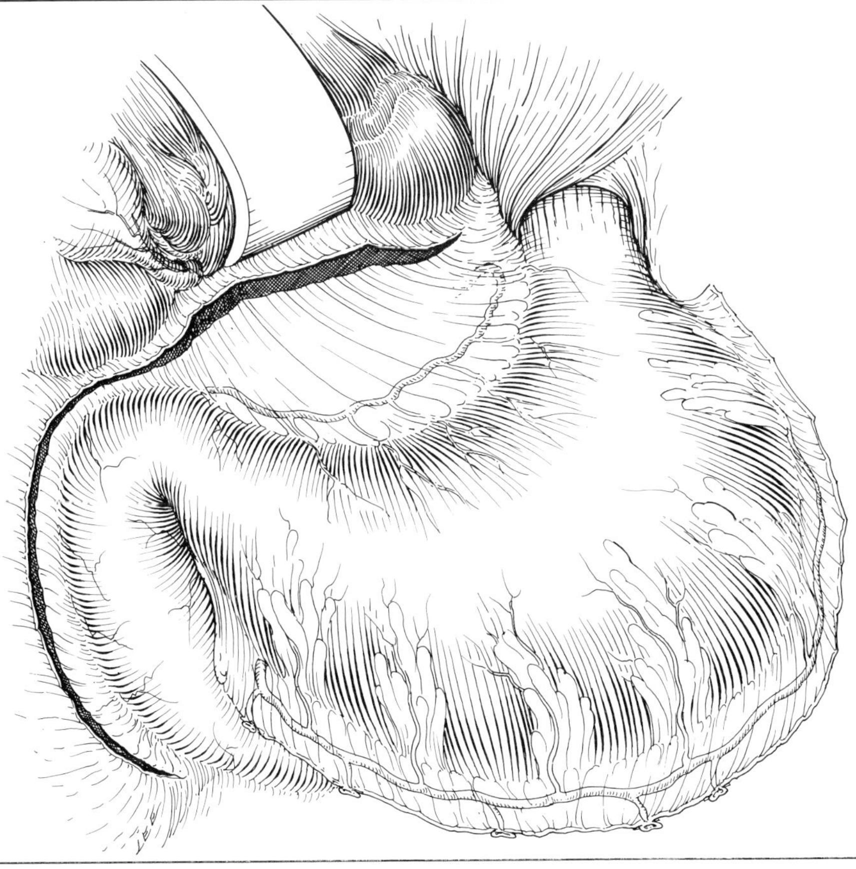

**Figure 58.7**

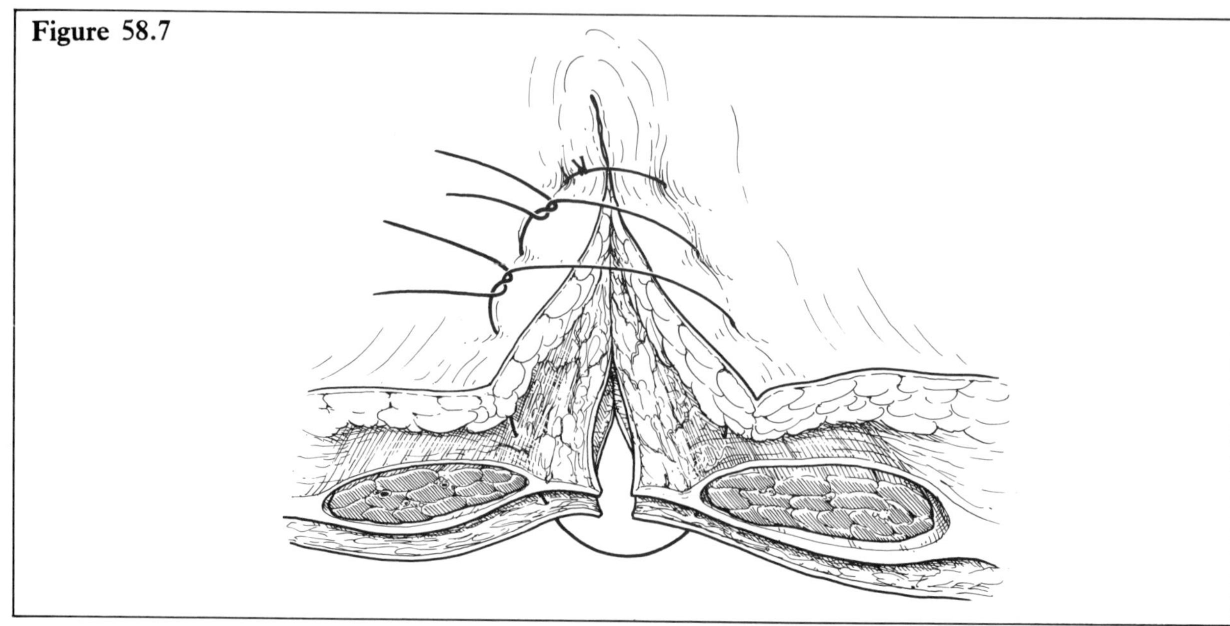

achieved. The abdomen is closed with a single layer looped nylon suture for the muscle and absorbable sutures for the fat and skin (**Fig. 58.7**). No drain is necessary.

## Thoracic stage

The patient is placed in the left lateral position and a right posterolateral thoracotomy is performed, stripping the periosteum from the lower border of the sixth rib. The lung is deflated and retracted forwards. The pulmonary ligament is divided and the mediastinal pleura incised over the whole length of the oesophagus (**Fig. 58.8**). The azygos vein is divided between ligatures (**Fig. 58.9**).

The oesophagus is mobilized from its bed and tapes are passed around it above and below the tumour (**Fig. 58.10**). Dissection proceeds centripet-

**Figure 58.8**

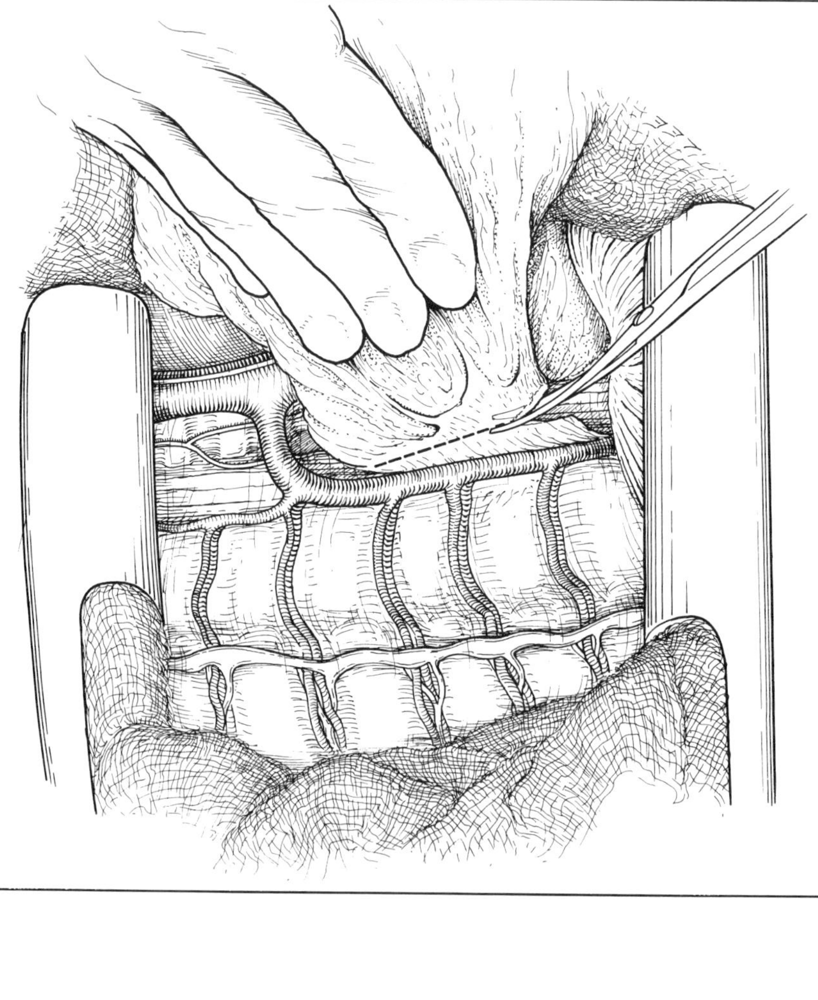

Figure 58.9

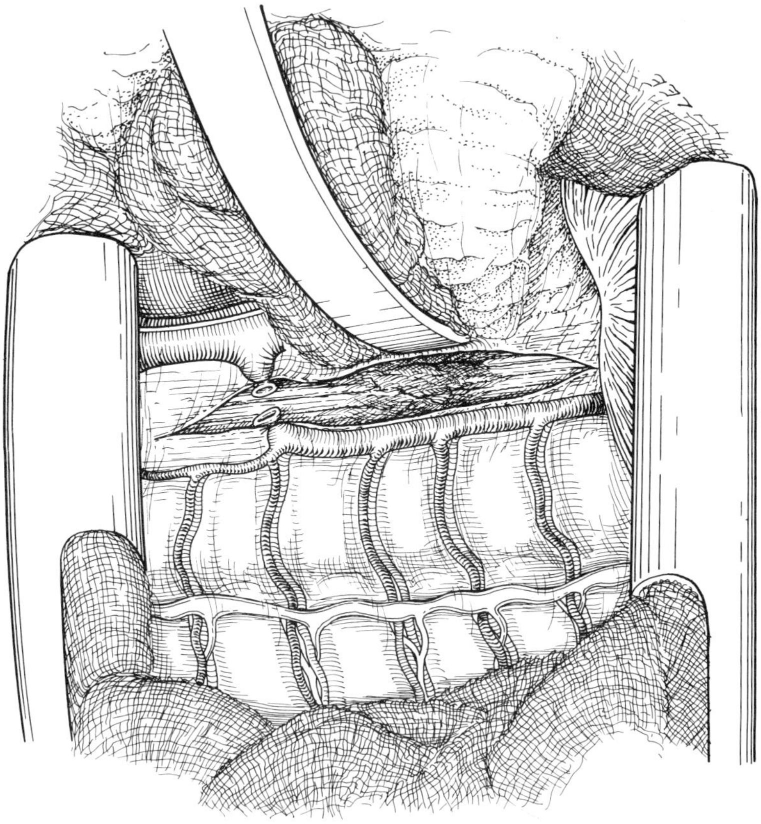

Figure 58.10

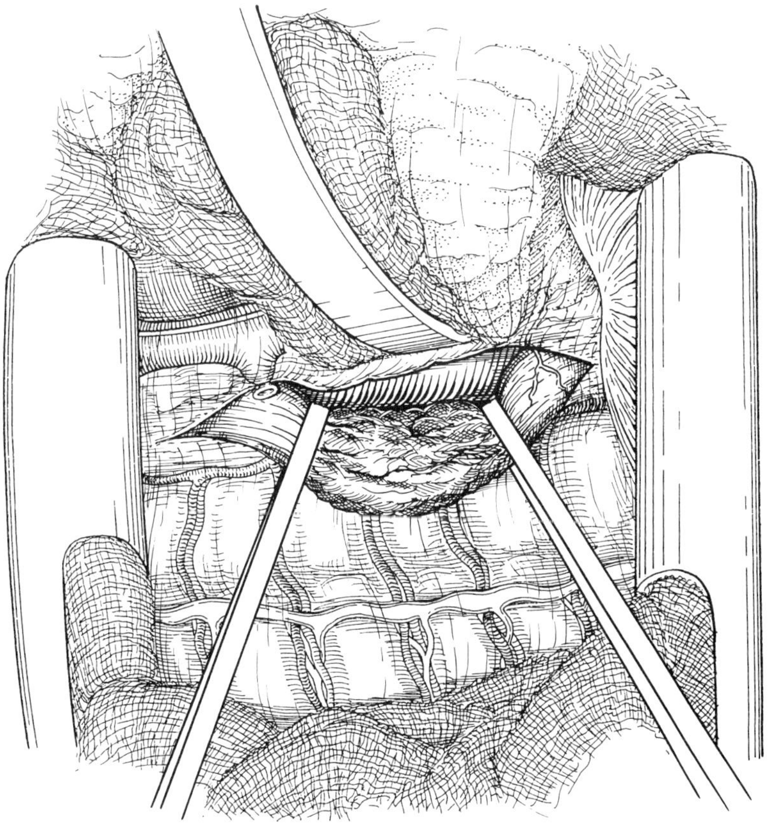

Figure 58.11

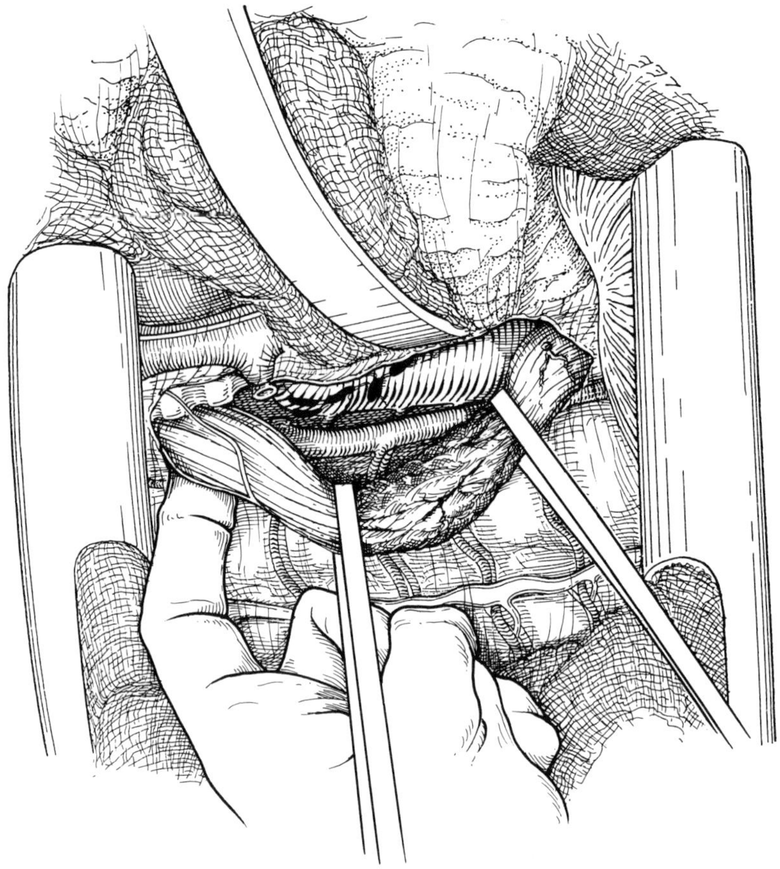

Figure 58.12

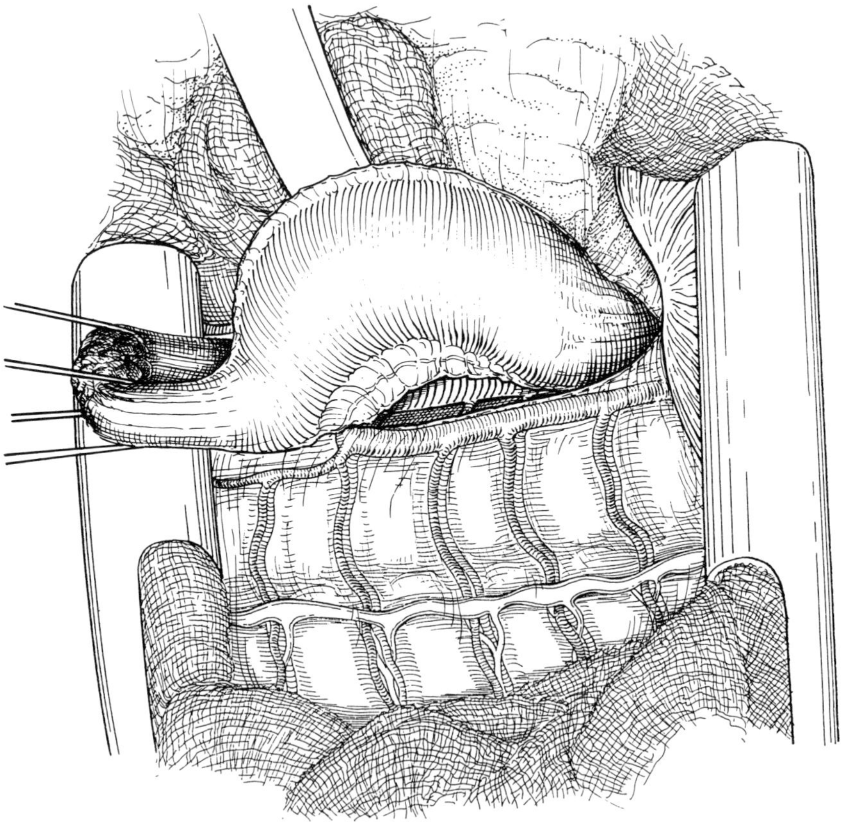

ally towards the tumour, which must be separated from the aorta, the trachea and main bronchi (**Fig. 58.11**). The carinal lymph nodes, which may contain metastases, are removed together with the oesophagus. The oesophageal vessels should be ligated as they are encountered. If one of them is torn from the aorta its origin should be secured with a 4/0 polypropylene stitch. The mobilization of the oesophagus should continue up to the root of the neck.

Traction on the oesophagus will now bring the stomach into view through the oesophageal hiatus. A few strands of mediastinal tissue may require division. After mobilization the stomach was left in the abdomen in its anatomical position, and this should be retained as it is drawn into the thorax, i.e. the greater curvature should remain to the patient's left and the lesser curvature to the right (**Fig. 58.12**).

The oesophagogastric anastomosis is then constructed as described on pp. 231–3. If the upper margin of the tumour is within 10 cm of the root of the neck an adequate clearance will not be obtained with an anastomosis in the chest. In such cases a cervical anastomosis is necessary.

### Cervical anastomosis

The oesophagus is mobilized by blunt dissection from the thoracic inlet as far as possible into the neck. If the tumour is too bulky to pass through the thoracic inlet, the stomach is transected as described on pp. 229–30 and the oesophagus is divided above the tumour. The tumour-bearing portion of oesophagus and stomach is then removed. The proximal end of the oesophagus is closed with a ligature, and the end of the stomach tube attached to the end of the oesophagus with two sutures which help to retain the anatomical position and prevent gastric torsion. Two drainage tubes are inserted into the pleural cavity and the thoracic incision is closed.

The patient is placed supine, and the cervical oesophagus exposed as described on pp. 248–51. When it has been fully mobilized, traction on it draws the end of the stomach into the cervical incision. The anastomosis is then carried out as described on pp. 231–3.

# Other methods of oesophageal reconstruction

# 59 Replacement of the oesophagus with a reversed gastric tube

## Indications

This procedure (also known as the Gavriliu–Heimlich operation) is a valuable alternative technique for bypassing the oesophagus in cases of corrosive or peptic strictures where the cardia cannot be retained. It has also been used for bypass of carcinomas of the middle third of the oesophagus, and for congenital anomalies such as oesophageal atresia where primary reconstruction has not proved feasible. It is particularly applicable in cases where the jejunum and colon have been rejected for oesophageal replacement, and also when thoracotomy is inadvisable, perhaps because of previous intrathoracic disease or operations.

The advantages of a reversed gastric tube are that it has a remarkably good blood supply; and since the vessels supplying it run parallel to its edge, they are less liable to torsion, kinking or obstruction from excessive tension, as may sometimes occur with mesenteric vessels when colon or jejunum is used.

A previous gastrostomy is not a contraindication to this technique. However, when a gastrostomy is planned as a preliminary to this operation it should be made towards the lesser curvature of the stomach.

## Procedure

The patient is placed in a supine position, and the abdomen is opened by an upper midline or transverse incision according to the shape of the subcostal arch (**Fig. 59.1**). The stomach is drawn out and the gastroepiploic arch inspected to ensure there is no interruption in its continuity.

The lienorenal ligament is now incised (**Fig. 59.2**), the spleen elevated into the wound and a splenectomy performed. The splenic vessels must be ligated deep in the hilum of the spleen so that the origins of the short gastric and left gastroepiploic arteries are preserved (**Fig. 59.3**). The tail of the pancreas is then mobilized from its bed; this increases the mobility of the fundus of the stomach.

The greater omentum is divided all the way along the greater curvature about 1 cm distal to the gastroepiploic arch. Branches from the gastroepiploic vessels supplying the omentum are ligated and divided. The right gastroepiploic artery is divided about 4 cm from the pylorus (**Fig. 59.4**).

**Figure 59.1**

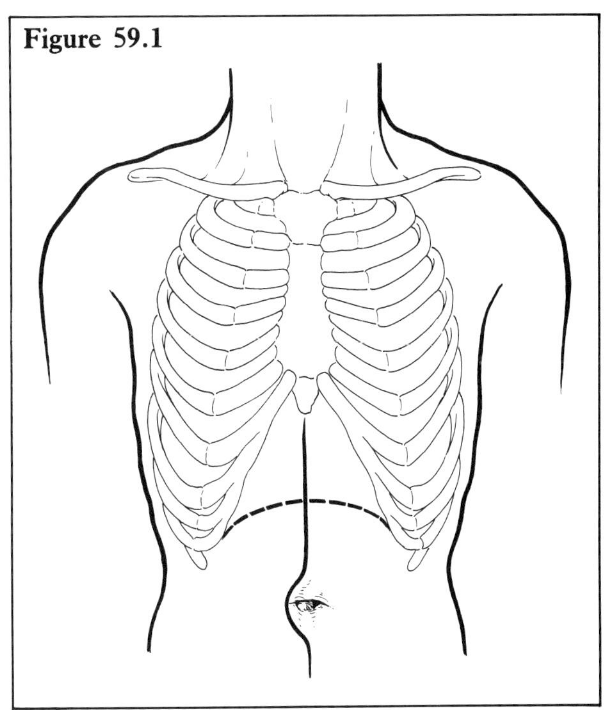

An incision is then made into the antrum at right angles to the greater curvature for a distance of 3 cm along each surface of the stomach. A size 40 Hurst–Maloney bougie is passed into the stomach, manipulated so that it lies along the greater curvature throughout its length, and fixed in this position by a few interrupted sutures (**Fig. 59.5**). An incision is then made parallel to the greater curvature of the stomach, between the tube and the remainder of the stomach as far as the fundus. The incision is made a short distance (3–4 cm) at a time, and both pairs of cut edges are closed with continuous 2/0 catgut sutures as the mobilization proceeds. Care must be taken that the incision is not made so close to the bougie that it creates tension when the cut edges are sutured around it (**Fig. 59.6**).

Formation of this gastric tube is greatly facilitated by the use of a GIA stapling device, which inserts two parallel rows of sutures and cuts between them.

Figure 59.2

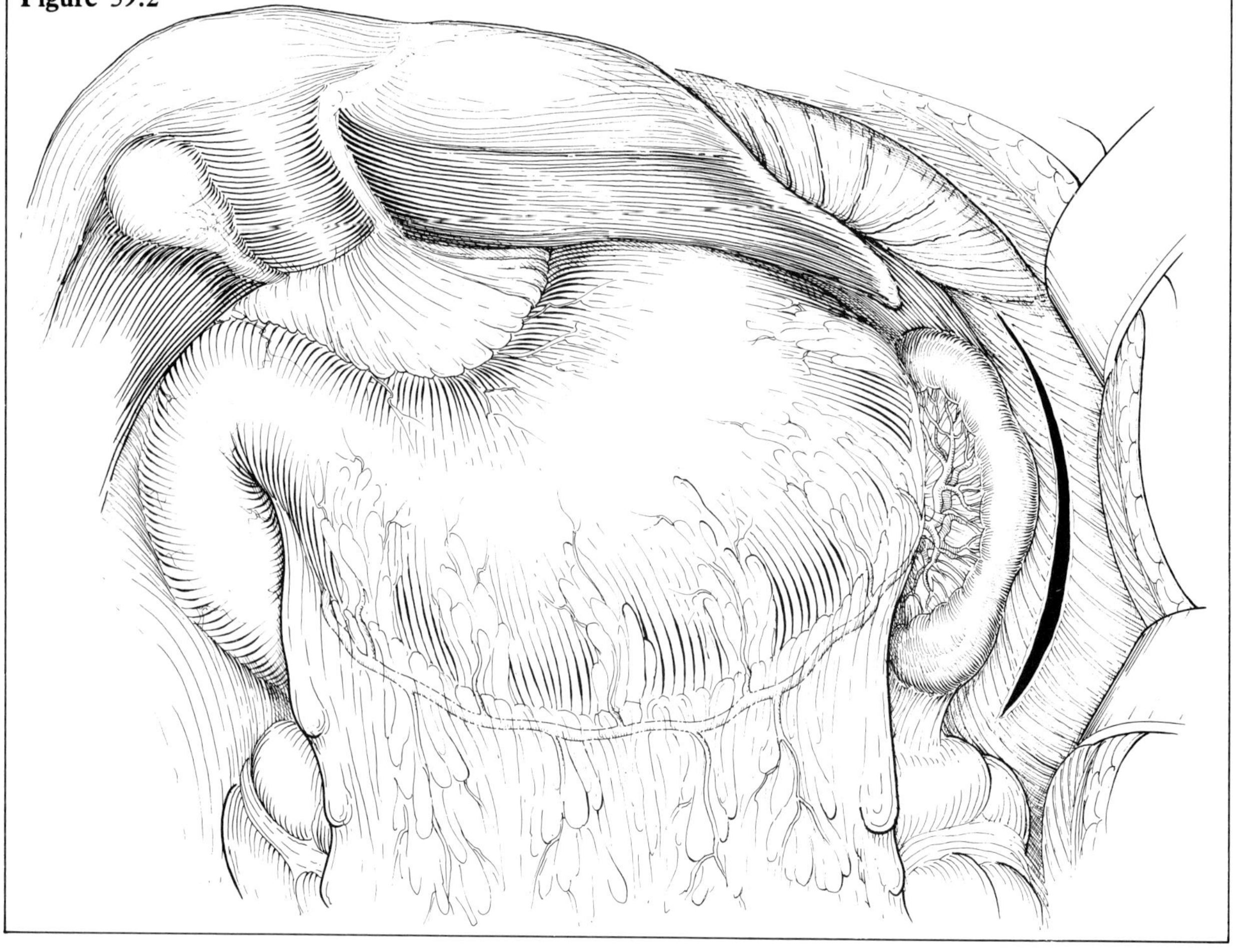

Figure 59.3

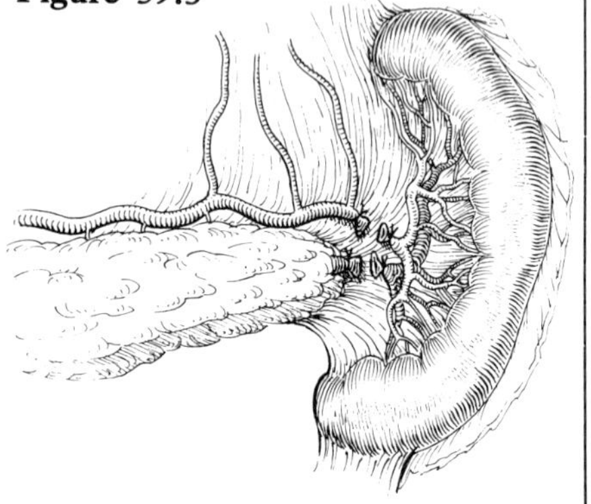

Figure 59.4

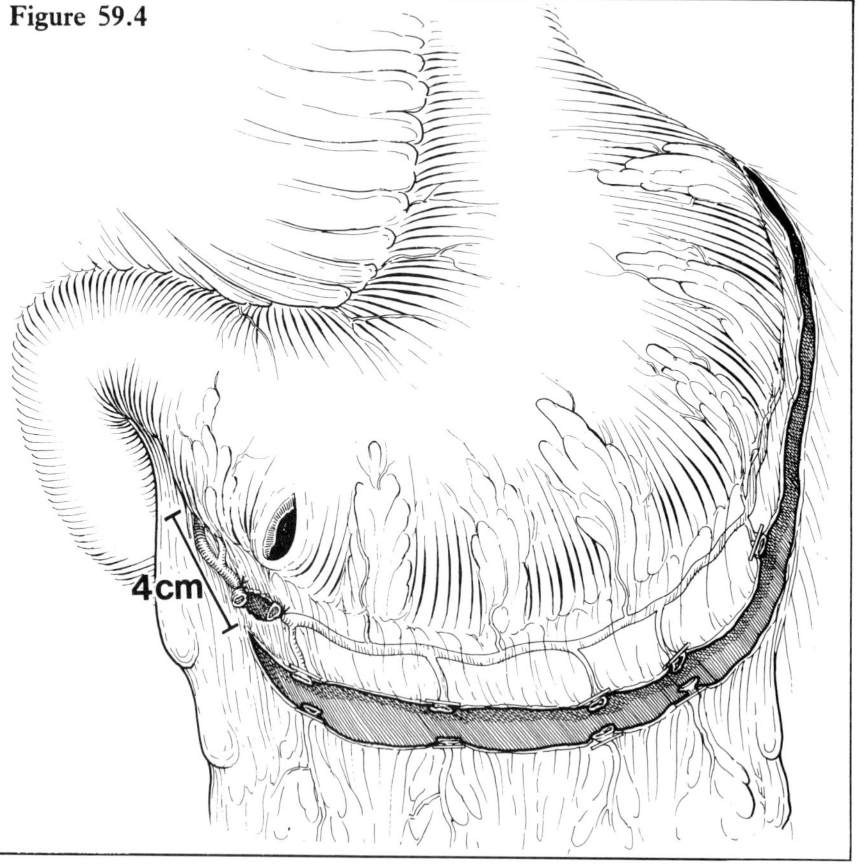

4cm

Figure 59.5

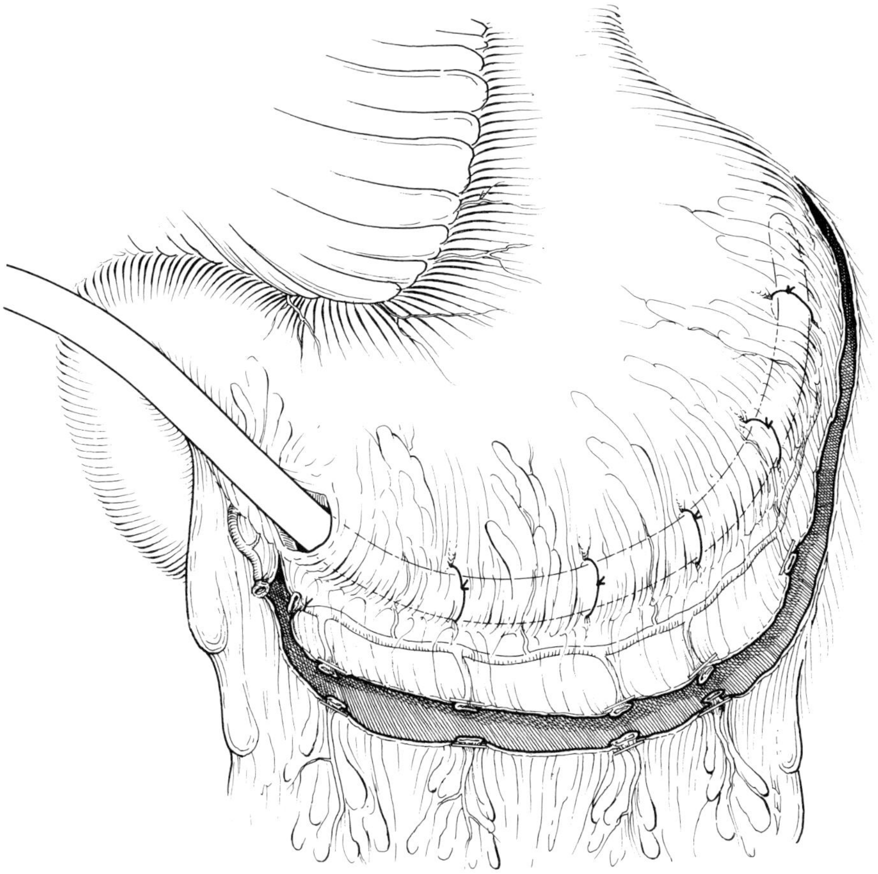

Figure 59.6

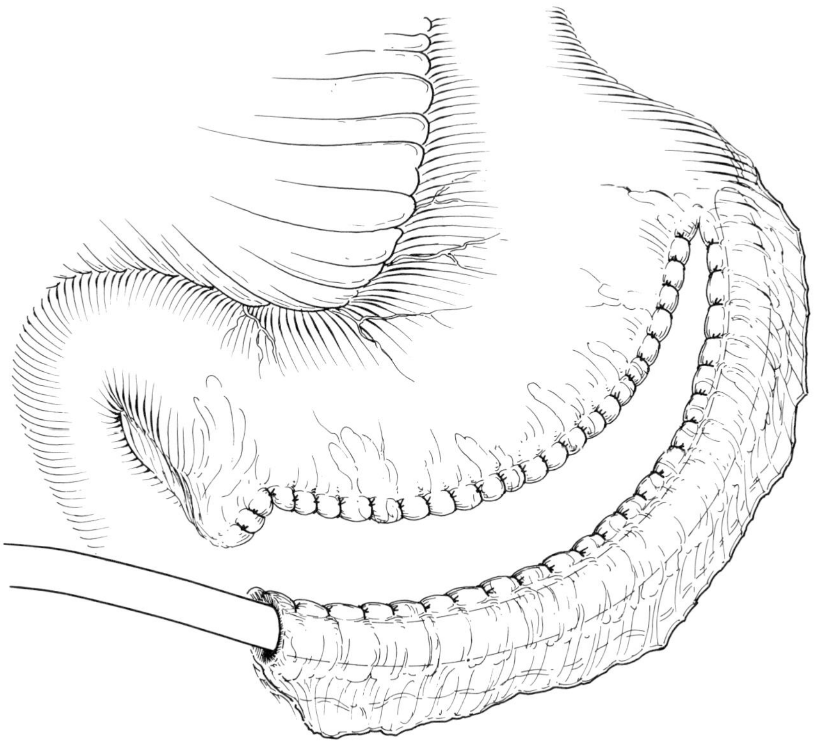

Figure 59.7

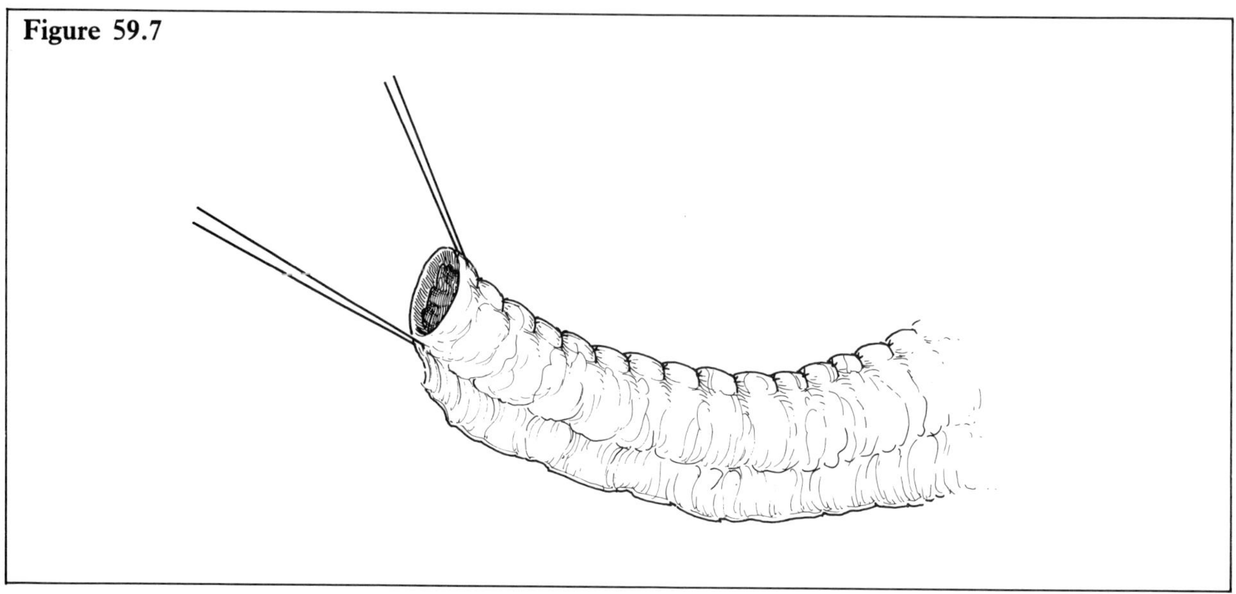

The tube length should be 30–35 cm; when this has been achieved the suture or staple line is oversewn with interrupted 3/0 polypropylene sutures to approximate the serous surfaces, but without producing invagination of the underlying continuous suture line. Interrupted sutures should be used to prevent shortening. The bougie is now removed. Two traction sutures are placed in the wall of the open end of the gastric tube, to draw the tube into the neck (**Fig. 59.7**).

The cervical incision, which can be right- or left-sided, is made in a skin crease about 4 cm above the suprasternal notch and reaches posteriorly just beyond the external jugular vein (**Fig. 59.8**). Anteriorly it crosses the midline by 1 cm. The platysma muscle is divided in the line of the incision, and the two flaps of skin and platysma are dissected downwards as far as the clavicle and suprasternal notch, and upwards to the level of the thyroid cartilage. This exposes the deep cervical fascia and the anterior border of the sternomastoid muscle (**Fig. 59.9**). The fascia is divided along the anterior border of this muscle which is retracted laterally, exposing the carotid sheath and the omohyoid muscle, which is divided (**Fig. 59.10**). The middle thyroid vein is identified entering the

Figure 59.8

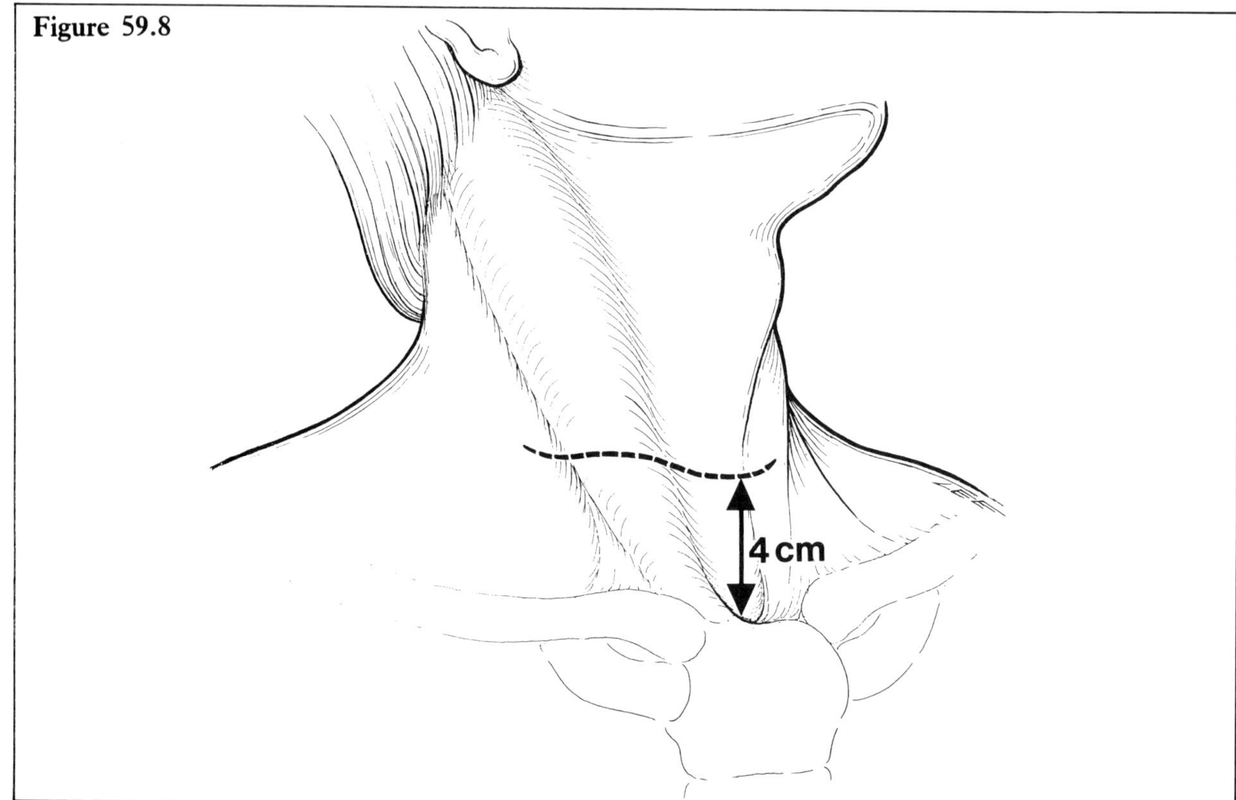

Figure 59.9

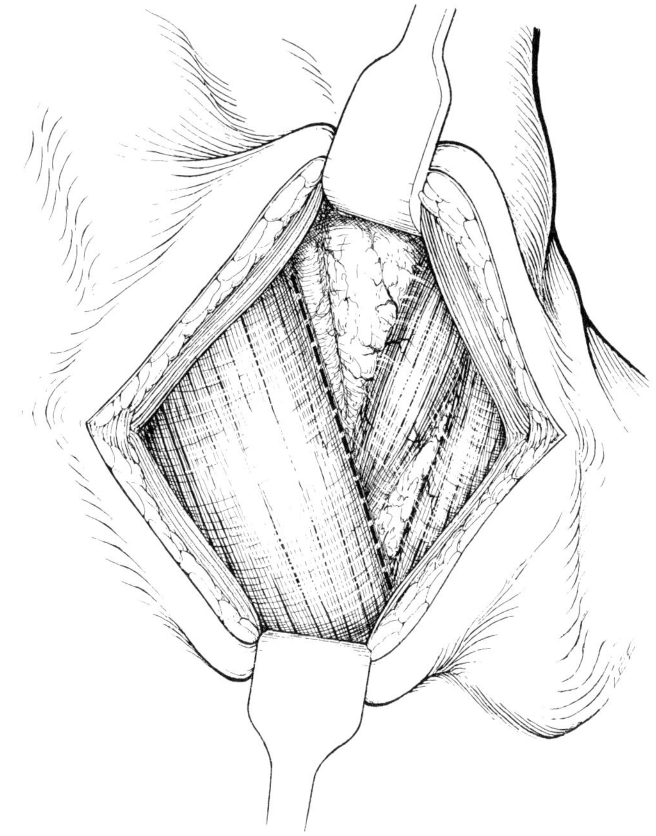

Figure 59.10

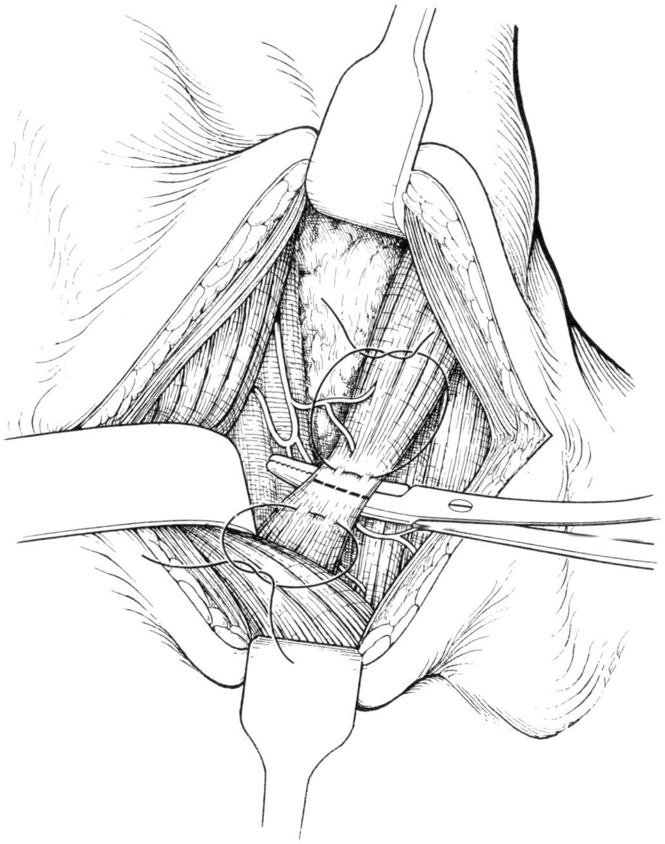

**Figure 59.11**

**Figure 59.12**

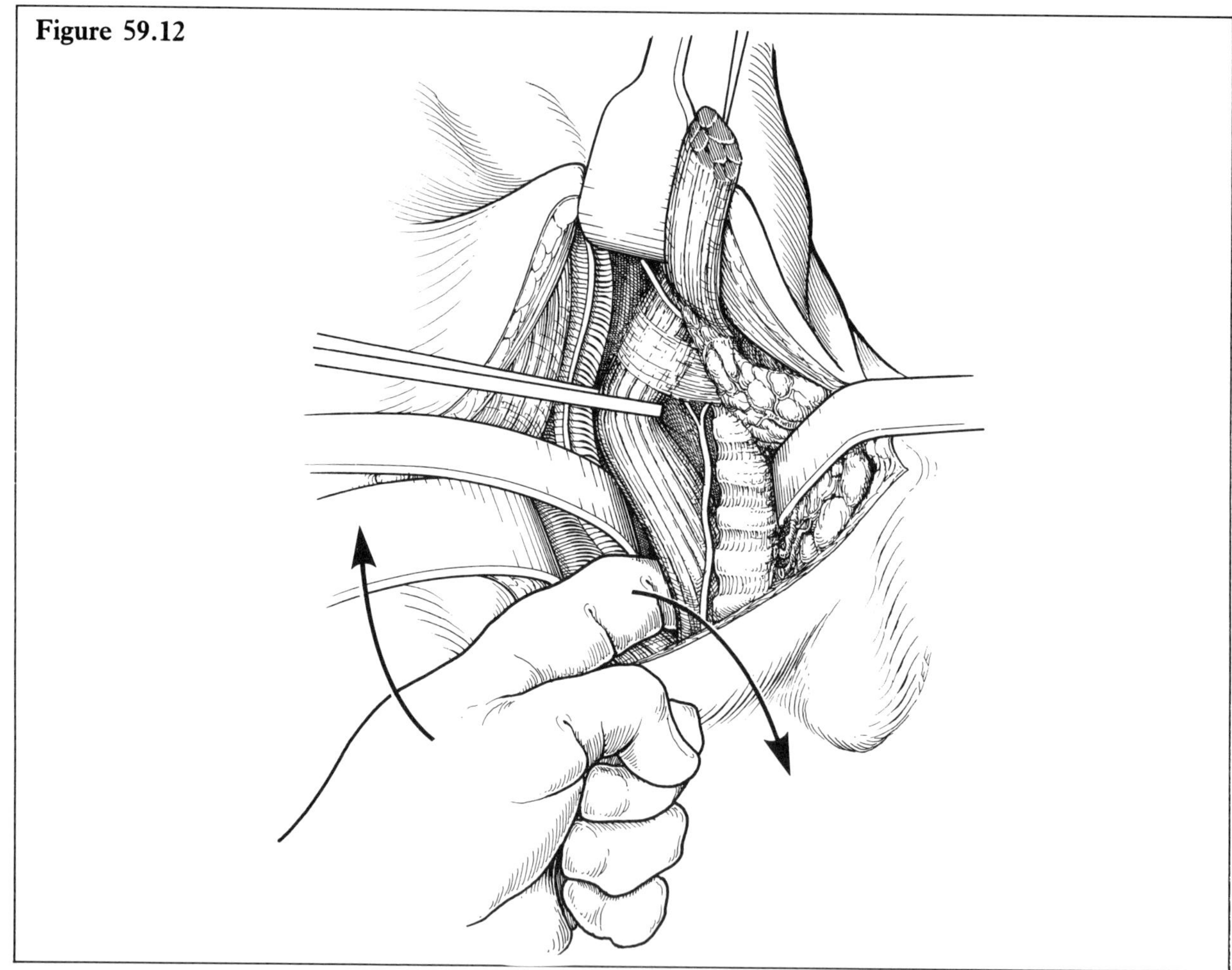

internal jugular vein, and divided between ligatures (**Fig. 59.11**). The right lobe of the thyroid gland is retracted medially, and the carotid sheath laterally. By blunt dissection between these two structures, the trachea and oesophagus are exposed with the recurrent laryngeal nerve lying in the groove between them (**Fig. 59.11**). This nerve should be identified and carefully preserved. The trachea is retracted medially and the whole circumference of the oesophagus gradually mobilized, leaving the recurrent laryngeal nerves behind. A tape is passed around the oesophagus, and by traction on it and blunt dissection with the index finger, the oesophagus is mobilized downwards and freed from the trachea (**Fig. 59.12**).

Attention is now turned to the abdomen; the two slips of diaphragm attached to the back of the xiphisternum are separated, the xiphisternum excised and a finger passed up beneath the sternum. The opening is gradually widened until two fingers can be passed up behind the sternum, separating the pleural sacs from it while taking great care to avoid opening them. At the same time a finger is passed downwards from the suprasternal notch exactly in the midline and between the strap muscles of the neck. It must pass anterior to the brachiocephalic artery, the arch of the aorta and brachiocephalic vein, and keep strictly and closely to the posterior surface of the sternum (**Fig. 59.13**). Two fingers are now inserted into each of the upper and lower incisions, and the retrosternal space is enlarged by sweeping the fingers from side to side until the fingers passed from above meet those passed from below, and the tunnel is completed.

Next, a 100 $cm^3$ Foley catheter is passed from above downwards in the retrosternal tunnel until the balloon end is in the abdomen. This end is tied to the stay sutures on the stomach tube, taking care to maintain the orientation (**Fig. 59.14**). If the balloon is then inflated and withdrawn into

**Figure 59.13**

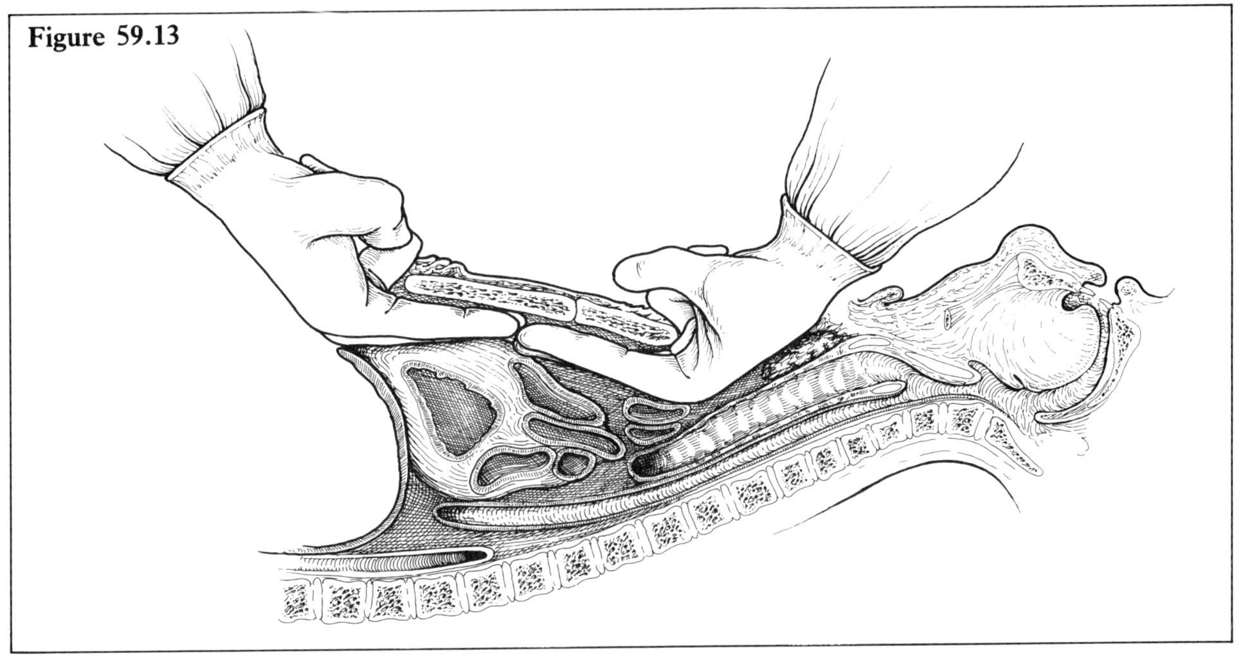

**Figure 59.14**

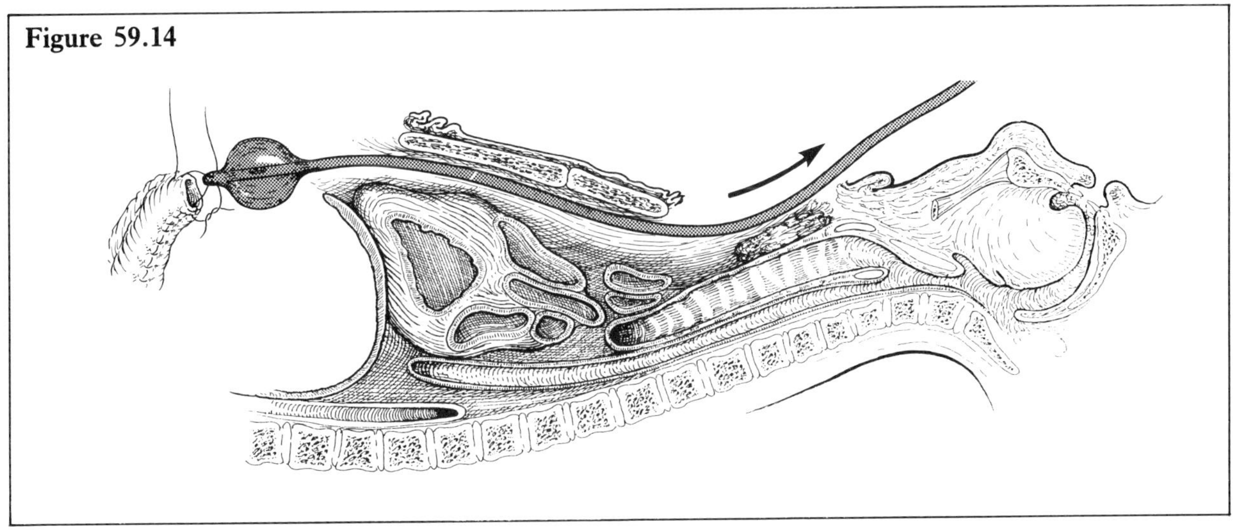

**Figure 59.15**

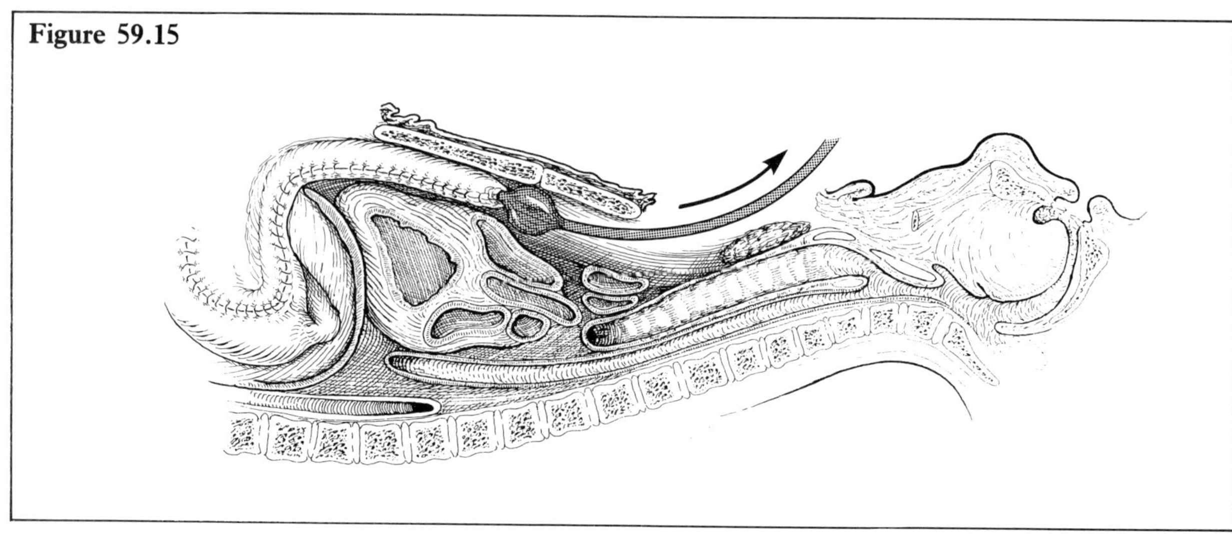

**Figure 59.16**

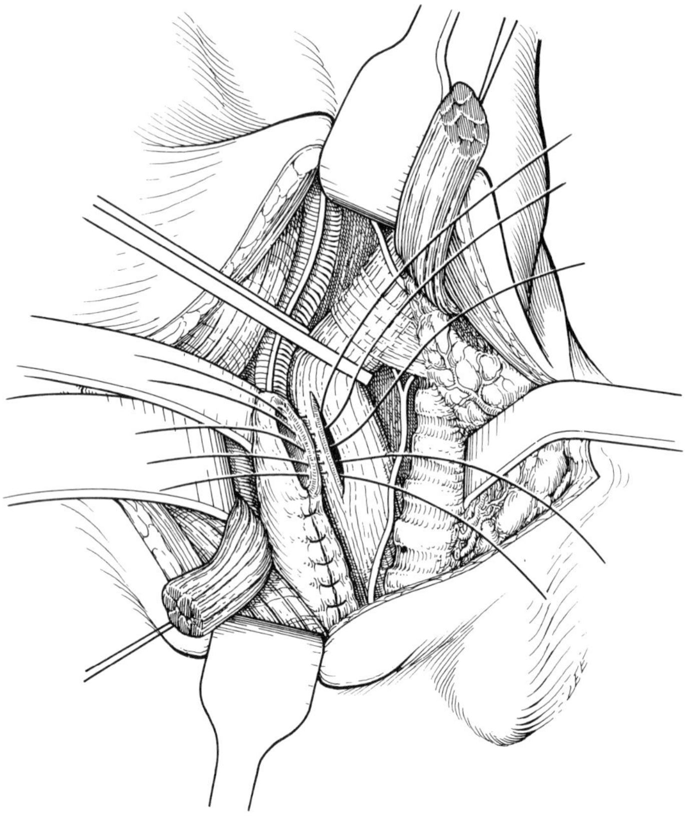

the suprasternal space, the stomach tube will be drawn behind it without compression (**Fig. 59.15**).

Cervical anastomosis

The upper end of the now reversed stomach tube is anastomosed in end-to-side fashion to the oesophagus. A longitudinal incision is made through all coats of the oesophagus, and the two structures are joined with interrupted, non-absorbable polypropylene sutures (**Fig. 59.16**).

Closure

The abdominal wound is closed with a looped monofilament nylon suture using the mass closure technique described on p. 238. The cervical incision is closed over a silicone drain sited close to the anastomosis. The omohyoid muscle is reconstructed with an absorbable suture such as chromic catgut or polygalactin. The platysma is closed with a further polygalactin suture, and the skin with skin clips or an interrupted polypropylene suture (**Fig. 59.17**). If skin clips are used, the clip remover must be kept at the patient's bedside at all times for speedy removal of the clips should bleeding occur.

**Figure 59.17**

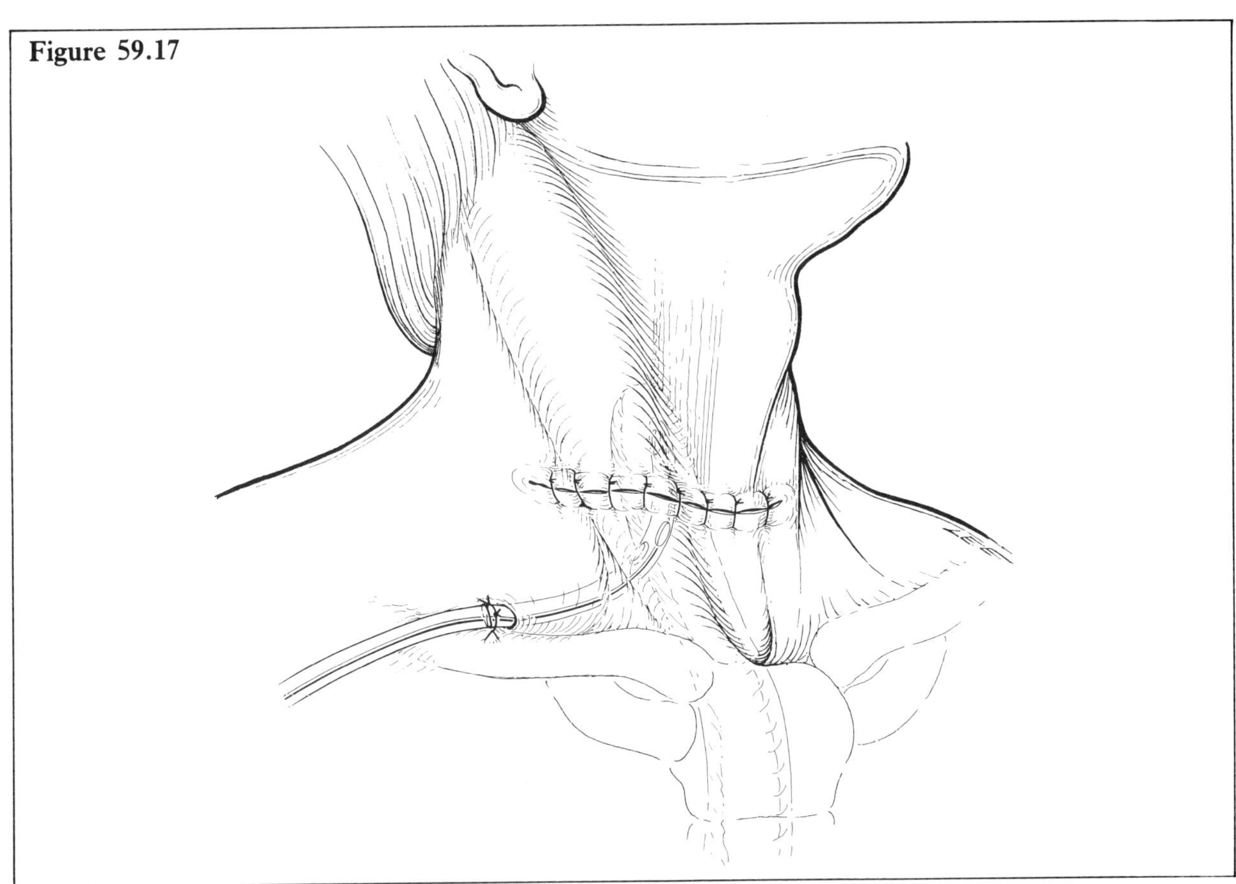

# 60 Colonic replacement of the oesophagus

The advantage of using colon for oesophageal replacement rather than the jejunum is that its vascular arcade is arranged in such a way that a long vascularized segment can be more easily mobilized. With the exception of rare cases of disease of the colic vessels, the colon can easily be advanced as far as the neck. The disadvantage is its slower and infrequent peristalsis, which delays the passage of food. Necrosis of a colonic transplant can be due to venous infarction as well as arterial occlusion, and therefore equal attention must be paid to the avoidance of any tension or kinking in the mobilized mesentery that could obstruct the veins. The indications include:

1. Caustic strictures of the oesophagus.
2. Restoration of continuity when oesophageal perforation has necessitated cervical oesophagostomy and gastrostomy.
3. Restoration of continuity in cases of oesophageal atresia where a primary anastomosis has proved impossible.
4. Restoration of continuity after resection of benign strictures.
5. Rare cases of gastro-oesophageal carcinoma where the stomach cannot be used for continuity, e.g. after a partial gastrectomy.

### Preoperative preparation

Preliminary arteriography is advisable to confirm the normality of the colonic blood supply.

The preparation of the colon requires only the administration of a low-residue diet for five days. At operation the contents of the colon will then be quite solid and can easily be squeezed out at the site of the incision without risk of fluid contents soiling the peritoneal cavity. The details of the operation vary according to the site of the anastomosis.

## Anastomosis below the level of the inferior pulmonary vein

The patient is placed in the right lateral position, with the chest and abdomen rotated backwards through 30 degrees. A left thoracotomy is performed through the seventh intercostal space. The anterior half of the diaphragm is detached from the chest wall, leaving a 1-cm margin for subsequent repair. The oesophagus and stomach are mobilized; the stomach is divided obliquely and the distal cut end closed as described on pp. 229–30.

The left half of the colon is now mobilized by incising the parietal peritoneal reflection (**Fig. 60.1**). The mesocolon with its accompanying vessels is dissected towards the midline. The greater omentum is detached from the transverse colon as far as the middle colic artery (**Fig. 60.2**). The colon is drawn up into the thoracic wound and the arterial supply inspected and palpated; identification of the arterial supply is facilitated by transillumination. The proposed lines of resection are illustrated in **Fig. 60.3**. The colon and vascular arcade are divided to the left of the middle colic artery, or further to the right after division of that artery if a greater length is necessary. The left colic artery now supplies the whole of the transposed colon via its marginal artery (**Fig. 60.4**). Any solid faecal material is squeezed out of the two ends of the colon into large packs and removed. The ends of the colon are wrapped in warm, moist swabs.

The oesophagus is now mobilized in the thorax up to the proposed level of the anastomosis and a tape is passed around it. Traction on the tape allows dissection of the cardia from the hiatus. The upper end of the stomach is then drawn into the thorax and turned upwards over the costal margin.

**Figure 60.1**

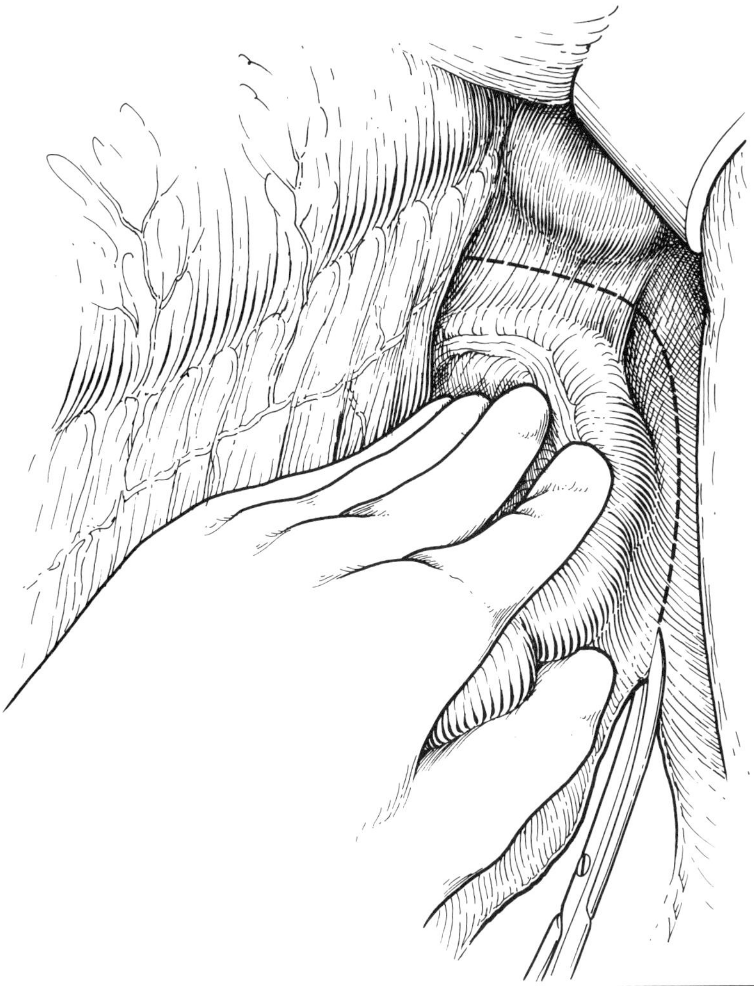

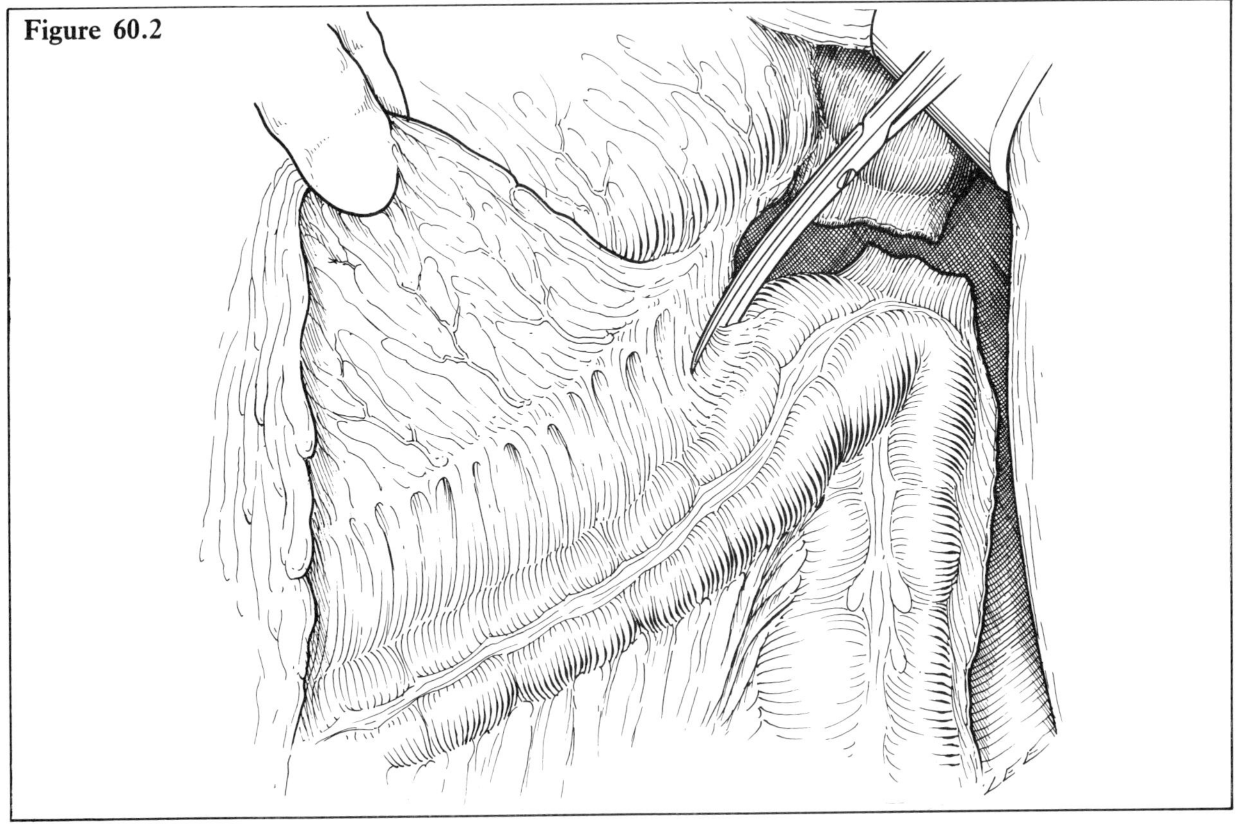

**Figure 60.2**

**Figure 60.3**

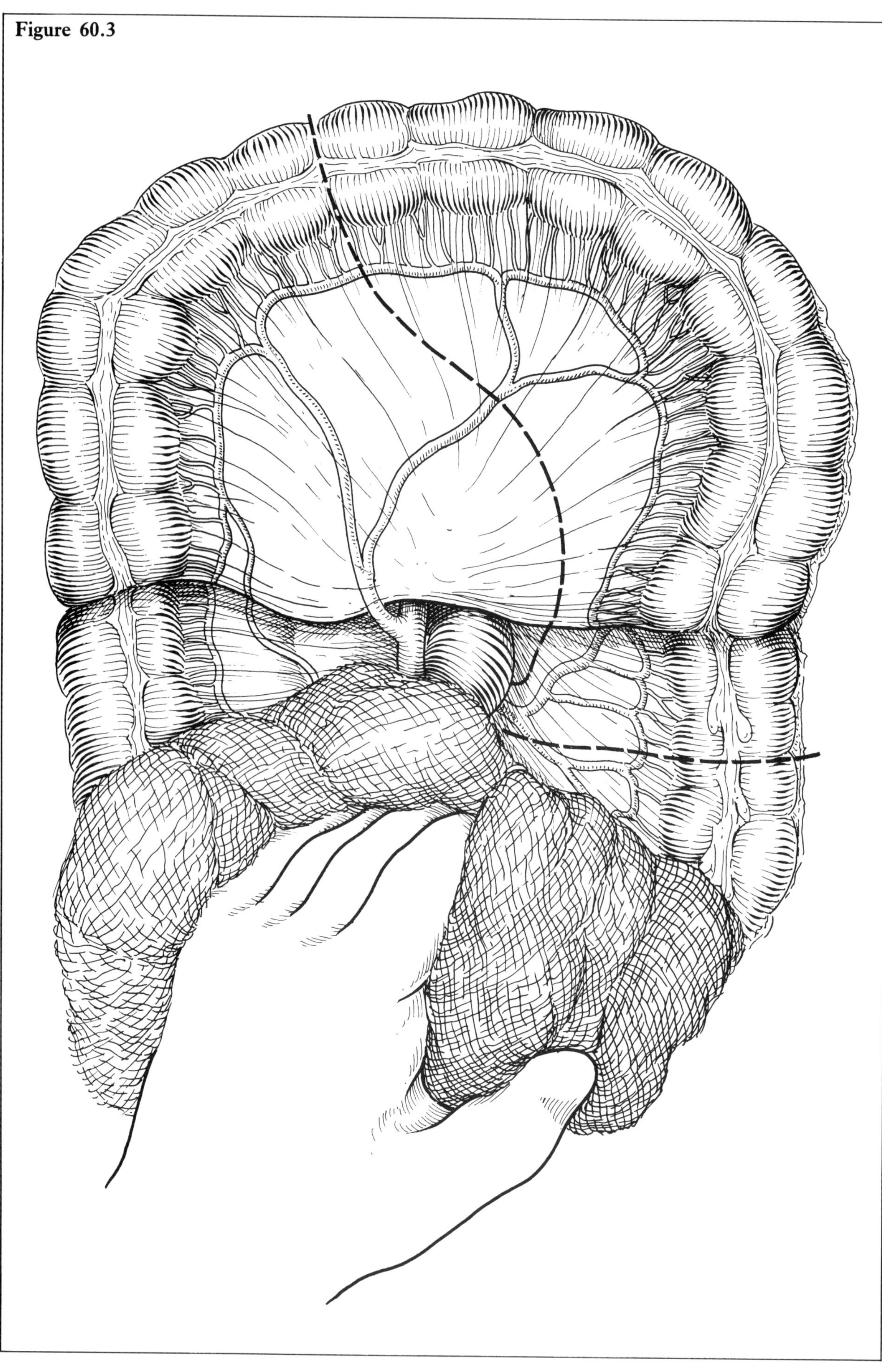

Figure 60.4

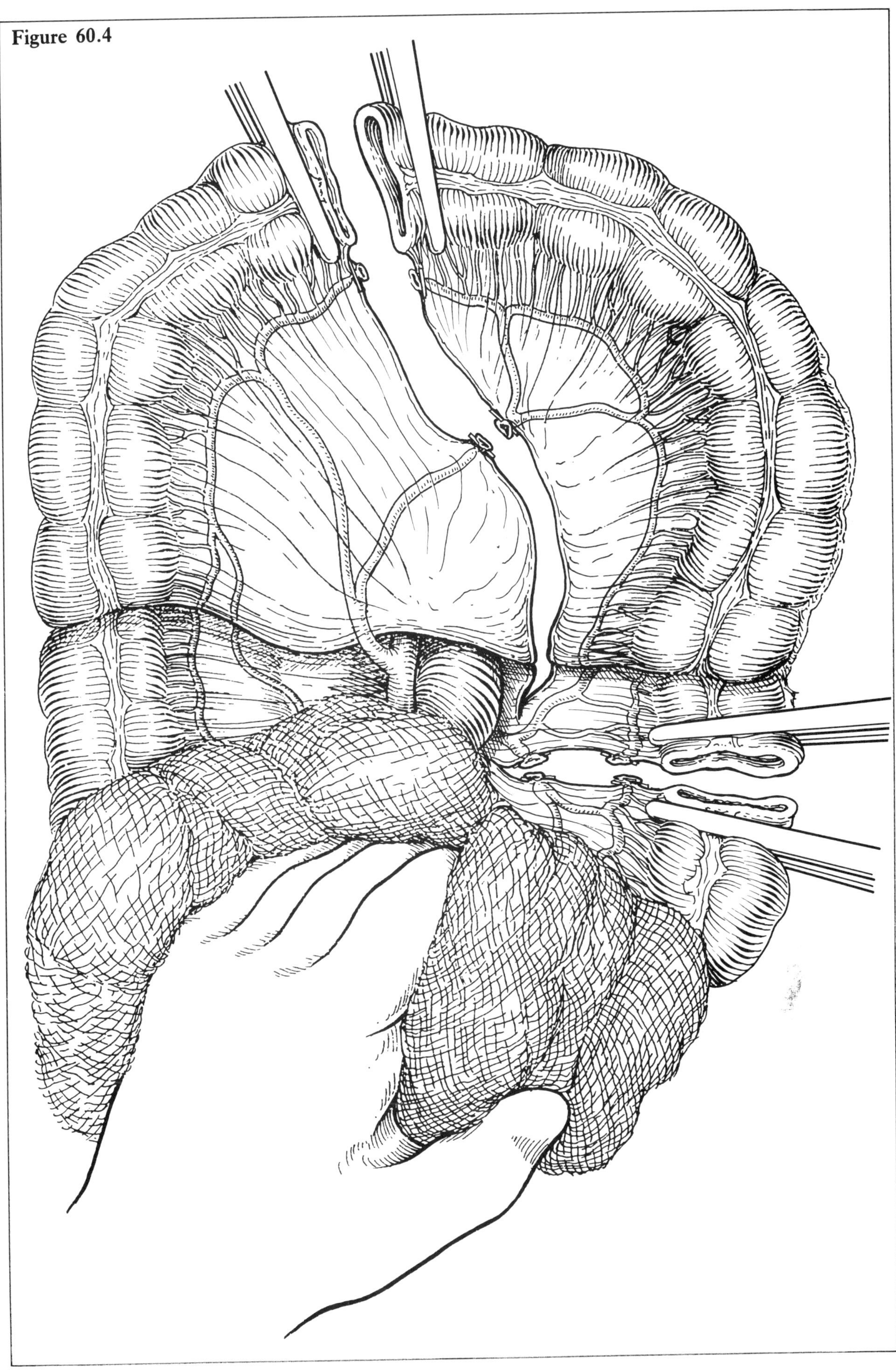

Figure 60.5

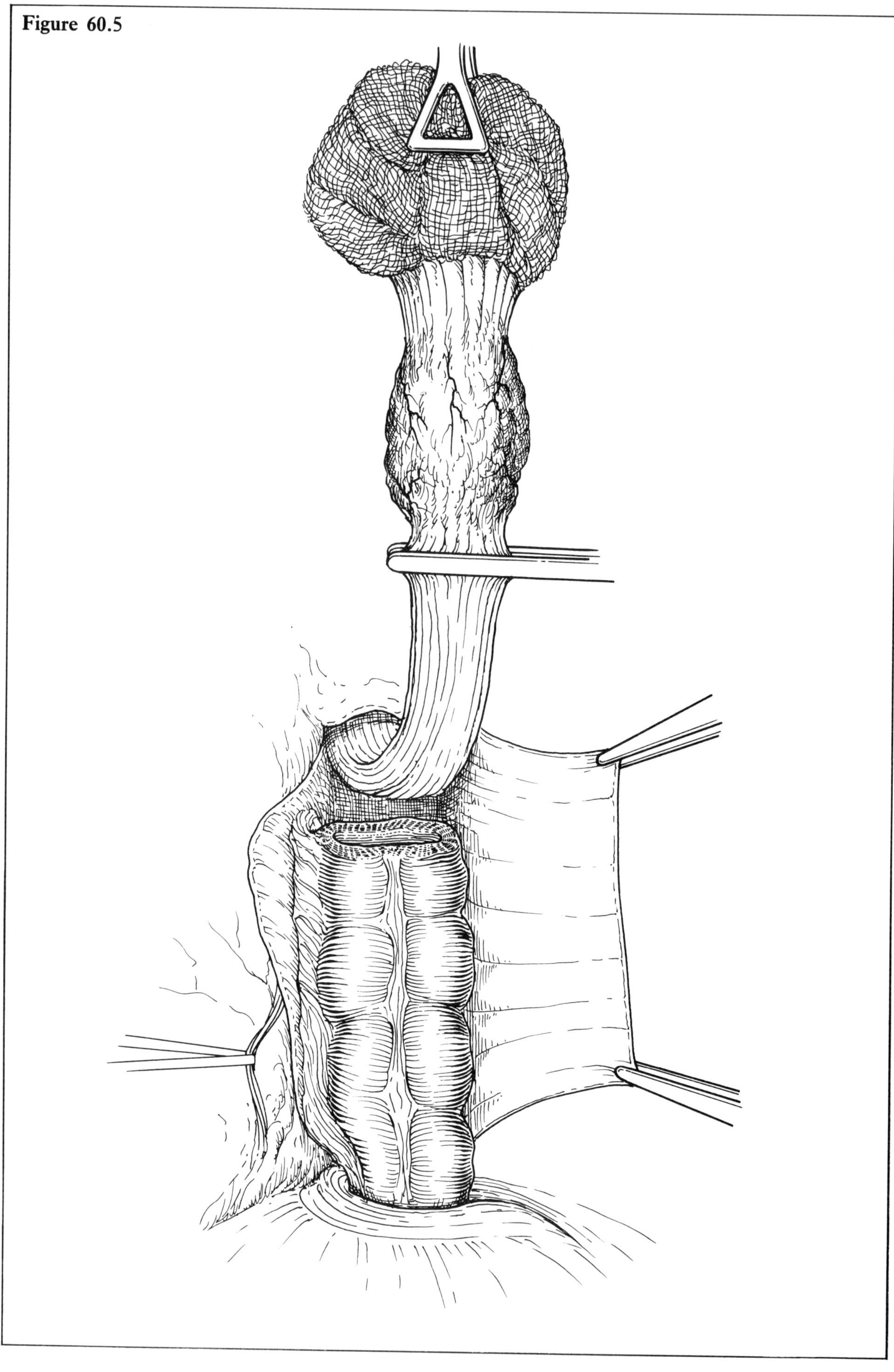

## Proximal anastomosis

The colon is inspected to ensure that it remains pink and that its marginal artery is pulsating. If not, it must be cut back to where the blood supply is adequate. The colon is then drawn upwards through the lesser sac, behind the stomach, in front of the pancreas, and through the oesophageal hiatus (**Fig. 60.5**). The colon is anastomosed to the oesophagus with a single-layer, interrupted, all-coats suture of non-absorbable material (see **Fig. 57.21**, p. 233). Alternatively, an annular stapling device may be used (pp. 270–73). The colon and particularly its pedicle must be quite relaxed and without tension.

## Distal anastomosis

The colon is transected just above the lowest point of the greater curvature of the stomach. A 5-cm incision is made in the posterior wall of the stomach near the greater curvature, and the gastric contents are sucked out. The colon is anastomosed to this opening using an inner continuous 3/0 polypropylene suture, and an outer interrupted layer of the same material (**Fig. 60.6**).

**Figure 60.6**

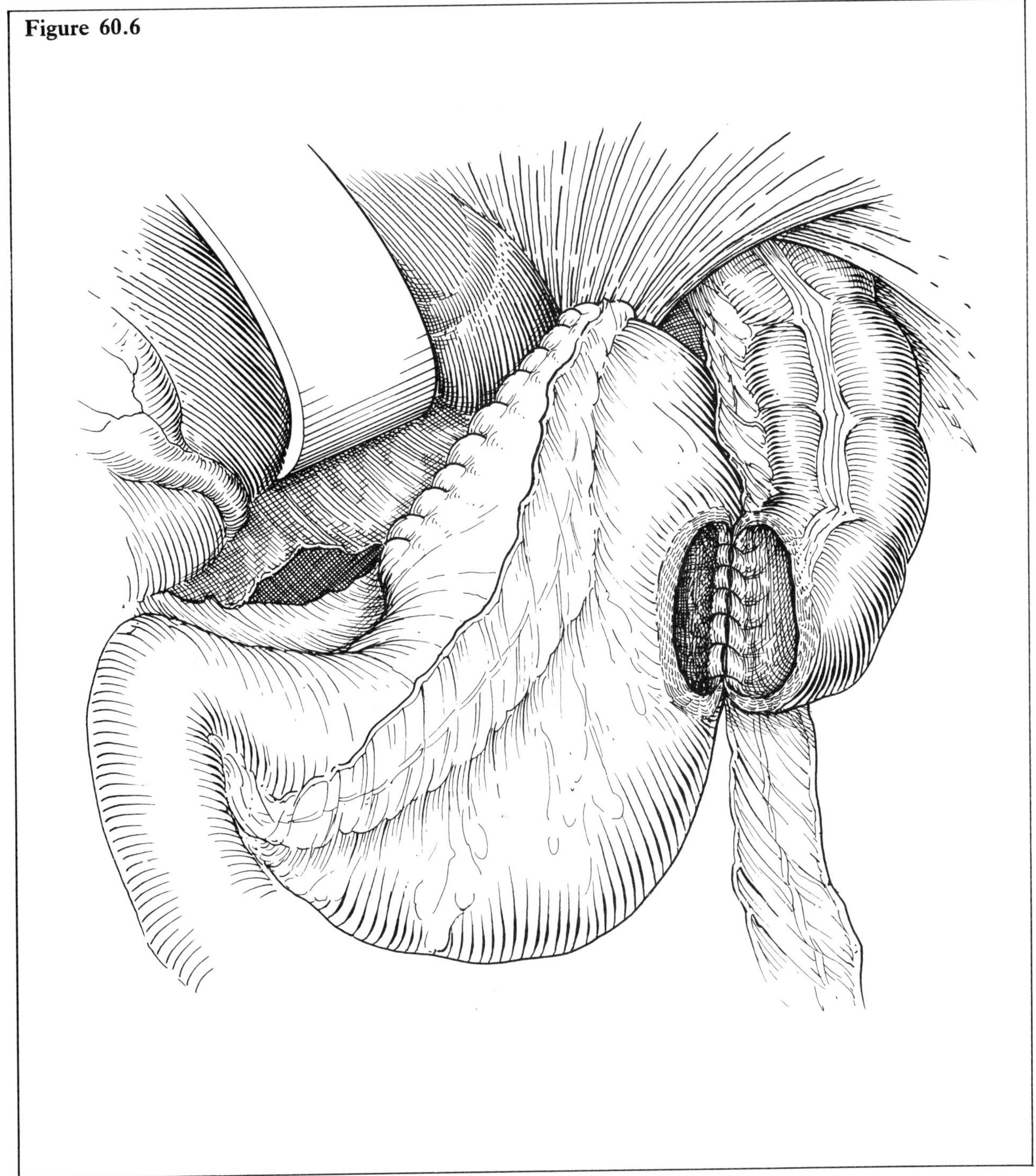

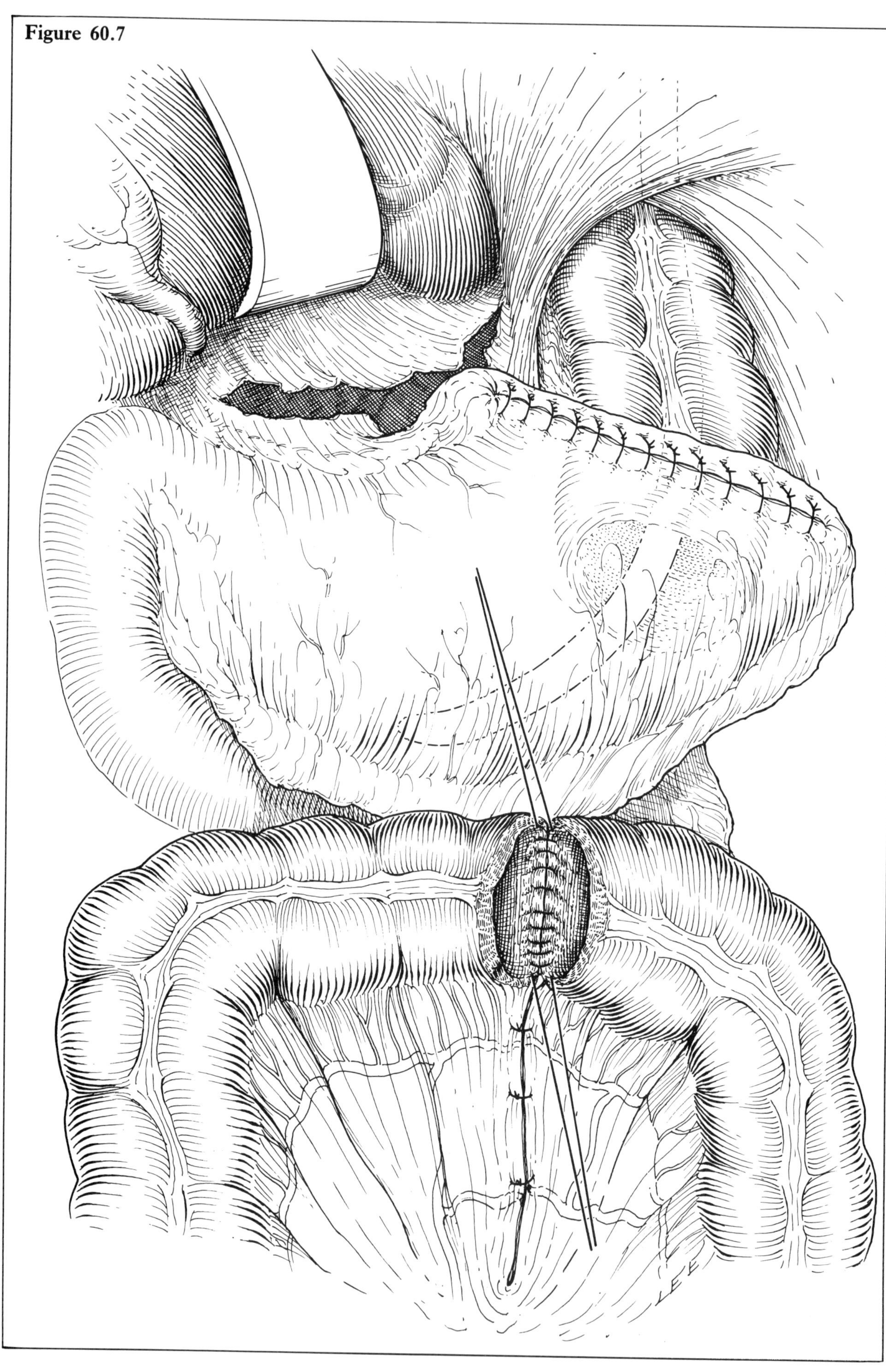
Figure 60.7

### Colocolic anastomosis

The two ends of the colon in the abdomen are united with a double row of fine interrupted sutures (**Fig. 60.7**) or with a circular stapler.

The margins of the hiatus are sutured to the colonic serosa with a few fine interrupted sutures to prevent herniation alongside the colon. When inserting the stitches, great care must be taken not to compress the vascular pedicle.

A nasogastric tube is passed into the stomach to prevent gastric dilatation postoperatively.

The diaphragmatic incision is repaired with interrupted non-absorbable mattress sutures. The incision is closed as described on pp. 27–8.

## Anastomosis at the level of the aortic arch

The patient is placed in the left lateral position with the pelvis rotated backwards 45 degrees. For the abdominal part of the operation the operating table is rotated to the patient's right to improve access.

### Abdominal procedure

A midline incision is made from the xiphisternum to the midpoint between the umbilicus and the pubic symphysis. The colon is mobilized as before, and the greater omentum is detached. The hepatic flexure and ascending colon, together with its blood supply, are then mobilized towards the midline. The splenic flexure is similarly mobilized. The stomach and cardia are mobilized as described on pp. 234–8, and the stomach is divided and closed.

Packs are placed in the abdominal incision while the table is rotated back to the neutral position to allow access to the chest.

### Thoracic procedure

The chest is opened via a left thoracotomy through the bed of the fifth rib. The oesophagus is mobilized and a tape passed around it. The cardia is drawn up from the abdomen.

The appropriate length of colon can now be estimated, and it is divided to the left of the middle colic artery or just above the right colic artery. The distal end is drawn up into the thorax through the hiatus and anastomosed to the end of the oesophagus. The lower end of the transplant now lies in front of the stomach, and is anastomosed to a 5-cm incision in the anterior wall close to the greater curvature using the technique described for the posterior cologastric anastomosis on pp. 233, 259.

The thoracic incision is then closed over two silicone drains. The two ends of the colon are united as described above, and a nasogastric tube is passed into the stomach. The abdomen is closed with a looped nylon suture to the muscle layers using the 'mass closure' technique.

## Cervical anastomosis

This procedure requires cervical and abdominal incisions. The mobilized colon is passed upwards through a retrosternal tunnel. The necessity for a right thoracotomy depends on whether the thoracic oesophagus is to be removed.

### Abdominal procedure

The patient lies supine and a midline incision is made. After division of the left triangular ligment, the left lobe of the liver is retracted medially and the cardia is mobilized. The stomach is divided and closed. If the oesophagus is to be left *in situ*, its distal end is sutured in two layers or closed with a stapler. The colon is mobilized as described above.

### Cervical procedure

The oesophagus is exposed through an incision parallel with the anterior border of the sternocleidomastoid muscle (**Fig. 60.8**), and mobilized in the neck as described on pp. 248–9. If there is an oesophagocutaneous fistula it is excised through a half-collar incision centred on the fistula. The oesophagus deep to the fistula is mobilized. Skin flaps are then dissected upwards and downwards to expose the sternomastoid muscle, which is divided close to its origin. The deep cervical fascia is incised and the carotid sheath retracted laterally after division of the middle thyroid vein. The trachea is retracted forward and the oesophagus mobilized from behind it, taking care to avoid damage to the recurrent laryngeal nerves.

The length of colon required is then estimated, and it is divided at the level of the right colic artery. The blood supply is maintained from the middle colic artery along the marginal artery.

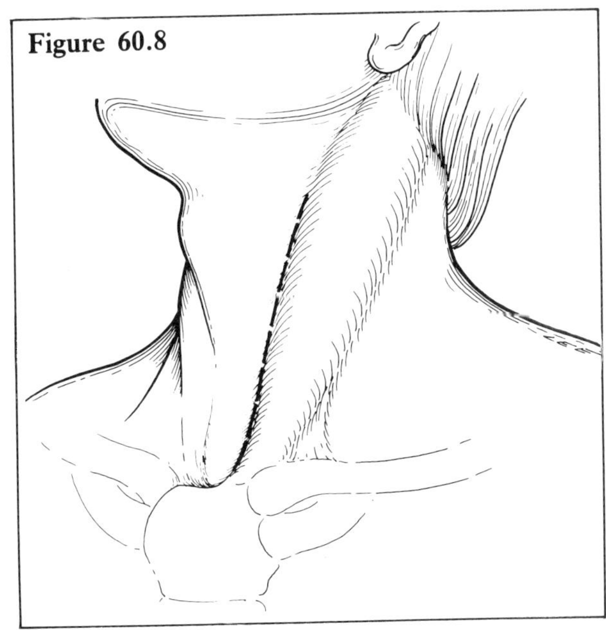

**Figure 60.8**

### Retrosternal tunnel

The two slips of diaphragm attached to the posterior surface of the sternum are separated, and a tunnel is created by blunt dissection behind the sternum, emerging anterior to the left subclavian artery. A tape is brought back through the tunnel to emerge at the abdominal incision. The passage of a large, moist pack through the anterior mediastinal space will enlarge it. A Foley catheter with a 100 $cm^3$ balloon is then drawn down into the abdomen from above. If the thoracic outlet is very narrow it may be necessary to resect the medial end of the clavicle and upper part of the manubrium.

Next, the colon is divided and the distal cut end is sutured to the distal end of the Foley catheter whose balloon has been maximally inflated. The proximal end of the catheter is then pulled and the colon drawn up into the cervical incision behind the balloon; this avoids damage to the colon, which can pass effortlessly into the neck. A two-layered anastomosis is constructed. A silicone corrugated drain is then brought out through a separate stab incision above the clavicle. The sternomastoid muscle is reattached and the wound closed with an absorbable suture to the fascial and platysmal layers. Metal clips are used to close the skin.

## Distal anastomosis

The distal limb of colon is divided and anastomosed to the anterior wall of the stomach near the greater curvature with a two-layer anastomosis. The two ends of colon in the abdominal cavity are similarly united. A nasogastric tube is passed into the stomach and the abdomen closed without drainage.

## Postoperative management

The patient is nursed in the intensive care unit for the first 24 hours. Urine flow, blood pressure and central venous pressure are monitored; intravenous fluids are administered at a rate in proportion to the patient's surface area, until bowel movement returns and oral fluids are allowed. Intravenous feeding is usually unnecessary. The nasogastric tube is allowed to syphon into an open bag which is secured at the level of the patient's shoulder and aspirated every two hours. Vigorous physiotherapy is given, and daily chest radiographs taken to detect atelectasis, pulmonary infiltrates or a hydropneumothorax.

Broad-spectrum antibiotics are given for 72 hours. We use penicillin, gentamicin and metronidazole. Ventilation is continued for the first 12 hours, after which the patient is allowed to breathe spontaneously. Supplementary oxygen is given via an MC mask until blood gas levels while the patient is breathing air are acceptable.

### Complications

Sputum retention and inhalation of gastric or intestinal contents may be responsible for atelectasis and pulmonary infection. If the patient is unable to cough, the elective insertion of a mini-tracheostomy tube through the cricothyroid membrane will allow easy access to the tracheobronchial tree for aspiration of secretions. If ventilation is inadequate, artificial ventilation should be resorted to without delay.

The most serious complication is necrosis of the colon secondary to thrombosis of its vascular pedicle. This may be recognized by the occurrence of fever, signs of peritonitis, and a bloodstained pleural effusion. Urgent removal of the necrosed colon is essential. A cervical oesophagostomy and gastrostomy are performed, and restoration of oesophageal continuity is deferred until infection has subsided and the patient's condition has improved. More common is leakage from the proximal anastomosis, giving rise to a fistula in the neck which will usually resolve with adequate drainage. When leakage occurs, prolonged intravenous feeding may be necessary.

# 61 Jejunal replacement of the oesophagus

A length of the jejunum instead of the colon or stomach may be used to replace the resected oesophagus.

To preserve the blood supply of the jejunum, a section of the appropriate length is mobilized outside the arterial arcade (**Fig. 61.1**). The diseased oesophagus is resected as previously described. The jejunum is brought into the chest and anastomosed with interrupted sutures. Great care must be taken to ensure that there is an adequate blood supply at the point of division, and that undue tension is not placed on the anastomosis. The proximal end of the jejunum left within the abdomen is anastomosed in end-to-side fashion to the distal jejunum, approximately 40 cm from the oesophagojejunal anastomosis (**Fig. 61.2**). If this distance is too short, bile reflux into the oesophagus will occur; if it is too long, then a blind loop syndrome may ensue.

**Figure 61.1**

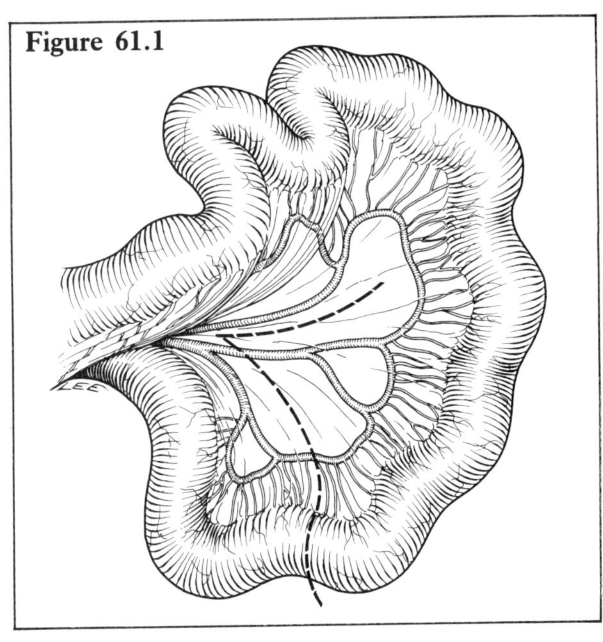

**Figure 61.2**

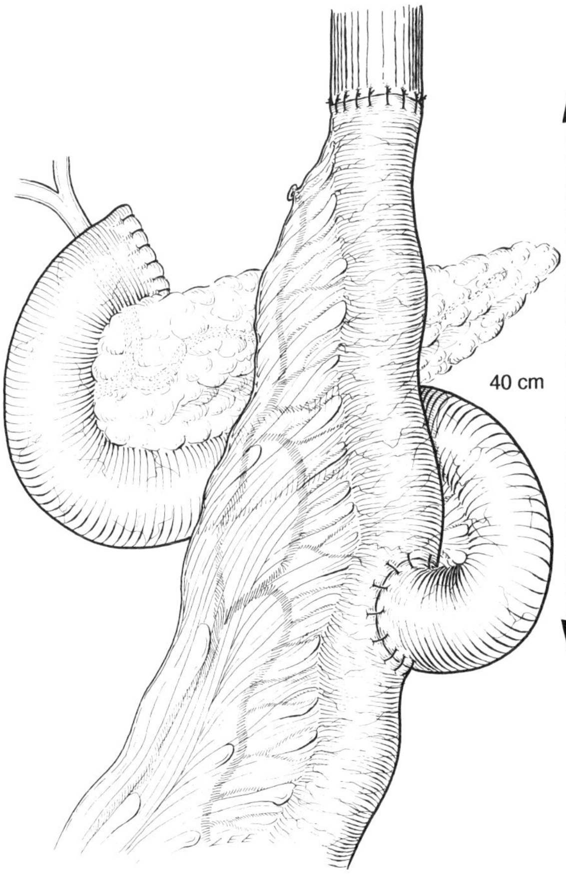

40 cm

# 62 Management of inoperable or irresectable carcinoma of the oesophagus

Many patients with carcinoma of the oesophagus present when their tumour has spread both locally and to other organs, the liver being the most common. In such cases surgical removal of the tumour is contraindicated because the patient's life expectancy is very short. However, relief from dysphagia (which may be absolute) is necessary. The options available to achieve this are:

1. Construction of a bypass conduit using colon, stomach or jejunum.
2. Intubation of the malignant stricture by antegrade or retrograde techniques.
3. Laser ablation with intermittent dilatation.
4. External beam radiotherapy, if the tumour is a squamous cell carcinoma.
5. Intracavitary radiotherapy: iridium wires or beads may be placed within the oesophagus at the site of the tumour. This technique has largely fallen into disuse with the advent of supervoltage external beam radiation; additionally, the equipment for this procedure is expensive and is not readily available.

Of these interventions, the use of laser equipment is the most recent advance, but only a few units possess the necessary equipment. Investigators within the field report that several treatments are usually required, in association with dilatation; but some good short-term palliative results are claimed.

The mainstays of treatment for this advanced stage of the disease remain, however, intubation or (in the younger or fitter patient) extra-anatomical bypass.

## Oesophageal intubation

In addition to its use in the management of malignant strictures, this technique is useful for the temporary management of patients who have suffered instrumental perforation during attempted dilatation of a difficult benign stricture. Long-term intubation in such patients is not recommended, however, as tube migration, reflux, aspiration pneumonia and ulceration with perforation are all recorded complications.

Intraluminal oesophageal tubes have also been employed to good effect in patients with malignant tracheo-oesophageal fistulae. They may be introduced by traction or pulsion techniques.

### Traction intubation

#### Procedure

The Celestin tube has most commonly been used for this technique. The patient lies supine. The abdomen is opened through a 10-cm upper abdominal incision. This may be a vertical midline incision, a left subcostal or a high left transverse incision, according to the shape of the subcostal arch (**Fig. 62.1**). In the latter two cases the muscles are divided in the line of the incision down to the peritoneum.

To reduce contamination of the wound by gastric contents a wound excluder may be used (**Fig. 62.2**). This consists of a sterile, flexible plastic ring, 10 cm in diameter, to the margin of which is attached a sheet of plastic. The ring is compressed, passed into the peritoneal cavity and allowed to expand. The attached sheet then drapes the edges of the wound, protecting them from gastric spillage.

**Figure 62.1**

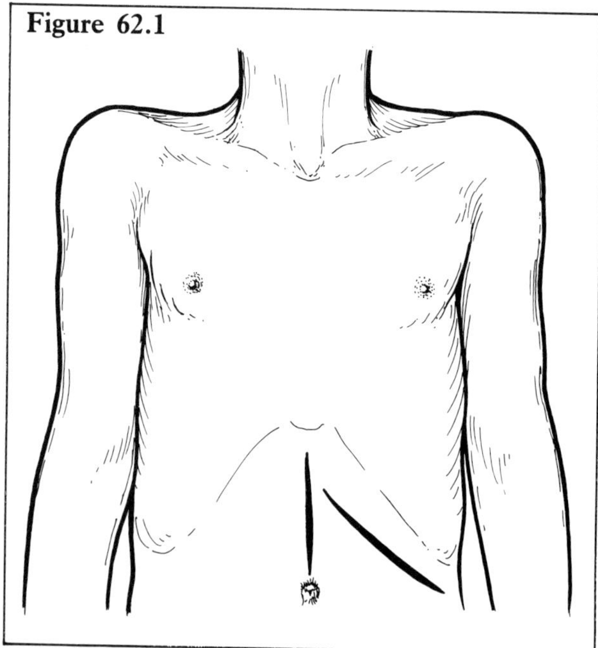

Figure 62.2

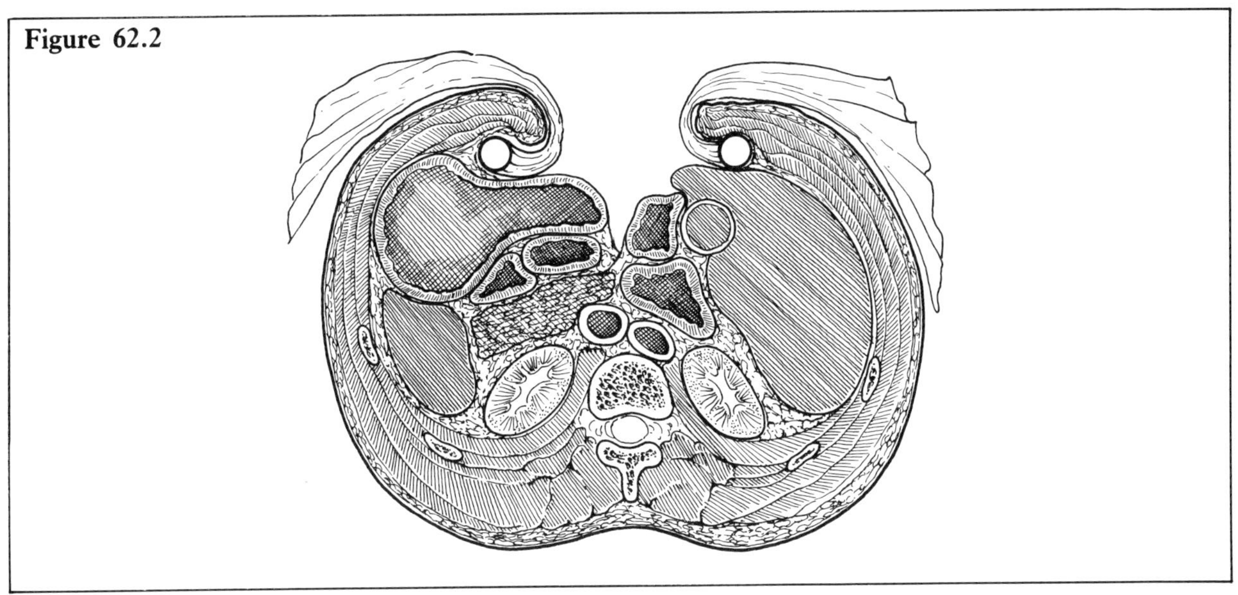

Supplied with the Celestin tube is a bougie, which the anaesthetist is asked to pass, well lubricated, into the oesophagus. In the majority of cases it requires only a little manipulation to persuade it to enter the stomach. Sometimes the surgeon's thumb and forefinger around the cardia will aid the passage of the bougie.

Two stay sutures are placed in the anterior wall of the stomach about halfway between the greater and lesser curvatures, 10–15 cm from the cardia. The stomach is incised between the stay sutures with diathermy down on to the tip of the bougie (**Fig. 62.3**). As the bougie emerges it is covered, and held with a sterile towel to reduce contamination.

The anaesthetist then attaches the Celestin tube to the bougie and fixes it firmly with a ligature in the groove provided (**Fig. 62.4**). By traction on the bougie the surgeon can draw the tube into the oesophagus. Meanwhile the anaesthetist guides the expanded proximal end through the mouth and

Figure 62.3

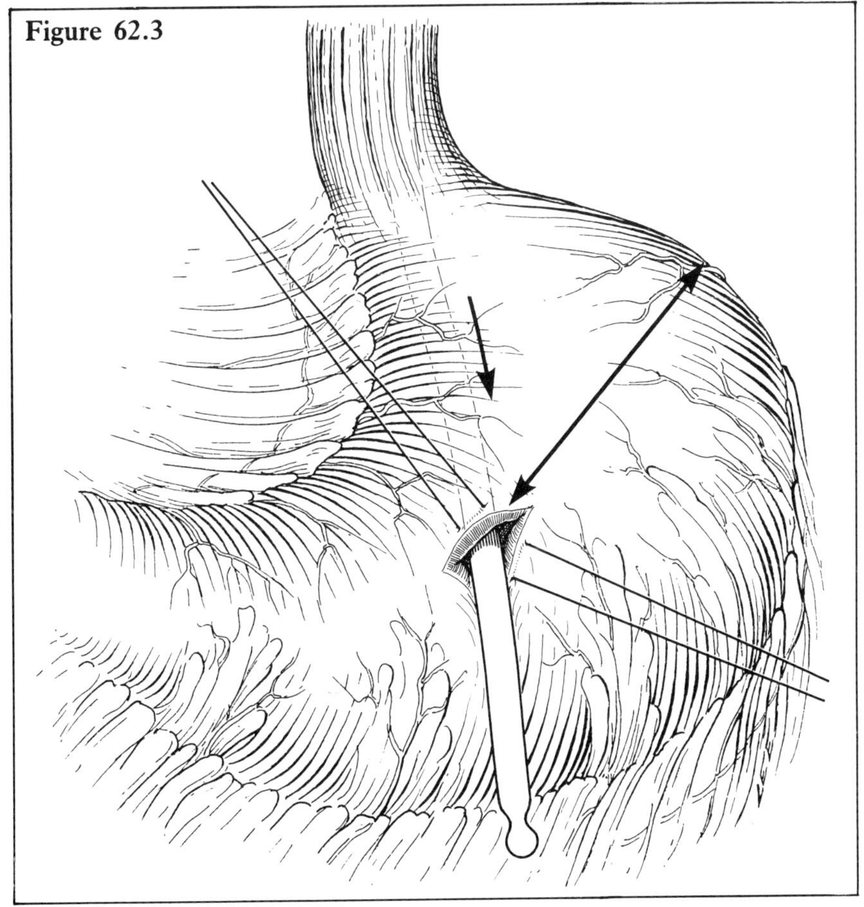

Figure 62.4

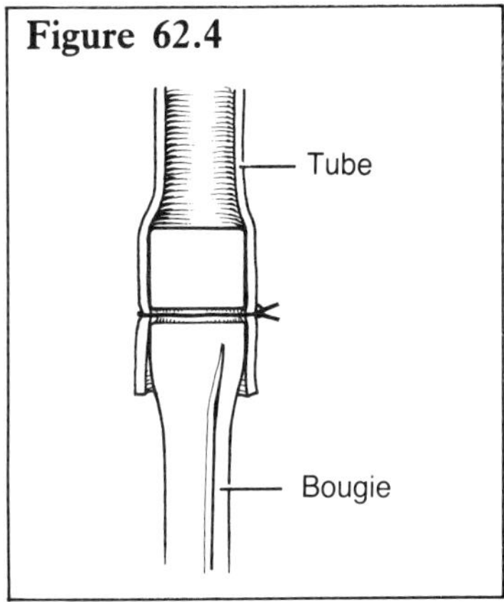

pharynx into the upper oesophagus. A steady increase in resistance informs the surgeon that the expanded end of the tube has lodged in the stricture and traction must now cease, otherwise the tube might be pulled past the obstruction into the stomach (**Fig. 62.5**). If there is doubt about the location of the expanded end of the tube in the oesophagus, its position is checked by oesophagoscopy before the tube is divided. At this stage the lower end of the Celestin tube will have emerged from the gastric wall, which is sleeved back along the tube until only about 10 cm of tube remains in the stomach. The tube is divided at this point with strong scissors (**Fig. 62.6**). The tube may be tacked to the anterior wall of the stomach with an absorbable suture, although this is not absolutely guaranteed to prevent migration.

The gastrotomy is closed with a continuous catgut suture, and the suture line buried with interrupted non-absorbable stitches, e.g. polypropylene (**Fig. 62.7**). The wound excluder is now removed, the edges of the incision liberally sprayed with antibiotic powder and the incision closed without drainage.

### Difficulty in bougie insertion

If the bougie will not negotiate the obstruction, there are several helpful techniques that may be

**Figure 62.5**

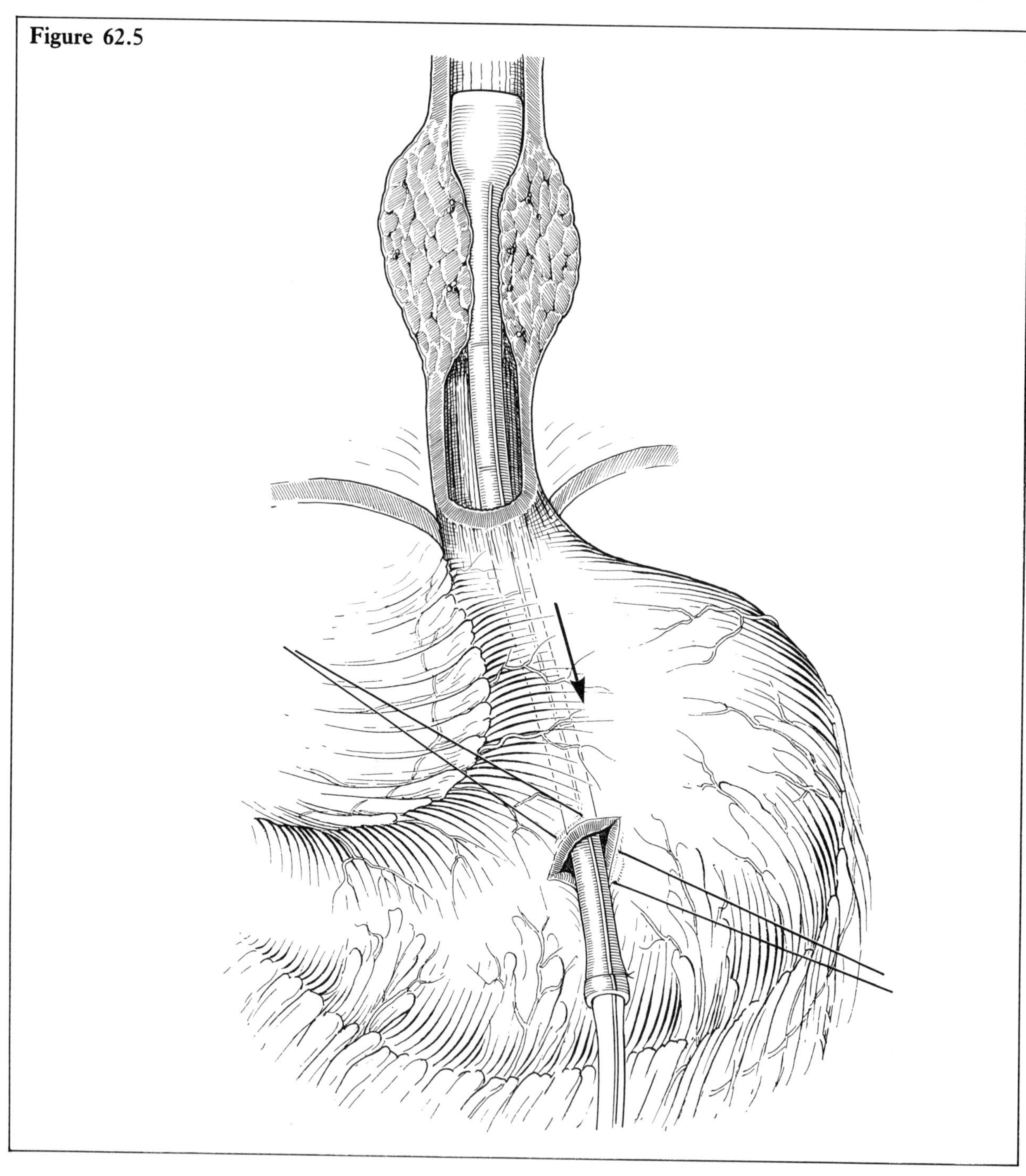

tried. An oesophagoscope is passed and an attempt made to pass the bougie under direct vision. If this fails, it may be possible to negotiate the stricture with a filiform or olivary-headed bougie. This is passed on into the stomach and made to emerge from the gastrotomy. A heavy ligature is then tied to its proximal end and to the lower end of the bougie, which is thus 'railroaded' into the stomach.

Another method is to make a larger gastrotomy, and to attempt to negotiate the cardia and the stricture from below with the aid of a finger passed into the stomach alongside the bougie.

When all else fails it may be possible to advance a long crocodile forceps through the tumour either from above or below. The bougie is then attached to this and drawn through the stricture. In these

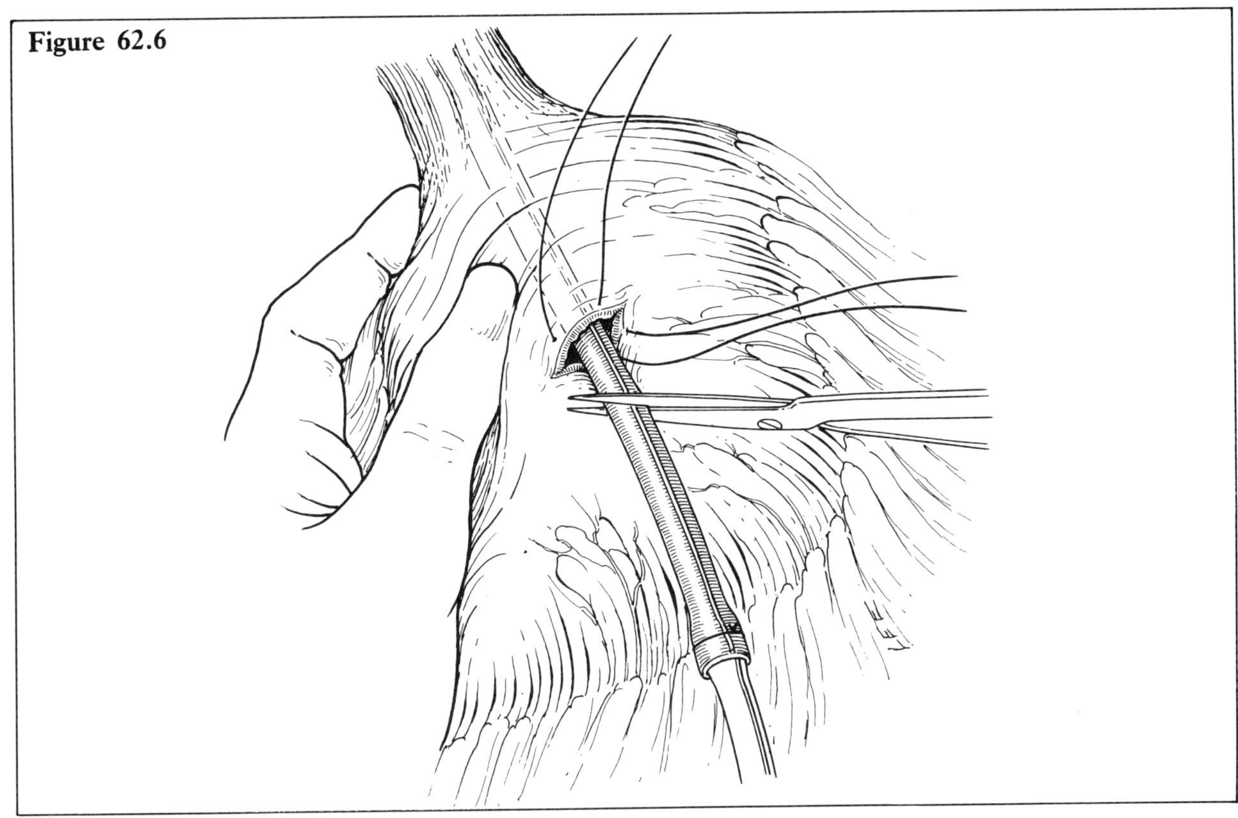

**Figure 62.6**

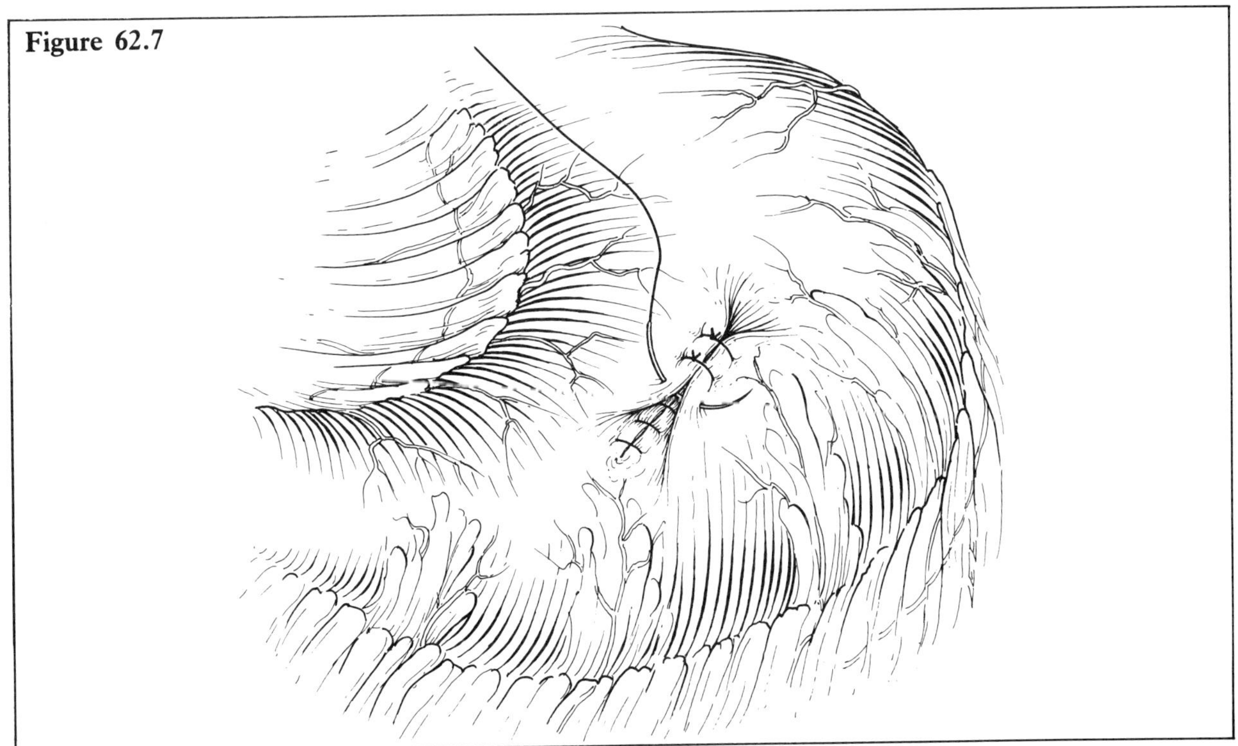

**Figure 62.7**

difficult cases one or more false passages may be made, but if a Celestin tube is ultimately fixed in place these rarely cause any trouble.

## Pulsion intubation

The attractions of this technique are obvious. A laparotomy is not needed, and all the attendant morbidity associated with it is obviated. Postoperative hospital stay is reduced when compared with transabdominal traction techniques.

X-ray control is desirable to ensure accurate tube placement and to reduce the risk of perforation.

A number of tubes and introducer systems are available. The principles guiding their use are the same.

### Procedure using the rigid oesophagoscope

First the lesion is identified and dilated with graduated bougies to size 40 (**Fig. 62.8**). A size 20 bougie is then passed through the tumour.

An appropriate tube is passed over the bougie and threaded into the pharynx. The rigid oesophagoscope is then used as a 'pusher' to place the tube across the stricture (**Fig. 62.9**).

### Procedure using the flexible endoscope

The site and length of the lesion is identified as accurately as possible using the flexible endoscope. A guide wire is passed through the stricture.

The appropriate introducer within the selected tube is passed over the guide wire, followed by the ramrod (**Fig. 62.10**). The tube is advanced into position, the introducer is withdrawn while the tube is held by the ramrod, and the ramrod is then removed.

The correct placement of the tube is checked endoscopically and with X-ray screening.

**Figure 62.8**

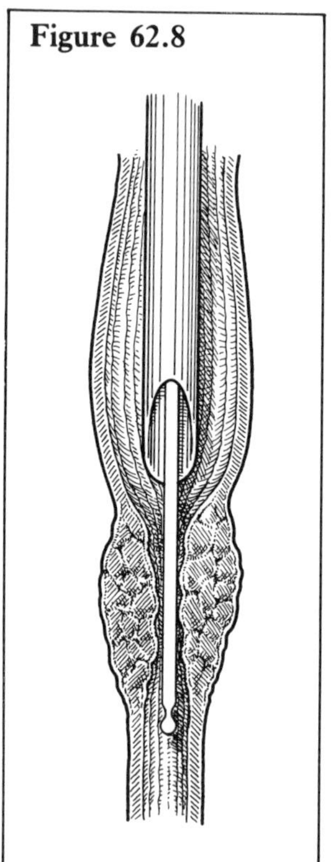

**Figure 62.9**

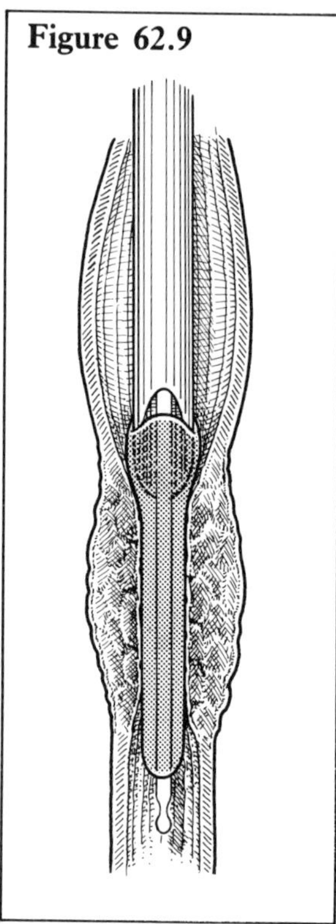

**Figure 62.10**

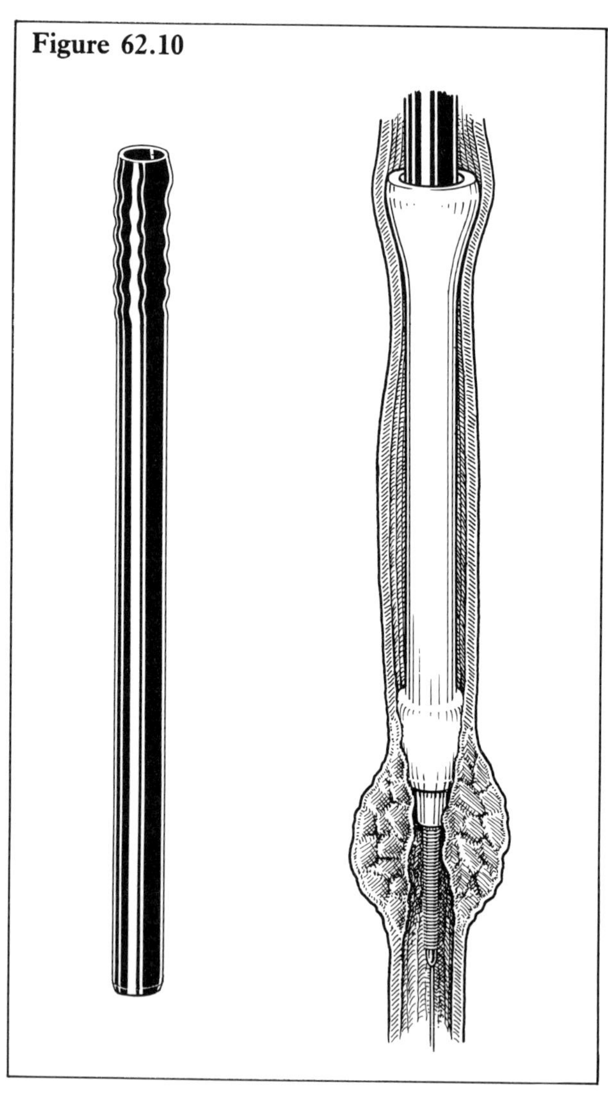

## Postoperative management

Antibiotics including metronidazole should be given for the first 72 hours after operation. The patient is mobilized on the first postoperative day and is allowed to drink freely. A liquefied diet is given from the second or third day, progressing to a semisolid diet over the ensuing week. The patient should be warned of the dangers of eating food that has not been well masticated and may block the tube. To ensure that this never occurs, all food should be puréed.

### Complications

If a tube is fixed with its upper limit too close to the cricopharyngeus it will cause persistent retching. It should therefore not be used for growths in the upper third of the oesophagus.

The tube may become displaced upwards, or more commonly downwards into the stomach. Disruption of the tube with perforation of the bowel has been described. In these circumstances the tube must be retrieved and replaced.

Generally speaking, although many patients derive considerable benefit from the placement of a feeding tube, it is a method of treatment that is less than ideal. In some cases, however, it may be all that a patient can withstand, and in those who have suffered absolute dysphagia, to be able to swallow at all is an enormous improvement.

## Extra-anatomic gastric bypass

These procedures are designed to restore swallowing without resecting the primary tumour. Colon, stomach or jejunum may be used. If stomach is to be used, e.g. for middle third tumours where the stomach is not involved, gastric mobilization is conducted as described on pp. 235–8. The distal oesophagus is transected at the gastro-oesophageal junction, and oversewn or stapled closed. The retrosternal plane is then developed as described on p. 250. A cervical incision is made on the left side of the neck as described on pp. 248–9. The stomach is then brought up into the neck and anastomosed to the cervical oesophagus. The proximal end of the divided thoracic oesophagus is oversewn or stapled.

Studies of this isolated mediastinal oesophageal segment have shown that occasionally sterile fluid collections develop, but these rarely, if ever, give rise to complications. Usually, however, the segment remains relatively empty.

It is often necessary to resect the head of the clavicle and a portion of the manubrium to accommodate the stomach in the thoracic inlet without compression. To do this the manubrium is split for 2–3 cm with a sternal saw. The head of the clavicle is then cut through with a Gigli saw. It is disarticulated from the manubrium and the costoclavicular ligament and removed. The upper half of the manubrium can then be removed by cutting transversely across it, to meet the midline incision (**Fig. 62.11**).

**Figure 62.11**

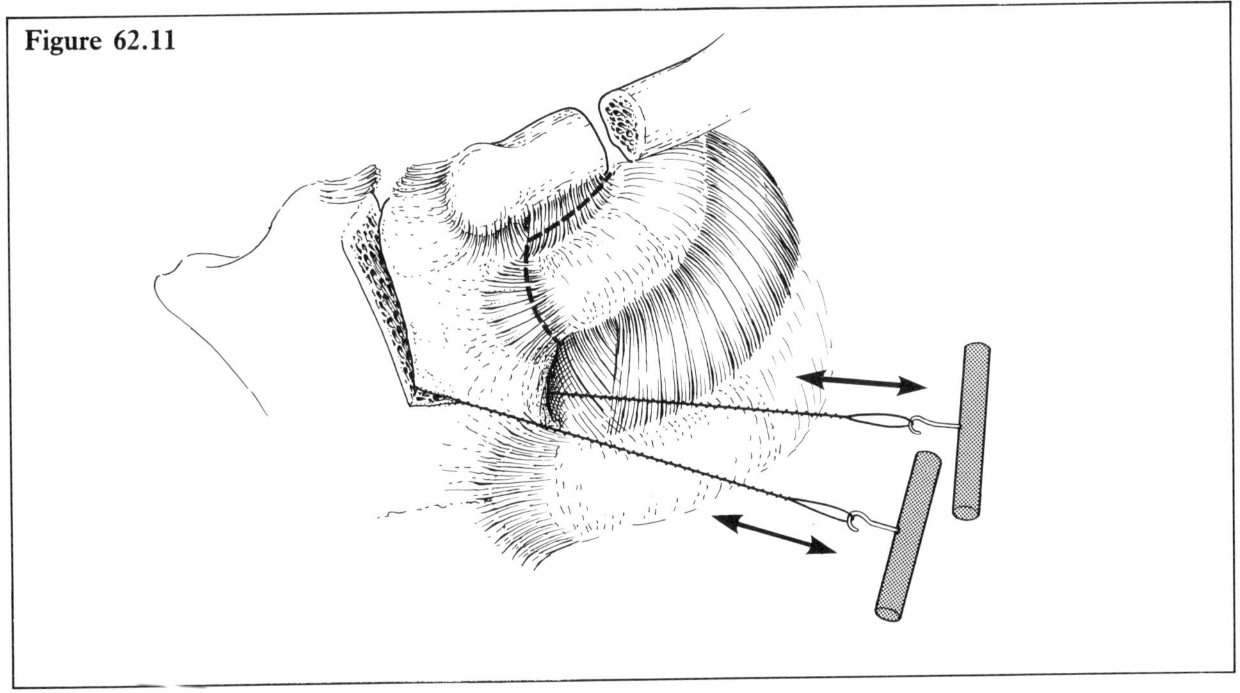

# 63 The use of staplers in oesophageal resections

Since the advent of stapling devices there has been a host of developments, culminating in a device for almost every stage of these operations. There are several published series of cases in which staplers have been used to construct oesophageal anastomoses with very low leak rates. However, whatever the method used to join two pieces of bowel, good arterial blood supply and venous drainage of the ends and minimal tension on the suture line are essential for sound healing.

## Use of staplers in oesophagogastrectomy

The stomach is mobilized as described on pp. 235–8. The division of the stomach is performed with a TA90 stapler loaded with 3.5 mm staples. Two parallel rows of staples are inserted and the stomach divided between them (**Fig. 63.1**). The cut distal end is invaginated with interrupted 3/0 polypropylene sutures (**Fig. 63.2**).

A circular stapling gun is now introduced into the stomach through a 25 mm incision made with diathermy about halfway between the pylorus and the proximal end of the stomach (**Figs. 63.2, 63.3**). The stapler, without the anvil, is passed into the stomach and directed proximally so that its tip marks the centre of the proposed anastomosis. A small incision is made over it and the central rod screwed out to its full extent so that it projects outside the stomach wall (**Fig. 63.4**). A 3/0 purse-

**Figure 63.1**

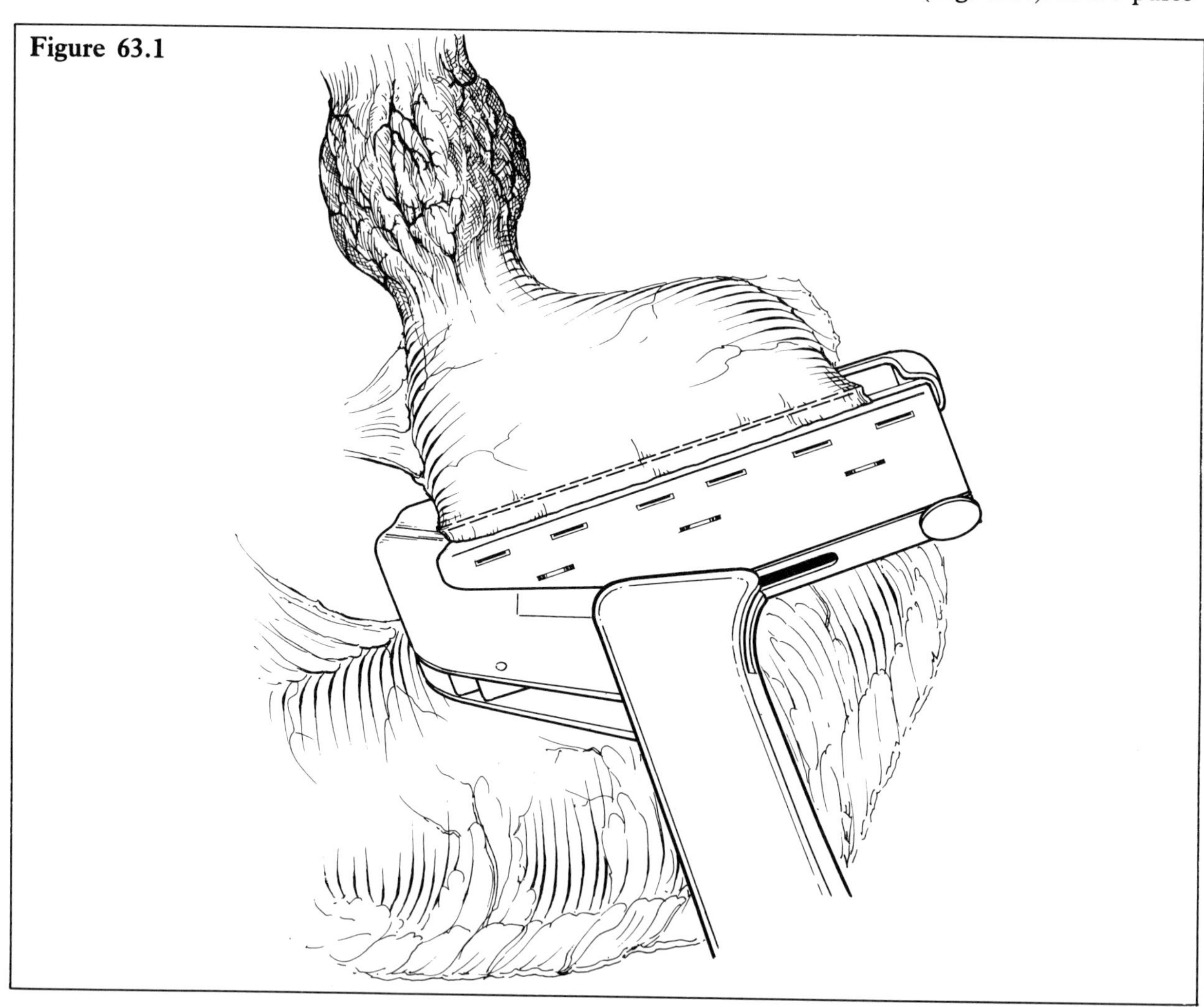

**Figure 63.2**

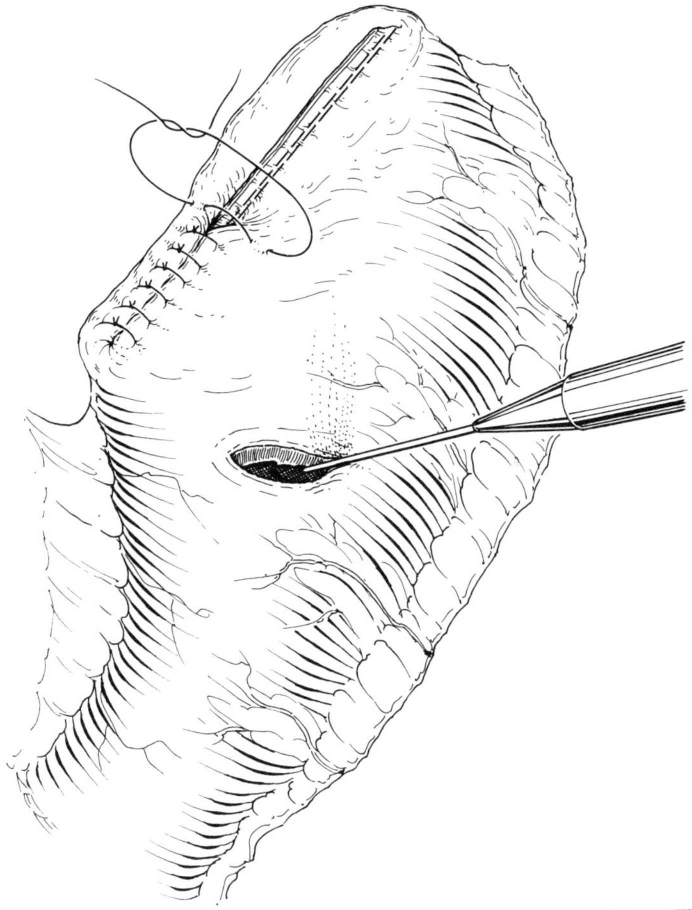

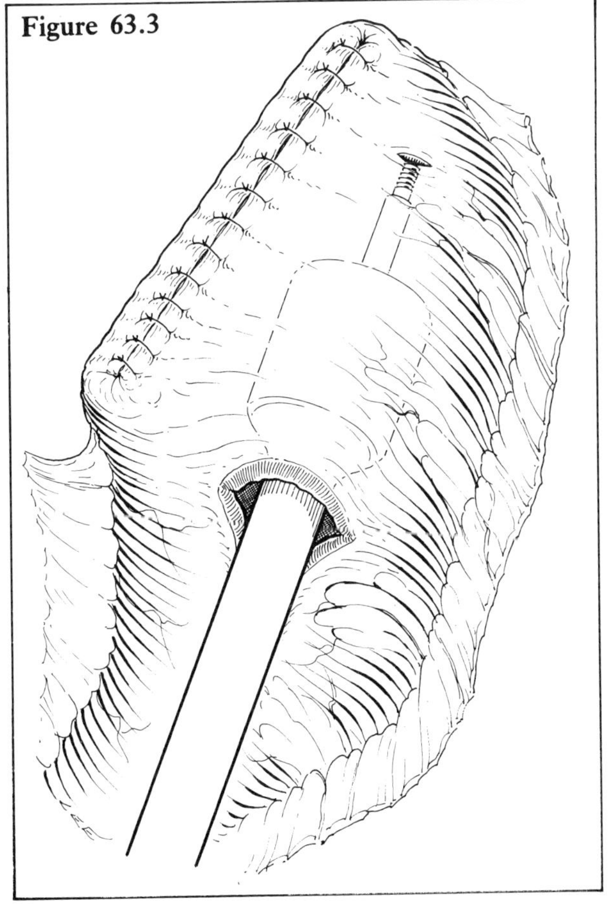

**Figure 63.3**

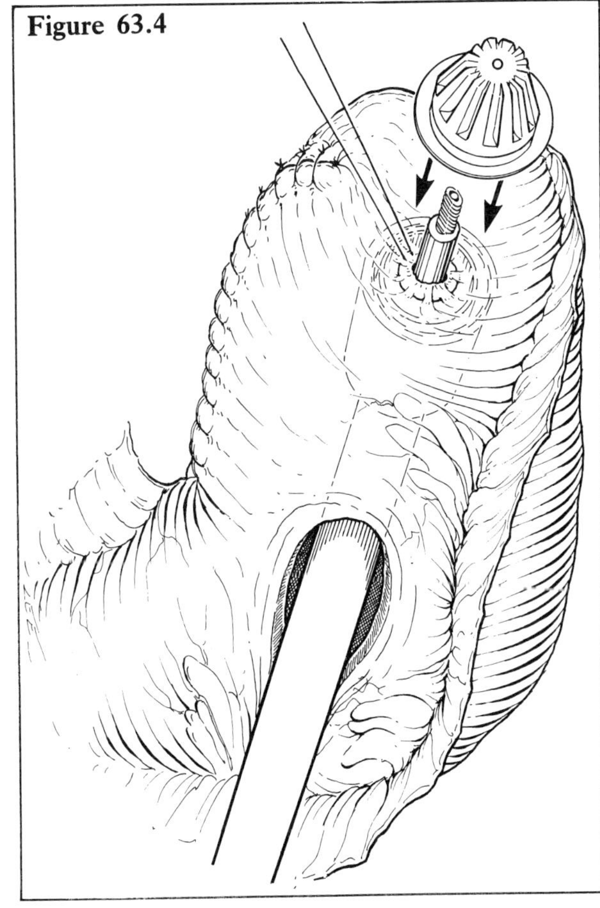

**Figure 63.4**

string suture is inserted through the full thickness of the gastric wall around the tip of the stapler, about 5 mm away from it, and tied. The anvil is now fixed into place at the end of the projecting rod (**Fig. 63.4**).

Next, a purse-string suture of 3/0 polypropylene is placed around the wall of the oesophagus at the site of the proposed anastomosis. The anterior wall of the oesophagus is incised at this level until the lumen can be seen (**Fig. 63.5**). Two stay sutures are inserted through the full thickness of the oesophageal wall to hold the incision open. Gentle dilatation with a finger, followed by the thumb, aids in the introduction of the anvil, which is liberally smeared with lubricant (**Fig. 63.6**). When the anvil has completely entered the oesophagus

**Figure 63.5**

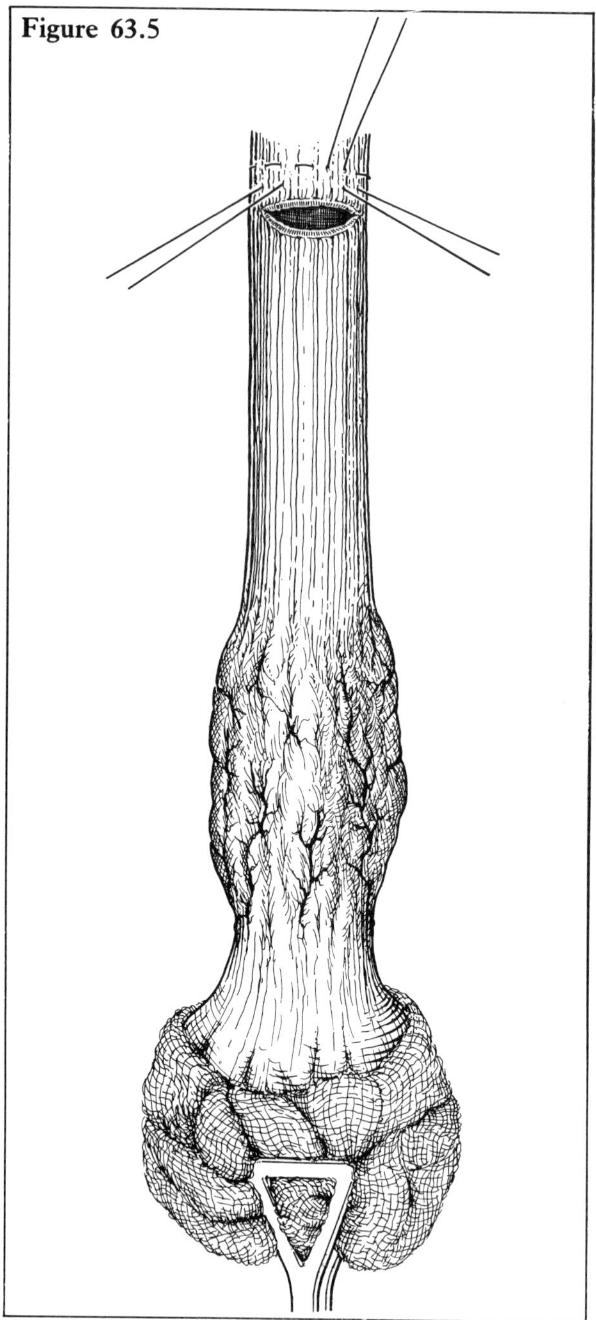

**Figure 63.6**

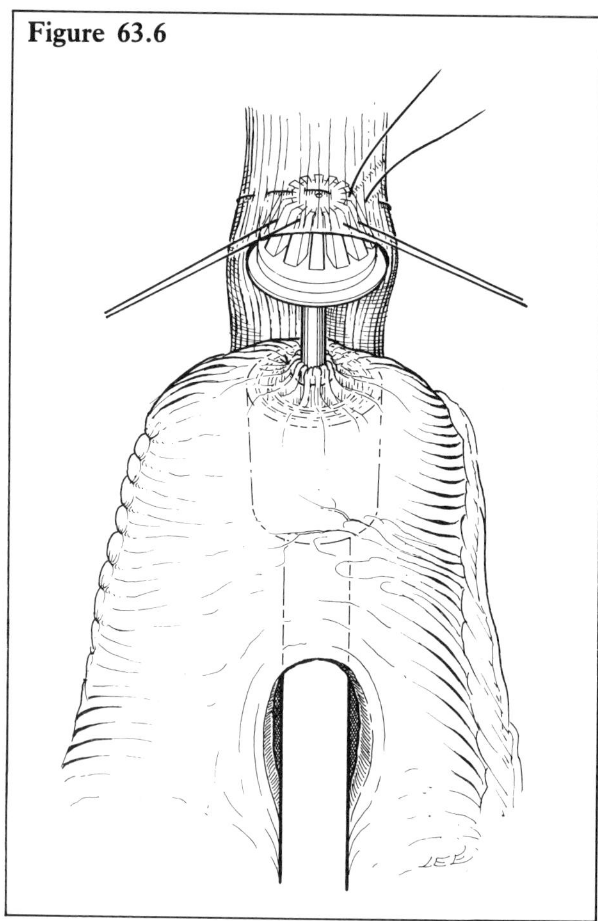


**Figure 63.7**

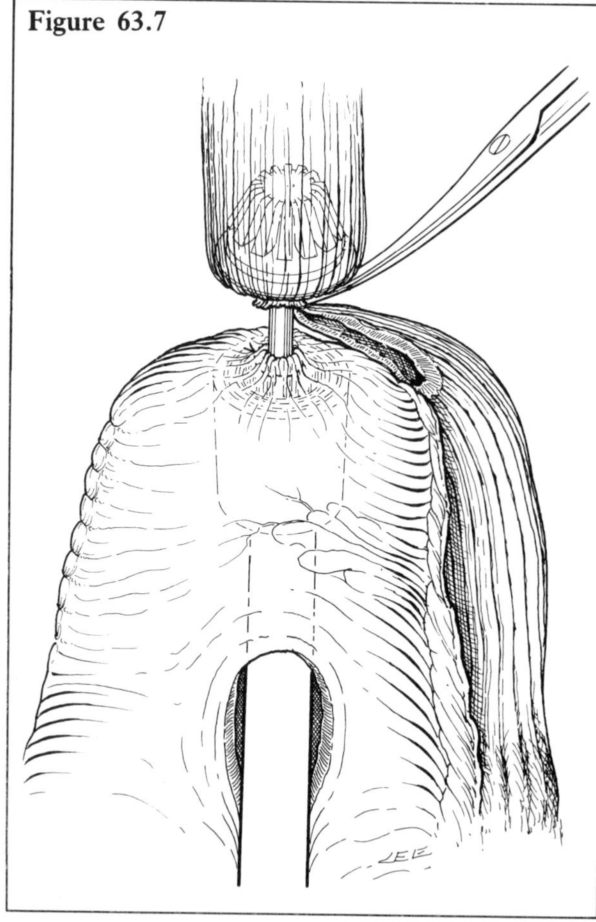

Figure 63.8

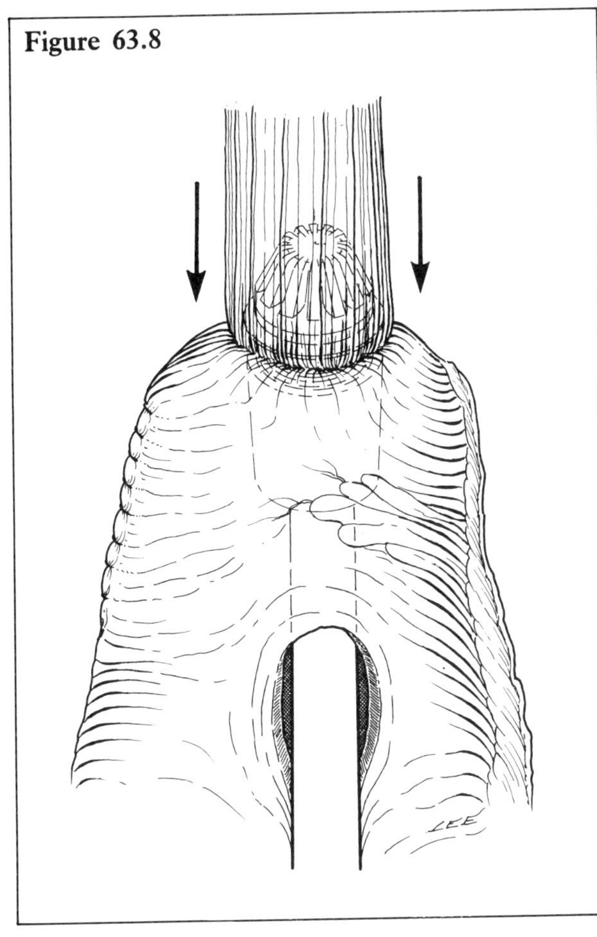

Figure 63.9

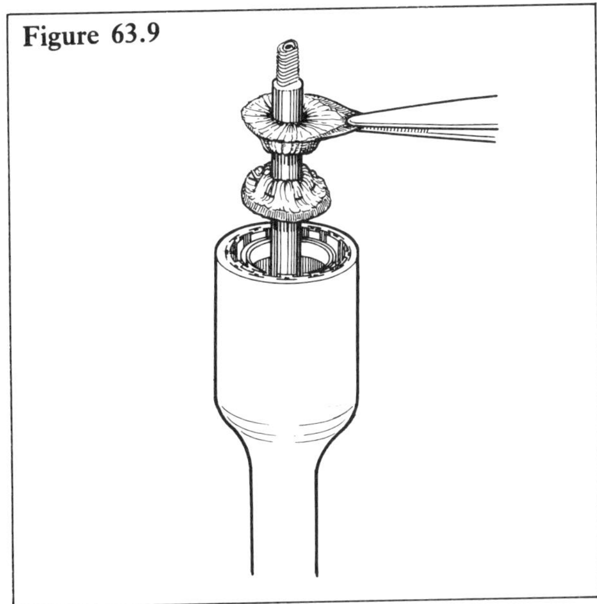

the proximal purse-string suture is tied, and the remaining posterior oesophageal wall divided with scissors (**Fig. 63.7**). The resected specimen is then removed.

The instrument is now fully tightened and fired (**Fig. 63.8**). This inserts a double circle of staples and cuts out the tissue between them. The instrument is unscrewed and carefully withdrawn, while the operator supports the anastomosis with the fingers of the left hand.

The anvil is removed and the excised tissue inspected. There should be two complete circles of mucosa (**Fig. 63.9**).

The anastomosis is now inspected all around to make sure that there are no gaps. A nasogastric tube is then passed into the stomach. The small gastrostomy is closed with a full-thickness polypropylene suture, followed by a serosal inverting stitch (**Fig. 63.10**).

Figure 63.10

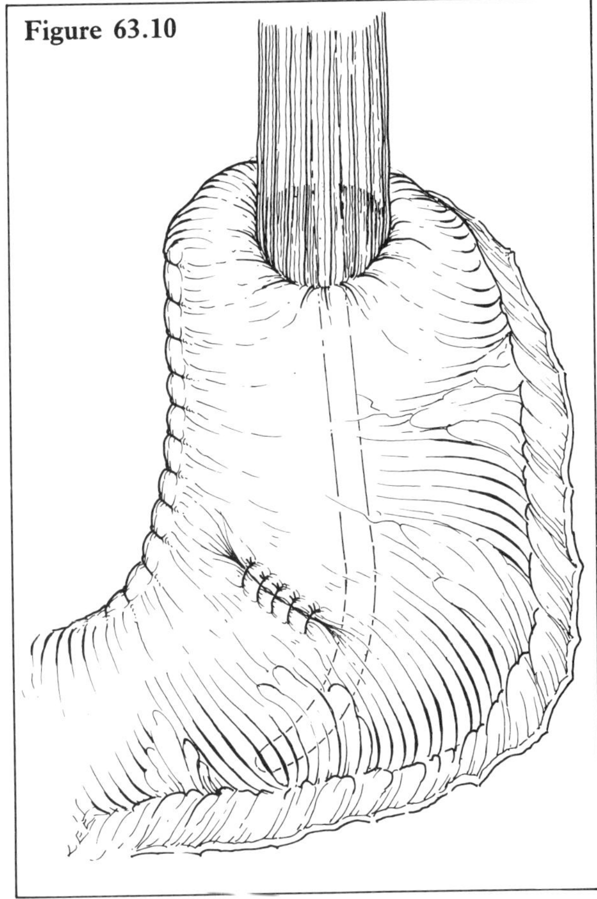

# Index